"This is an excellent book not only for those who are new to the area of neonatal nursing but also for those undertaking their qualification in specialty. It sets topics out in an easy to understand and logical fashion, identifies where the following text will impact and encourages students and readers to test themselves at the end of each chapter. It is also evidenced throughout ensuring that readers are signposted to further information. An updated and essential part of neonatal nurses' toolkits."

— *Dr Lynne Paterson, Nurse Lead, NHS Northern Neonatal Network*

T0246313

NEONATAL INTENSIVE CARE NURSING

Thoroughly revised and updated, this new edition of *Neonatal Intensive Care Nursing* is a comprehensive, evidence-based text for nurses and allied health professionals caring for sick newborn infants.

This user-friendly text focuses on the common problems and related care occurring within the neonatal specialty. All previous chapters have been thoroughly updated and new content includes chapters on, for example, organisation of neonatal care, assessment of the neonate, the premature and low birth weight neonate as well as palliative care. In addition, the book now includes a broad and in-depth web-based companion comprising online resources, case studies with answer guides and learning activities. This accessible and interactive approach enables nurses to recognise, rationalise and understand clinical problems using an evidence-based approach. Divided into four parts, the book provides an overview of neonatal care, and a detailed look at the physical and emotional wellbeing of the neonate and family, a range of clinical aspects of neonatal care, and key practices and procedures.

Neonatal Intensive Care Nursing will be essential reading for both new and experienced nurses, allied health professionals and students learning about neonatal care including those undertaking qualifications in the neonatal specialism and pre-registration students taking relevant modules or placements.

Glenys Boxwell was an Advanced Neonatal Nurse Practitioner for Plymouth Hospitals NHS Trust. She was previously a senior lecturer at Homerton College, Cambridge, and has now retired from clinical practice.

Julia Petty worked as a neonatal and children's nurse clinical educator and neonatal course leader prior to her current role as senior lecturer in children's nurse education at the University of Hertfordshire.

Lisa Kaiser qualified as an Advanced Neonatal Nurse Practitioner in 2014 and is currently practising at Glan Clwyd Hospital in North Wales. She completed her MSc in Advanced Clinical Practice at Brighton and Sussex University Hospitals NHS Trust, which involved research on noradrenaline infusion stability.

NEONATAL INTENSIVE CARE NURSING
THIRD EDITION

Edited by Glenys Boxwell,
Julia Petty and Lisa Kaiser

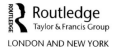
Routledge
Taylor & Francis Group

LONDON AND NEW YORK

Third edition published 2020
by Routledge
2 Park Square, Milton Park, Abingdon, Oxon, OX14 4RN

and by Routledge
52 Vanderbilt Avenue, New York, NY 10017

Routledge is an imprint of the Taylor & Francis Group, an informa business

First edition published by Routledge 2010
Second edition published by Routledge 2015

British Library Cataloguing-in-Publication Data
A catalogue record for this book is available from the British Library

Library of Congress Cataloging-in-Publication Data
A catalog record has been requested for this book

ISBN: 978-1-138-55683-6 (hbk)
ISBN: 978-1-138-55684-3 (pbk)
ISBN: 978-1-315-15045-1 (ebk)

Typeset in Akzidenz Grotesk
by Newgen Publishing UK

Visit the companion website: www.routledge.com/cw/nicnursing
Visit the eResources: www.routledge.com/9781138556843

CONTENTS

PART 4: PRACTICES AND PROCEDURES IN NEONATAL CARE

19 Medication practice in the neonatal unit

KAREN HOOVER

LIST OF FIGURES

LIST OF TABLES

LIST OF BOXES

LIST OF CONTRIBUTORS

Breidge Boyle is a general and children's nurse and an ANNP, specialising in neonatal surgery. She was lead nurse for neonates for North Central London, worked on the BOOST II UK trial and has a doctorate in perinatal epidemiology. She lectures in Children's and Neonatal Nursing at Queens University Belfast.

Liam Brennan is a consultant paediatric anaesthetist at Cambridge University Hospitals NHS Trust. He has a strong commitment to education and training, lecturing and publishing widely on a range of subjects including paediatric obesity, consent in children and maintaining clinical competency. He now combines clinical practice with the role of Deputy Medical Director in Cambridge.

Alexandra Connolly holds the role of a Highly Specialist Speech and Language Therapist at Barts Health NHS Trust in London. She has a specific interest in the field of neonatal care in relation to enhancing feeding skills and supporting parents in this field, in which she has received specialist training.

Jo Cookson is a midwifery/neonatal lecturer at Keele University and works for a neonatal network one day a week as a practice educator. Her work at the University involves leading on post-registration neonatal education and developing the neonatal component of pre-registration midwifery. Jo completed her MA in Medical ethics and law in 2016 and has a keen interest in neonatal ethics.

Yvonne Cousins was a neonatal surgical nurse specialist at the neonatal unit, Evelina London Children's Hospital and held that role for ten years. Prior to this role, she worked within a range of neonatal units; namely, Great Ormond Street NHS Trust, King's College Hospital and Mayday University Hospital. She has previously published on the topic of wound care considerations in neonates in which she has a particular interest along with stoma care.

Liz Crathern works in freelance consultancy in neonatal care; education and practice. She has been a neonatal nurse in the UK since 1980 which has involved research and education interests in parenting, family dynamics, grief and loss including her doctoral research that focused on first-time fathers of preterm infants. Prior to her current role, she led and developed the curriculum for Advanced neonatal and paediatric nursing practice (MMedSci ANNP/APNP) programme at the University of Sheffield.

Erica Everett has been practicing in neonatal care for 27 years and has worked as a neonatal nurse and ANNP on level 3 neonatal units and neonatal transport. She has worked as neonatal lecturer at Anglia Ruskin University and is currently working as the lead nurse for practice development East of England ODN. She is a resuscitation council NLS and GIC instructor and Fellow of the Institute of Higher Education.

Sarah Fitchett was appointed as a neonatal lecturer at the University of Salford in 2016 and works within the midwifery team. She has been a practicing nurse for over 25 years of which 20 years have been spent working within neonatal care. Sarah has experience of working within the "Making it Better" programme team for the transformation of neonatal services across Greater Manchester and currently leads the Emergency and Intensive Care of the Newborn module.

Karen Hoover is an ANNP at Brighton and Sussex University Hospitals NHS Trust. After several years as a neonatal nurse, in the UK and overseas, she completed a Master's degree in Advanced Clinical Practice (neonatal) and has worked in her current Trust since 2010. Her particular interests are genetics and congenital heart disease.

Tracey Jones has had a career in neonatal nursing since 1996 progressing to a senior nurse role. Tracey now works as a senior lecturer in neonatal education at the University of Manchester. She sits on the Council of International Neonatal Nursing executive board and chairs the education committee. She is a published author and has a large portfolio of peer-reviewed publications. Tracey is part of the editorial board for the *Journal of Neonatal Nursing*.

Lesley Kilby qualified as an ANNP in 2004 and currently works at Milton Keynes University Hospital. She has also worked in both level 2 and level 3 units within this role in London and the East of England. In 2011 she began working with the University of Bedfordshire to develop and deliver QIS training across the East of England. Lesley is a recognised instructor for the S.T.A.B.LE program, a Fellow of the Institute of Higher Education and is currently completing a Masters in Medical Education.

Emma Kyte is an experienced neonatal nurse and qualified ANNP having worked in tertiary neonatal centres and on neonatal transport. Recently, she has worked within the Neonatal Network as Quality Improvement lead nurse and now works at Liverpool Women's Neonatal Unit as Neonatal Nurse Consultant.

Marie Lindsay-Sutherland works as the Lead ANNP in the neonatal unit in Poole, England. Since qualifying as an ANNP, she has developed a special interest in caring for neonates born to women with mental health problems and has completed postgraduate programmes in neonatal studies, advanced clinical practice and a doctorate examining the effect of antenatal exposure to SSRIs on the neonatal QT interval.

Nicky McCarthy works for Brighton and Sussex University Hospitals NHS Trust, on the neonatal unit and the neonatal transfer service as an ANNP. She is currently undertaking a doctoral degree in health sciences at the University of Southampton comprising an ethnographic study of the neonatal and midwifery teams in the neonatal golden hour. Her special interests include human factors and simulation.

Linda McDonald established her nursing career as a critical care children's nurse in Australia, before relocating to London where she took a neonatal nursing role at St Thomas' Hospital. She has subsequently worked in a number of roles, including senior sister, Clinical Educator, Neonatal Transport nurse and Lecturer Practitioner. She is currently based in Worcester practising as an ANNP and NLS instructor.

Heather Maxwell at the time of writing her chapter was a Neonatal Sister/Education and Engagement Lead at Barnsley Hospital NHS Foundation Trust and had recently continued her clinical and education role in Northern Ireland. She is passionate about standardising neonatal nursing practice and empowering neonatal nurses.

Alli Mitchell is a Midwifery lecturer and Programme lead MSc Advanced Practice (Neonates) at the University of Salford. As neonates are a vulnerable population, she believes strongly in the importance of developing and upholding evidence-based, gold standards of medical and nursing care to optimise their wellbeing.

Debra Nicholson is a Neonatal Clinical Facilitator at Lancashire Teaching Hospitals NHS Foundation Trust and has worked in neonatal care since qualifying as a children's nurse in 2001, completing both her BSc (hons) and MA Neonatal Studies. Debra facilitates simulation training on NICU as part of the nursing and medical teaching programme and has recently completed a secondment with the North West Neonatal Network on the education team.

Katherine Noble (Katie) is a Neonatal Sister and Clinical Facilitator at Lancashire Teaching Hospitals NHS Foundation Trust and has worked in neonatal care since qualifying as a children's nurse in 2002, completing both her BSc (hons) and MA Neonatal Studies. Her MA involved developing a teaching portfolio based upon classroom teaching in the university and clinical settings. As part of this, she focused on parental involvement in decisions when considering withholding and withdrawing life-sustaining treatments in NICU.

Sharon Nurse works as a Senior Lecturer (Education) at the School of Nursing & Midwifery in Belfast. She currently lectures in a range of midwifery and neonatal topics and is Chair of the Neonatal Nurses Association (Northern Ireland group). She has a particular interest in palliative neonatal care.

Katie O'Connell-Binns is a Registered Children's Nurse and at the time of contributing to the book was a Transitional Care and Neonatal Staff Nurse at Burnley General Hospital.

Alison O'Doherty is a Registered Children's Nurse and has worked in Neonatal Nursing since qualifying from the University of Bradford in 2005. She has undertaken a number of roles in her career, including education and practice development. She currently works as a Matron on the Neonatal Unit at St Mary's Hospital, Manchester.

Louise Oduro-Dominah is a consultant paediatric anaesthetist working at Cambridge University NHS Foundation Trust.

Ella Porter is a fifth year student doctor, Riga Stradens University, Latvia. Ella has an interest in foetal medicine and neonatology along with family support due to the importance she places on the value of parent–infant attachment and good mental health for newborns as they grow and develop, facilitated by high-quality, multidisciplinary care.

Katy Powis has worked as a neonatal nurse in Northampton from 2001, after completing her nursing degree in New Zealand, and left her post as Clinical Educator in 2017 to pursue her career in teaching. She now is primarily a Lecturer on the QIS modules at the University of Bedfordshire, where she also contributes to the midwifery, paramedic and nursing degrees in relation to neonatal care. Katy is an NLS instructor and a Fellow of the Higher Education Academy and is currently completing a Masters in Medical Education.

Annette Rathwell is a Teaching Fellow at the Florence Nightingale School of Nursing and Midwifery, King's College, London.

Kaye Spence is a clinical nurse consultant in neonatal research at the Children's Hospital at Westmead in Sydney and holds an Adjunct Associate Professor appointment at Western Sydney University. She was the inaugural clinical nurse consultant in neonatology and worked in the role for 30 years. Kaye is a NIDCAP Professional and is Co-director of the Australasian NIDCAP Training Centre and is a FINE Preceptor for the international foundation developmental care program.

Patrick Turton is currently the Lead Nurse for the Newborn Emergency Stabilisation and Transport (NEST) Team based in St Michael's Hospital, University Hospitals Bristol NHS

Foundation Trust. Patrick has experience of working in both neonatal and paediatric intensive care, as well as for neonatal and paediatric critical care transport teams.

Lynne Wainwright is a general and children's nurse who specialised in neonatal care. She has worked in neonatal units as a staff nurse and practice development nurse and is now a senior teaching fellow in the Child & Family Health department at King's College London where she teaches Children's and Neonatal Nursing. Lynne is undertaking a PhD considering the impact on the whole family including siblings when a baby is admitted to a neonatal unit.

Debbie Webster is a neonatal Educator employed at Liverpool Women's Hospital and teaches the QIS programme in collaboration with Liverpool John Moore's University. Currently, she is seconded to Northwest Neonatal Network as Quality Improvement Lead Nurse for Education.

PREFACE

This is the 3rd edition of *Neonatal Intensive Care Nursing*, first published in 2000, with the previous edition published in 2010 edited by Glenys Boxwell. Since 2010, many areas of practice have remained the same, while certain new areas have emerged. What has *not* changed is the recognition and value placed on the family, regarding them as essential partners in the care of their baby. In addition, the fundamental principle of sound nursing care practice based on evidence has remained steadfast and of vital importance. What *has* emerged over the last ten years since the 2nd edition, however, are findings from a vast amount of new research, undertaken in all the key areas covered in this book which have, and continue to have, an impact on practice. Examples are: Family Integrated Care (FICare), timing of cord clamping, high flow oxygen administration, less invasive ventilation strategies, the first hour of care, to name but a few. Therefore, it is imperative that a reputable book such as this, which is widely referenced and used by those both learning and working within the clinical area nationally and internationally, is updated to ensure that readers have the most current information to apply to their nursing care practice.

However, regardless of whether there has been change or not, does not detract from the importance of ensuring any book content is updated in line with the most recent research-based evidence and *current* practices. The new editors were mindful of this in the planning of the new edition. The majority of previous chapters have remained with their original titles and are presented in updated forms and re-ordered. Other chapters are new and have been added in response to the peer review of the 2nd edition, detailed below.

In summary, the *new* features of this 3rd edition are: new sections, new chapters, the addition of reflective practice, new case studies with answer guides and a web-based companion. Taking on board the suggestions from a robust peer review of the need for a 3rd edition, further detail of these new areas is as follows:

- **New sections**: the chapters in their entirety are divided into four sections:
    - **Part 1**: An overview of neonatal care, which sets the broad context of care, how it is organised and where it sits in the wider arena of the baby and family's future.
    - **Part 2**: The physical and emotional wellbeing of the neonate and family, which places importance on psycho-emotional care as well as the more physical, clinically based care.
    - **Part 3**: Clinical aspects of neonatal care which includes the majority of the previous chapter topics in the context of a systems approach.

- ■ **Part 4**: Practices and procedures in neonatal care, which focuses on some of the more procedural-based content relevant to practice.
- ■ **New chapters:** New content added comprises; Organisation of neonatal care, Assessment of the neonate, The premature and low birth weight baby, and Palliative care.
- ■ **Reflective practice:** Reading through the chapters in the new edition, you are encouraged to reflect on the key points and content relating to your practice and engage with this and the relevant literature in an enquiring way. Specific pointers to consider, and questions to reflect on, are therefore posed at the start of each chapter.
- ■ **New case studies:** These are at the end of each chapter as before but in this edition there will be the opportunity to view suggested answer guides (by referring to the relevant web page, on the companion website for each chapter).
- ■ **Web-based companion:** This includes the following:
  - ■ **Case study answer guides** (with signposting to additional information and resources as applicable)
  - ■ **Supplementary information** – any extra information relevant to the chapter that is not included in the actual book
  - ■ **'Test your knowledge'** – multiple-choice quizzes and a combination of other self-testing formats for learning reinforcement (such as crosswords, word searches, short-answer quizzes) related to each chapter
  - ■ **Web-based resources** – a selection of open-access articles and web resources is provided for each chapter.

Finally, we feel it is vital to emphasise some key, underpinning principles that are relevant to each and every chapter in this book – the baby and family together, parents as key members of the multidisciplinary team, and the value and inclusion of allied health professionals who significantly contribute to the best care for babies and families.

It has been a real privilege to edit this valuable textbook that plays an important role in the joint learning about the vital elements of current, high-quality neonatal nursing practice.

Julia Petty and Lisa Kaiser

PART 1

AN OVERVIEW OF NEONATAL CARE

An overview of neonatal care: The parent voice

Going into neonatal care was like entering another world. The highs and lows and hurdles along the way. We went from intensive care to high dependency and then to special care but then had to go back again to intensive care when he got an infection. Everything seemed to start all over again … the uncertainty and another bumpy ride.

He then got transferred to another hospital for his heart which was very different, and we returned three days later.

Eventually, we were transferred back to our home unit, another new experience, but it was still weeks before we could finally go home.

Going home was a like a miracle almost – we couldn't believe the day had finally arrived. It was difficult and so daunting, but we knew it had to happen and we had to cope without the pillars of the neonatal staff supporting us.

Of all the different transitions though the different parts of the neonatal unit and the different hospitals, going home was the hardest step for the first couple of years. He needed to be re-admitted a couple of times with infections and breathing problems.

But we got there and can look back at the challenges, knowing that he overcame them all.

Voice of a mother of a 24-week gestation baby, Tom (pseudonym), who spent four months in neonatal care within three different hospitals.

Adapted from Petty et al., 2019a; 2019b

See chapter 4 reference list for full citations.

1 ORGANISATION OF NEONATAL CARE

Heather Maxwell and Katie O'Connell-Binns

CONTENTS

GUIDANCE ON HOW TO ENHANCE PERSONAL LEARNING FROM THIS CHAPTER

Key points covered in this chapter

■ Definitions of the different care categories infants fall under within neonatal services, and the structure of neonatal care in the United Kingdom (UK).

■ Neonatal nursing education, continuous professional development and career progression.

■ Various roles of the multidisciplinary team and their contribution to a baby's journey through the neonatal unit.

Reflection

Reading through the chapter, you are encouraged to engage with the key points and related literature in an enquiring way. Ask these questions:

■ Why are categories of care important and how do they impact on the planning and delivery of neonatal care?

■ What are the advantages of extended and enhanced nursing roles? Do they form part of your unit's structure?

■ Which specialities of the multidisciplinary team are available for your unit, and how can they benefit your patients?

Implications for nursing care

■ Finally: this chapter should facilitate your understanding of how neonatal care is organised in the UK. Consider how you can contribute towards the effectiveness of your own neonatal network, and what this means for the individual babies you look after on a day-to-day basis.

INTRODUCTION AND BACKGROUND

Approximately 750,000 babies are born in England, Scotland and Wales each year. Of these, 95,000, or 1 in 8 of these infants, will be admitted to a neonatal unit (Royal College of Paediatrics and Child Heath (RCPCH), 2018a), while in Northern Ireland 1,800 babies are born prematurely or sick, requiring care in one of NIs' seven neonatal units (TinyLife and Bliss, 2018). Neonatology is a relatively small speciality but, owing to continual medical advancements, the survival rates of small, sick and extremely premature babies have improved. Numerous stakeholders from national organisations and government bodies, such as the National Institute for Health and Care Excellence (NICE), Department of Health (DH), British Association of Perinatal Medicine (BAPM), Neonatal Nurses Association (NNA), Royal College of Nursing (RCN), Scottish Neonatal Nurses Group (SNNG), Bliss and TinyLife among others, help shape neonatal care and provide guidance and support for staff and families. Recently, the new National Health Service (NHS) plan (NHS, 2019) lays out recommendations for neonatal and maternity care moving forward for the next ten years. This chapter will explore how neonatal services are structured and coordinated in the UK by outlining the BAPM Categories of Care and levels of service provision, describing the function of operational delivery networks (ODN), and finally examining the role of the neonatal nurse and the multidisciplinary team.

CATEGORIES OF NEONATAL CARE

Newborn infants are admitted to the neonatal unit (NNU) for a variety of clinical conditions and treatment, including having been born too early, having a low birth weight or a medical or surgical condition that needs specialist treatment (RCPCH, 2018a). These will determine the levels of care different infants require, and thus the staff who may safely look after them. In 2011 BAPM defined criteria for four categories of care for neonatal patients to ensure every baby is assigned appropriate care levels. These are transitional care, special care, high dependency care and intensive care. Throughout an infant's stay within neonatal services, the category of care may vary due to changes in their condition, e.g. clinical improvement or deterioration (NHS Improvement, 2018).

Transitional care

The concept of transitional care (TC) was originally developed by Whitby (1983) and has proven its value by preventing unnecessary separation of mother and baby (Duddridge, 2001; Miah, 2013; Battersby et al., 2017). It serves infants who require support but do not require NNU admission (see p. 6 for criteria), until they may be discharged home. This model confers benefits such as reduced length of stay on the NNU, allowing for optimised use of neonatal cots, improved parental confidence, bonding, establishment of breastfeeding with higher success rates and an overall improvement of the family experience including promotion of sibling bonds (Duddridge, 2001; BAPM, 2017). As reported by Boyle et al. (2015) in a paper on late and moderately **preterm** infants, a substantial amount of specialist input is provided in postnatal wards, beyond normal newborn care. Therefore, appropriate expertise and early planning are essential if such infants are managed away from specialised neonatal settings.

TC can be delivered in two service models: on a dedicated TC ward, or within a postnatal ward and is facilitated via close cooperation of neonatal and midwifery staff. This may include maternity care assistants, nursery nurses and other nursing support roles. In either case, the mother must be resident and caring for her baby as the primary caregiver. The mother is supported with care activities above those required normally (BAPM, 2017).

Criteria for TC could include:

- Prematurity (≥34 weeks or ≥33 weeks if discharged from the neonatal unit)
- Low birth weight (but >1600 grams)
- Nasogastric tube feeding (≥3 hourly)
- Babies on IV antibiotics, if otherwise stable
- Hypothermia (<36°C) requiring intervention
- Haemolytic jaundice requiring phototherapy
- Maternal substance misuse resulting in the baby's need for oral medication and/or feeding support
- Palliative care following multidisciplinary team discussion with parental agreement
- Congenital malformations resulting in feeding problems, e.g. cleft lip/palate
- Newborn babies readmitted from home with excessive weight loss and requiring nasogastric tube feeding
- Babies transferred from the neonatal unit for further support/observation prior to discharge home.

Other areas of care provision, above routine postnatal care of mother and baby may be observation of infants at risk of deteriorating health, blood glucose monitoring for infants at risk of hypoglycaemia, feeding support, monitoring jaundice and meeting care needs arising from a baby's social background. These are classed as 'normal care' and should ideally be provided by midwifery staff on the postnatal ward (BAPM, 2017; National Maternal and Perinatal Audit, 2017).

Despite the need for TC, there is variation in the provision of facilities nationally alongside care delivery, classification and commissioning (Davies, 2014; Bliss, 2015; Battersby et al., 2017). While many maternity and neonatal services provide elements of TC, these may not always be formally recognised (BAPM, 2017). Davies (2014), in a UK survey on behalf of the Neonatal Clinical Reference Group, found that of the responding units (85% nationally) only 46% had access to any kind of designated TC area. Investing in appropriately staffed TC facilities should be viewed as a priority by commissioners and NHS Trusts, as otherwise numbers of admissions to NNUs resulting in separation of mother and baby will continue to rise in England. Admissions of **term** infants in particular were the focus of NHS Improvement (2017) who identified avoidable admissions to neonatal care. These include the number of full-term babies who did not have serious birth defects or disorders, thus leading to stress and trauma for the families and additional financial pressures on neonatal services with finite resources.

The following three levels of care require admission to the NNU and therefore result in separation of mother and baby until the infant is fit for discharge home, to the postnatal ward or a TC ward.

Special care

Special care (SC) is defined as any care in which a baby does not fulfil the criteria for intensive or high dependency care.

Criteria for special care include:

- Oxygen by nasal cannula
- Feeding by nasogastric/nasojejunal tube or gastrostomy
- Continuous physiological monitoring (excluding apnoea monitors only)
- Care of a stoma
- Presence of IV cannula
- Baby receiving phototherapy
- Special observation of physiological variables at least four-hourly.

High dependency care

Infants under the high dependency (HD) care category should be looked after by highly skilled staff but they have lower demands than those under intensive care, from a perspective of nurse-to-patient ratios. Any day where a baby does not fulfil the criteria for intensive care is classed as a high dependency day, and may include the following:

- Any form of non-invasive respiratory support (e.g. nasal continuous positive airway pressure (nasal CPAP), biphasic positive airway pressure (BiPAP), humidified high flow nasal cannula (HHFNC))
- Any day receiving any of the following:
  - Parenteral nutrition
  - Continuous infusion of drugs (except prostaglandin and/or insulin)
  - Presence of a central venous or percutaneous central venous catheter
  - Presence of a tracheostomy
  - Presence of a urethral or **suprapubic** catheter
  - Presence of a transanastomotic tube following oesophageal **atresia** repair

- ■ Presence of nasopharyngeal airway/nasal stent
- ■ Observation of seizures/cerebral function monitoring
- ■ Barrier nursing
- ■ Need for ventricular taps.

Intensive care

This is provided for the most unwell or unstable infants with the greatest needs in relation to staff skills and staff-to-patient ratios. An intensive care day is defined as:

- ■ Any day where a baby receives any form of mechanical respiratory support via a tracheal tube
- ■ *Both* non-invasive ventilation (e.g. nasal CPAP, BiPAP, HHFNC) and parenteral nutrition (PN)
- ■ Day of surgery (including laser therapy for retinopathy of prematurity)
- ■ Day of death
- ■ Any day receiving where any of the following applies:
  - ■ Presence of an umbilical arterial line
  - ■ Presence of an umbilical venous line
  - ■ Presence of a peripheral arterial line
  - ■ Insulin infusion
  - ■ Presence of a chest drain
  - ■ Exchange transfusion
  - ■ Therapeutic hypothermia
  - ■ Prostaglandin infusion
  - ■ Presence of a Replogle tube
  - ■ Presence of an epidural catheter
  - ■ Presence of a silo for gastroschisis
  - ■ Presence of an external ventricular drain
  - ■ Dialysis (any type).

LEVELS OF SERVICE PROVISION

Factors such as gestation, weight, clinical condition and co-morbidities determine the category of care each individual infant requires (BAPM, 2018). Due to numerous potential clinical conditions discussed throughout this book, levels of care may mean an infant cannot be safely nursed in the NNU at the hospital in which the mother has booked to deliver, or clinical deterioration may result in a need for transfer to another specialist neonatal unit. According to the Toolkit for High-Quality Neonatal Services (Department of Health, 2009), neonatal care provision can be categorised as outlined in table 1.1.

TABLE 1.1 CATEGORIES OF NEONATAL CARE

Level 1 **Special Care Unit (SCU)**	Units provide SC (usually to the hospital's local population) but do not aim to provide any continuing HD or IC.
Level 2 **Local Neonatal Unit (LNU)**	Units provide HD care and some short-term IC (as agreed locally), but infants who require complex or longer-term IC would be transferred to a neonatal intensive care unit.
Level 3 **Neonatal Intensive Care Unit (NICU)**	Units provide the entire range of medical neonatal care, including IC. In some units, specialist services such as neonatal surgery are available. These units also provide additional care for babies and their families referred from the neonatal network in which they are based, and from other networks when necessary to deal with peaks of demand or requests for specialist care not available elsewhere.

(adapted from BAPM, 2010)

Thus, an infant born at 33 weeks' gestation who needs no respiratory support but is clinically well, requiring solely nasogastric feeds while progressing to oral feeding, would be placed under the SC category and could be nursed at a level 1, 2 or 3 NNU. However, if there is a need for respiratory support such as CPAP, this infant would fall under the HD category of care and would thus not be eligible to be nursed on a level 1 Special Care Unit (SCU), requiring transfer to either a level 2 Local Neonatal Unit (LNU) or a level 3 NICU. In another instance, if an infant was born at 24 weeks' gestation with an anticipated ongoing need for mechanical ventilation (i.e. not short-term IC), this infant should be delivered and cared for at a level 3 NICU. However, not all mothers whose infants require level 3 NICU admission book to deliver at such hospitals, so that transfer to a suitable hospital is required, ideally antenatally (Musson and Harrison, 2016). Once the infant's progress and clinical condition allow, transfer back to the home unit may be appropriate.

NEONATAL TRANSPORT

Neonatal services depend on the availability of reliable transport facilities to bring babies and their mothers to the most appropriate care setting to meet their needs. Prior to birth, if admission to neonatal services is deemed necessary, ideally the level of care required can be anticipated and transport can be *in utero*. This is safer than *ex utero* transfer after a baby is born and is seen as a necessary component of contemporary obstetrics to ensure better health outcomes for the mother and the foetus (Porcellato et al., 2015). However, many problems only become apparent at delivery or later, and this may necessitate stabilisation and transport to a higher-level NNU from the place of delivery (Mears and Chalmers, 2005; Chang et al., 2015) or thereafter, hence the need for an *ex utero* transfer (chapter 22).

Neonatal transport services in the UK have previously been criticised for a lack of standardisation and understanding of the effect of transport on neonatal physiology (Teasdale and Hamilton, 2008). This highlights the importance of ensuring that transfers are appropriately managed, based on the clinical need to improve outcomes. Prior to the advent of centralised transport services, problems identified in relation to transport included:

■ Staff having to leave units to accompany babies in transit
■ Availability and response times from the ambulance service
■ Journey times affecting outcomes
■ In the case of transfers for cot capacity issues, an impact on the ability of the receiving unit to cope with the demands on their service.

Chapter 22 (neonatal transportation) will explore this subject in more depth in line with the current perspective.

THE ROLE OF OPERATIONAL DELIVERY NETWORKS

Over recent decades, the survival rate of preterm infants has rapidly increased with advances in healthcare and medical technology. The EPICure study highlighted the rise in survival rates of the extremely premature infant (Costeloe, 2000; EPICure, 2012) and still continues to inform our knowledge in this area (Marlow et al., 2014; Linsell et al., 2017). Following this research, the Department of Health (2003) formulated and published the 'Neonatal Intensive Care Review: Strategy for Improvement' document which placed all NNUs within geographically determined groups known as a neonatal network or operational delivery network (ODN). As a result, every NNU in the UK is part of an ODN, and each network oversees multiple NNUs within their allocated region, with a responsibility for estimating their population's neonatal care needs. There are allocated numbers of SC, HD and IC beds in each ODN, which are coordinated with the aim of ensuring that babies receive their required care as close to home as possible where this can be anticipated. Cot capacity issues within an ODN may sometimes result in a baby being transferred to the nearest available cot outside their geographical network, to be cared for there until a cot within the network is available and the infant is stable enough for the journey.

ODNs have a duty to benchmark and audit their practice, as well as monitoring their workforce with regard to sustainability of neonatal services (Department of Health, 2012; NHS Improvement, 2018). The continuous drive towards improving care standards and efficiency is facilitated by projects such as the Commissioning for Quality and Innovation (CQUINs) framework and the National Neonatal Audit Programme (NNAP) delivered by the RCPCH. By evaluating data obtained through the BadgerNet UK system, the aim of the NNAP is to establish whether there is consistency with regard to the standards of care received by infants admitted to UK NNUs (RCPCH, 2018b). The web-based companion contains a number of relevant links for additional information.

STAFFING OF NEONATAL UNITS

Appropriate nurse, medical and allied health professional staffing on all NNUs is essential to meet the needs of babies at various care levels. It is, however, well documented that there are issues both in recruiting and retaining neonatal nurses (National Audit Office, 2007; Department of Health, 2009; BAPM, 2010; NICE, 2010; RCN, 2011; BAPM, NNA and SNNG, 2012; Bliss, 2015). Based on professional consensus, recommendations for minimum staffing levels are as follows (BAPM, 2010; BAPM, 2018; NHS Improvement, 2018).

Intensive Care: Due to the complex needs of both the baby and their family the ratio of neonatal nurses who are qualified in specialty (QIS) to baby should be one nurse: one baby. This nurse should have no other (including managerial) responsibilities during the time of clinical care but may be involved in the support of a less experienced nurse working alongside him/her in caring for the same baby, e.g. a nurse undertaking the QIS course.

High Dependency Care: The ratio of neonatal nurses QIS responsible for the care of babies requiring HD care is recommended as one nurse: two babies. The more stable and less dependent babies may be cared for by registered nurses not QIS, but who are under the direct supervision and responsibility of a neonatal nurse QIS.

Special Care: At a minimum, a ratio of one nurse: four babies is required for infants categorised as SC. It is essential that staffing in SC is sufficient to ensure all discharges are carefully planned and organised, including rigorous parental support. Registered nurses and non-registered clinical staff may care for these babies under the direct supervision and responsibility of a neonatal nurse QIS.

Transitional Care: The ratio of neonatal nurses caring for TC babies should be at least one nurse: four babies, while midwifery support must also be available for the mother. There must be joint working between midwifery and neonatal nursing to determine appropriate staffing for the transitional care service (BAPM, 2017).

THE NEONATAL NURSE

In 2018, NHS Improvement on behalf of the National Quality Board validly summarised the neonatal nursing function in their statement:

> Neonatal nurses play a key role in the planning and delivery of care to babies and their families. They require a wide skill base as their work ranges from providing care for the sick or premature neonate to teaching parents how to care for their baby, gradually handing over responsibility for this in the lead up to discharge. They also provide care across a whole spectrum of care needs, from intensive care, high dependency care, special care and eventually to care in the home environment.
>
> (NHS Improvement, 2018, p. 22)

This wide skill base is a combination of undergraduate study, ever-growing experience as well as personal characteristics and postgraduate education.

Education and continuing professional development

Neonatal nursing offers the opportunity for a nurse to undertake postgraduate study and become a 'QIS' neonatal nurse. On successful completion, this allows neonatal nurses to provide care for HD and IC patients and to supervise non-QIS nurses. Recommendations for the achievement of this qualification outlined by BAPM (2012) and the Royal College of Nursing (RCN) (2015) include consistent competency within nursing practice and a preceptorship period including defined foundation knowledge within the neonatal specialty. Undertaking postgraduate study towards QIS neonatal nursing involves combining theory, which is delivered and fully assessed at a higher educational institute (HEI), and acquiring competency within clinical practice.

The QIS course should include:

(A) Theory modules relating to the care of the neonate and their family within SC, HD care and IC.
(B) Achievement of the core skills set, level 2 undertaken with supervision of an experienced qualified neonatal nurse, assessed in practice and supported by evidence of learning.
(C) Appropriate clinical decision-making skills (SNNG, 2005).

Furthermore, all neonatal nurses with acquired QIS must demonstrate competency in a core skill set (BAPM, 2010; RCN, 2015):

■ Respiratory and cardiovascular management
■ Fluid, electrolyte, nutrition and elimination management
■ Neurological and pain management
■ Skin and hygiene, and infection prevention management
■ Management of health, safety and security for neonates and their families, including complex medicine management
■ Investigations and procedures
■ Temperature management
■ Breastfeeding support
■ Supporting the family.

All infants have individual needs, which can often be complex. In addition to core competencies, neonatal nurses QIS must undertake assessment in clinical practice and acquire clinical skills to provide high-quality care for infants (Spence et al., 2016; Turrill, 2014) who meet the following criteria:

- Birth weight ranging from **extremely low birth weight** (<1000g), **very low birth weight** (<1500g), **low birth weight** (<2500g), to normal birth weight and large for **gestational age**
- Physical condition: identification of continuing improvement or deterioration
- Care of the extremely premature infant to post-term
- Infants requiring surgical intervention
- Infants with congenital abnormalities
- Preparation for discharge (BAPM, 2010).

Standardising neonatal nurse QIS education is a current development given the variations that have been reported nationally in competency and training (Gallagher, 2013; Health Education England, 2017). In order to provide a consolidated career pathway for neonatal nurses, which would aid recruitment and retention, a national professional body should ideally regulate QIS education and continuous professional development. This is still a work in progress at the time of printing. Irrespective of the level at which a neonatal nurse functions, he/she is obliged to have evidence of continuous professional development and conform to Nursing and Midwifery Council (NMC) revalidation requirements (NMC, 2019).

CAREER PROGRESSION

Following completion of postgraduate neonatal nursing QIS study, there will be the opportunity for career progression and the potential to develop skills beyond QIS level, as well as to undertake additional study to work within further neonatal roles. BAPM (2010) outline a variety of established nursing roles; these are not all utilised in every NNU but integrated to match an individual unit's requirements.

Extended nursing roles

Senior QIS nurses may have the opportunity to undertake and lead additional non-clinical activities, such as:

- Breastfeeding support
- Family support
- Infant development
- Discharge planning
- Safeguarding children
- Bereavement support and palliative care
- Health, safety and risk management
- Education and practice development (BAPM, 2010).

Neonatal outreach nurse

Following discharge from the neonatal unit some infants have ongoing care needs (Petty et al., 2018), e.g. due to requiring nasogastric tube feeding at home. The role involves providing nursing care, practical and emotional support, parental education and growth monitoring in the home environment (BAPM, 2017).

Enhanced Neonatal Nurse Practitioner (ENNP)

Enhanced practice roles can be undertaken by QIS nurses following additional education and clinical skills, such as venepuncture, cannulation etc. A pathway for acquisition and maintenance of agreed competencies should be defined within the ODN.

Advanced Neonatal Nurse Practitioner (ANNP)

The role of the ANNP was introduced in the UK approximately 25 years ago (Smith and Hall, 2003). Advanced nursing practice is based on the four pillars of advanced practice (see figure 1.1).

From a clinical perspective, following education at master's level, ANNPs may autonomously and independently manage their own caseload through assessment, diagnosis and instigation of treatment within the neonatal population. This includes activities such as the attendance of high-risk deliveries and delivery room resuscitation, stabilisation, independent prescribing, ordering and evaluation of investigations and complex procedures, among other aspects (Department of Health, 2010; RCN, 2018a; RCN, 2018b). With regard to education, ANNPs are frequently involved in teaching junior doctors as well as members of the neonatal nursing team (BAPM, 2010), and should furthermore participate in quality

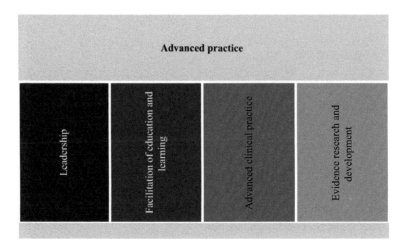

Figure 1.1 Four pillars of advanced practice

improvement activities such as audit, research and the implementation of **evidence-based practice** as part of their role (DH, 2010; RCN, 2018a).

As yet there is no national register of ANNPs/Advanced Nurse Practitioners, but an accreditation pathway is now in place (RCN, 2018c).

Neonatal Nurse Consultant

The role of nurse consultant is structured around

- Expert practice
- Professional leadership and consultancy
- Education, training and development
- Practice and service development, research and evaluation.

As with advanced nursing practice, postgraduate education underpins highly specialist clinical expertise and non-clinical functions. The nurse consultant role has been described as being 'at the pinnacle of the clinical career ladder' (RCN, 2012, p. 97).

THE MULTIDISCIPLINARY TEAM

Neonatology involves working within a multidisciplinary team to achieve the best neonatal outcomes. Both medical and nursing teams have various roles and responsibilities, each designed to work in collaboration with the extended multidisciplinary team. These roles have been defined through *Service Standards for Hospitals Providing Neonatal Care* (BAPM, 2010).

Pharmacy

Pharmacists play a vital role in the monitoring and optimisation of neonatal drug therapy and have an important advisory function with regard to safe delivery of complex and often unlicensed medications. Issues unique to the neonatal population such as patient size, limited intravenous access, and uncertain **pharmacodynamics** and **pharmacokinetics** mean that specialist training is required before the role of neonatal pharmacist can be safely assumed (BAPM, 2010). Medication practice in the neonatal unit is further discussed in chapter 19.

Dietetics

Neonatal dieticians play an integral role for assessing and improving the nutrition of premature infants (Sneve et al., 2008) and work in collaboration with medical and nursing teams as well as families. There is a requirement for all NNUs to have access to a dietician who has undergone specialist education in neonatal nutrition (BAPM, 2010). Please refer to chapter 17 for nutritional management in the NNU for more information.

Radiography

NHS Improvement (2018) highlights the need for all neonatal units to be able to draw on the expertise of diagnostic imaging staff with the ability to interpret neonatal imaging.

Occupational therapy

The role of the neonatal occupational therapist involves neurobehavioural assessment, advice on sensory issues and parental education for response to infant behavioural cues. The role of the occupational therapist often overlaps with that of the physiotherapist, both being vitally important for the wellbeing of infant and family (BAPM, 2010).

Physiotherapy

The neonatal physiotherapist will usually be a very experienced individual who has undertaken master's level education to enable autonomous, evidence-based and innovative practice. Physiotherapy in the form of movement and postural intervention has a positive impact on the development of infant musculoskeletal and motor coordination and thus outcomes. Furthermore, physiotherapists have an educational role for parents and staff with regard to optimising infant support relating to these aspects (Brady & Smith, 2015).

Speech and language therapy

The speech and language therapist is responsible for the assessment of infant feeding and swallowing and formulation of individualised management plans. This is vital to promote successful oral feeding and reduce aversion to feeding. Additionally, the role involves providing feeding education for all staff on general and complex feeding and swallowing problems, as well as supporting parents (BAPM, 2010).

Psychological support

It is recognised that emotional outcomes are improved by providing appropriate support for parents and families (Hall et al., 2016; Patel et al., 2018). The POPPY Project found that although NNUs usually provide outstanding clinical care, less consistent attention has been paid to non-clinical issues and how these affect a family's journey through neonatal care and the transfer from hospital to home (POPPY Steering Group, 2009). Furthermore, Woodroffe (2006) found parents whose infants are admitted to the NNU may experience significant post-traumatic stress symptoms. Unfortunately, not all NNUs have around-the-clock access to psychological support for parents. Neonatal charities such as Bliss may assist parents throughout their neonatal journey, and ensuring access to psychological support for families is a criterion for achieving accreditation to the Bliss Baby Charter (Bliss, 2015). Thus, the future should see an increase in psychological support facilities for families and a reduction of post-traumatic stress symptoms following neonatal admission. This aspect will be covered in more detail in chapter 4, families in the NNU.

CONCLUSION

The organisation of neonatal care in the UK is governed by nationally universal standards. The aim of this organisational structure is to ensure that each infant is looked after as close to home as possible in the clinical environment their level of care requirement necessitates, by appropriately skilled and educated staff. ODNs have been created to facilitate this and work on improving outcomes by benchmarking, standardising and optimising practice in their respective neonatal units. The neonatal nurse plays a pivotal role in a baby's progress on the neonatal unit, not only through the clinical aspects of his/her responsibilities, but also by identifying potentially changing care needs and communicating these where necessary to appropriate hospitals within the ODN, enhancing care by collaborating within the multidisciplinary team and supporting families on their journey.

CASE STUDIES

Case study 1: The 27-week infant in a LNU

You have just commenced your shift at your unit, which is a level 2 LNU. Dylan, the baby you have been allocated today, was born only 2 hours before at 27 weeks' gestation, weighing 1085 grams. He was delivered via emergency C-section due to concerns about foetal wellbeing.

Having received surfactant in the delivery room, he is now stable on CPAP with acceptable blood gases. His other parameters are satisfactory. Dylan is receiving PN via an umbilical venous catheter.

Q.1.   Which care category does Dylan fall under in accordance with BAPM guidelines? Is it suitable for him to be cared for on your unit in the longer term – what is the rationale behind your answer?

Q.2.   What does the nurse in charge have to consider with regard to distribution of the workload among staff, and whom she allocates to look after Dylan?

CASE STUDY

The decision is made for Dylan to be transferred to a level 3 NICU for his ongoing care.

Q.3. How would you prepare for Dylan's transfer? Who needs to be contacted to facilitate this happening?

Case study 2: The journey of an extremely preterm infant transferred *ex utero*

Pavneet was born unexpectedly at 23^{+2} weeks' gestation without having received antenatal corticosteroids. The level 1 SCU at her mother Rashmi's booking hospital stabilised Pavneet and had her transferred to the regional level 3 NICU.

Q.1. Could anything have been done to prevent Pavneet's being delivered in an inappropriate setting for her care requirements?
Pavneet is now nine weeks old and has multiple problems: she is still requiring HHFNC, has suffered significant intraventricular haemorrhages likely to affect her long-term neurodevelopment, and is failing to thrive with her current weight on the 0.4th percentile. However, as Pavneet is now stable, there is a plan to transfer her back to the SCU at her booking hospital. Rashmi and her husband Manjunath are feeling extremely anxious about this and express a wish for Pavneet to remain on the NICU instead.

Q.2. In your opinion, is it appropriate for Pavneet to be repatriated to her local SCU, considering the level of care she is now receiving?

Q.3. How would you approach a conversation with Rashmi? Do you think it would be feasible for Pavneet to be discharged from the NICU instead of her booking hospital's SCU?

Q.4. What are your considerations for Pavneet's ongoing care? Which members of the multidisciplinary team will most likely need to be involved?

For suggested answer guides to the questions posed in these case studies, please refer to the web-based companion site specific to this chapter (see URL below).

WEB-BASED RESOURCES

For further information, online resources and greater detail on the case studies featured in this chapter go to www.routledge.com/cw/nicnursing

References

Battersby, C., Michaelides, S., Upton, M., & Rennie, J. M. (2017). Term admissions to neonatal units in England: a role for transitional care? A retrospective cohort study. *BMJ Open, 7*(5), e016050.

Bliss. (2015). Bliss Family Friendly Accreditation Scheme: Helping to make family-centred care a reality on your neonatal unit. www.bliss.org.uk/health-professionals/bliss-baby-charter/what-is-the-bliss-baby-charter

Boyle, E. M., Johnson, S., Manktelow, B., Seaton, S. E., Draper, E. S., Smith, L. K., Dorling, J., Marlow, N., Petrou, S., & Field, D. J. (2015). Neonatal outcomes and delivery of care for infants born late preterm or moderately preterm: a prospective population-based study. *Archives of Disease in Childhood. Fetal and Neonatal Edition, 100*(6), F479–485.

Brady, A., & Smith, P. (2015). *A Competence Framework and Evidenced-Based Practice Guidance for the Physiotherapist working in the Neonatal Intensive Care and Special Care Unit in the United Kingdom.* Huntingdon: Association of Paediatric Chartered Physiotherapists .

British Association of Perinatal Medicine. (2010). *Service Standards for Hospitals Providing Neonatal Care.* (3rd Edition) London: BAPM.

British Association of Perinatal Medicine, Neonatal Nurses Association and Scottish Neonatal Nurses' Group (2012). *Matching skills and knowledge for Qualified in Speciality (QIS) Neonatal nurses: A core syllabus for clinical competency.* London: British Association of Perinatal Medicine.

British Association of Perinatal Medicine. (2017). *Neonatal Transitional Care – A Framework for Practice.* www.bapm.org/resources/framework-neonatal-transitional-care

British Association of Perinatal Medicine. (2018). Optimal arrangements for Local Neonatal Units and Special Care Units in the UK including guidance on their staffing: A Framework for Practice. London: BAPM.

Chang, A. S. M., Berry, A., Jones, L. J., & Sivasangari, S. (2015). Specialist teams for neonatal transport to neonatal intensive care units for prevention of morbidity and mortality. *Cochrane Database of Systematic Reviews*, Issue 10. Art. No.: CD007485. DOI: 10.1002/14651858.CD007485.pub2

Costeloe, K., Hennessy, E., Gibson, A. T., Marlow, N., Wilkinson, A. R., & EPICure Study Group. (2000). The EPICure study: outcomes to discharge from hospital for infants born at the threshold of viability. *Pediatrics, 106*(4), 659–671.

Davies, A. (2014). *Transitional Care Report.* www.wmscnsenate.nhs.uk/index.php/download_file/view/205/971/

Department of Health. (2003). *Neonatal Intensive Care Review: Strategy for Improvement.* London: Department of Health.

Department of Health. (2009). *Toolkit for High Quality Neonatal Services.* London: Department of Health.

Department of Health. (2010). *Advanced Level Nursing: A Position Statement.* London: Department of Health.

Department of Health. (2012). *Developing Operational Delivery Networks. The Way Forward.* London: Department of Health.

Duddridge, E. (2001). What are the advantages of transitional care for neonates? *British Journal of Midwifery, 9*(2), 92–98.

EPICure. (2012). www.epicure.ac.uk

Gallagher, K. (2013). Neonatal nursing education provision in the United Kingdom. *Journal of Neonatal Nursing, 19*(5), 224–232.

Hall, S. L., Phillips, R., & Hynan, M. T. (2016). Transforming NICU care to provide comprehensive family support. *Newborn and Infant Nursing Reviews, 16*(2), 69–73.

Health Education England. (2017). *Exploring New Ways of Working in the Neonatal Unit.* www.londonpaediatrics.co.uk/wp-content/uploads/2017/11/ExploringNewWaysofWorkinginthe NeonatalUnitv4.pdf

Linsell, L., Malouf, R., Morris, J., Kurinczuk, J. J., & Marlow, N. (2017). Risk factor models for neurodevelopmental outcomes in children born very preterm or with very low birth weight: a systematic review of methodology and reporting. *American Journal of Epidemiology, 185*(7), 601–612.

Marlow, N., Bennett, C., Draper, E. S., Hennessy, E. M., Morgan, A. S., & Costeloe, K. L. (2014). Perinatal outcomes for extremely preterm babies in relation to place of birth in England: the EPICure 2 study. *Archives of Disease in Childhood: Fetal and Neonatal Edition, 99*(3), F181–F188.

Mears, M., & Chalmers, S. (2005). Neonatal pre-transport stabilisation–caring for infants the STABLE way. *Infant, 1*(1), 34–37.

Miah, R. (2013). Does transitional care improve neonatal and maternal health outcomes? A systematic review. *British Journal of Midwifery, 21*(9), 634–646.

Musson, R. E., & Harrison, C. M. (2016). The burden and outcome of in utero transfers. *Acta Paediatrica, 105*(5), 490–493.

National Audit Office. (2007). *Caring for Vulnerable Babies: The reorganisation of neonatal services in England.* London: The Stationery Office.

National Health Service (NHS). (2019). *Maternity and neonatal services.* www.longtermplan.nhs.uk/online-version/chapter-3-further-progress-on-care-quality-and-outcomes/a-strong-start-in-life-for-children-and-young-people/maternity-and-neonatal-services/

National Institute for Health and Care Excellence. (2010). *Neonatal Specialist Care: Quality Standard.* NICE.

NHS Improvement on behalf of the National Quality Board. (2018). *Safe, sustainable and productive staffing. An improvement resource for neonatal care.* London: NHS Improvement. https://improvement.nhs.uk/resources/safe-staffing-neonatal-care-and-children-and-young-peoples-services/

NHS Improvement. (2017). *Reducing admission of full term babies to neonatal units.* London: NHS Improvement. https://improvement.nhs.uk/resources/safe-staffing-neonatal-care-and-children-and-young-peoples-services/

National Maternal and Perinatal Audit. (2017). *Definitions used in the second organisational survey.* www.maternityaudit.org.uk/pages/ResourcesUnitTypeDef

Nursing and Midwifery Council. (2019). *Revalidation.* http://revalidation.nmc.org.uk/

Patel, N., Ballantyne, A., Bowker, G., Weightman, J., Weightman, S., & Helping Us Grow Group (HUGG). (2018). Family integrated care: Changing the culture in the neonatal unit. *Archives of Disease in Childhood, 103*(5), 415–419.

Petty, J, Whiting, L., Green, J., Fowler, C., Rossiter, C., & Elliott, D. (2018). Parents' views on preparation to care for extremely premature infants at home. *Nursing Children and Young People. 30*(4), 22–27.

POPPY Steering Group. (2009). *Family-centred care in neonatal units: A summary of research results and recommendations from the POPPY project.* London: NCT.

Porcellato, L., Masson, G., O'Mahony, F., Jenkinson, S., Vanner, T., Cheshire, K., & Perkins, E. (2015). 'It's something you have to put up with' – service users' experiences of in utero transfer: A qualitative study. *BJOG: An International Journal of Obstetrics & Gynaecology, 122*(13), 1825–1832.

Royal College of Nursing. (2011). *Competence, education and careers in neonatal nursing: RCN guidance.* Canterbury: Royal College of Nursing.

Royal College of Nursing. (2012). *Becoming and being a nurse consultant: towards greater effectiveness through a programme of support.* London: Royal College of Nursing.

Royal College of Nursing. (2015). *Career, education and competence framework for neonatal nursing in the UK.* London: Royal College of Nursing.

Royal College of Nursing. (2018a). *Advanced Level Nursing Practice Section 1: The registered nurse working at an advanced level of practice.* London: Royal College of Nursing.

Royal College of Nursing. (2018b). *Standards for Advanced Level Nursing Practice.* London: Royal College of Nursing.

Royal College of Nursing. (2018c). *Advanced Level Nursing Practice Section 3: RCN accreditation and credentialing.* London: Royal College of Nursing.

Royal College of Paediatrics and Child Health & Healthcare Quality Improvement Partnership. (2018a). *National Neonatal Audit Programme 2018 Annual Report on 2017 data.* Royal College of Paediatrics and Child Health.

Royal College of Paediatrics and Child Health. (2018b) *About the National Neonatal Audit Programme.* Retrieved from www.rcpch.ac.uk/work-we-do/quality-improvement-patient-safety/national-neonatal-audit-programme-nnap/about

Scottish Neonatal Nurses Group (2005). *The Competency Framework and Core Clinical Skills for Neonatal Nurses.* Unpublished. Scotland: Scottish Neonatal Nurses Group.

Smith, S. L., & Hall, M. A. (2003). Developing a neonatal workforce: role evolution and retention of advanced neonatal nurse practitioners. *Archives of Disease in Childhood: Fetal and Neonatal Edition, 88*(5), F426–F429.

Sneve, J., Kattelmann, K., Ren, C., & Stevens, D. C. (2008). Implementation of a multidisciplinary team that includes a registered dietitian in a neonatal intensive care unit improved nutrition outcomes. *Nutrition in Clinical Practice, 23*(6), 630–634.

Spence, K., Sinclair, L., Morritt, M. L., & Laing, S. (2016). Knowledge and learning in speciality practice. *Journal of Neonatal Nursing, 22*(6), 263–276.

Teasdale, D., & Hamilton, C. (2008). Baby on the move: issues in neonatal transport. *Paediatric Nursing, 20*(1), 20.

TinyLife & Bliss (2018). *Northern Ireland Baby Report 2018.* http://TinyLife.org.uk/dloads/17071_bliss_northern_ireland_baby_report_aw_lr_single_pages.pdf

Turrill, S. (2014). The education of UK specialised neonatal nurses: Reviewing the rationale for creating a standard competency framework. *Nurse Education in Practice, 14*(5), 504–511.

Whitby, C. A. (1983). Moving forward in neonatal care–transitional care. *Midwives Chronicle, 96*(1149), suppl. 17.

Woodroffe, I. (2006). Multiple losses in neonatal intensive care units. *Journal of Neonatal Nursing, 12*(4), 144–147.

2 ASSESSMENT OF THE NEONATE

Linda McDonald and Lisa Kaiser

CONTENTS

GUIDANCE ON HOW TO ENHANCE PERSONAL LEARNING FROM THIS CHAPTER

Key points covered in this chapter

■ How history taking, including a background of maternal health problems in pregnancy, can improve the quality of an assessment.

■ A systematic approach to assessment of the neonate.

■ Practical considerations for neonatal assessment.

Reflection

Reading through the chapter, you are encouraged to engage with the key points and related literature in an enquiring way. Ask these questions:

■ How do you incorporate assessment into your daily nursing care and the planning of this?

■ Do you understand the potential implications of maternal health problems, or health problems of the wider family, for the health of your patient on the neonatal unit?

■ Following a systems approach, which aspects do you need to incorporate into the assessment of your patients to ensure this is thorough and complete?

Implications for nursing care

■ Finally: how will this chapter enable you to plan your approach to assessment of the neonate? Will what you learn affect your current practice?

INTRODUCTION AND BACKGROUND

Assessment of the neonate is a fundamental aspect of nursing in the neonatal unit (NNU). Familiarisation with the clinical status of a baby at the beginning of a shift, and continuous re-evaluation throughout, is crucial and frequently occurs unconsciously. Yet it facilitates the detection of often subtle changes, and thus makes the neonatal nurse role crucial in the timely recognition, escalation and management of the deteriorating infant. This chapter aims to provide a theoretical background as well as a practical approach to the comprehensive assessment of the neonate. As individual pathologies commonly seen in the NNU are explored in the following chapters, it should be considered how the principles discussed over the next few pages can be applied in the context of these various conditions.

HISTORY TAKING

The foremost aim of history taking is to identify infants who may be at risk of difficulties following birth and even health issues extending into childhood, which require ongoing monitoring and management (Ingram, 2017). Good-quality history taking has thus been suggested to contribute positively to short- and long-term outcomes, and even impact on mortality (Evans, 2015). Whether history taking and assessment take place in chronological sequence will depend on the immediate needs of the baby. For example, attending to a hypoxic baby requiring resuscitation at delivery will take precedence over acquiring an in-depth family history. The nature and depth of details explored will also depend on the situation – while clinicians caring for a term infant born in poor condition just admitted from the labour ward need to establish the salient elements of maternal, familial, antenatal and perinatal history, such details will be already known and less relevant to the six-week-old preterm infant in the NNU at the point in time when he/she is deteriorating with sepsis (see table 2.1 for the components of a comprehensive history).

Thus, history taking may occur at various points in a baby's care episode:

■   At delivery through midwives and obstetricians.
■   On admission to the NNU (whether from labour ward or the postnatal ward).
■   Following a referral from the community or another NNU.
■   During antenatal screening for probable neonatal admission post birth.
■   Specialist consultation referral to a tertiary or surgical centre.
■   During daily ward rounds.
■   At any time, a change in the neonate's condition requires reassessment.

Several sources may be consulted to complete a baby's history (see table 2.1 and figure 2.1).

Particularly in the context of the newborn infant physical examination (NIPE; Public Health England, 2018), the process of history taking may furthermore help to establish a rapport between parents and practitioner (Evans, 2015). While the order of history taking may differ, each element outlined above should be established to form a comprehensive understanding of the baby's background, facilitating the formation of an appropriate care plan (Tappero and Honeyfield, 2014; Lomax, 2015).

Maternal conditions and their potential impact

It is not within the scope of this chapter to discuss every maternal condition that may result in planned or unplanned NNU admission. There are however, several medical problems which commonly precipitate the need for neonatal care. Having a basic understanding of these is essential to correctly place assessment findings into context. The list of antenatal and perinatal issues with the potential of impacting on the neonate outlined in table 2.2 is not exhaustive; some will be covered in more depth in subsequent chapters.

TABLE 2.1 HISTORY TAKING COMPONENTS

Identification	Name, sex, date of birth, gestational age, corrected gestational age
Presenting problem(s)	What are the primary concerns with this baby at this time?
History of current illness or presenting problem(s)	When did current problem(s) commence?
Current treatment	Current diagnoses/treatments?
Previous medical history	Using a systems approach (see below), inquire about the baby's journey so far; any previous diagnoses/treatments?
Medications	Relevant medications the baby has received in the past? What medication is the baby currently receiving and why? Any known drug allergies/reactions?
Maternal history	Long-term conditions or medications? (Maternal problems are further discussed in table 2.2)
Antenatal history	Maternal health during pregnancy? Results of investigations – blood group, serology, ultrasound scans? Problems in pregnancy/hospital admissions?
Perinatal history: Labour	Onset of labour – spontaneous/induced/none? Signs of infection? Antenatal corticosteroids/magnesium sulphate received?
Perinatal history: Birth	Presentation? Mode of delivery (vaginal/instrumentally assisted/caesarean section)? Condition at birth? Resuscitation required?
Family history	Is there a family history of note, particularly of first-degree relatives during infancy or early childhood? Any known genetic abnormalities in the family?
Social concerns	Are there any social concerns including maternal substance misuse, other children in care, parental disability?
Parents	Asking parents to share their baby's journey can provide vital information about the baby as well as their understanding of the current care plan.

(adapted from Evans, 2015)

ASSESSMENT AT BIRTH

Virginia Apgar was an anaesthesiologist who developed the Apgar tool to assess well infants' recovery from anaesthesia (Apgar et al., 1958). Despite it being designed for term babies, Apgar scoring remains the most universally used tool in the assessment of all new-born babies regardless of gestation. Scored at 1 minute, 5 minutes and 10 minutes of age, 10 is the highest score whereas a score of 0 would indicate a baby requiring emergency assistance (see table 2.3). The system has been recognised to have major limitations – usually scores are recorded retrospectively and are very subjective (O'Donnell et al., 2006; Bashambu et al., 2012; Wyllie et al., 2016). Furthermore, various research studies have identified poor correlation between low Apgar scores and cord gases reflecting perinatal

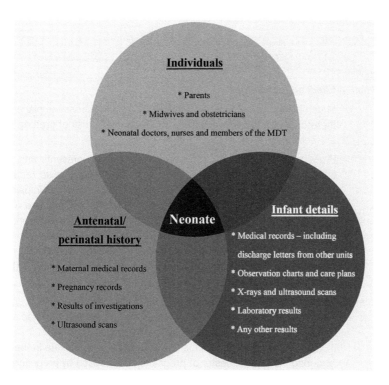

Figure 2.1 Sources for history taking

compromise (Sykes et al., 1982), or adverse neurodevelopmental outcome (Nelson and Ellenberg, 1981). It is generally now accepted that the Apgar score should be used in conjunction with other assessment criteria (American Academy of Pediatrics, 2015) such as cord blood gases and clinical signs.

When using this scoring system, it is important to recognise that adaptation of the evaluation criteria is necessary when assessing preterm infants. For example, the tone of a preterm baby is less **flexed** than that of a term baby. Therefore, in an extremely preterm infant, flexed arms and legs would be abnormal.

PHYSICAL ASSESSMENT AFTER BIRTH – A SYSTEMS APPROACH

There are many approaches to physical assessment, and these may vary dependent on the situation (Petty, 2015). For example, an Airway, Breathing, Circulation, Disability, Exposure approach and NLS algorithm would be appropriate during an emergency situation (see chapter 10 for details). A systems approach is useful in providing a **holistic** and comprehensive assessment of a baby. Having access to resources to update knowledge on

TABLE 2.2 COMMON MATERNAL HEALTH PROBLEMS WITH THE POTENTIAL TO AFFECT BABY

Maternal condition	Effect on foetus/infant
Hypertension	Maternal high blood pressure reduces blood flow across the placenta, therefore slowing foetal growth and increasing the risk of preterm labour and pre-eclampsia.
Pre-eclampsia	Pre-eclampsia occurs after 20 weeks' gestation and presents with hypertension and proteinuria. It can lead to foetal compromise, reduced foetal growth, **oligohydramnios**, maternal coagulopathy and organ impairment, and may progress to convulsions (eclampsia). When this is diagnosed, a woman is carefully monitored and treated with antihypertensive medication; this may have an impact on the newborn baby's glucose **homeostasis** following birth. Not infrequently, the baby will have to be delivered prematurely, as the condition can become life-threatening to both mother and foetus (National Institute for Health and Care Excellence (NICE), 2019).
Diabetes mellitus (Type 1, type 2 or gestational)	Type 1 diabetes typically presents in childhood, but may develop up until 40 years old, and is usually insulin-dependent; type 2 usually has a later onset and can be non-insulin-dependent. Gestational diabetes mellitus (GDM) usually presents late in the second or during the third trimester of pregnancy. It is caused by pregnancy-related hormonal changes resulting in reduced pancreatic insulin secretion, or suboptimal response to insulin. As a result, the foetus is exposed to excessive glucose levels. The foetal pancreas will secrete high levels of insulin to combat maternal high blood sugar, while storing excess glucose as fat (macrosomia). After birth, the maternal blood sugar supply ceases, resulting in a decrease in neonatal blood sugar levels. High levels of insulin, however can continue until the pancreas adjusts, resulting in short-term but potentially severe hypoglycaemia.
Infection	Infection is one of the most common causes for NNU admission. Within the neonatal period, infection is classified as early onset (EOS) or late onset sepsis (LOS). EOS is defined as presenting within the first 72 hours of life. *E. coli* and *S. agalactiae* (Group B streptococcus) can lead to chorioamnionitis, resulting in preterm delivery, and are the most common causative organisms of term EOS (NICE, 2014).
Maternal substance (mis)use	Improved obstetric practices have made it possible for women with complex health issues to have children, who may previously not have been able to. This means that maternal polypharmacy may pose just as much of a challenge as substance misuse in pregnancy, resulting in similar issues to the foetus and neonate, such as neonatal abstinence syndrome (NAS). NNU admission sometimes results from maternal substance (mis)use, and a safeguarding referral, if not in place antenatally, may be indicated. A detailed history is imperative, so that families can be adequately supported in the postnatal period, and feeding choices discussed, as in rare cases breastfeeding may be contraindicated.

Maternal condition	Effect on foetus/infant
Antepartum haemorrhage and placental abruption	Antepartum haemorrhage (APH) is associated with placenta praevia (placenta is near or overlying the cervical opening) or, more seriously placental abruption. APH can be life-threatening for mother and baby. In placental abruption, the placenta partially or completely separates from the uterine wall before delivery. Significant or prolonged blood loss can result in a hypoxic-ischaemic event for the foetus, potentially leading to compromise at birth and secondary encephalopathy, or death.
Instrumental delivery	Owing to improved obstetric care, injury related to instrumental delivery (ventouse/forceps) has significantly decreased. However, there remains a risk of bruising with associated discomfort and increased likelihood of hyperbilirubinaemia, or, in more severe cases, intracranial haemorrhage.
Cord prolapse	Umbilical cord prolapse is a complication that occurs before or during delivery of the baby. The umbilical cord drops (prolapses) through the open cervix into the vagina ahead of the baby. The cord can then become occluded by the baby's body during delivery, obstructing any blood flow from the placenta. Umbilical cord prolapse occurs in approximately 1 in every 300 births and is an obstetric emergency.
Shoulder dystocia	Shoulder dystocia is a complication that occurs during delivery when an infant's shoulders become lodged in the mother's pelvis, often because the baby's size is disproportionate to that of the birth canal. This can result in an emergency situation, as once again pressure from the baby's body may obstruct the umbilical cord, leading to severe compromise. A less serious complication is injury to the brachial plexus nerves secondary to excessive traction on the baby's head and neck. This can result in temporary paralysis of certain nerves, seen with Erb's palsy.
Malpresentation	Malpresentation, such as breech presentation, can cause an issue when this results in protracted delivery, compromising the baby.
Preterm pre-labour rupture of the membranes (PPROM)	Pre-labour rupture of membranes can be defined as uterine membranes that rupture before the onset of contractions, creating a higher risk for EOS. Preterm pre-labour rupture of membranes is when this takes place before the 37th week of pregnancy. Alongside the increased risk of infection, this can also result in pulmonary hypoplasia, as the presence of amniotic fluid is required for 'practice breathing' *in utero* which enables normal lung development.
Multiple pregnancies	Pregnancies involving twins, triplets etc. commonly result in preterm delivery, and can be associated with other conditions including maternal hypertension, placental abruption, twin-to-twin transfusion, infants who are **small for gestational age**, **polyhydramnios** and malpresentation.

(adapted from Baston and Durward, 2016)

TABLE 2.3 APGAR SCORING

Score	0	1	2
Colour	Pale/blue	Pink centrally, blue extremities	Pink
Heart rate	Absent	Below 100bpm	Above 100bpm
Response to stimulation	None	Some movement	Cry
Muscle tone	Floppy	Some flexion of extremities	Well flexed
Respiratory effort	Absent	Slow and irregular	Vigorous cry/regular respiratory effort

(adapted from Apgar et al., 1958)

neonatal-specific anatomy and physiology is also helpful to guide assessment (Petty, 2011a; 2011b; 2011c). As discussed in the history taking section, it also provides a systematic method for collecting and communicating information between staff members and family members (Petty, 2018).

Table 2.4 suggests a practical approach to assessment of the neonate.

Respiratory system

Respiratory problems soon after birth may be due to delayed adaptation to extrauterine life, congenital pneumonia, congenital (surgical) conditions, meconium aspiration, but also non-respiratory causes such as cardiac conditions. Normal neonatal breathing may be periodic with bilateral chest movement and clear chest sounds. No extra oxygen should be required, and saturations should be within the normal range. Signs of respiratory distress may include tachypnoea (with a breathing rate above 60 breaths per minute), nasal flaring, chest recession, apnoea, oxygen requirement, cyanosis, abnormal chest sounds including stridor or wheezing (Reuter et al., 2014), and 'grunting' – a noise occurring during exhalation resulting from the baby's breathing against a partially closed glottis. Abnormal respiratory rate (RR) is a key symptom of disease in the newborn (Tveiten et al., 2016). In the presence of any of these signs, the baby needs to be reviewed urgently; oxygen saturations, a blood gas, chest X-ray and screen for infection usually form the baseline investigations (Gallacher et al., 2016). If ventilation is required, bilateral chest movement should be visible and clear breath sounds with no audible secretions should be heard. Increased oxygen requirement with poor oxygen saturation must be observed for and escalated. Absent breath sounds on one or both sides may be indicative of air leaks or other conditions such as diaphragmatic hernia (Pober et al., 2010).

Cardiovascular system

It is not just auscultation of the heart and determination of the heart rate which give information about the baby's cardiovascular system status. A full assessment, as is carried out for example during the NIPE, takes into account several other aspects. Easily and quickly

TABLE 2.4 THE LOOK-LISTEN-FEEL APPROACH TO ASSESSING THE NEONATE

Look

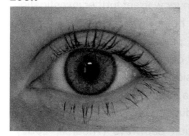

LOOK: Looking first without disturbing the baby can provide a valuable starting point for assessing at rest. Examples: Is the baby's posture appropriate for gestation? Are there visual signs of increased work of breathing? Is the colour pale, jaundiced or plethoric? Does the abdomen appear full, loopy or discoloured? Is there evidence of distress or pain?

Listen

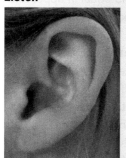

LISTEN: Complete an auditory assessment without and then with a stethoscope.
Examples: Are there audible noises such as grunting or stridor that you can hear without a stethoscope? A stethoscope should be used to listen to the baby's breath sounds, heart sounds and abdomen for active or absent bowel sounds.

Feel

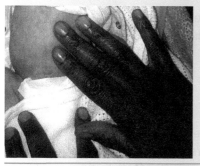

FEEL: Finally, assess the baby by gentle purposeful touch. Examples: Does the baby feel warm, hot or cold to touch? Is the **anterior** fontanelle tense/normotensive/sunken? Does the abdomen feel soft or firm? Is there hepatomegaly or a palpable spleen?

appreciated is the baby's colour. Facial congestion and peripheral cyanosis of the hands and feet are common in the early postnatal period, but must be differentiated from central cyanosis, which is evident as blue discolouration of the mucous membranes and indicates the presence of blood insufficiently saturated with oxygen. As this can be a sign not only of congenital heart defects (Puri et al., 2017) but respiratory problems, the immediate management of checking saturation levels (ideally pre- and post-ductally) and oxygen supplementation as indicated is the same for both cases (Baston and Durward, 2016). Pulse oximetry is a safe, non-invasive, inexpensive, and reasonably sensitive test that will detect many cases of critical congenital heart disease (Swenson et al., 2012).

Abnormal work of breathing may not only reflect respiratory problems, but underlying cardiac pathology, so that this forms part of the cardiovascular assessment and must be borne in mind as a potential cause (Gallacher et al., 2016). On auscultation, the baby's heart rate, heart rhythm and heart sounds can be appreciated. This may reveal murmurs, additional noises caused by the blood flowing through the heart. Murmurs warrant further investigation as they may be indicative of congenital heart defects. The heart rhythm should be regular, although dysrhythmias are not uncommon in the neonatal period and often benign. More detail about both can be found in chapter 13, management of cardiovascular disorders.

Multiple reasons may be causative of a heart rate outside normal limits (see table 2.5): **tachycardia** can be secondary to stress, pain, hyperthermia, congestive heart failure, but is also a common side effect of inotrope infusions. **Bradycardia** can be a sign of hypothermia, significant acidosis or problems in the cardiac conduction pathways (Theorell, 2002). When the baby's pulses are palpated, they should be easy to feel, and equal in upper and lower limbs on both sides. Weak, 'thready' pulses are indicative of shock, while a 'bounding' quality can be noted in the presence of a ductus arteriosus (ibid).

Blood pressure (BP) evaluation is very liable to measurement errors, so that it is important to ensure that the infant is at rest, and the correct cuff size is selected; the BP will appear high if the cuff is too small, while inappropriately large cuffs will give falsely low readings. Normal limits for the BP vary depending on the baby's gestational and postnatal age. The historically suggested cut-off of the baby's gestational age for mean BP has been more recently suggested to be inappropriate (Dasgupta and Gill, 2003; Noori and Seri, 2015), but is still widely used in many NNUs (Bhojani et al., 2010). The management of hypotension is discussed in chapter 13.

Finally, abdominal palpation also forms part of the cardiovascular assessment: hepatomegaly, a liver edge palpable more than 1cm below the costal margin is a sign of cardiac failure (Diehl-Jones and Askin, 2002).

Gastrointestinal system

The neonate's abdomen should be pink, soft, not distended, and non-tender with active bowel sounds present. Dusky or erythematous discolouration, or periumbilical erythema are abnormal and may indicate necrotic/inflamed bowel or omphalitis. On palpation, no enlargement of the abdominal organs should be noted (Baston and Durward, 2016). The majority of term infants will pass meconium within 24 hours of birth. In comparison, this is delayed in preterm infants, whose transition to changed/normal stools also occurs later (Bekkali et al., 2008). If a gastric tube is in situ, stomach aspirates should be clear and minimal in volume. Poor feed tolerance as indicated by abnormal gastric aspirates or vomiting, as well as an abnormal abdominal examination may be indicative of infection or surgical problems, further discussed in chapter 21. Assessment of nutritional status is also important in relation to inclusion of weight and other growth parameters (Johnson et al., 2015) which will be covered in chapter 17.

Hepatic system

Assessment of jaundice is a core nursing role in neonatal care and early recognition of jaundice is vital for treatment of any underlying condition (Rennie et al., 2010). Bilirubin is a product of red blood cell decay, and is conjugated in the liver prior to excretion. An increased turnover of foetal erythrocytes compared to adult red blood cells, combined with hepatic immaturity at birth, makes jaundice – the deposition of yellow pigment in the neonate's sclera and skin – a common occurrence. This should usually become apparent from 48 hours of age and resolve by the end of two weeks. Infants who are bruised following delivery are more likely to develop jaundice. Serum and/or transcutaneous bilirubin levels may need to be acquired to identify infants who require treatment. Pathological jaundice is defined as jaundice occurring during the first 24 hours of life and is not normal. Physiological jaundice does not usually require intervention, whereas pathological jaundice should trigger investigation and treatment for possible sepsis, congenital infections or haemolytic causes of jaundice (Turnbull and Petty, 2012).

While many breastfed infants remain jaundiced beyond two weeks, pathological causes for prolonged jaundice need to be excluded. Conjugated hyperbilirubinaemia is commonly seen in preterm infants who have received parenteral nutrition but must be excluded in any infant presenting with jaundice which has not resolved after two weeks, as it can be indicative of biliary atresia. In any baby with conjugated hyperbilirubinaemia, it is vital to observe for signs of biliary atresia, such as dark urine and pale stools (Siew and Kelly, 2016). At this stage, it may again be indicative of **haemolysis**, or galactosaemia (Ives, 2011).

Renal system

The renal tract is not functioning fully at birth, meaning that neonates have poor urine concentration ability in the early postnatal period (Abitbol et al., 2016). In preterm infants particularly, this can result in dehydration necessitating careful fluid balance assessment and individualised fluid management plans based on clinical hydration status as well as biochemical indicators such as serum sodium. Many newborns do not pass urine in the first 24 hours of life, but this needs to be closely observed. Evaluation of renal health on the NNU may furthermore include dipstick urinalysis to monitor glycosuria, haematuria and proteinuria and determination of specific gravity. This substitutes measurements of urine osmolality, which indicates whether fluid intake is adequate by reflecting hydration status and urine concentration. Normal specific gravity in the neonate is 1020–1030. Colour should also be documented – dark appearance of urine may be due to conjugated hyperbilirubinaemia or haematuria. If urine output falls below 1mL/kg/hour, this could be indicative of acute renal failure, which can result from sepsis, respiratory disease, necrotising enterocolitis or following a perinatal hypoxic-ischaemic event. This requires further investigation and careful management (Modi, 2012). Fluid management will be covered later in chapter 16.

TABLE 2.5 VITAL SIGNS ASSESSMENT

Measurement: Respiratory	Method: Visual, ECG, stethoscope	Preterm Values: 40–60 resp. rate/min	Term Values: 40–60 resp. rate/min

Respiratory assessment: Observe the movement of the chest for symmetry and bilateral air entry via stethoscope. Work of breathing should also be assessed, making note of the rate per minute and any substernal or intercostal recession.

Measurement: Heart rate	Method: ECG, pulse oximetry, auscultation	Preterm values: 120–180	Term values: 90–160

Cardiac assessment: Place bell of the stethoscope to the immediate left of sternum between the originating from the sinoatrial node located in the right atrium of the heart, this electrical impulse travels throughout the heart causing the heart to contract thus creating each heartbeat.

Measurement: Blood pressure	Method: cuff or invasive via arterial access. The transducer should be zeroed to the right atrium of the heart before measurement.	Preterm values: Mean: > current gestational age (note: evidence for this is poor, yet still mainstay in most UK NNUs) Systolic: 50–62mmHg Diastolic:25–47mmHg	Term values: Mean: > current gestational age (note: evidence for this is poor, yet still mainstay in most UK NNUs) Systolic: 46–94mmHg Diastolic: 31–63mmHg

Blood pressure assessment: Recorded measurements are **systole**, mean and **diastole**. The systolic pressure reflects the arterial pressure resulting from the ejection of blood during ventricular contraction. The diastolic pressure represents the arterial pressure of blood during ventricular relaxation. Mean blood pressure is of particular significance within the neonatal period as desirable blood pressure should be gestational age or greater.

Measurement: capillary refill time (CRT)	Method: apply gentle pressure by the pad of a finger to sternum	Term values: <3seconds indicates adequate perfusion	Preterm values: <3seconds indicates adequate perfusion

Perfusion assessment: Apply gentle pressure by the pad of the finger onto the middle chest and hold for 5 seconds. Release and count seconds the area takes to return to normal colour. This will be the capillary refill time. It is important to remember that many factors can influence perfusion particularly in the newborn period, including immature or changing pulmonary, cardiac and renal function.

Measurement: Oxygen saturation	Method: pulse oximetry probe on foot, hand or wrist	Preterm values: 91%–100% Titrate supplemental O_2 as indicated	Term values: 95%–100% Titrate supplemental O_2 as indicated

Oxygen saturation assessment: Analysis of how much the haemoglobin is saturated with oxygen. Measurement is taken from capillary blood which provides a close representation of arterial blood oxygen saturation.

TABLE 2.5 (Cont.)

Measurement: Carbon dioxide and oxygen	Method: transcutaneous probe, end-tidal CO_2, blood gas	Preterm values: pO_2 7.5–10kPa pCO_2 4.5–6.5kPa	Term values: pO_2 8–12kPa pCO_2 4.5–6kPa

Both oxygenation and carbon dioxide can be assessed by application of a calibrated heated skin probe applied to skin preferably the abdomen. Another alternative to blood gases is the use of end-tidal CO_2 monitoring attached to endotracheal tubes. If neither of these equipment options is available, blood gases continue to provide the most common form of pCO_2 and pO_2 measurement.

Measurement: Temperature	Method: Tempa DOT™ (single use), axilla, abdominal and rectal probe	Preterm values: 36.5–37.5°C	Term values: 36.5–37.5°C

Assessment of temperature: While Tempa DOT™ or axilla thermometers may be appropriate for stable babies, continuous monitoring may be useful for babies that are unwell or for servo-control modes. Toe-core gap monitoring provides a useful indicator for perfusion. While hyperthermia indicates a higher than normal body temperature, hypothermia forms part of the three H triangle for metabolic adaption (hypoxia, hypothermia, hypoglycaemia).

Measurement: Blood sugar	Method: Glucometer, blood gas or laboratory	Preterm values: 2.6–6mmol/L	Term values: 2.6–6mmol/L

Assessment of blood sugar: Ensure a neonatal lancet is used choosing the appropriate puncture depth for a preterm or term baby. Frequency of blood sugar assessment may differ between units and on infant's individual needs, therefore check local guidelines for instruction.

Measurement: Urine output	Method: calculate all fluid intake and output, including insensible water losses	Preterm values for urine output: >1ml/ kg/hr	Term values for urine output: >1ml/kg/hr

Assessment of fluid status: Expected urine output is dependent on time since birth, gestational age and underlying condition. For example; perinatal hypoxia can reduce renal function, as can prematurity.

(adapted from Rennie, 2012)

Neurological system

Inspection alone of the baby's posture, tone and movements can be very helpful in the evaluation of an infant's neurological status. A normal response to external stimuli should be observable and this includes alertness such as waking for feeds and/or crying when in pain. Infants should be observed for excessive wakefulness and irritability as well as excessive quiet, as both are indicative of neurological problems. Unresponsiveness or subdued response to stimuli may indicate neurological dysfunction or injury (Lomax, 2015) as does hypotonia (Ahmed et al., 2016). Depending on the baby's gestational age at time of assessment, reflexes such as suck, gag and moro reflex may be evaluated as part of a neurological examination. This would however, not be appropriate for very preterm infants.

In any gestation, there should be no signs of pain or stress and the baby should appear comfortable and be able to sleep for long periods. The presence of pain or stress will be exhibited by tense continual movements, facial expressions, excessive crying, grimacing, changes to vital signs, colour change, apnoea and desaturations. The mainstay of neurological assessment remains the Dubowitz Neurological Examination (Dubowitz et al., 2005) or alternatively, the Ballard's score (Ballardscore.com). Differentiating premature infants from those born small-for-dates is an essential aspect to anticipate different clinical scenarios and intervene accordingly (Nandy et al., 2018). The web-based companion has various links to resources on assessment tools including neurological, including diagrams.

Skin and general appearance

Issues with regard to skin integrity and variations are discussed in more detail in chapters 3 and 18. Essentially, maturity of the skin should match the baby's gestational age. Breakdown of the skin is abnormal, yet there are several normal skin variations and rashes which occur particularly in the term population and must be differentiated from abnormal skin lesions.

In infants with indwelling cannulas and central venous catheters, the insertion sites must be regularly observed for swelling and erythema, or evidence of **extravasation.**

Immunology

Signs of infection may be non-specific and difficult to distinguish from other situations; for example, changes to vital signs such as increased respiratory rate and heart rates may be indicative of infection but may also be signs of pain and/or thermal stress. Neonatal infection should always be considered as part of holistic assessment of the neonate due to the potential impact both short- and long-term. It is discussed in detail in chapter 18.

Thermal control

Temperature fluctuations may be difficult to interpret in the first few hours after birth, as they can be subject to environmental conditions. Persistently abnormal or unstable temperature measurements, however, warrant further investigation as they may be indicative of infection or intracranial haemorrhage (Tappero and Honeyfield, 2014). Assessment of thermal stability and temperature is a fundamental area of assessment, as establishment of such is an essential part of transition and adaptation to extrauterine life at birth and thereafter. This will be covered in greater depth in chapter 11.

Metabolism

Following birth, the neonatal metabolism must adapt to the intermittent nutritional delivery having been accustomed to a constant placental supply of glucose and other nutrients. In well term babies, the utilisation of fatty fuels and ketones compensates for interruptions in glucose availability. However, in preterm and low birth weight infants, the immaturity of such metabolic processes results in a propensity for hypoglycaemia. Similarly, unwell term babies may not be able to meet their heightened metabolic demands with such alternative fuels. As a result, glucose levels need to be carefully monitored in NNU patients.

Hyperglycaemia is commonly transient, and an issue more commonly observed in the extremely preterm and low birth weight population. This may be due to immaturity-related insulin resistance or the inability to down-regulate **gluconeogenesis** in the presence of the infusion of glucose solutions such as parenteral nutrition. While the above-mentioned postnatal changes affect the neonatal metabolic system and must contend with the necessity for close observation of glucose levels early on, it is also important to recognise changes in glucose homeostasis, as they can indicate problems such as sepsis (Hawdon, 2012).

It is essential to place the time of systems observations in the context of events preceding assessment. Ideally, the assessment should take place when the baby has not been disturbed recently as this will provide a baseline of observations when the baby is at rest. Parents' views must be incorporated into any assessment, as they can provide valuable information about their baby's normal status quo and any changes that may have occurred.

NEWBORN INFANT PHYSICAL EXAMINATION

The NIPE programme is endorsed by the UK Screening Committee (Public Health England, 2018) and aims to reduce mortality and morbidity through the identification of infants with congenital abnormalities of four key areas (see below). All eligible infants should be examined within the first 72 hours of life, unless they are too unwell, or an examination would not be appropriate in this time period, as may be the case with preterm infants. The examination can be carried out by a doctor, nurse or midwife who has undertaken a university-accredited NIPE module.

The minimum of the examination constitutes these four key areas:

■ *Eyes* These are primarily assessed for congenital cataracts, but conditions such as aniridia, coloboma or retinoblastoma are also excluded. This is achieved by inspection of the eyes and eliciting the red reflex with the aid of an ophthalmoscope.

■ *Heart* Examination of the cardiovascular system aims to identify critical or major serious heart defects which require timely (surgical) intervention. Inspection, palpation and auscultation as described above complete the cardiovascular assessment.

■ *Hips* Developmental dysplasia of the hips is a congenital problem associated with serious long-term morbidity. Dislocated or dislocatable hips found on examination need to be referred for ongoing management to allow for normal mobility later in life. The condition is identified by performing the Barlow and Ortolani manoeuvres. If the screen is positive, an urgent hip ultrasound and orthopaedic review is arranged. Infants with certain risk factors will automatically be referred for a non-urgent ultrasound of the hips, as well as undergoing the examination.

■ *Testes* Both testes are assessed to determine whether they have descended into the scrotum at birth. Bilaterally undescended testes (cryptorchidism) must raise the possibility of ambiguous genitalia and trigger relevant investigations. As cryptorchidism has been associated with reduced fertility and the potential for malignancies, even unilaterally undescended testes must be referred for ongoing monitoring and possibly intervention.

The NIPE is repeated at 6–8 weeks of age, at which point previously undetected issues may have emerged (Public Health England, 2018).

CONCLUSION

Assessment of the infant on the postnatal ward or NNU forms the basis of neonatal nursing care. While this is a continuous and sometimes unconscious process, timely identification of potentially serious problems affecting newborns can be facilitated through meticulous assessment, which includes history taking as well as physical observations. As the cornerstone of practitioner–patient interface, the neonatal nurse therefore plays a crucial role in promoting neonatal wellbeing and improving outcomes which includes an understanding of the theory and practice behind sound assessment principles.

CASE STUDY

CASE STUDIES

Case study 1: Term baby with respiratory distress

Archie has been admitted from the postnatal ward with tachypnoea and grunting. You are asked to undertake an initial assessment.

Q.1. What are your immediate steps, and which investigations would you like to do?

Q.2. What would you like to know about Archie's history?

Q.3. Can you think of any aspects of Archie's mum's history that may be important to know?

Q.4. What could be the possible causes for Archie's presentation?

Case study 2: Distended abdomen

Amy was born at 27 weeks and is now 3 days old. She developed a distended abdomen today.

Q.1. What information would you like to know from Amy's history?
Q.2. What information would you like to know about Amy's current care?
Q.3. Using the vital signs parameters and a look, listen and feel approach, how would you undertake a physical assessment of Amy?
Q.4. Reviewing the information you have collected, list possible causes (differential diagnoses) for Amy's distended abdomen.

For suggested answer guides to the questions posed in these case studies, please refer to the web-based companion site specific to this chapter (see URL below).

WEB-BASED RESOURCES

For further information, online resources and greater detail on the case studies featured in this chapter go to www.routledge.com/cw/nicnursing

References

Abitbol, C. L., DeFreitas, M. J., & Strauss, J. (2016). Assessment of kidney function in preterm infants: life-long implications. *Pediatric Nephrology*, *31*(12), 2213–2222.

Ahmed, M. I., Iqbal, M., & Hussain, N. (2016). A structured approach to the assessment of a floppy neonate. *Journal of Pediatric Neurosciences*, *11*(1), 2–6.

American Academy of Pediatrics (2015). *The Apgar Score*. www.acog.org/Clinical-Guidance-and-Publications/Committee-Opinions/Committee-on-Obstetric-Practice/The-Apgar-Score?IsMobileSet=false

Apgar, V., Holaday, D. A., James, L. S., Weisbrot, I. M., & Berrien, C. (1958). Evaluation of the newborn infant-second report. *Journal of the American Medical Association*, *168*(15), 1985–1988.

Bashambu, M. T., Whitehead, H., Hibbs, A. M., Martin, R. J., & Bhola, M. (2012). Evaluation of interobserver agreement of apgar scoring in preterm infants. *Pediatrics*, *130*(4), e982–7.

Baston, H., & Durward, H. (2016). *Examination of the newborn: a practical guide (3rd edition)*. Oxford and London: Routledge.

Bekkali, N., Hamers, S. L., Schipperus, M. R., Reitsma, J. B., Valerio, P. G., Van Toledo, L., & Benninga, M. A. (2008). Duration of meconium passage in preterm and term infants. *Archives of Disease in Childhood: Fetal and Neonatal Edition*, *93*(5), F376–F379.

Bhojani, S., Banerjee, J., & Rahman, M. (2010). Management of neonatal hypotension–a national questionnaire survey. *Infant*, *6*(5), 152–154.

Dasgupta, S. J., & Gill, A. B. (2003). Hypotension in the very low birthweight infant: the old, the new, and the uncertain. *Archives of Disease in Childhood: Fetal and Neonatal Edition*, *88*(6), F450–F454.

Diehl-Jones, W., & Askin, D. F. (2002). The neonatal liver, Part 1: embryology, anatomy, and physiology. *Neonatal Network, 21*(2), 5–12.

Dubowitz, L., Ricciw, D., & Mercuri, E. (2005). The Dubowitz neurological examination of the full-term newborn. *Mental retardation and developmental disabilities research reviews, 11*(1), 52–60.

Evans, C. (2015). History taking and the newborn examination: an evolving perspective. In Lomax, A. (2015). Examination of the Newborn: An Evidence Based Guide (2nd Edition). London and New York: John Wiley & Sons.

Gallacher, D. J., Hart, K., & Kotecha, S. (2016). Common respiratory conditions of the newborn. *Breathe, 12*(1), 30–42.

Hawdon, J. (2012). Disorders of Metabolic Homeostasis in the Neonate. In Rennie, J. M. (Ed.) *Rennie & Roberton's Textbook of Neonatology* 5th Edition. London and New York: Elsevier Health Sciences.

Ingram, S. (2017). Taking a comprehensive health history: learning through practice and reflection. *British Journal of Nursing, 26*(18), 1033–1037.

Ives, N. K. (2011). Management of neonatal jaundice. *Paediatrics and Child Health, 21*(6), 270–276.

Johnson, M. J., Wiskin, A. E., Pearson, F., Beattie, R. M., & Leaf, A. A. (2015). How to use: nutritional assessment in neonates *Archives of Disease in Childhood: Education and Practice.*100: 147–154.

Lomax, A. (2015). *Examination of the newborn: An evidence-based guide* (2nd Edition). New York: John Wiley & Sons.

Modi, N. (2012). Renal Function and Renal Disease in the Newborn. In Rennie, J. M. (Ed.) *Rennie & Roberton's Textbook of Neonatology 5th Edition*. London and New York: Elsevier Health Sciences.

Nandy, A., Guha, A., Datta, D., & Mondal, R. (2018). Evolution of clinical method for new-born infant maturity assessment. *The Journal of Maternal-Fetal & Neonatal Medicine*, 18:1–181. doi:10.1080/14767058.

National Institute for Health and Care Excellence (NICE). (2019). *Hypertension in pregnancy: diagnosis and management*. NICE.

National Institute for Health and Care Excellence (2014). *Neonatal infection (early onset): antibiotics for prevention and treatment*. NICE.

Nelson, K. B., & Ellenberg, J. H. (1981). Apgar scores as predictors of chronic neurologic disability. *Pediatrics, 68*(1), 36–44.

Noori, S., & Seri, I. (2015). Evidence-based versus pathophysiology-based approach to diagnosis and treatment of neonatal cardiovascular compromise. *Seminars in Fetal and Neonatal Medicine, 20*(4), 238–245.

O'Donnell, C. P., Kamlin, C. O. F., Davis, P. G., Carlin, J. B., & Morley, C. J. (2006). Interobserver variability of the 5-minute Apgar score. *The Journal of Pediatrics, 149*(4), 486–489.

Petty, J. (2011a). Fact Sheet; Neonatal Biology – An Overview Part 1. *Journal of Neonatal Nursing*, 17, 1, 8–10.

Petty, J. (2011b). Fact Sheet; Neonatal Biology – An Overview Part 2. *Journal of Neonatal Nursing,* 17, 3, 89–91.

Petty, J. (2011c). Fact Sheet; Neonatal Biology – An Overview Part 3. *Journal of Neonatal Nursing,* 17, 4, 128–131.

Petty, J. (2015). *Bedside Guide for Neonatal Care: Learning Tools to Support Practice*. London: Palgrave.

Petty, J. (2018). Chapter 3: Principles of systematic assessment. In Gormley-Fleming, E., & Martin, D. (Eds.) *Children and young people's nursing skills at a glance* (pp. 6–7) Newark: John Wiley & Sons.

Pober, B. R., Russell, M. K., & Ackerman, K. G. (2010). Congenital diaphragmatic hernia overview. In *GeneReviews®[Internet]*. University of Washington, Seattle.

Public Health England (2018). *Newborn and infant physical examination screening programme handbook*. Public Health England.

Puri, K., Allen H. D., & Quureshi, A. M. (2017). Congenital Heart Disease. *Pediatric Reviews, 38*(10), 471–486.

Rennie, J., Burman-Roy, S., & Murphy, M. S. (2010). Neonatal jaundice: summary of NICE guidance. *BMJ, 340*, c2409.

Rennie, J. M. (2012). *Rennie & Roberton's Textbook of Neonatology* (5th Edition). London and New York: Elsevier Health Sciences.

Reuter, S., Moser, C., & Baack, M. (2014). Respiratory distress in the newborn. *Pediatrics in review*, *35*(10), 417–428.

Siew, S. M., & Kelly, D. A. (2016). Evaluation of jaundice in children beyond the neonatal period. *Paediatrics and Child Health*, *26*(10), 451–458.

Sykes, G., Johnson, P., Ashworth, F., Molloy, P., Gu, W., Stirrat, G. M., & Turnbull, A. C. (1982). Do Apgar scores indicate asphyxia? *The Lancet*, *319*(8270), 494–496.

Swenson, A. K., Brown, D., & Stevermer, J. J. (2012). Pulse oximetry for newborns: Should it be routine? *The Journal of Family Practice*, *61*(5), 283.

Tappero, E. P., & Honeyfield, M. E. (2014). *Physical assessment of the newborn: A comprehensive approach to the art of physical* examination (5th Edition). New York: Springer Publishing Company.

Theorell, C. (2002). Cardiovascular assessment of the newborn. *Newborn and Infant Nursing Reviews*, *2*(2), 111–127.

Turnbull, V., & Petty, J. (2012). Early onset jaundice in the newborn: understanding the ongoing care of mother and baby. *British Journal of Midwifery*, *20*(9), 615–622.

Tveiten, L., Diep, L. M., Halvorsen, T., & Markestad, T. (2016). Respiratory rate during the first 24 hours of life in healthy term infants. *Pediatrics*, *137*(4), e20152326.

Wyllie, J., Ainsworth, S., Tinnion, R., & Hampshire, S. (2016). *Newborn Life Support*. (4th Edition). London: Resuscitation Council UK.

3 THE PRETERM AND LOW BIRTH WEIGHT INFANT

Lesley Kilby, Erica Everett, Katy Powis and Emma Kyte

CONTENTS

GUIDANCE ON HOW TO ENHANCE PERSONAL LEARNING FROM THIS CHAPTER

Key points covered in this chapter

- An overview of prematurity and low birth weight.
- Common conditions affecting premature infants, their underlying pathophysiology and clinical management.
- Aspects to be considered antenatally, on the neonatal unit and in preparation for discharge when caring for infants born prematurely.

Reflection

Reading through the chapter, you are encouraged to engage with the key points and related literature in an enquiring way. Having cared for a range of infants born prematurely or at a low birth weight, ask these questions:

- What are your considerations when caring for an extremely/very preterm infant? How do these differ from when you are planning your care of a late preterm infant?
- Are you confident in recognising presenting signs of most of the issues preterm infants can encounter during their journey through the neonatal unit?
- How do you need to focus your support to the parents depending on the gestation their baby was born at?

Implications for nursing care

- Finally: how will this chapter enable you to approach the assessment, management and nursing care of neonates born prematurely or at a low birth weight? Consider the implications of what you learn for your daily practice relating to this area.

INTRODUCTION AND BACKGROUND

The World Health Organisation (WHO, 2018) define prematurity as birth before 37 weeks completed gestation. This, however, is a broad definition, as outcomes and management can vary significantly across this spectrum. Infants who are small for their gestation may experience issues not unlike those faced by preterm infants, so that there are similarities in the approach to their care. This chapter will identify the causes, clinical presentation and key physiological aspects of prematurity and low birth weight. It will also explore the impact this may have on the infant and form a basis for topics discussed in subsequent chapters.

ASSESSMENT OF GESTATIONAL AGE

Gestational age (GA) refers to the time elapsed since the beginning of the last menstrual period and is counted in weeks and days. Antenatally, GA is most accurately determined by menstrual history or ultrasound scanning in the first trimester. However, not all mothers have a regular cycle, and some may not receive antenatal care, so exact information regarding GA may not be available at the time of delivery. Weight can be a useful indicator but does not predict GA accurately. Infants who are small for gestational age (SGA) may initially appear to be more premature, and conversely infants who are large for GA may appear more mature (Petty, 2017). Preterm infants and infants who are SGA differ in their characteristics and primary problems in the neonatal period (see table 3.1).

Tools to determine GA accurately in the immediate postnatal period are useful in situations where there is uncertainty. The New Ballard Score (Ballard et al., 1991) has widely replaced the Dubowitz Assessment of Gestational Age (Dubowitz et al., 1970) and the original Ballard Score (Ballard et al., 1979) to encompass preterm infants born before 28 weeks GA. It enables the practitioner to estimate GA through the assessment of neuromuscular control as well as physical characteristics. A link to this can be found on the companion website.

PREMATURITY AND ITS CAUSES

In acknowledgement of the broad spectrum of prematurity as indicating births before 37 weeks' completed GA, the WHO definition of this includes further sub-categories: extremely preterm (<28 weeks), very preterm (born between 28 and 32 weeks), and moderate to late preterm (32–36 weeks). Although rare (incidence of 0.3% of all deliveries), infants delivered at the borderline of viability – defined as an infant born before 24 completed weeks' gestation – pose an ethical dilemma due to poor survival rates and adverse neurological outcome. There is a 50% or less chance of survival for those infants born at the borderline of viability (Nuffield Council on Bioethics, 2014).

TABLE 3.1 CHARACTERISTICS OF SGA AND PRETERM INFANTS

	SGA/IUGR infant	Preterm infant
Weight	< 10th centile	Appropriate for gestational age
Cry	Strong	Weak
Eyes	Open	May be fused
Skin	Mature / dry	Keratinised
Lanugo	Absent	+++
Breast tissue	Tissue buds	No breast tissue palpable
Genitalia	Scrotum well developed and testes in the scrotal sac / labia majora fully developed	Undescended testes / prominent clitoris and poorly developed labia majora
Tone	Good muscle tone	Hypotonia
Head circumference	Disproportionately large for trunk (asymmetrical)	Appropriate for gestational age
Primary problems	Thermoregulation Hypoglycaemia	Thermoregulation Hypoglycaemia Immature respiratory system

The outcome for infants delivered prematurely has been investigated widely. The most robust studies are EPICure and EPICure 2 (Costeloe et al., 2000; Marlow, 2006). These collected information on all infants born in England between 22 and 26^{+6} weeks' gestation. The findings showed that deliveries and admissions of infants in this gestational range are increasing, with significantly improved survival for infants born between 24 and 25 weeks. However, despite improvements in survival, the number of infants leaving neonatal units (NNUs) with abnormalities on cranial ultrasound scan, respiratory and abdominal issues remains similar to the first study.

Follow-up data at 2–3 years of age shows that the incidence of outcome with no disability ranges from 20% at 22–23 weeks to 50% at 26 weeks. The main categories of disability are

- Cerebral palsy
- Other motor problems
- Visual or hearing impairment
- Learning difficulties
- Behavioural problems
- Respiratory problems
- Growth problems.

There is thus a global drive to continuously enhance antenatal care, monitor the incidence of preterm deliveries, investigate their causes and implement evidence-based strategies to avoid premature births and improve the outcomes of infants born too early (WHO, 2015; WHO, 2018). Common causes of prematurity include pregnancy-induced hypertension, multiple pregnancy, maternal health (including weight, drug misuse, smoking and stress), infection/chorioamnionitis, uterine abnormality and cervical incompetence among others. However, most commonly the underlying cause is unknown, although genetic abnormalities have been suggested (WHO, 2018).

THE LOW BIRTH WEIGHT INFANT

With regard to birthweight (BW), the WHO (2018) differentiate extremely low birth weight (ELBW) <1000g, very low birth weight (VLBW) 1000g–1500g, and low birth weight (LBW) <2499g.

It is important to recognise that these weight categories can relate to any gestation. LBW can be the result of premature birth, genetic abnormalities or intrauterine growth restriction (IUGR). Small for GA (SGA) refers to infants with a birth weight <10th percentile and includes infants who are constitutionally small; i.e. taking into account mother's size and ethnicity (Royal College of Obstetricians and Gynaecologists (RCOG), 2013). The group of SGA infants also includes those with IUGR, which means that for a number of possible reasons a baby may not achieve his/her growth potential *in utero*. While the terms SGA and IUGR are often used synonymously, they are in fact not interchangeable but refer to different conditions (RCOG, 2013).

Causes of intrauterine growth restriction

IUGR infants are further subcategorised into symmetrical and asymmetrical IUGR. Symmetrical IUGR means weight, length and head circumference are all below the 10th percentile, and this accounts for approximately 30% of all infants with IUGR. This usually results from early problems *in utero* associated with reduced oxygen delivery impacting on foetal development.

Asymmetrical IUGR is defined as weight below the 10th percentile but head circumference and length preserved within the normal range, and this accounts for >60% of IUGR infants. It tends to occur later within the pregnancy, caused by placental compromise, and resulting in clinical features of malnutrition which are absent in the SGA infant (Sharma et al., 2016). IUGR occurs when demands for oxygen and nutrition outstrip placental supply. The main causes are congenital infections, maternal hypertension, suboptimal maternal health and weight gain, drug misuse/smoking, chromosomal and genetic factors, and multiple pregnancy. Outcome is dependant on the type and severity of IUGR, with asymmetrical growth restriction being favourable.

Monitoring the quality of placental blood flow has been beneficial in identifying foetal wellbeing and early detection of IUGR. A Cochrane meta-analysis showed that the monitoring of umbilical artery blood flow reduces the risk of perinatal deaths as it detected those at risk of developing reduced foetal growth and compromise (Alfirevic et al., 2017). Figure 3.1 depicts the typical appearance of a growth-restricted neonate.

CARE IN THE DELIVERY SETTING

Pre-delivery considerations

Attempts to optimise maternal and foetal health should start before conception and continue throughout a woman's pregnancy. Adequate antenatal management is of crucial

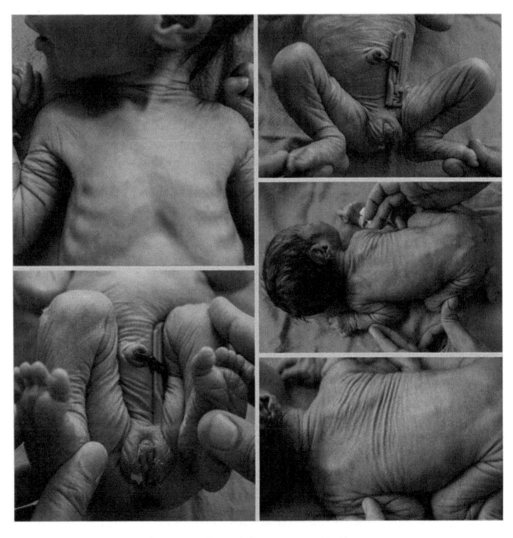

Figure 3.1 The IUGR infant (Source: Dr Deepak Sharma et al., 2016)

importance particularly for the preterm population, and has a direct impact on long-term outcomes (Beaino et al., 2010; Schmid et al., 2011; Chang, 2015).

The British Association of Perinatal Medicine (BAPM) has recently updated guidance for perinatal management at less than 27 weeks' gestation based on steadily improving outcomes over the past decade. It is acknowledged that care should be individualised and led by senior, experienced neonatal, midwifery and obstetric staff. Decision-making for babies born at extremely low gestational ages should not be based on gestational age alone, but on assessment of the baby's prognosis taking into account multiple factors which are associated with an increased or decreased risk of absolute survival and survival without severe impairment. These factors include:

■ *Foetal factors* which may increase risk include male sex, multiple pregnancy, congenital anomaly, and poor foetal growth.

■ *Clinical conditions* which pose additional risk and have been associated with increased mortality and morbidity are prolonged pre-labour rupture of membranes before 24 weeks' gestation and clinical evidence of chorioamnionitis.

■ *Therapeutic strategies* Administration of antenatal steroids and magnesium sulphate are associated with improved survival, neonatal outcomes and reduced risk of childhood impairment, even before 24 weeks gestation.

■ *Clinical setting* Survival is highest at these low gestations in centres with experienced staff and higher patient numbers. A strategy of antenatal transfer < 27 weeks of gestation for delivery in a maternity unit with co-located neonatal intensive care unit (NICU) is recommended (BAPM, 2019).

Following full history taking and assessment of both foetal and maternal health, the chances of unacceptably poor outcome if life-sustaining care is provided for the baby will generally fall into one of the following categories: extremely high risk; moderate to high risk; lower risk. Discussion with the family should be led by a senior neonatologist where possible and decisions for active management or palliative care based on prognosis should be agreed and documented fully prior to the delivery.

Where delivery at borderline viability is likely, the role of the joint neonatal and obstetric team under the guidance of the most senior clinician is to discuss the likely outcome with the family, and to provide support in their informed decision-making. A prognosis can be determined using an outcomes calculator, such as the Prognosis for Average Gestations Equivalent infant framework (PAGE; see table 3.2), or the National Institute of Child Health and Human Development (NICHD) prognosis calculator (South Australian Perinatal Practice Guidelines Workgroup and Wilkinson, 2013).

At present, EPICure data on long-term developmental outcomes of babies born at the borderline of viability remains the best available evidence for counselling parents on their individualised prognosis.

TABLE 3.2 THE PAGE FRAMEWORK FOR DECISION-MAKING

Chance of poor outcome if intensive care is provided	PAGE	Treatment category	Obstetric management
90%	<22 weeks' gestation	Comfort care (life-sustaining treatment should not be provided under usual circumstances)	Maternal focused
50–90%	22–23 weeks' gestation	Optional (Life-sustaining treatment a possibility in consideration of parental wishes)	Exploration of parents' wishes
<50%	24 weeks' gestation	Usual (life-sustaining treatment should be provided under usual circumstances)	Maternal/foetal focused

(adapted from South Australian Perinatal Practice Guidelines Workgroup and Wilkinson, 2013)

Corticosteroid and magnesium sulphate administration

Respiratory morbidity including respiratory distress syndrome (RDS) is a serious and often fatal complication of preterm birth, being the primary cause of early neonatal mortality and disability. Antenatal corticosteroids are the most powerful health intervention introduced to neonatal care to improve survival and outcomes. Corticosteroids are administered to women who are in confirmed or suspected early labour, to stimulate foetal surfactant production. A Cochrane review by Roberts et al. (2017) found treatment with antenatal corticosteroids had a positive impact on the incidence of a number of serious adverse outcomes associated with prematurity, such as perinatal and neonatal death, moderate/ severe RDS, intraventricular haemorrhage, necrotising enterocolitis and a reduction in the need for ventilation. According to a standard set by the National Neonatal Audit Programme (NNAP) 85% of mothers in threatening preterm labour at 23–33 weeks' gestation should receive at least one dose of antenatal steroids.

Magnesium sulphate administration in the 24 hours prior to delivery for women at risk of preterm labour has been shown to have a dramatic positive impact on outcomes. Its neuroprotective properties have been associated with a 30% reduction of cerebral palsy (Doyle et al., 2009). It is endorsed by the Royal College of Obstetricians and Gynaecologists (RCOG, 2011) and has been implemented as a national guideline (National Institute of Health and Care Excellence (NICE), 2019).

Delivery room management

Most preterm infants require support with transition to extrauterine life rather than resuscitation at birth (O'Donnell and Stenson, 2008). The team attending deliveries of preterm

TABLE 3.3 ACCEPTABLE PRE-DUCTAL SATURATIONS

2 minutes	60%
3 minutes	70%
4 minutes	80%
5 minutes	90%
10 minutes	95%

(adapted from Dawson et al., 2010)

infants should be experienced in this support. Breathing and heart rate should be assessed immediately following delivery, and every 30 seconds until stable. The use of electrocardiogram (ECG) as the most accurate way to obtain rapid and continuous heart rate monitoring is recommended (Katheria et al., 2012). However, in the absence of ECG monitoring on the resuscitaire, most units use pulse oximetry to obtain both heart rate and oxygen saturation levels. As assessment of colour as a proxy for saturation is usually inaccurate, pre-ductal saturations should be obtained by placing the probe on the right hand or wrist. Hyperoxaemia is particularly damaging to the preterm infant, therefore a low concentration of oxygen (21–30%) should be used in the first instance and until oxygen saturation levels can be assessed (Resuscitation Council UK, 2016). Table 3.3 contains acceptable pre-ductal saturations for infants in the delivery room.

Delaying clamping of the umbilical cord by 1–5 minutes has been recommended in the term population (with the initial heart rate >60bpm and not requiring positive-pressure ventilation) by NICE and the UK Resuscitation Council, and is known to increase neonatal blood volume and increase iron stores (NICE, 2015; Resuscitation Council UK, 2016). In preterm infants, delayed cord clamping (DCC) of 30–60 seconds has been shown to reduce the risk of intraventricular haemorrhage (IVH) and late onset sepsis (Mercer et al., 2006; Rabe et al., 2012; Backes et al., 2014) and is now common practice. Contraindications to delayed clamping include bradycardia, major congenital abnormality and significant particulate meconium where patency of the airway is undetermined. Experimental studies have demonstrated positive effects if respiratory support is initiated prior to clamping of the cord, however this remains controversial due to the practical considerations. An alternative to DCC is milking of the cord (the physical expression of blood from the cord), which may be quicker and easier to facilitate than DCC. Trials have shown that cord milking also improves systemic blood flow and confers benefits in the short term, while long-term benefits similar to DCC have yet to be established (Al-Wassiah and Shah, 2015). Practice varies across the UK, and local guidelines should be followed.

There is a strong association between hypothermia on admission and increased mortality in preterm infants (de Almeida et al., 2014; Mank et al., 2016; Wilson et al., 2016). It may furthermore have a significant impact on long-term outcomes, as hypothermia is known to increase the risk of morbidities such as RDS, IVH, sepsis, and disturbances of haemostasis among others (Costeloe et al., 2000; International Liaison Committee on

Resuscitation 2006; Laptook et al., 2007; Miller et al., 2011). Heat loss can be rapid without intervention due to a large surface area to weight ratio; thin, unkeratinised skin leading to evaporative losses and reduced brown fat stores.

However, hypothermia is an easily preventable condition and many different initiatives have been introduced to neonatal care to combat this issue. A Cochrane review in 2018 found the use of plastic bags or wraps were effective at reducing heat loss at delivery for infants of less than 28 weeks' gestation and improved temperature on admission to the NNU (McCall et al., 2018). Other interventions in the delivery setting to maintain normothermia include maintenance of ambient temperature >26°C, removal of wet towels, the use of a radiant warmer, warmed, humidified gases and warm towels or mattress. Thermoregulation of the infant during transfer to the neonatal setting should be considered and a transport incubator is often chosen to prevent convective heat loss and facilitate warming of respiratory gases during transfer.

This is an area where the experienced neonatal nurse can proactively contribute to the optimisation of the neonate's start to life and his or her individual risk of mortality and morbidity. At delivery, the neonatal nurse may be better placed to remind the team in attendance about the baby's temperature control than the practitioners focused on the management of airway and cardiovascular system. In spontaneously breathing preterm infants, non-invasive respiratory support such as continuous positive airway pressure (CPAP) or humidified high flow nasal cannula (HHFNC) rather than tracheal intubation should be offered. The use of CPAP (with a pressure of 6cm H_2O) has been found to maximise functional residual capacity (FRC) of the lungs, reduce numbers of infants receiving oxygen at 28 days (Morley et al., 2008) and to reduce the use of surfactant without increasing the incidence of bronchopulmonary dysplasia (BPD).

HHFNC has been reported to be as effective as CPAP as primary intervention for respiratory distress syndrome (RDS) in infants >28 weeks' gestation and compared to CPAP reduced abdominal distension and nasal trauma (Wilkinson et al., 2016). In the infant <28 weeks' gestation, if intubation is required for insufficient respiratory effort, surfactant should be administered prophylactically in the delivery room, preferably within 15 minutes of birth. Less invasive methods of administration of surfactant have been found to be effective for those infants with RDS who are spontaneously breathing and requiring surfactant, such as infants with increasing oxygen requirements on CPAP (Aldana-Aguirre et al., 2017). Delivery room management is discussed in further detail in chapter 10, early care of the newborn.

COMMON CONDITIONS ASSOCIATED WITH PREMATURITY

Premature and some LBW infants are at risk of conditions which can affect long-term health or be life-limiting. The more preterm the infant, the more likely there is a lasting impact; each physiological system will be affected by the interruption of normal embryological development. The following is a brief overview of these potential conditions; more detailed information can be found within the relevant chapters.

Surfactant insufficiency

Surfactant insufficiency is one of the major causes of RDS associated with prematurity. Surfactant is produced from approximately 25 weeks within Type II Pneumocytes and continues to term (Nkadi et al., 2009) The more prematurely a baby is born, the more likely surfactant deficiency is to occur. Other risk factors include maternal diabetes in pregnancy, perinatal asphyxia, and LBW. The lack of surfactant availability results in increased surface tension and alveolar **atelectasis**. Clinical presentation includes worsening signs of respiratory distress and respiratory acidosis, which result in ventilation/perfusion mismatch that may require management with varying levels of ventilatory support. The advent of exogenous surfactant administration has resulted in a reduction of mortality and morbidity. Refer to chapter 12, management of respiratory disorders, for more details about RDS and its management.

Chronic lung disease

Chronic lung disease (CLD), or bronchopulmonary dysplasia (BPD) is commonly seen in preterm infants who have required mechanical ventilation and oxygen therapy for treatment of respiratory distress (Davidson and Berkelhamer, 2017). It is widely acknowledged that CLD can result in longer hospitalisation, increased healthcare costs, and impacts quality of life for the infant and family (Trembath and Laughon, 2012). There have been significant changes in practice with regard to antenatal corticosteroid administration, surfactant administration, a move to early extubation and the use of non-invasive respiratory support over the past few decades. Despite this, however, CLD remains a persistent issue (Trembath and Laughon 2012), and National Neonatal Audit programme (NNAP) data from 2016 showed that in the UK 31% of infants born at less than 32 weeks' gestation developed significant CLD, with the occurrence of the condition varying from 26% to 39% across all neonatal networks (Royal College of Paediatrics and Child Health (RCPCH), 2017). Further information about CLD can be found in chapter 12, management of respiratory disorders.

Retinopathy of prematurity

Retinopathy of prematurity (ROP) is recognised as one of the preventable causes of childhood blindness. The highest-risk group constitutes infants born at less than 32 weeks GA or less than 1500g BW; further risk factors are the need for supplemental oxygen, intraventricular haemorrhage (IVH), RDS, sepsis, a white ethnic background, and multiple births. Most premature infants will develop some degree of ROP, which will resolve spontaneously. Some, however, will develop a more severe form of the disease which requires intervention (RCPCH et al., 2008).

To function adequately, the retina requires a constant supply of blood to provide oxygen. The blood vessels supplying this usually develop between weeks 16 and 36 of pregnancy. During the last 12 weeks of a pregnancy, the eye develops rapidly. When a baby is born at full term, the retinal blood vessel growth is mostly complete (the retina usually finishes growing a few weeks to a month after birth). Vascularisation begins at the optic nerve and branches out to the edge of the retina. In infants born prematurely, normal vessel growth, which is modulated by the retinal vascular endothelial growth factor (VEGF) and interleukin growth factor (ILGF), is disturbed. The infant is exposed to higher oxygen levels than would have been experienced *in utero*, which affects the balance of VEGF and ILGF. Vascular development is subsequently delayed so that the retinal blood supply does not meet the requirements of the growing retina. The consequence of this is abnormal vasoproliferation. This area of pathological vascularisation can cause a ridge within the retina (commonly in the temporal zone). If this growth continues, the blood vessels can migrate to areas that are not usually vascularised, such as the vitreous humour or the surface of the retina. This may then go on to produce scarring and traction that will result in the detachment of the retina, and thus blindness (Fleck and McIntosh, 2008).

ROP is categorised in stages 1–4 and the presence of Plus disease (see table 3.4). Plus disease is an indicator of the activity of the blood vessels. It is recognisable by tortuosity and engorgement of the blood vessels, and, if left untreated, will result in partial or total detachment of the retina.

Treatment of ROP depends on disease progression. It will be required if stage 1–2 is present with Plus disease, or stage 3 with or without Plus disease. The most effective proven treatments for ROP are cryotherapy or laser therapy, although more recent evidence is favourable towards the latter (Connolly et al., 2002; O'Keefe and Kirwan, 2006). The underlying concept for both is destruction of a small area of avascular retina adjacent to the region of abnormal vessel growth, to prevent disease progression. The difference is that this is achieved via a freezing probe in the case of cryotherapy. The Cryotherapy for Retinopathy of Prematurity Outcome Study (CRYO-ROP) demonstrated that this treatment reduced the rate of retinal detachment in approximately 50% of cases (Cryotherapy for Retinopathy of Prematurity Cooperative Group, 1988).

Follow-up results for CRYO-ROP at 10 years of age proved conclusively that peripheral retinal ablation significantly reduces the incidence of blindness compared to controls, with at least equal if not better visual acuity of 20/40 found in the control group (Cryotherapy for Retinopathy of Prematurity Cooperative Group, 2001). While these treatments can be effective at preserving central vision required for activities such as reading or driving, the treatments unfortunately have been shown to severely reduce peripheral vision. The longer-term side effects are still unknown.

The Early Treatment for Retinopathy of Prematurity Study (ETROP) examined whether earlier treatment was more beneficial to the overall visual outcome compared to treatment

TABLE 3.4 CATEGORIES OF ROP

Stage One	A demarcation line within the plane of the retina between vascularised and avascularised regions
Stage Two	Ridge or elevation at the junction of vascular and avascular regions of the retina
Stage Three	Ridge with extraretinal fibrovascular proliferation, continuous with the ridge, **posterior** but disconnected to the ridge or within the vitreous humour
Stage Four	Subtotal retinal detachment
Stage Five	Total retinal detachment

(adapted from RCPCH et al., 2008)

at the later conventional disease threshold point used in the CRYO-ROP study. The study found early treatment of high-risk pre-threshold ROP significantly improved outcomes (Good et al., 2004). A further treatment modality, which has recently been investigated (BEAT-ROP study), is the injection of anti-VEGF antibodies (bevacizumab) into the vitreous cavity. While long-term side effects are yet unknown, this therapy appears to reduce the incidence of myopia later on, but carries the same risk of subsequent retinal detachment, unless it is provided in conjunction with laser ablation, which has shown a reduction in this risk (Sankar et al., 2018).

Outcomes for infants with ROP can be greatly improved locally, by the implementation of strict oxygen saturation guidelines. A number of research trials have shown that the safest target range for oxygen saturations which affect patient morbidity and mortality, as well as a reduction of ROP, appears to be 90–95% (Lloyd et al., 2003; SUPPORT Study Group of the Eunice Kennedy Shriver NICHD Neonatal Research Network, 2010; BOOST II UK, Australia, and New Zealand Collaborative Groups, 2013; Schmidt et al., 2013). High oxygenation increases the risk of severe ROP, believed to be a result of oxygen-induced vascular closure and hypoxic stress, which increases VEGF.

Due to the importance of timely diagnosis and treatment, robust pathways of referral, which ensure on-time screening and treatment of ROP, need to be implemented and adhered to. Worryingly, the 2017 NNAP report demonstrated the standard set of 100% compliance, based upon guidance from the RCPCH, Royal College of Ophthalmologists, BAPM and Bliss, was not being achieved nationally, with only 94% of babies being screened on time for ROP (RCPCH, 2017). This is one aspect where the neonatal nurse can contribute towards improving ROP-related morbidity. Perhaps more importantly, it is the nurse's responsibility to continuously ensure that his or her patients' oxygen saturations are within normal (evidence-based) limits, which means close observation, prompt response to monitor alarms and often frequent adjustments to supplemental oxygen delivery rates for infants on respiratory support.

Anaemia of prematurity

Haemoglobin (Hb) production *in utero* is regulated by the cytokine **erythropoietin**. This is released by the liver and kidneys in response to tissue hypoxia. Hepatic production predominates in antenatal and perinatal life, but reduces throughout childhood. Erythropoietin binds to the circulating red blood cells (RBC), and if there is a low number of RBC in circulation, the relatively high level of unbound erythropoietin stimulates the production of RBC within the bone marrow (Palis and Segel, 1998).

Following delivery, a term infant has a natural drop in Hb levels at 10–14 weeks' postnatal age. This is referred to as physiological anaemia and does not require treatment. However, this event occurs earlier and with a more dramatic decline at around 4–6 weeks for the preterm infant. The process is exacerbated by frequent blood samples, the missed opportunity of transplacental iron transfer which occurs in the third trimester, and the rapid growth requiring good oxygenation undergone by infants born prematurely (Strauss, 2010). Furthermore, the erythropoietin response to reduced RBC in the plasma is slower than that of the term infant. Chapter 15 discusses the management of anaemia of prematurity.

Intraventricular haemorrhage and periventricular leukomalacia

The pathophysiology, management and prognosis of this significant sequela of prematurity is described in chapter 14, neonatal brain injury.

Suboptimal postnatal growth

Optimising postnatal nutrition and growth has been a constant challenge in preterm and LBW infants while aiming to avoid complications such as necrotising enterocolitis (NEC). Many studies have demonstrated that poor nutrition in the early stages will impact long-term development and brain growth (Su, 2014). Therefore, it is vital to ensure the correct amount of protein and energy is delivered, in order to promote growth and good developmental outcome in the preterm/LBW population. A major risk factor for the most concerning complication, NEC, identified in the 1990s was thought to be early feeding with formula as opposed to breast milk. However, in more recent studies it has been shown that there has been no increased risk of NEC in early fast feeding of breast milk or formula, compared to slow delayed introduction of enteral feeds (Kumar et al., 2017). Early enteral feeding has been associated with improved gut development and metabolic adaptation and optimised postnatal weight gain. There have been varying views regarding the speed at which full enteral feeds should be established, with the SIFT (Speed of Increasing Milk Feeds Trial) currently still ongoing (National Perinatal Epidemiology Unit, 2018). Studies using breast milk and formula have shown that fast steady increases shorten the duration of time it takes to achieve full enteral feeds and regain birth weight (Oddie et al., 2017).

In circumstances where enteral feeding is not appropriate, parenteral nutrition (PN) is a useful adjunct while enteral nutrition is achieved. It is now common practice to commence

PN within a few hours of life in both term and preterm infants where enteral feeding is not likely to be achieved within a reasonable timeframe (BAPM, 2016). The majority of preterm infants are thought to undergo a period of rapid growth, which tends to occur in the first 6–12 months of life. However, this may not specifically constitute bone growth, but a higher proportion of body fat, which has been suggested may contribute to health issues into adulthood (Ong et al., 2015). It has been suggested that catch-up growth within the first two years of life is beneficial for both renal and general health, whereas catch-up growth after this period may be detrimental to future health (Lapillonne and Griffin, 2013). Ongoing monitoring of growth and development in the early years is therefore vital for the preterm and LBW population. For more detail on nutrition and feeding in the NNU, see chapter 17.

Immunological immaturity

Like many body systems, the immune system is not fully functional at birth. It is particularly immature in infants born prematurely or at LBW, predisposing them to a high risk of infection. One hypothesis with regard to this risk is related to the immunosuppressive environment of the womb, which is followed by overwhelming exposure after delivery. The immune system subsequently reduces its response in order to prevent excessive reactivity to benign inflammatory processes (Basha et al., 2014). Once born, the preterm infant is exposed to a multitude of invasive medical procedures, such as insertion of central lines, cannulas and intubation, all of which increase the risk of infection. The mechanisms of the immune system and immunity in the neonate are discussed in more detail in chapter 18, neonatal infection.

Skin integrity issues

Keratinisation of the skin commences at 18 weeks, but only becomes effective at 34 weeks (Modi, 2004). Preterm birth results in an accelerated adaptation of the skin due to the differences between the *in utero* environment and the dry *ex utero* environment. The stratum corneum is layered with epithelial cells filled with keratin, and prevents transepidermal water loss. In order for skin to function as a protective barrier, there is a need for robust cohesion in the epidermis, which consists of the stratum corneum and dermis layers of the skin (figure 3.2). Not only are these layers thinner in the preterm infant than in the term population, but there is also a reduction in the elastin fibres, and a lack of cohesion between the two layers. This and incomplete keratinisation impacts on the skin's ability to prevent transepidermal water loss (TEWL) and contribute to thermoregulation.

Skin integrity assessment tools are important in the recognition of potential issues such as dry, cracked skin, which can increase the risk of infection, as well as repeated puncturing of the skin and friction injuries from the use of adhesive dressings and tapes. Optimising humidity within the incubator can prevent the drying of the skin, limit TEWL and aid in thermoregulation. For infants born at 28 weeks' GA, humidity should commence at

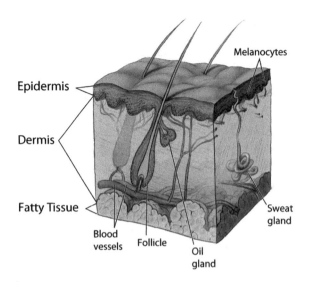

Figure 3.2 Layers of the skin

80% and remain at this level for the first 7 days. If at this point the baby's temperature is stable, humidity can gradually be reduced to 50%, with an aim to discontinue humidification after 21 days or 32 weeks' corrected GA, whichever occurs sooner (Sinclair et al., 2009).

THE 'LATE PRETERM INFANT'

Babies born between 34^{+0} to 36^{+6} weeks' gestation are referred to as late preterm infants. In 2011, this group was noted to constitute 83% of all preterm births in England (Office for National Statistics, 2015). This large percentage may be due to elective preterm deliveries and advances in obstetric care. Historically, the late preterm infant was referred to as 'near term', but this was misleading. There has been documented evidence of increasing incidence of RDS, hypothermia, hypoglycaemia, jaundice, poor feeding and suspected sepsis within the late preterm population, along with increased risk of readmission following discharge, and long-term neurodevelopmental problems (Engle et al., 2007). Thus, the late preterm baby is at increased risk of morbidity requiring admission to the NNU. Otherwise, these infants may be managed on postnatal wards with specialist input by the multidisciplinary postnatal team, in order to keep mother and baby together. The implementation of transitional care (TC) is one such model, which enables the mother to provide normal care to her baby with support from professionals in relation to, for example, nasogastric feeding, establishing breastfeeding, or observation for sepsis etc.

It is now well recognised that the late preterm infant should not be treated in the same way as a well term infant, as doing so can increase the risk of neonatal morbidity and thus NNU admission (Boyle et al., 2015).

THE IMPACT OF PREMATURITY ON PARENTAL BONDING

The significantly improved survival of premature and LBW infants necessitates an acknow-ledgement of the impedance of parental bonding with a potential impact on the socio-emotional stress regulation of the infant as a result (Provenzi et al., 2017). Increased survival rates have gone hand in hand with an increased incidence of morbidities in the extremely preterm infant (Glass et al., 2015); this can cause distress, negative feelings and fear for the parents, especially as there is limited ability to predict outcomes. Mothers and fathers can feel overwhelmed by the physical condition of their baby (Hoffenkamp et al., 2015).

The set-up and routines of the neonatal unit affect interactions between parent and baby, so that it is crucial for the neonatal nurse to facilitate parental sharing in what they regard as important events; such as first-time attending to care activities, integrating the baby into the family, and experiencing a feeling of closeness and interaction with their baby (Baylis et al., 2014). The disruption parents face starts at delivery, as the bonding process, which begins in pregnancy, would ordinarily be cemented in the first hour of life with skin-to-skin contact. However, many preterm and LBW infants require medical stabilisation and intervention that mean this critical time is replaced by a traumatic and sometimes life-altering experience (Fernández Medina et al., 2018). This then leads to a potentially long-term physical separation, which can have a significant negative impact on a mother's mental health (Misund et al., 2016). It has furthermore been suggested that the child is up to 6 times more likely to experience Disorganised Attachment Disorder (Pennestri et al., 2015).

Parents have to relinquish sole responsibility of their child to strangers in an instant. Effective and empathetic communication is, therefore, vital to rapidly formulating a partner-ship that enables the parents to maintain a sense of involvement and empowerment. Equally, the communication between staff should aim to minimise any separation that could disrupt parent bonding during a critical period of brain organisation (Purdy et al., 2015). Attentive communication is seen by parents as a relief from the burdens of the trying times which they are experiencing and, in contrast, lack of communication can contribute to feelings of loneliness and abandonment (Wigert et al., 2014).

There are now many video contact technologies that can support and enhance par-ental communication and contact. These include Skype, FaceTime, Angel Eye, and NICView Webcams and, overall, have demonstrated a positive impact on stress reduction for the parents (Weems et al., 2016; Epstein et al., 2017; Flores et al., 2017).

Fundamentally, parents need to be recognised as important collaborative members of the neonatal team and as facilitators of the developmental needs of their babies. This can have long-lasting positive effects on parental bonding and the life-changing experience of having a baby on the NNU. This topic will be covered in more detail in chapter 4.

DISCHARGE PLANNING

The key to effective discharge means that planning towards this must commence soon after admission. Studies have shown that barriers in the transition from the NNU to home stem from poor communication and lack of parental involvement in the decision-making process and care planning for their infant (Purdy et al., 2015). Identifying readiness for discharge is paramount. Many units will have varying factors highlighting infants suitable for the transition of care from the hospital to home. These may include: ability to maintain their temperature in a normal environment, respiratory stability, consistent ability to feed by whichever means (bottle, breast or nasogastric tube), and consistent weight gain (Jefferies, 2014).

The development of a supportive relationship with the family will facilitate parental teaching enabling the parents to care for their baby. NNU graduates have been found to disproportionately contribute to demands on out-of-hours services (Harijan and Boyle 2012), mainly due to parental uncertainty in how to respond to changes in their babies' conditions or minor illnesses (Brett et al., 2011). Therefore, parental education must include the recognition of normal behaviours as well as identifying signs of illness or deterioration. The opportunity for the parents to 'room in' with their baby may help build confidence, as it allows them to take responsibility for them with the support of the nursing team, should it become necessary. While this is seen as a positive experience and milestone for most parents, it is important to note that not all parents will wish to take advantage of this, and they should not feel obliged or pressured into doing so (Bennet and Sheridan, 2005).

A coordinated approach to discharge planning will ensure that health promotion has been addressed, ensuring that risk factors for sudden infant death and similar issues are discussed. Due to the complexity of care that has been required, it is key to ensure that follow-up with the neonatal outreach team if available, neonatal clinics and relevant specialists is well coordinated.

CONCLUSION

The use of technology and innovative research has given many opportunities to improve the outcomes for sick and preterm infants. This ongoing advancement in the management of the preterm infant not only affects the baby but the family as well. In order to provide appropriate care and support, there must be appreciation of the preterm infant's unique physiology, even within the broad gestational age range that defines prematurity. An understanding of the impact premature birth and LBW can have on physiological processes and systems is a vital part of neonatal nursing. This chapter has outlined the key issues which need to be considered antenatally, in the delivery room and on the NNU, including some conditions commonly seen in the preterm and LBW population. The following chapters will explore a variety of problems seen in the NNU in more detail.

CASE STUDIES

Case study 1: Impending birth of a preterm infant

Labour ward has contacted your unit to alert them to a new admission. Leonora is a 26-year-old primigravida who is 27 weeks pregnant, and has attended the assessment unit with ruptured membranes and tightenings.

Q.1. What else would you like to know at this stage?

Q.2. Leonora is not able to attend the NNU for a look around, so you go and speak to her on the labour ward. What information does Leonora require at this stage? Is there anything in particular you would like to discuss with her?
Leonora's labour is progressing rapidly. She is expected to deliver within the next 30 minutes, but has only received one dose of corticosteroids 2 hours ago. Magnesium sulphate was commenced soon after admission.

Q.3. Consider the prematurity-associated problems Leonora's baby is likely to encounter, both based on gestation and antenatal events. How can you contribute to their early recognition and minimisation of their impact on outcomes in the short term and long term?

Case study 2: management of an IUGR infant

Sarah is a 34-week gestation infant born via normal vaginal delivery with a birth weight of 1.1 kg. Her mother Angela had been well throughout her pregnancy with the exception of pregnancy-induced hypertension from 26 weeks' gestation, for which she was treated with labetalol. Foetal growth began to slow from 28 weeks' gestation. This was noted to be static in the week prior to delivery, with normal diastolic flow noted on ultrasound.

There were no risk factors for sepsis identified. Sarah's mother wishes to breastfeed.

Q.1. What could be potential causes for Sarah's poor growth?

Q.2. How would Sarah's care differ from infants at 34 weeks who are born at an appropriate weight for gestational age?

Q.3. What are your thoughts about Angela's wish to exclusively breastfeed Sarah? Will this be feasible?

Case study 3: at the borderline of viability

Alice is a 42-year-old woman who was admitted to the labour ward with abdominal pain at 22^{+5} weeks' gestation. She is a 'gravida 4, para 0^{+2}', having had 2 early miscarriages and 2 extremely preterm babies, both of whom survived less than 24 hours. This pregnancy is the result of *in vitro* fertilisation using a donor egg. On admission Alice is assessed to be in established labour. Alice and her partner Liam agree that they would like the neonatal team to attempt full resuscitation following delivery.

Q.1. What are your thoughts about Alice's and Liam's wishes? Do you think this is in the best interest of their baby?

Q.2. Using one or more available prognostic tools, try and establish their baby's prognosis for survival and long-term outcomes. How would you counsel Alice and Liam?

For suggested answer guides to the questions posed in these case studies, please refer to the web-based companion site specific to this chapter (see URL below).

WEB-BASED RESOURCES

For further information, online resources and greater detail on the case studies featured in this chapter go to www.routledge.com/cw/nicnursing

References

Aldana-Aguirre, J. C., Pinto, M., Featherstone, R. M., & Kumar, M. (2017). Less invasive surfactant administration versus intubation for surfactant delivery in preterm infants with respiratory distress syndrome: a systematic review and meta-analysis. *Archives of Disease in Childhood: Fetal and Neonatal Edition, 102*(1), F17–F23.

Alfirevic, Z., Stampalija, T., & Dowswell, T. (2017). Fetal and umbilical Doppler ultrasound in high-risk pregnancies. *Cochrane Database of Systematic Reviews,* Issue 6. Art. No.: CD007529. DOI: 10.1002/14651858.CD007529.pub4

Al-Wassia, H., & Shah, P. S. (2015). Efficacy and safety of umbilical cord milking at birth: A systematic review and meta-analysis. *JAMA Pediatrics, 169*(1), 18–25.

Backes, C. H., Rivera, B. K., Haque, U., Bridge, J. A., Smith, C. V., Hutchon, D. J., & Mercer, J. S. (2014). Placental transfusion strategies in very preterm neonates: a systematic review and meta-analysis. *Obstetrics & Gynecology, 124*(1), 47–56.

Ballard, J. L., Novak, K. K., & Driver, M. (1979). A simplified score for assessment of fetal maturation of newly born infants. *The Journal of Pediatrics, 95*(5), 769–774.

Ballard, J. L., Khoury, J. C., Wedig, K. L., Wang, L., Eilers-Walsman, B. L., & Lipp, R. (1991). New Ballard Score, expanded to include extremely premature infants. *The Journal of pediatrics*, *119*(3), 417–423.

Basha, S., Surendran, N., & Pichichero, M. (2014). Immune responses in neonates. *Expert review of clinical immunology*, *10*(9), 1171–1184.

Baylis, R., Ewald, U., Gradin, M., Nyqvist, K. H., Rubertsson, C., & Blomqvist, Y. T. (2014). First-time events between parents and preterm infants are affected by the designs and routines of neonatal intensive care units. *Acta Paediatrica*, *103*(10), 1045–1052.

Beaino, G., Khoshnood, B., Kaminski, M., Pierrat, V., Marret, S., Matis, J., … & Zupan-Simunek, V. (2010). Predictors of cerebral palsy in very preterm infants: the EPIPAGE Prospective population-based cohort study. *Developmental Medicine & Child Neurology*, *52*(6), e119-e125.

Bennett, R., & Sheridan, C. (2005). Mothers' perceptions of 'rooming-in'on a neonatal intensive care unit. *Infant*, *1*(5), 171–174.

BOOST II UK, Australia, and New Zealand Collaborative Groups. (2013). Oxygen saturation and outcomes in preterm infants. *New England Journal of Medicine*, *368*(22), 2094–2104.

Boyle, E. M., Johnson, S., Manktelow, B., Seaton, S. E., Draper, E. S., Smith, L. K., … & Field, D. J. (2015). Neonatal outcomes and delivery of care for infants born late preterm or moderately preterm: a prospective population-based study. *Archives of Disease in Childhood: Fetal and Neonatal Edition*, *100*(6), F479–F485.

Brett, J., Staniszewska, S., Newburn, M., Jones, N., & Taylor, L. (2011). A systematic mapping review of effective interventions for communicating with, supporting and providing information to parents of preterm infants. *BMJ Open*, *1*(1), e000023.

British Association of Perinatal Medicine (2016). *The Provisions of Parenteral Nutrition within Neonatal Services – A Framework for Practice*. London: British Association of Perinatal Medicine.

British Association of Perinatal Medicine (2019). *Perinatal Management at less than 27 weeks' Gestation. A Framework for Practice*. London: British Association of Perinatal Medicine.

Chang, E. (2015). Preterm birth and the role of neuroprotection. *BMJ, 350*, g6661.

Connolly, B. P., Ng, E. Y., McNamara, J. A., Regillo, C. D., Vander, J. F., & Tasman, W. (2002). A comparison of laser photocoagulation with cryotherapy for threshold retinopathy of prematurity at 10 years: Part 2. Refractive outcome1. *Ophthalmology*, *109*(5), 936–941.

Costeloe, K., Hennessy, E., Gibson, A. T., Marlow, N., Wilkinson, A. R., & EPICure Study Group. (2000). The EPICure study: outcomes to discharge from hospital for infants born at the threshold of viability. *Pediatrics*, *106*(4), 659–671.

Cryotherapy for Retinopathy of Prematurity Cooperative Group. (1988). Multicenter trial of cryotherapy for retinopathy of prematurity: Preliminary results. *Pediatrics*, *81*(5), 697–706.

Cryotherapy for Retinopathy of Prematurity Cooperative Group. (2001). Multicenter Trial of Cryotherapy for Retinopathy of Prematurity: Ophthalmological outcomes at 10 years. *Archives of ophthalmology (Chicago, Ill.: 1960)*, *119*(8), 1110.

Davidson, L., & Berkelhamer, S. (2017). Bronchopulmonary dysplasia: Chronic lung disease of infancy and long-term pulmonary outcomes. *Journal of Clinical Medicine*, *6*(1), 4 doi:10.3390/jcm6010004.

Dawson, J. A., Kamlin, C. O. F., Vento, M., Wong, C., Cole, T. J., Donath, S. M., … & Morley, C. J. (2010). Defining the reference range for oxygen saturation for infants after birth. *Pediatrics*, *125*(6), e1340-7.

de Almeida, M. F. B., Guinsburg, R., Sancho, G. A., Rosa, I. R. M., Lamy, Z. C., Martinez, F. E., … & de Cássia Silveira, R. (2014). Hypothermia and early neonatal mortality in preterm infants. *The Journal of Pediatrics*, *164*(2), 271–275.

Doyle, L. W., Crowther, C. A., Middleton, P., Marret, S., & Rouse, D. (2009). Magnesium sulphate for women at risk of preterm birth for neuroprotection of the fetus. *Cochrane Database of Systematic Reviews*, Issue 1. Art. No.: CD004661. DOI: 10.1002/14651858.CD004661.pub3

Dubowitz, L. M., Dubowitz, V., & Goldberg, C. (1970). Clinical assessment of gestational age in the newborn infant. *The Journal of Pediatrics*, 77(1), 1–10.

Engle, W. A., Tomashek, K. M., & Wallman, C. (2007). 'Late-preterm' infants: A population at risk. *Pediatrics*, 120(6), 1390–1401.

Epstein, E. G., Arechiga, J., Dancy, M., Simon, J., Wilson, D., & Alhusen, J. L. (2017). Integrative Review of Technology to Support Communication With Parents of Infants in the NICU. *Journal of Obstetric, Gynecologic & Neonatal Nursing*, 46(3), 357–366.

Fernández Medina, I. M., Granero-Molina, J., Fernández-Sola, C., Hernández-Padilla, J. M., Camacho Ávilae, M., & López-Rodríguez, M. (2018). Bonding in neonatal intensive care units: experiences of extremely preterm infants' mothers. *Women and Birth*, 31(4), 325–330.

Fleck, B. W., & McIntosh, N. (2008). Pathogenesis of retinopathy of prematurity and possible preventive strategies. *Early Human Development*, 84(2), 83–88.

Flores, N. I., Friedlich, P., Belfort, M., Vanderbilt, D. L., Williams, R., Kipke, M. D., & Lakshmanan, A. (2017). Access to Technology for Communication Improves Health-Related Quality of Life for Low Income Families after NICU Discharge. *Pediatrics, 140*(1) Meeting Abstract.

Glass, H. C., Costarino, A. T., Stayer, S. A., Brett, C., Cladis, F., & Davis, P. J. (2015). Outcomes for extremely premature infants. *Anesthesia and Analgesia*, 120(6), 1337–1351.

Good, W. V., & Early Treatment for Retinopathy of Prematurity Cooperative Group. (2004). Final results of the Early Treatment for Retinopathy of Prematurity (ETROP) randomized trial. *Transactions of the American Ophthalmological Society*, 102, 233.

Harijan, P., & Boyle, E. M. (2012, June). Health outcomes in infancy and childhood of moderate and late preterm infants. In *Seminars in Fetal and Neonatal Medicine*, 17(3), 159–162.

Hoffenkamp, H. N., Braeken, J., Hall, R. A., Tooten, A., Vingerhoets, A. J., & van Bakel, H. J. (2015). Parenting in complex conditions: Does preterm birth provide a context for the development of less optimal parental behavior? *Journal of Pediatric Psychology*, 40(6), 559–571.

International Liaison Committee on Resuscitation. (2006). The International Liaison Committee on Resuscitation (ILCOR) consensus on science with treatment recommendations for pediatric and neonatal patients: pediatric basic and advanced life support. *Pediatrics, 117*(5), e955-e977.

Jefferies, A. L. (2014). Going home: facilitating discharge of the preterm infant. *Paediatrics & Child Health*, 19(1), 31–36.

Katheria, A., Rich, W., & Finer, N. (2012). Electrocardiogram provides a continuous heart rate faster than oximetry during neonatal resuscitation. *Pediatrics*, 130(5), e1177–1181.

Kumar, R. K., Singhal, A., Vaidya, U., Banerjee, S., Anwar, F., & Rao, S. (2017). Optimizing nutrition in preterm low birth weight infants–Consensus summary. *Frontiers in Nutrition*, 4, 20.

Lapillonne, A., & Griffin, I. J. (2013). Feeding preterm infants today for later metabolic and cardiovascular outcomes. *The Journal of Pediatrics*, 162(3), S7–S16.

Laptook, A. R., Salhab, W., & Bhaskar, B. (2007). Admission temperature of low birth weight infants: Predictors and associated morbidities. *Pediatrics*, 119(3), e643–e649.

Lloyd, J., Askie, L. M., Smith, J., & Tarnow-Mordi, W. O. (2003). Supplemental oxygen for the treatment of prethreshold retinopathy of prematurity. *Cochrane Database of Systematic Reviews,* Issue 2. Art. No.: CD003482. DOI: 10.1002/14651858.CD003482

McCall, E. M., Alderdice, F., Halliday, H. L., Vohra, S., & Johnston, L. (2018). Interventions to prevent hypothermia at birth in preterm and/or low birth weight infants. *Cochrane Database of Systematic Reviews,* Issue 2. Art. No.: CD004210. DOI: 10.1002/14651858.CD004210.pub5

Mank, A., van Zanten, H. A., Meyer, M. P., Pauws, S., Lopriore, E., & te Pas, A. B. (2016). Hypothermia in preterm infants in the first hours after birth: Occurrence, course and risk factors. *PloS One*, 11(11), e0164817.

Marlow, N. (2006). Outcome following extremely preterm birth. *Women's Health Medicine*, 3(5), 197–201.

Mercer, J. S., Vohr, B. R., McGrath, M. M., Padbury, J. F., Wallach, M., & Oh, W. (2006). Delayed cord clamping in very preterm infants reduces the incidence of intraventricular hemorrhage and late-onset sepsis: A randomized, controlled trial. *Pediatrics*, *117*(4), 1235–1242.

Miller, S. S., Lee, H. C., & Gould, J. B. (2011). Hypothermia in very low birth weight infants: Distribution, risk factors and outcomes. *Journal of Perinatology*, *31*(S1), S49–56.

Misund, A. R., Bråten, S., Nerdrum, P., Pripp, A. H., & Diseth, T. H. (2016). A Norwegian prospective study of preterm mother–infant interactions at 6 and 18 months and the impact of maternal mental health problems, pregnancy and birth complications. *BMJ Open*, *6*(5), e009699.

Modi, N. (2004). Management of fluid balance in the very immature neonate. *Archives of Disease in Childhood: Fetal and Neonatal Edition*, *89*(2), F108–F111.

Morley, C. J., Davis, P. G., Doyle, L. W., Brion, L. P., Hascoet, J. M., & Carlin, J. B. (2008). Nasal CPAP or intubation at birth for very preterm infants. *New England Journal of Medicine*, *358*(7), 700–708.

National Institute for Health and Care Excellence (2015). *Intrapartum care. Quality standard QS105*. NICE.

National Institute for Health and Care Excellence (2019). *Preterm labour and birth. Quality Standard. NICE Guidelines*. NICE.

National Perinatal Epidemiology Unit (2018). SiFT: Speed of increasing milk feeds trial. Retrieved from www.npeu.ox.ac.uk/sift

Nkadi, P. O., Merritt, T. A., & Pillers, D. A. M. (2009). An overview of pulmonary surfactant in the neonate: genetics, metabolism, and the role of surfactant in health and disease. *Molecular Genetics and Metabolism*, *97*(2), 95–101.

Nuffield Council on Bioethics (2014). *Critical care decisions in fetal and neonatal medicine: ethical issues*. London: Nuffield Council on Bioethics.

O'Donnell, C. P., & Stenson, B. J. (2008). Respiratory strategies for preterm infants at birth. In *Seminars in Fetal and Neonatal Medicine*, 13(6), 401–409.

O'Keefe, M., & Kirwan, C. (2006). Diode laser versus cryotherapy in treatment of ROP. *British Journal of Ophthalmology*, 90(4): 402–403.

Oddie, S. J., Young, L., & McGuire, W. (2017). Slow advancement of enteral feed volumes to prevent necrotising enterocolitis in very low birth weight infants. *Cochrane Database of Systematic Reviews*, Issue 8. Art. No.: CD001241.DOI: 10.1002/14651858.CD001241.pub7

Office for National Statistics (2015) *Pregnancy and ethnic factors influencing births and infant mortality: 2013*. www.ons.gov.uk/peoplepopulationandcommunity/healthandsocialcare/causesofdeath/bulletins/pregnancyandethnicfactorsinfluencingbirthsandinfantmortality/2015-10-14

Ong, K. K., Kennedy, K., Castañeda-Gutiérrez, E., Forsyth, S., Godfrey, K. M., Koletzko, B., ... & Van Der Beek, E. M. (2015). Postnatal growth in preterm infants and later health outcomes: a systematic review. *Acta Paediatrica*, *104*(10), 974–986.

Palis, J., & Segel, G. B. (1998). Developmental biology of erythropoiesis. *Blood Reviews*, *12*(2), 106–114.

Pennestri, M. H., Gaudreau, H., Bouvette-Turcot, A. A., Moss, E., Lecompte, V., Atkinson, L., ... & Mavan Research Team. (2015). Attachment disorganization among children in neonatal intensive care unit: Preliminary results. *Early Human Development*, *91*(10), 601–606.

Petty, J. (2017). The preterm baby and the small baby. In MacDonald, S. & Johnson, G. (Eds) *Mayes Midwifery* (15th Edition), Edinburgh, London & New York: Elsevier.

Provenzi, L., Fumagalli, M., Bernasconi, F., Sirgiovanni, I., Morandi, F., Borgatti, R., & Montirosso, R. (2017). Very Preterm and Full-Term Infants' Response to Socio-Emotional Stress: The Role of Postnatal Maternal Bonding. *Infancy*, *22*(5), 695–712.

Purdy, I. B., Craig, J. W., & Zeanah, P. (2015). NICU discharge planning and beyond: recommendations for parent psychosocial support. *Journal of Perinatology*, *35*(S1), S24–28.

Rabe, H., Diaz-Rossello, J. L., Duley, L., & Dowswell, T. (2012) Effect of timing of umbilical cord clamping and other strategies to influence placental transfusion at preterm birth on maternal and infantoutcomes.

Cochrane Database of Systematic Reviews, Issue 8. Art. No.: CD003248.DOI: 10.1002/14651858. CD003248.pub3

Resuscitation Council UK (2016). *Newborn Life Support.* (4th Edition), London: Resuscitation Council (UK).

Roberts, D., Brown, J, Medley, N., & Dalziel, S. R. (2017). Antenatal corticosteroids for accelerating fetal lung maturation for women at risk of preterm birth. *Cochrane Database of Systematic Reviews,* Issue 3. Art. No.: CD004454. DOI: 10.1002/14651858.CD004454.pub3

Royal College of Obstetricians and Gynaecologists. (2011). Magnesium Sulphate to Prevent Cerebral Palsy following Preterm Birth. Scientific Impact Paper No. 29. London: Royal College of Obstetricians and Gynaecologists.

Royal College of Obstetricians and Gynaecologists. (2013). Small for Gestational age Fetus: Investigation and Management. London: Royal College of Obstetricians and Gynaecologists.

Royal College of Paediatrics and Child Health, Royal College of Ophthalmologists, British Association of Perinatal Medicine & Bliss. (2008). UK Retinopathy of Prematurity Guideline. RCPCH, RCOphth, BAPM & Bliss.

Royal College of Paediatrics and Child Health & Healthcare Quality Improvement Partnership. (2017). National Neonatal Audit Programme 2017 Annual Report on 2016 data. Royal College of Paediatrics and Child Health.

Sankar, M. J., Sankar, J., & Chandra, P. (2018). Anti-vascular endothelial growth factor (VEGF) drugs for treatment of retinopathy of prematurity. *Cochrane Database of Systematic Reviews,* Issue 1. Art. No.: CD009734. DOI: 10.1002/14651858.CD009734.pub3

Schmid, M., Kasprian, G., Kuessel, L., Messerschmidt, A., Brugger, P. C., & Prayer, D. (2011). Effect of antenatal corticosteroid treatment on the fetal lung: a magnetic resonance imaging study. *Ultrasound in Obstetrics & Gynecology, 38*(1), 94–98.

Schmidt, B., Whyte, R. K., Asztalos, E. V., Moddemann, D., Poets, C., Rabi, Y., ... & Canadian Oxygen Trial (COT) Group. (2013). Effects of targeting higher vs lower arterial oxygen saturations on death or disability in extremely preterm infants: A randomized clinical trial. *Jama, 309*(20), 2111–2120.

Sharma, D., Shastri, S., & Sharma, P. (2016). Intrauterine growth restriction: antenatal and postnatal aspects. *Clinical medicine insights: Pediatrics, 10,* 67–83.

Sinclair, L., Crisp, J., & Sinn, J. (2009). Variability in incubator humidity practices in the management of preterm infants. *Journal of Paediatrics and Child Health, 45*(9), 535–540.

South Australian Perinatal Practice Guidelines Workgroup, & Wilkinson, D. (2013) *Perinatal Care at the Threshold of Viability.* Retrieved from www.sahealth.sa.gov.au/wps/wcm/connect/ 8ddf798042ac004d9f11bfad100c470d/Perinatal%2Bcare%2Bat%2Bthreshold%2Bviability-WCHN-PPG-09122013.pdf?MOD=AJPERES

Strauss, R. G. (2010). Anaemia of prematurity: pathophysiology and treatment. *Blood Reviews, 24*(6), 221–225.

Su, B. H. (2014). Optimizing nutrition in preterm infants. *Pediatrics & Neonatology, 55*(1), 5–13.

SUPPORT Study Group of the Eunice Kennedy Shriver NICHD Neonatal Research Network. (2010). Target ranges of oxygen saturation in extremely preterm infants. *New England Journal of Medicine, 362*(21), 1959–1969.

Trembath, A., & Laughon, M. M. (2012). Predictors of bronchopulmonary dysplasia. *Clinics in Perinatology, 39*(3), 585–601.

Weems, M. F., Graetz, I., Lan, R., DeBaer, L. R., & Beeman, G. (2016). Electronic communication preferences among mothers in the neonatal intensive care unit. *Journal of Perinatology, 36*(11), 997–1000.

Wigert, H., Blom, M. D., & Bry, K. (2014). Parents' experiences of communication with neonatal intensive-care unit staff: An interview study. *BMC Pediatrics, 14,* 304. doi:10.1186/s12887-014-0304-5.

Wilkinson, D., Andersen, C., O'Donnell, C. P. F., De Paoli, A. G., & Manley, B. J.(2016) High flow nasal cannula for respiratory support in preterm infants. *Cochrane Database of Systematic Reviews,* Issue 2. Art. No.: CD006405.DOI: 10.1002/14651858.CD006405.pub3

Wilson, E., Maier, R. F., Norman, M., Misselwitz, B., Howell, E. A., Zeitlin, J., ... & Pryds, O. (2016). Admission hypothermia in very preterm infants and neonatal mortality and morbidity. *The Journal of Pediatrics, 175*, 61–67.

World Health Organization. (2015). *WHO recommendations on interventions to improve preterm birth outcomes*. World Health Organization

World Health Organization (2018) *Preterm birth.* Retrieved from www.who.int/en/news-room/fact-sheets/detail/preterm-birth

PART 2

THE PHYSICAL AND EMOTIONAL WELLBEING OF NEONATE AND FAMILY

The physical and emotional wellbeing of neonate and family: The parent voice

My baby was whisked away as soon as he was born … I only had a quick glimpse as he was so unwell and so was I. The separation was so awful, and I couldn't make sense of what was happening.

But the neonatal staff made sure I got to see him as soon as possible and encouraged me and my husband to touch and hold him very early so we could get to know him. Looking back, I now know how important that was to all of us.

Voice of a mother of a 31-week gestation baby, Leo (pseudonym), who spent four weeks in neonatal care.

The staff helped us to be involved in every aspect of her care right from the start. We felt we had a role and eventually started to feel like her parents even though she was so sick and covered in wires and tubes.

It was vital that we were involved in the decisions about her care … We are her parents and our voice was heard. This was especially important because of the emotional toll the experience had on us all.

Voice of a father of a 26-week gestation baby, Fatima (pseudonym), who spent three months in neonatal care.

Adapted from Petty et al., 2019a; 2019b

See chapter 4 reference list for full citations.

4

NURTURING SUPPORTIVE FAMILY AND INFANT RELATIONSHIPS IN THE NEONATAL ENVIRONMENT

Liz Crathern

CONTENTS

GUIDANCE ON HOW TO ENHANCE PERSONAL LEARNING FROM THIS CHAPTER

Key points covered in this chapter

■ The significant emotional impact of having a baby in neonatal care on parents/families.

■ The parents' need for support from neonatal staff and participate in the care of their baby as part of the multidisciplinary team.

■ The emerging importance and value of Family Integrated Care.

Reflection

Reading through the chapter, you are encouraged to engage with the key points and related literature in an enquiring way. Ask these questions:

■ Does the content, relating to the emotional effects of neonatal care on families, have resonance with me? If not, why not?

■ Is it likely to make me want to change personal practice? If not, why not?

■ Do I want to change how my work environment provides family support?

Implications for nursing care

■ Finally: how will this chapter enable me to support and nurture the relationship of a family with their baby from any or all these perspectives: personal; practice; policy; education and research? Consider the implications of what you learn for your nursing care relating to families.

INTRODUCTION AND BACKGROUND

When updating this chapter, it was encouraging to note the evolving emphasis on supporting and nurturing of family-and-baby relationships within the literature; not only in those frameworks that underpin the recent focus on integrating the family more meaningfully within the neonatal unit (NNU), but also based on the drivers and standards that inform and reform family-focused clinical practice (Bliss, 2011; Health Foundation, 2014; Bliss, 2015a; Royal College of Nursing (RCN), 2015; British Association of Perinatal Medicine (BAPM), 2017; Royal College of Paediatrics and Child Health (RCPCH), 2017). It is not possible to do justice to the plethora of recent developments in one chapter, such as Family Integrated Care (FIC; Lee and O'Brien, 2018), the Family and Infant Neurodevelopmental Education (FINE) teaching package (Warren, 2017), and the Bliss Family Friendly Accreditation scheme (Bliss, 2015b) to name some examples. However, all healthcare practitioners should be aware of these developments when supporting families in the NNU.

It is worth reconsidering at the beginning of this chapter that one of the most challenging aspects of caring for the infant in the NNU is the management and support of parents and the wider family, particularly for novice neonatal nurses. The emergence of neonatal care as a specialist discipline has brought with it recognition of the critical role of the family in the recovery of their infant, and the psychosocial importance of providing opportunities for families and their infant to develop a close relationship in an environment alien to them (Warren, 2000; Gerhardt, 2004; Bliss, 2011; Flacking et al., 2016). The technological advances in supportive care has presented a range of dilemmas and challenges for both novice and expert nurses that could be summarised as a balancing act: the attunement of parental hope for the future with realism of the present (Crathern, 1997; 2004) and the expert nurse's role as both protector and advocate for the vulnerable infant (Crawford and McLean, 2010). For some families, this support may well involve caring for their dying infant (Robichaux and Clark, 2006), which will be covered in chapters 7 and 8.

It is clear that in setting aside a chapter on families and their babies, there will be overlap with other topics such as developmental care, pain, feeding, and end-of-life care, all of which are discussed in other chapters, aspects of which should be considered in conjunction with this one. Moreover, recognition of the family as a part of the wider multidisciplinary team should be applied throughout this book in relation to all areas of care.

HISTORICAL JOURNEY OF FAMILY INVOLVEMENT IN NEONATAL UNIT CARE

When considering how to improve family support in the NNU, it is key that both historical and contemporary perspectives are explored, and in doing so an understanding of internal and external factors that influence this unique family picture increased. There is a need to acknowledge and critique the past and present of neonatal care.

Particular emphasis will and should be given to facilitating a participant role for both parents. The definition of what constitutes family in neonatal care is diverse and at times challenges personal perspectives on this. Neonatal staff may hold an image of what the 'happy family unit' is, while families do not conform to stereotype. Healthcare practitioners require a non-judgemental acceptance that it is up to the family to define the members of their family unit (Whyte, 1997). Personal values and judgements must not impede the ability to care unconditionally and non-judgementally. This involves encompassing and embracing diversity in relation to ethnic background, social status, religious beliefs, sexual orientation, and any other individual attributes that families may possess.

It is also important to reflect upon the historical basis of caring for families in NNUs, as it is impossible to ignore that the present dynamic of parenting in neonatal care has been shaped by our history, and any future potential to best support families means that we must learn from our past.

From the 1930s, when the first Special Care Baby Unit in the UK was opened (Crosse, 1957), through the postwar era, there emerged a social trend for hospital rather than home delivery, as midwifery care and pregnancy were increasingly under the supervision of obstetricians. Thus care surrounding birth was directed from a medical rather than a family perspective (Dunn, 2007). Importantly, the social acceptance of doctors' authority at this time inhibited a questioning culture from both nurses and parents, either into the specifics of care or their roles as caregivers. Understandably, this had a huge impact on the parenting role in the NNU.

In a pre-antibiotic era, parents were potential carriers of disease, and consequently, to reduce the risk of infection, were almost always discouraged from visiting the nursery, and, if permitted inside, had to wear a gown at all times (see figure 4.1) and were prohibited from physical contact (Davis et al., 2003). While the principles of such austere care were driven by a genuine concern for the vulnerable infant and focused on sterility and cleanliness (Crosse, 1957), the discovery that hospital-acquired (**nosocomial**) infection was spread more rapidly by staff was yet to emerge. Fear of death from infection was an overriding driver in the policy of exclusion, and despite improving survival rates of preterm infants, the separation of mothers from their infants in this era increased (Davis et al., 2003). As a result, the 1960s saw many special care units permitting parents access to their babies only through the glass windows of viewing corridors, these being built to prevent families from entering the unit while still allowing them to see their baby.

Many parents who were living further distances from increasingly specialised centres, may not have touched their infant for the first time until they were allowed to take the baby home from hospital. This was to have consequences beyond the neonatal period. The phenomena of 'failure to thrive' and abuse among infants separated from their parents in this way started to emerge with recognition of a clear risk of physical and emotional neglect (Klaus and Kennell, 1976). Further evidence relating to the negative impact of minimum mother touch in some infants was being reported in the 1990s (Polan and Ward, 1994).

Firsthand experience of neonatal care in the late 1970s exclusively saw parents allowed to visit during strictly enforced time slots, nurses having completed most of a baby's care before visiting time. As early as 1980, taking an infant in their incubator or cot to the window of a viewing corridor, so that grandparents and siblings could see the new addition to the family, was commonplace. It is clear that the visiting polices in neonatal care were draconian.

Throughout the 1960s and 1970s, the volume of research findings stressing the importance of a secure infant attachment continued to influence neonatal practice and encouraged nurses to promote greater parental participation in care (Thomas, 2008). Thus research, although slow to impact practice, was beginning to support the nurses' intuitive knowledge.

During the 1970s, the arrival of neonatal intensive care units (NICUs), with increasing numbers of infants receiving respiratory support, heralded a rapid change in technology and supportive therapies. With the increased level of medical interventions and the consequent lengthening of hospital stays for smaller, sicker babies came the beginning of further integration of parents, a practice now regarded as necessary for future family functioning (Sophie et al., 2009; Bliss, 2011; Roué et al., 2017; Banerjee et al., 2018).

The 1980s also saw the emergence of social developments in healthcare, such as consumer and maternity pressure groups – the latter promoting the importance of support for the mother and breastfeeding in the neonatal period. This also contributed to the recognition of a need to humanise the neonatal environment (Davis et al., 2003).

Arguably, the 1990s could be perceived as the time when neonatal nursing began to flourish and find its voice. This was aided no doubt by emanating research evidence which had contributed to the introduction of both family-centred and developmental approaches to care within many NNUs, promoting not only physical care, but also the family as a central tenet of this (Raeside, 1997; Turrill, 1999). These models of care had a basis in family wellbeing. Barriers, both physical and emotional, which had previously been created by healthcare professionals and accepted – or more than likely tolerated – by parents, started

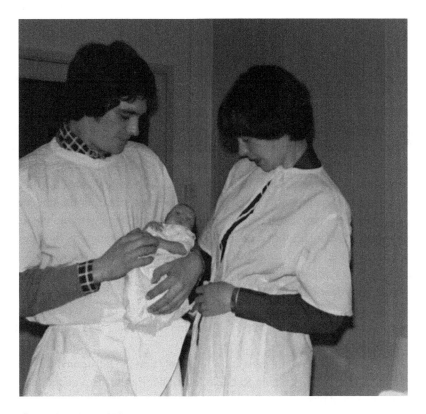

Figure 4.1 Parenting circa 1970

to be broken down. This involved professionals relinquishing control while encouraging wider family participation. The Audit Commission (1997) recommended maternity services that valued women and recognised the importance of communication with professionals looking after them.

More recently, infants' psychological outcomes have become the focus of attention in research, highlighting the importance of 'nurturing' and stability (Warren, 2017), thus recognising the critical role of parental love and attachment in shaping the baby's brain and the effect this has on later psychological functioning. However, it took some time to recognise the role of the father as essential to the family relationship, being viewed at that time as solely a support to the mother (Crathern, 2009a). Gerhardt (2004, p. 3), observing the importance of parents' involvement in the immediate postnatal period, when an infant's social skills begin to develop, cautions 'when these influences are less than benign, the groundwork is laid for a variety of later social and emotional difficulties'.

PARENTING IN THE NEONATAL UNIT ENVIRONMENT

To put the contents of this chapter into context, it is worth recalling some figures discussed in chapter 1, organisation of neonatal care. To summarise, European countries' preterm birth rates range from between 5 and 10% among live births, dependent primarily on the level of healthcare provided in that country. In the UK this figure ranges from 4.1 to 8.2% (Delnord et al., 2015; Jacob et al., 2017). Survival rates and health outcomes are inversely related to gestational age and birth weight. Those infants born ≤28 weeks' gestation, and/or ≤1.5kg are at the highest risk of adverse outcome.

Thus a significant number of families are facing the early days of their baby on the NNU, a place with little privacy, where the practitioners can be very busy. Parents feel that this is a challenging environment, where life is fragile, which is exacerbated by adverse environmental factors, such as noise, heat, and seeing their baby surrounded by multiple pieces of equipment. The NNU has been described as resembling a large fish bowl, designed to enable staff to have 100% sight and access to the infants in their care, thus creating the feeling that a crisis could occur at any moment, heightening parental stress and awareness (Drew, 2006; Petty et al., 2019a). More recently, neonatal care environments are adapting to provide a more family friendly setting that is meeting parents' needs. Yet despite these advances, the admission of a preterm infant to the NNU is still a stressful event and can create strong feelings of inadequacy and loss of confidence for parents (Gulla et al., 2017; Thomson-Salo et al., 2017; Lee and O'Brien, 2018; Premji et al., 2018).

Nurses who work in neonatal care know intuitively that the environment is not conducive to fostering a stable environment to begin family life. Parents express a perception of being strange and out of place in an alien world of alarms and machinery (Gulla et al., 2017).

Mothers report feeling intimidated, like outsiders, tolerated at best (Reid et al., 2007; Gulla et al., 2017; Lee and O'Brien, 2018), while fathers describe feeling alienated and out of control. (Crathern, 2009b; Thomson-Salo et al., 2017; Stefana et al., 2018).

To provide care for their baby, both parents must adapt to this strange, uninviting environment, which creates strong feelings of inadequacy and anxiety (Kynø et al., 2013; Petty et al., 2019b). The great paradox of birth and potential death are occurring simultaneously, meaning that families are exposed to a myriad of emotions.

Neonatal nurses are best placed to provide support through this time of crisis. However, the environment can still often be dominated by a medical and technical focus. This has been changing since the turn of the century, but there is still much to do to support families better. Nurses must recognise that institutional constraints within their healthcare systems may curtail their ability to integrate family-focused research into practice. Nevertheless, neonatal nurses have an important focal role in alleviating the impact of this environment and in shifting the balance of power towards the needs of the family, enabling them to navigate their parenting role in a more meaningful way.

This requires a good insight into the dynamic and complex parent–staff relationship with an awareness of social and personal aspects impacting on parents' NNU journey (Reid, 2007; Lyndon et al., 2017).

BECOMING A PARENT

Becoming a parent for the first time represents a mixture of joy and stress for both parents. It cannot be underestimated that the arrival of a new baby is, for most couples, one of the single most important events in their lives and is normally viewed, while being stressful, as a very positive experience (Gross and Van den Akker, 2004; Hall, 2005). It signifies the end of one single relationship as a couple (dyad) and the beginning of multiple relationships (dyads and triads) to adjust to, in terms of family functioning.

Learning to understand their baby's behaviours, cries and grimaces is all part of developing the individual bond parents have with their baby (Kerr et al., 2017). This process takes time and closeness to develop, even with healthy babies where there is no need of separation from their parents. Physical and emotional needs are provided for in a relationship that, while including adjustment and disruption of previous norms, allows for healthy attachment processes to begin (Benoit, 2004). Both mothers and fathers have unique, individual roles that contribute as a whole in developing the family unit. These roles are not fixed and will vary between couples, based on their personalities as well as diverse cultural, religious and economic backgrounds. Traditionally, in heterosexual relationships, mothers have been carers with fathers taking on the role of provider (Crathern, 2009a; 2009b; 2011; Thomson-Salo et al., 2017). Although these roles have become more blurred, the symbiotic nature of the two remains very important. Understanding each other's roles is part of the strength of a couple. Consequently, the breakdown of one role can lead to the unit falling apart.

The birth of a sick or preterm infant represents a time of major stress for both parents (Ballantyne et al., 2018; Garfield et al., 2018; Petty et al., 2018).

Transition to parenthood on a NNU is a particular challenge, so that the postnatal period is experienced by both parents as stressful (Provenzi and Santoro, 2015). Neonatal staff have an important role in supporting parents to make that transition to parenthood less traumatic (Sophie et al., 2009; Crathern, 2012). Parenting in the NNU is likened to a crisis with reactions and anxieties similar to those seen in acute and post-traumatic stress disorders (Aftyka et al, 2017; Fowler et al, 2019). It is therefore important to consider the different and specific effects on both mothers and fathers of babies admitted to the NNU to understand further the pressure this may put on the successful functioning of each parent and their ability to cohesively create a strong family unit (Crathern, 2009b; Matricardi et al., 2013).

Becoming a mother

For a woman having given birth to a healthy baby, transition to motherhood is complex. New mothers must establish their parenting role at a time when they feel fragile and unsure, and they experience disempowerment when they most need to be in control (Emmanuel and St John, 2010). The concept of motherhood has a basis in contact rather than separation. The interaction between mother and baby begins during pregnancy and, with the birth of a well baby, the development of this attachment is strengthened by the physical contact immediately following delivery.

In addition to this, the experience of attachment can be affected in different ways by each mother's individual situation, for example health during pregnancy, type of delivery, social and family support network, work commitments, self-identity, and relationships with significant others (Aagaard and Hall, 2008; Gulla et al., 2017).

Four attributes of maternal distress as responses to the transition to motherhood have been identified: '(1) stress; (2) adapting; (3) functioning and control; and (4) connecting' – each attribute response occurring along a continuum of intensity (see figure 4.2).

The triggers for maternal distress include: '(1) becoming a mother, (2) role changes, (3) body changes and functioning, (4) increased demands and challenges, (5) losses and gains, (6) birth experiences, and (7) changes to relationships and social context' (Emmanuel and St John, 2010, p. 2104). As importantly, it was found that maternal distress could lead to '*a compromised mental health status and maternal role development, compromising quality of life and relationships and ability to function, finally also affecting quality of relationships and social engagement*' (Emmanuel and St John, 2010, p. 2104).

It follows that if the mother of a healthy term infant can undergo such experiences, then the mother of a preterm infant has the potential for even greater distress (see box 4.1).

BOX 4.1 A MOTHER'S EXPERIENCE OF HAVING A PREMATURE BABY IN NNU

Giving birth to a premature baby is something you never prepare for.

A way for staff to help parents who have a baby facing a NNU stay is to show them around the unit, welcoming them and being confident while doing so. Resources in the form of leaflets or booklets which can be processed later helped me understand the situation more too.

Walking into the NNU at 3am clutching a syringe of 0.5ml of colostrum, clad in pyjamas can leave you feeling vulnerable, however I was always greeted with a 'Well done Mummy, brilliant work'.

I felt part of a team helping my baby survive, it spurred me on and gave me a real feeling that I was contributing.

The practical support when guiding the baby from the incubator to my chest with all the wires was helpful, at first it is very daunting. As time went on the staff encouraged my husband and I to be able to do it ourselves. Having a team who promoted the benefits of kangaroo care was very positive too. Kangaroo care helped us bond, it regulated my son's breathing and heart rate, as well as boosting my milk supply.

Having neonatal nurses and doctors who were calm, professional, warm and knowledgeable really helped us feel safe during a very nerve-wracking time.

Vanessa, Mother to Owen born at 26^{+4} weeks

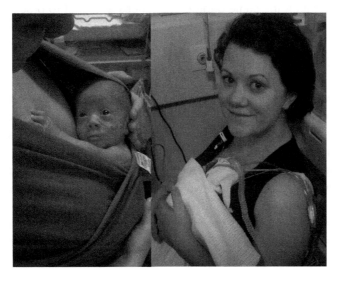

Figure 4.2 Mothering in the NNU

Women having given birth to a premature baby have been noted to experience a delay in feelings associated with becoming a mother due to 'hovering around the edge of motherhood' (Shin and White-Traut, 2007). There are recognised factors which have a dramatic impact on the planned trajectory to 'normal' motherhood following admission to neonatal care, causing a sudden change in expectations and a need to renegotiate a 'new kind of mothering':

■ *Separation* Being unable to take important first steps to attachment is seen as the most difficult aspect of having a baby in the NNU for mothers (Wigert et al., 2006; 2014; Gulla et al., 2017). Feelings of exclusion where their infant is cared for by experts with the consequent reduced physical contact, loss of identity as a mother, and lacking a sense of belonging to either the NNU or the maternity wards, leads to perceptions of inadequacy. The need to start again in redefining their role to include separation from their baby can be too difficult for many mothers and leave them floundering in a state of limbo.

■ *Feelings of guilt and shame* Pregnant women develop expectations of delivering a normal, healthy baby to add to their family. Once this picture is broken, they report shame at not meeting their own and, what they perceive to be, others' expectations including those of their partners, parents and society. In addition to this, feelings of guilt appear as they feel they have caused the unwanted situation their child is exposed to.

■ *Loss and grief* This cannot be underestimated and should not be associated only with the death of a baby. Once a baby is admitted to NNU, the parents lose the baby they had dreamt of. Images of taking the baby home, holding, feeding, and changing nappies have disappeared. While this is not a tangible loss, it nevertheless carries with it the same degree of sadness and grief to process and come to terms with. This is complicated by a real concern and worry that the baby may not survive, or if the baby does, will be handicapped in some way (Emmanuel and St John, 2010).

In conjunction with these personal barriers to healthy attachment, mothers have identified the lack of empowering information, contradictions from different healthcare professionals, and omission of information as compounding their feelings of lack of control (Fleury et al., 2014; Fowler et al., 2019; Petty et al., 2019a; 2019b). The mother also has to cope with sharing the care of their baby with another person – the normal mother–infant dyad becomes a three-way mother–infant–nurse relationship due to the inevitability of the infant's needs. In order to regain this authority over their baby's care, mothers have been shown to feel the need to 'work hard' with healthcare staff to learn about the routines and 'rules' which surround their baby (Fenwick et al., 2008), including navigating their voice and speaking up in the NNU (Lyndon et al., 2017). In other words, mothers become torn between caring for their baby, speaking up as their parent advo-cate and convincing professionals of their ability to do so. A sense of biographical dis-ruption feeds into this narrative where what was once expected is no more (Williams et al., 2018).

Becoming a father

Transition to fatherhood is also a complex phenomenon. It is now viewed as a time of emotional, physical and financial challenges (Fletcher et al., 2017) and can be a major upheaval in a man's life, being described as 'destabilising, decentering and disturbing' while challenging a man's sense of purpose (Crathern, 2009a; 2009b; Noergaard et al., 2017). Fathers of well newborn infants find conforming to a 'new fatherhood' role more difficult and distressing than they had anticipated before the birth. They can also take a 'back seat' to the needs of mothers during the antenatal and early postnatal period (Crathern, 2011).

Historically, there has been a gender-focus within parenting research on mothers' experiences of having a preterm infant, with many findings on fathers' experiences spe-cifically having emerged as an addition, or an afterthought, to mother-focused studies. By the turn of the century there was an evidence-based understanding of a need to explore parenting from the father's perspective, and recognition of the importance of establishing a loving father–child relationship from birth in both the home and neonatal environment (Pohlman, 2005).

Fathers, like mothers, experience feelings of isolation, fear and stress. They are confused about their role in NNU. One study saw men pay only one or two visits to NNU without their partners during the first week of their baby's stay in hospital; after that time they always spoke of visiting the NNU as a couple (Crathern, 2011). This finding has implications for attachment and fostering of the father-infant-dyad. Nurses can play a key role in enhancing the quality of time that fathers have with their babies to foster commitment, reciprocity and interaction, which are key components of attachment (Fegran et al., 2008). This may be difficult if men are never alone with their baby, so nurses need to create oppor-tunities for men to parent in NNU (see figure 4.3).

Some fathers reported feeling undervalued by staff, which can have an impact on father and baby getting to know each other (Arockiasamy et al., 2008; Crathern, 2012). Early father–infant involvement improves the baby's emotional and cognitive sta-bility in the long term, highlighting the need to nurture the relationships between men and their babies (Shaw et al., 2006). One study reported that holding their baby was a defining moment in feeling like a father; one father waited three weeks for this experience (Crathern, 2011).

Fathers found room moves between different levels of acuity of care a 'double-edged sword', making them anxious about their babies having less intensive monitoring; see figure 4.4. Furthermore, a lack of communication about room moves is a source of parental stress (POPPY Steering Group, 2009; Crathern, 2012). Several researchers reported that fathers wanted easier access to neonatal consultants at either end of their working day to discuss their baby's care (Arockiasamy et al., 2008; Harvey, 2010; Hollywood and Hollywood,

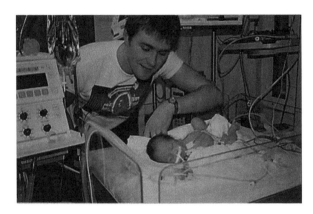

Figure 4.3 Fathering in the NNU

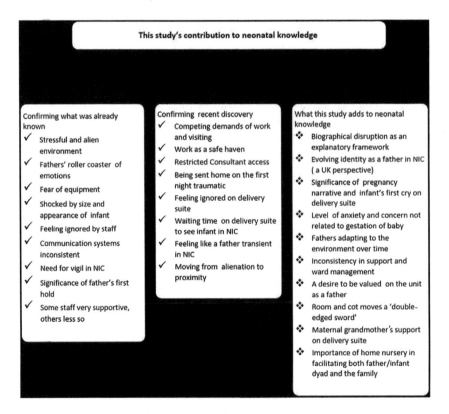

Figure 4.4 Disrupted biographies (Crathern, 2012)

TABLE 4.1 IMPLICATIONS FOR PARENTS: POLICY, PRACTICE, EDUCATION AND RESEARCH

Policy	Practice	Education	Research
Audit the quality of care for fathers in midwifery and neonatal services and link with user/carer groups. National strategy: Provision of overnight accommodation for fathers in neonatal intensive care.	Improve access to neonatal consultants for working fathers. Neonatal nurses need to nurture the father–infant relationship on the neonatal unit. Ensure that fathers have the opportunity to hold their infant as soon as the infant is stable. Inform fathers about transfer between rooms, including explanation about the acuity level of care and expected care regimes. Supplement with written information/leaflet. Adopt a flexible approach to parent craft teaching to meet the needs of working fathers.	Provide informal teaching sessions for all levels of midwifery and neonatal staff on improving the psychosocial care of fathers on delivery suite and neonatal intensive care. Higher education institutions curricula for neonatal qualified in specialty-programmes need to provide continuing education and training on support for fathers in delivery suite and the neonatal unit.	Further exploration of the pregnancy narrative of first-time fathers of preterm infants. Further exploration of the key concept of biographical disruption in neonatal studies on fathers in neonatal intensive care Explore the needs of fathers following their preterm baby's discharge home. Explore the impact of a preterm birth on grandparents within the neonatal environment.

(from Crathern, (2012) The lived experiences of first-time fathers with a preterm infant in a neonatal intensive care unit. Bliss Briefings November 2012)

2011; Harvey and Pattison, 2012. The need for more conversations between the medical team and both parents was highlighted in a recent audit (RCPCH, 2017); see also table 4.1.

Same-sex parenting in neonatal care

Sexual orientation and gender will also inform the parent dyad/triad, including the following: same-sex parenting, transgender couples, bisexual individuals in same-sex relationships/not in same-sex relationship, homosexual men and surrogacy, and 'donor dads' including differing perspectives on the role of a biological parent in such couplings. According to a briefing paper for the House of Commons, same-sex cohabiting had risen from 16,000 in 1976 to 101, 000 in 2017, and that it could be estimated that around 20,000 dependent children were living in a same-sex relationship (all types) in 2017, an increase of 530% (Fairbairn, 2018). The key message for institutions is that, in terms of family processes, conflict between same-sex parents was more likely to be concerned with the division of labour and work over and above gender and sexuality. Arguably this is similar to that of a heterosexual couple in NNU who have one designated 'working parent'.

It is now clear that same-sex coupling is increasing in prevalence around the globe (Hammond, 2014) and that this is beginning to filter through to maternity services and neonatal care. When homosexual women have been interviewed about their experiences of maternity services, they report feeling marginalised, or 'not fitting in' (Dibley, 2009). More recently, lesbian parents report positive experiences of maternity care overall, but that some subtle judgements among practitioners still exist (Hammond, 2014).

'Parents want to be treated no differently to heterosexual parents but with special recognitions of their diverse family constellation' (Hammond, 2014, p. 495). It is therefore important to examine the culture of neonatal care and consider if heterosexism and homophobia are part of that institution's definition of parenthood. Simple measures of inclusivity could be the addition of 'civil partner' or 'other' to relationship status on official hospital forms, as this offers an opportunity for discussion; the use of inclusive language; avoidance of assumptions; and provision of equal standards for physical and emotional support (Dibley, 2009). Care of the co-mother on NNU must be treated as equally important as support of the biological mother (Hammond, 2014).

A working paper on same-sex parenting in Australia highlighted that parents in transition from their biological sex definition faced a lack of family and community acceptance (Dempsey, 2013). According to an American review on transgender men and pregnancy, the acceptance of their gender diversity from preconceptual care through to the postnatal phase was crucial in the promotion of feelings of being cared for by clinicians in an inclusive and non-judgemental way (Obedin-Maliver and Makadon, 2016).

What we know of the NNU as a stressful environment is applicable to any parent, irrespective of their gender or sexual orientation. However, while midwifery research has begun moving forward on this issue, the NNU lags behind, and more work is needed.

SIGNS OF PARENTAL STRESS AND COPING

The psychological impact of having a baby admitted to the NNU cannot be underestimated. Figure 4.5 shows some of the descriptors highlighted by parents of babies admitted to neonatal units over the past 20 years. Shaw et al. (2006) explored parenting stress in more detail, specifically acute and post-traumatic stress disorder in neonatal care, and concluded that parents exhibit acute stress disorder similar to parents of other critically ill children. Importantly, families with an underlying level of conflict and those who tried to suppress feelings seemed to develop yet more stress.

Neonatal nurses may be perceptive to parents exhibiting the following signs: being unable to process information and requiring repetition of facts, difficulty thinking clearly and problem-solving, being unable to prioritise, mastering tasks becomes impossible and

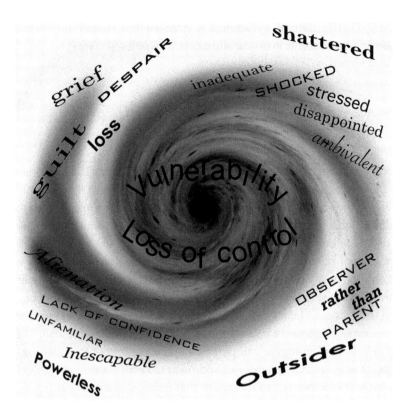

Figure 4.5 The whirlpool of parents' feelings on admission to the NNU

frustrating leading to feelings of ineffectiveness as a person, increasingly missing cues due to shutting off from the environment, withdrawal or irritability.

Parents also demonstrate recognisable stages in their initial coping strategies: Immobility on entering the NNU, performing a visual survey of machinery and layout, withdrawal from the environment and staff, over-protectiveness, hyper-vigilance and focusing on small things, e.g. tapes, blood stains on sheets or clothing (Shaw et al., 2006). Parents subsequently move on to try to intellectualise reality, i.e. understanding how machinery works, trying to interpret blood results, or showing a greater interest in the pathology of diseases (Pinelli, 2000). These behaviours will have resonance with neonatal nurses, mindful that withdrawal from the environment can be wrongly misconstrued as a lack of emotional connection with their baby.

Having drawn upon their initial and early coping strategies, some parents begin to feel more confident in being a part of their baby's care and will negotiate management with nurses, starting as an observer and eventually moving towards taking a lead in their baby's care.

This has been described in two ways; as moving from an outsider to partner position and from alienation to familiarity, or from dependence to independence (Skene et al.,

2012). In addition to this, parents will attempt to increase their support networks by building relationships with other parents in similar situations, as well as gathering support from immediate family and friends.

FAMILY NURSING AND SUPPORT: CARING FOR THE WHOLE FAMILY

Understanding the influence of the family on each individual infant's development, and the uniqueness the infant brings to the family, is key to understanding the principles of family nursing. However, the sick or preterm infant has a limited repertoire in engaging with parents and carers due to the level of their physical development, the severity of their illness and the constraints of their environment. This in itself may precipitate a lack of emotional attachment and investment from parents as they struggle to understand their baby. The impact that these limitations can have on developing family relationships should not be underestimated, nor should the positive way family-nursing strategies can influence the situation.

Central to successful family nursing are the skills nurses portray in being able to step aside from personal judgements and values and accepting the family unit. The notion of families having individual strengths and personal resources, rather than deficits, should be the starting point when planning a tailored approach to family care.

Increasingly, it is important to recognise that families span several generations, and these multigenerational relationships can be a source of strength for all family members. Bengtson (2001, p. 1) suggests three reasons why these relationships are important: (1) the demographic changes of population ageing resulting in longer years of shared lives between generations; (2) the increasing importance of grandparents and other kin in fulfilling family functions; (3) the strength and resilience of intergenerational solidarity over time.

Yet intergenerational households have been described as having the potential to be polarised into two camps: cohesive or dysfunctional (Pain, 2005). It is likely that, given the struggle young parents have regarding affordable housing, that intergenerational living will increase. Neonatal nurses need to ascertain who will be a baby's primary and secondary carer in such households, with grandparents taking on more of the burdens of childcare when a child is disabled in any way. Consideration needs to be given to the potential stresses of such a role and how the NNU can support them.

Siblings are also an important component of the family and should not be ignored (Morrison and Gullon-Rivera, 2017). They will have concerns about their baby brother or sister, whether they are encouraged to visit or not. The implications of not including them in care planning could have longer-term repercussions on family dynamics and function.

A family nursing perspective challenges nurses to adopt an even more collaborative approach to care. The emphasis is on using a style which reflects a whole family's strengths and assists them in finding solutions to the problems they themselves identify. In doing so, responsibility and therefore ownership of the situation increase for the family, which in turn improves their sense of control. '*Being a family unit is what gives most families the ability to endure the emotional upheaval and suffering that come with the critical illness experience*' (Eggenberger and Nelms, 2007, p. 1618).

Looking beneath the surface of 'apparent coping' and creating the opportunities for families to demonstrate their capabilities and identify their strengths requires a skilled approach. The foundations of this understanding for nurses are based on the concept of family systems and how the diverse complexities of family dynamics can both hinder and support family wellbeing. Literature consistently supports the notion of true, constant family-centered care as being essential (Ballantyne et al., 2017; Roué et al., 2017; Segers et al., 2018; Skene et al., 2019) that includes clear and consistent communication with families (Enke et al., 2017; Petty et al., 2019a; 2019b).

NURTURING SUPPORTIVE FAMILY AND INFANT RELATIONSHIPS IN THE NEONATAL ENVIRONMENT: THE NURSE'S ROLE

It is not within the remit of this chapter to dictate a family strategy to the neonatal nursing community, but rather to provide the tools to begin those discussions and map across to a unit philosophy and agreed standards. As mentioned at the beginning of this chapter, from a historical perspective, caring for the family has improved radically since the development of neonatal care across the globe. It is up to individual units or collective networks to decide on the best evidence available on what best suits their environment(s). This chapter finally turns to recommended strategies to enhance the family experience based on key evidence.

To nurture is closely linked with the descriptor '*to nurse*' and can be associated with several concepts: to touch and be close; to sustain, feed and nourish; to be attentive and listen; to provide care and train; to respect and encourage the individual and their family.

Importantly, babies must be invited to participate in human interaction via sounds, smell, touch, holding or containment (Altimier and Phillips, 2016). The neonate's brain continues to form and develop with each human interaction, and an infant's ability to respond to human interaction requires a continuous stimulus that shapes their understanding of social interaction. This process is a potential capacity for social interaction and requires nurturing from birth – how the orbitofrontal cortex develops is entirely experience-dependent (Gerhardt, 2004).

However, for parents to hold their baby and help him or her to feel secure, they need to feel secure themselves – they need to experience being psychologically held/contained in an alien environment to feel secure holding their own infant; this is a two-way process (Warren, 2000). Taking care with language used (e.g. being 'allowed' to visit and to see their baby) and the avoidance of parents feeling like visitors are vital. Both physical and psychological space is needed to ensure parenting roles are maintained (Petty et al., 2019a). Holding their baby close is a key part of the journey of nurturing (Flacking et al., 2016).

The FINE programme encompasses many of these issues. It provides a family-centred developmental approach that is suitable for anyone working in neonatal care (Warren, 2017) and is offered at three levels dependent upon role and working environment (see website for link).

Bliss, the UK charity for supporting families of sick and preterm newborns has recommended key elements that define a family-centred care focus emanating from the POPPY study (Sophie et al., 2009; see box 4.2).

Roué et al. (2017) have summarised eight evidence-based principles of sound family-centered care, see box 4.3.

BOX 4.2 ESSENTIAL ELEMENTS OF FAMILY-CENTRED CARE IN THE NEONATAL UNIT

- Recognising and valuing the role of parents, siblings and other family members
- Developing awareness of parents' needs, the emotional impact of preterm birth and individual differences in parental responses and needs
- Recognising critical steps for parents on the care pathway
- Maximising opportunities for communication with parents and local communities
- Providing practical help with infant care and parent interaction, including behavioural cues
- Increasing confidence in role as a parent and supporting the parent–infant relationship
- Providing psychological support
- Valuing and supporting mother's ability to nurture their baby through expressing breast milk and breastfeeding
- Providing appropriate family friendly facilities.

What do parents need?

- To get to know their baby
- Emotional support
- Involvement in care and decision-making
- Effective communication between the family and the healthcare team
- Family friendly facilities in neonatal care
- Support at time of transitions, including going home
- Positive closeness
- Positive touch, contact, skin-to-skin, nappy changing and general care, giving own feed.

(adapted from POPPY Steering Group, 2009)

BOX 4.3 EIGHT PRINCIPLES OF FAMILY-CENTRED CARE

■   24-hour parental access with no limitations during shift changes or rounds

■   psychological support for parents

■   effective pain management

■   environmental care

■   postural support

■   skin-to-skin contact (see figure 4.6)

■   facilitation of breastfeeding and lactation support

■   sleep protection.

(adapted from Roué et al., 2018)

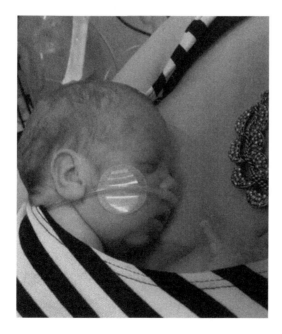

Figure 4.6 Skin-to-skin care

Historically, NNUs have been built to be efficient in technological care and may not be optimal for growth and development of the sick and preterm child and their family. Equally, a family-centred care vision or philosophy does not guarantee family-centered care exists in everyday practice. For a detailed analysis and discussion on standards for neonatal care refer to both the POPPY report (POPPY Steering Group, 2009) and the Bliss standards for best practice.

A more recent development, supported by the Bliss charity, has been the family-integrated care (FIC) programme in the UK. This was developed in Canada for use on NNU, with its origins embedded in neonatal care in Estonia, where a healthcare system is challenged with limited practitioners and intensive care technology. In the NNUs of this Eastern European country, families were active participants in many aspects of their baby's care (Lee and O'Brien, 2018).

The four pillars of FIC are defined as: (1) staff education and support; (2) parent education; (3) NNU environment; and (4) psychological support (Lee and O'Brien, 2018). Outcomes suggest that true parent participation in care improves breastfeeding rates, parental confidence and reduces anxiety (Ottosson and Lantz, 2017; Banerjee et al., 2018).

Some caution is needed in interpreting results that have originated in NNUs that are not similar to neonatal intensive care in the UK. A recent audit of parental experiences of FIC in one NNU in the UK, that has harnessed parent narratives to explore their experiences, does show positive outcomes for those parents (Aloysius et al., 2018). The audit findings from the UK are encouraging, but more research is needed, particularly into parent satisfaction with the role and environment in which to carry out FIC.

Table 4.2 summarises the tenets of FIC in the UK. A change in culture is required as described by Patel et al. (2018), for NNUs who have not yet done so,

TABLE 4.2 SUMMARY OF THE TENETS OF FIC

Staff education	Structured training empowers healthcare professionals to be coaches, mentors and counsellors for parents.
Parent education	Clear training curriculum and competency assessment for parents.
Parent visiting policy	Encouraged to be present on the unit for at least 6–8 hours per day and assume most of the primary care of their infant – facilities in place to support this (kitchen, family room, accommodation for every parent).
Routine cares	Parents are encouraged to be involved in daily and enhanced care for their baby with a level of autonomy following competency training.
Medical rounds	Parents are encouraged to be active participants on the ward round and present their baby to the health professionals.
Administration of medications	Identify the purpose of routine medication. Administer approved oral medication under supervision of nursing staff.
Psychosocial support	Availability of psychosocial support and peer support from trained veterans.

(adapted from Banerjee et al., 2018)

to really embrace and take parental involvement to a new level, placing families at the centre of care and empowering them as primary caregivers.

The previous discussion has focused on what is needed for family nurturing and support and how to do this. The next two figures below should enable an enquiry into personal practice on how much the family are involved in the NNU and how much the unit philosophy adheres to its principles.

It would be useful to use these in tandem with local, regional, and national standards for neonatal care on how far the NNU involves families. Clearly, full participation is a much more integrated way of working (figure 4.7; adapted from Department of Health, UK (DoH, UK), 2008), as is delegating control as opposed to informing (figure 4.8). New models such as FIC may be a way forward in improving experiences for families.

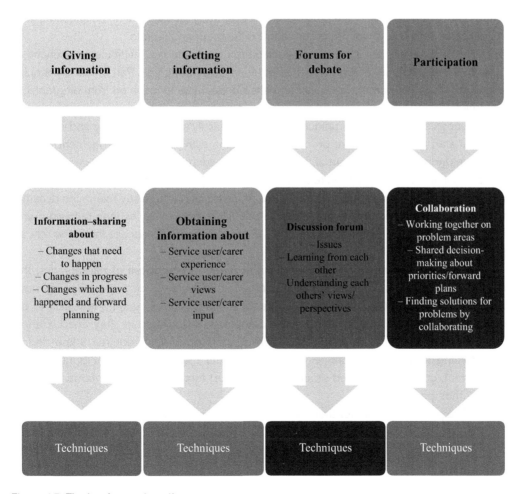

Figure 4.7 The involvement continuum

Consider where your unit fits in this matrix	Strategic policy making	Whole service change	Treatment processes at team level	Individual care
Informing				
Consulting				
Partnership				
Delegating control				

Figure 4.8 Types and levels of participation

CONCLUSION

It is easy to recognise when evaluating the literature that parents must quickly learn to adapt to the overwhelming NNU environment to be able to develop the confidence and competence both to care for their vulnerable baby and eventually take control of the situation, thus successfully completing their transition to this different parenting role.

Neonatal nurses are in the prime position to coordinate this multifaceted scenario in order to assist the family in achieving their potential as a strong unit. Part of this will require a realignment of the parents' personal and shared identities to move on from biographical disruption.

Recognising the infant's uniqueness and the family's individual entity and strengths is a vital start to this important process. This begins with the acknowledgement of both parents as individuals and as part of the caring team, taking into account their own stressors and emotional burden. In addition to this, the wider family network spanning the generations from siblings to grandparents must also be considered as having a key role in the dynamic family unit. Babies themselves play a part in this altered structure, as their behaviour and responses need to be learnt and reinforced to enable parents to accept their new role as parents in critical care.

Being able to anticipate and plan for the differing responses of parents, and the effect of interactions between family members and nurses, by understanding both the concept of family systems and the practicalities of family nursing, is a skill to be developed to ensure families receive the complex level of support they need. Caring for families who have experienced the birth of a preterm infant requires a knowledge of parenting and family dynamics, of psychological theory in terms of bonding and attachment, grief and loss, and strategies to support families and their infants that help nurture their parenting.

It is a privilege to care for them at their most vulnerable time.

CASE STUDIES

Case study 1: Addressing family challenges

Olive has been delivered at 26 weeks' gestation by vaginal delivery, first baby to a young mother Eve who is 18 years old. Eve's partner, Tom is away on military duties as he is in the Army and is not returning home for another 3 weeks. Eve's mother is present with her. Olive is admitted to intensive care and placed within an incubator onto bi-level continuous positive airway pressure after a brief period of ventilation but remains unstable and her oxygen requirement is 50%. She is currently 20 hours old.

   With reference to the key points within the chapter, consider the following questions:

Q.1. What are the possible challenges and emotions that Eve and her mother are likely to be experiencing?

Q.2. What early nursing interventions are required so that Eve can experience bonding with her daughter?

When Olive is 2 weeks old, she develops a suspected bowel obstruction and experiences complications with her respiratory status requiring referral and transfer to a tertiary centre for further management

Q.3. How will this situation impact on the emotional wellbeing of Olive and her family?

Q.4. Again, what strategies can be employed to enhance the wellbeing of Olive and Eve, including psycho-emotional and practical considerations?

After a 3-week period in the receiving neonatal unit, Olive is transferred back to her referring unit and plans are commenced to work towards discharge home.

Q.5. What factors need to be considered when planning discharge for this family and what strategies are needed for the transition home to go smoothly?

Case study 2: Cultural considerations

Amar and Fatima are married parents who have recently arrived in the UK from Pakistan with their three children, all girls aged 18 months, three and eight years old. They speak Bengali and only Amar has some very basic, rudimentary English. Soon after arrival to the country, Fatima went into premature labour at 23 weeks + 5 days and delivered a baby boy called Asif. He is currently 6 hours old and is fully oxygenated with a high oxygen requirement. Fatima suffered an antepartum bleed during labour and is still in the delivery suite. Amar has just arrived at the neonatal unit to visit his son and is very distressed. They have no other family in the UK and are practicing Muslims.

With reference to the key points within the chapter, consider the following questions:

Q.1. What are the immediate challenges faced by these parents?

Q.2. What strategies should be put in place to reduce the father's anxiety?

Fatima finally is able to visit Asif later that day.

Q.3. What strategies should be put in place to enable her to bond with her son?
In addition,

Q.4. What cultural issues need considering? How would you integrate these into your care?

Q.5. How can the staff support the whole family during this time? Identify the most appropriate roles for all members of the team.

Case study 3: A father's story

Read the extract below about a father's experience and with reference to the key points within the chapter, consider the task that follows, below:

Jack was 22 years old and lived with his partner Rose at his parents' home while they were decorating their new home in preparation for the new arrival. They were both first-time parents. Jack worked full time. He had no prior experience of hospitals. Jack is now the father of a baby boy called Henry who was born 5 weeks early at 35 weeks' gestation by normal delivery weighing 2.75kg. The experience of transition to fatherhood in this situation was very traumatic for Jack, it was not a nice experience, an unanticipated event and not what he was expecting or prepared for; consequently a major a disruption in his life. His newborn son Henry was whisked away to the neonatal unit immediately, the neonatal staff briefly telling Jack and Rose that their baby was *fine*. Having had no communication from the midwifery or neonatal staff for three hours he spent his time during and after the delivery in a kind of limbo, a not-knowing period. This was very stressful for Jack, a first-time father, as he tried to be a comfort and support for Rose. He was concerned about revealing his emotions to Rose and at the same time he says he *felt scared as hell inside*, worrying about his son Henry, trying not to think the worst but also trying to prepare for the fact that he might die. No one had told him where he could find his son and not knowing the hospital layout this was an additional stress. He described the whole labour experience *as going from the best day to the worst day of my life in hours.*

Going to visit Henry in NICU was equally traumatic, walking into the room and seeing tubes, wires and machinery around his infant son was scary. He said the next few hours were all a blur and he couldn't remember anything the staff had told him. He does remember feeling angry at that point, feeling helpless, willing the staff to do something to save his son.

TASK: Identify the key issues and strategies you would employ in this situation. What potential situations may occur that might mean you will need to revise your plan?

For suggested answer guides to the questions posed in these case studies, please refer to the web-based companion site specific to this chapter (see URL below).

WEB-BASED RESOURCES

For further information, online resources and greater detail on the case studies featured in this chapter go to www.routledge.com/cw/nicnursing

References

Aagaard, H., & Hall, E. O. (2008). Mothers' experiences of having a preterm infant in the neonatal care unit: a meta-synthesis. *Journal of Pediatric Nursing, 23*(3), e26–e36.

Aftyka, A., Rybojad, B., Rosa, W., Wróbel, A., & Karakuła-Juchnowicz, H. (2017). Risk factors for the development of post-traumatic stress disorder and coping strategies in mothers and fathers following infant hospitalisation in the neonatal intensive care unit. *Journal of Clinical Nursing, 26*(23–24), 4436–4445.

Aloysius, A., Platonos, K., Theakstone-Owen, A., Deierl, A., & Banerjee, J. (2018). Integrated family delivered care: Development of a staff education programme. *Journal of Neonatal Nursing, 24*(1), 35–38.

Altimier, L., & Phillips, R. (2016). The neonatal integrative developmental care model: Advanced clinical applications of the seven core measures for neuroprotective family-centered developmental care. *Newborn and Infant Nursing Reviews, 16*(4), 230–244.

Arockiasamy, V., Holsti, L., & Albersheim, S. (2008). Fathers' experiences in the neonatal intensive care unit: A search for control. *Pediatrics, 121*(2), e215–e222.

Audit Commission. (1997). *First class delivery: improving maternity services in England and Wales.* London: Audit Commission.

Ballantyne, M., Orava, T., Bernardo, S., McPherson, A. C., Church, P., & Fehlings, D. (2017). Parents' early healthcare transition experiences with preterm and acutely ill infants: a scoping review. *Child: Care, Health and Development, 43*(6), 783–796.

Banerjee, J., Aloysius, A., Platonos, K., & Deierl, A. (2018). Family centred care and family delivered care– What are we talking about? *Journal of Neonatal Nursing, 24*(1), 8–12.

Bengtson, V. L. (2001). Beyond the nuclear family: The increasing importance of multigenerational bonds: The burgess award lecture. *Journal of Marriage and Family, 63*(1), 1–16.

Benoit, D. (2004). Infant-parent attachment: Definition, types, antecedents, measurement and outcome. *Paediatrics & Child Health, 9*(8), 541–545.

Bliss. (2011). *The Bliss Baby Charter Standards*. London: Bliss UK.

Bliss. (2015a). *Bliss baby report 2015: Hanging in the balance*. London: Bliss UK.

Bliss. (2015b). *Bliss Family Friendly Accreditation Scheme. Helping to make family-centred care a reality on your neonatal unit* London: Bliss UK.

British Association of Perinatal Medicine & Bliss. (2017). *Neonatal Service Quality Indicators. Standards relating to Structures and Processes supporting Quality and Patient Safety in Neonatal Services.* London: British Association of Perinatal Medicine.

Crathern, L. (1997). 'Walking the tightrope'. The nature and scope of expert neonatal nursing when caring for the neonate on the edge of viability. (Unpublished doctoral Dissertation). University of Huddersfield.

Crathern, L. (2004). Walking the tightrope: Experiences of nurses caring for extremely small neonates. *Bliss Newborn News Spring:* 12–13.

Crathern, L. (2009a). Men becoming fathers: From the perspective of transition to fatherhood in a neonatal intensive care environment. *Midirs Midwifery Digest, 19*(4), 555–561.

Crathern, L. (2009b). Dads matter too: A review of the literature focusing on the experiences of fathers of preterm infants. *MIDIRS Midwifery Digest, 19*(2), 159–167.

Crathern, L (2011). Disrupted Biographies: The lived experiences of first time fathers with a preterm infant in a neonatal intensive care unit. (Unpublished doctoral dissertation). University of Sheffield.

Crathern, L. (2012). Bliss research briefing: The lived experiences of first time fathers with a preterm infant in a neonatal intensive care unit. London: Bliss UK.

Crawford, D., & McLean, M. (2010). The care of the pre-viable and questionably viable infant–A midwife and a neonatal nurse dilemma. *Journal of Neonatal Nursing, 16*(2), 53–57.

Crosse, V. M. (1957). *The Premature Baby* (4th Edition). London: Churchill.

Davis, L., Mohay, H., & Edwards, H. (2003). Mothers' involvement in caring for their premature infants: An historical overview. *Journal of Advanced Nursing, 42*(6), 578–586.

Delnord, M., Blondel, B., & Zeitlin, J. (2015). What contributes to disparities in the preterm birth rate in European countries? *Current Opinion in Obstetrics & Gynecology, 27*(2), 133–142.

Dempsey, D. (2013). Same-sex parented families in Australia. Melbourne: Australian Institute of Family Studies.

Department of Health, UK (DoH, UK). (2008). Real involvement: Working with people to improve health services.

Dibley, L. B. (2009). Experiences of lesbian parents in the UK: Interactions with midwives. *Evidence-Based Midwifery, 7*(3), 94–101.

Drew, D. (2006). Mark. *Midirs Midwifery Digest, 16*(2), 257.

Dunn, P. M. (2007). The birth of perinatal medicine in the United Kingdom. In *Seminars in Fetal and Neonatal Medicine, 12*(3), 227–238.

Eggenberger, S. K., & Nelms, T. P. (2007). Being family: The family experience when an adult member is hospitalized with a critical illness. *Journal of Clinical Nursing, 16*(9), 1618–1628.

Emmanuel, E., & St John, W. (2010). Maternal distress: A concept analysis. *Journal of Advanced Nursing, 66*(9), 2104–2115.

Enke, C., y Hausmann, A. O., Miedaner, F., Roth, B., & Woopen, C. (2017). Communicating with parents in neonatal intensive care units: The impact on parental stress. *Patient Education and Counseling, 100*(4), 710–719.

Fairbairn, C. (2018). "Common law marriage" and cohabitation. *Home affairs section, House of Commons library SN/HA/3372, 6.*

Fegran, L., Helseth, S., & Fagermoen, M. S. (2008). A comparison of mothers' and fathers' experiences of the attachment process in a neonatal intensive care unit. *Journal of Clinical Nursing, 17*(6), 810–816.

Fenwick, J., Barclay, L., & Schmied, V. (2008). Craving closeness: a grounded theory analysis of women's experiences of mothering in the Special Care Nursery. *Women and Birth, 21*(2), 71–85.

Flacking, R., Thomson, G., & Axelin, A. (2016). Pathways to emotional closeness in neonatal units – a cross-national qualitative study. *BMC Pregnancy and Childbirth, 16*(1), 170. doi:10.1186/s12884-016-0955-3.

Fletcher, R., Kay-Lambkin, F., May, C., Oldmeadow, C., Attia, J., & Leigh, L. (2017). Supporting men through their transition to fatherhood with messages delivered to their smartphones: A feasibility study of SMS4dads. *BMC Public Health, 17*(1), 953. doi: 10.1186/s12889-017-4978-0.

Fleury, C., Parpinelli, M. A., & Makuch, M. Y. (2014). Perceptions and actions of healthcare professionals regarding the mother-child relationship with premature babies in an intermediate neonatal intensive care unit: A qualitative study. *BMC Pregnancy and Childbirth, 14*, 313. doi: 10.1186/1471-2393-14-313.

Fowler, C., Green, J., Elliott, D., Whiting, L., & Petty, J. (2019). The forgotten mothers of extremely premature babies: Need for increased psychosocial support. *Journal of Clinical Nursing 28*(11–12), 2124–2134.

Garfield, C. F., Simon, C. D., Rutsohn, J., & Lee, Y. S. (2018). Stress from the neonatal intensive care unit to home: Paternal and maternal cortisol rhythms in parents of premature infants. *The Journal of Perinatal & Neonatal Nursing, 32*(3), 257–265.

Gerhardt, S. (2004). *Why love matters: How affection shapes a baby's brain*. London and New York: Routledge.

Gross, H., & Akker, V. D. (2004). The importance of the postnatal period for mothers, fathers and infant behaviour. *Journal of Reproductive and Infant Psychology, 22*(1), 3–4.

Gulla, K., Dahlø, R., & Eilertsen, M. E. B. (2017). From the delivery room to the neonatal intensive care unit: Mothers' experiences with follow-up of skin-to-skin contact after premature birth. *Journal of Neonatal Nursing, 23*(6), 253–257.

Hall, E. O. (2005). Being in an alien world: Danish parents' lived experiences when a newborn or small child is critically ill. *Scandinavian Journal of Caring Sciences, 19*(3), 179–185.

Hammond, C. (2014). Exploring same sex couples' experiences of maternity care. *British Journal of Midwifery, 22*(7), 495–500.

Harvey, M. E. (2010). The experiences and perceptions of fathers attending the birth and immediate care of their baby (Doctoral dissertation, Aston University).

Harvey, M. E., & Pattison, H. M. (2012). Being there: a qualitative interview study with fathers present during the resuscitation of their baby at delivery. *Archives of Disease in Childhood: Fetal and Neonatal Edition, 97*(6), F439–F443.

Health Foundation. (2014). Person-centred care made simple: What everyone should know about person-centred care. Health Foundation.

Hollywood, M., & Hollywood, E. (2011). The lived experiences of fathers of a premature baby on a neonatal intensive care unit. *Journal of Neonatal Nursing, 17*(1), 32–40.

Jacob, J., Lehne, M., Mischker, A., Klinger, N., Zickermann, C., & Walker, J. (2017). Cost effects of preterm birth: a comparison of health care costs associated with early preterm, late preterm, and full-term birth in the first 3 years after birth. *The European Journal of Health Economics, 18*(8), 1041–1046.

Kerr, S., King, C., Hogg, R., McPherson, K., Hanley, J., Brierton, M., & Ainsworth, S. (2017). Transition to parenthood in the neonatal care unit: a qualitative study and conceptual model designed to illuminate parent and professional views of the impact of webcam technology. *BMC Pediatrics, 17*(1), 158.

Klaus, M. H., & Kennell, J. H. (1976). *Maternal-infant bonding: The impact of early separation or loss on family development*. St Louis: Mosby.

Kynø, N. M., Ravn, I. H., Lindemann, R., Smeby, N. A., Torgersen, A. M., & Gundersen, T. (2013). Parents of preterm-born children; sources of stress and worry and experiences with an early intervention programme: A qualitative study. *BMC Nursing, 12*(1), 28.

Lee, S. K., & O'Brien, K. (2018). Family integrated care: Changing the NICU culture to improve whole-family health. *Journal of Neonatal Nursing, 24*(1), 1–3.

Lyndon, A., Wisner, K., Holschuh, C., Fagan, K. M., & Franck, L. S. (2017). Parents' perspectives on navigating the work of speaking up in the NICU. *Journal of Obstetric, Gynecologic & Neonatal Nursing, 46*(5), 716–726.

Matricardi, S., Agostino, R., Fedeli, C., & Montirosso, R. (2013). Mothers are not fathers: Differences between parents in the reduction of stress levels after a parental intervention in a NICU. *Acta Paediatrica*, *102*(1), 8–14.

Morrison, A., & Gullón-Rivera, A. L. (2017). Supporting Siblings of Neonatal Intensive Care Unit Patients: A NICU Social Story™ as an Innovative Approach. *Journal of Pediatric Nursing*, *33*, 91–93.

Noergaard, B., Ammentorp, J., Fenger-Gron, J., Kofoed, P.-E., Johannessen, H., & Thibeau S. (2017). Fathers' needs and masculinity dilemmas in a neonatal intensive care unit in Denmark. *Advances in Neonatal Care*, *17*(4), E13–E22.

Obedin-Maliver, J., & Makadon, H. J. (2016). Transgender men and pregnancy. *Obstetric Medicine*, *9*(1), 4–8.

Ottosson, C., & Lantz, B. (2017). Parental participation in neonatal care. *Journal of Neonatal Nursing*, *23*(3), 112–118.

Pain, R. (2005). Intergenerational relations and practice in the development of sustainable communities. Paper for the Office of the Deputy Prime Minister from ICRRDS, Durham University.

Patel, N., Ballantyne, A., Bowker, G., Weightman, J., & Weightman, S. (2018). Family Integrated Care: Changing the culture in the neonatal unit. *Archives of Disease in Childhood*, *103*(5), 415–419.

Petty, J., Jarvis, J., Thomas, R. (2019a). Listening to the parent voice to inform person-centred neonatal care. *Journal of Neonatal Nursing*, *25*(3), 121–126.

Petty, J., Jarvis, J., Thomas, R. (2019b). Understanding parents' emotional experiences for neonatal education: A narrative, interpretive approach. *Journal of Clinical Nursing*, *28*(9–10), 911–1924.

Petty, J., Whiting, L., Green, J., & Fowler, C. (2018). Parents' views on preparation to care for extremely premature infants at home. *Nursing Children and Young People*, *30*(4), 22–27.

Pinelli, J. (2000). Effects of family coping and resources on family adjustment and parental stress in the acute phase of the NICU experience. *Neonatal Network*, *19*(6), 27–37.

Pohlman, S. (2005). The primacy of work and fathering preterm infants: Findings from an interpretive phenomenological study. *Advances in Neonatal Care*, *5*(4), 204–216.

Polan, H. J., & Ward, M. J. (1994). Role of the mother's touch in failure to thrive: A preliminary investigation. *Journal of the American Academy of Child & Adolescent Psychiatry*, *33*(8), 1098–1105.

POPPY Steering Group. (2009). Family-centred care in neonatal units. A summary of research results and recommendations from the POPPY project. London: NCT.

Premji, S. S., Pana, G., Currie, G., Dosani, A., Reilly, S., Young, M., … & Lodha, A. K. (2018). Mother's level of confidence in caring for her late preterm infant: A mixed methods study. *Journal of Clinical Nursing*, *27*(5–6), e1120–e1133.

Provenzi, L., & Santoro, E. (2015). The lived experience of fathers of preterm infants in the Neonatal Intensive Care Unit: A systematic review of qualitative studies. *Journal of Clinical Nursing*, *24*(13–14), 1784–1794.

Raeside, L. (1997). Perceptions of environmental stressors in the neonatal unit. *British Journal of Nursing*, *6*(16), 914–923.

Reid, T., Bramwell, R., Booth, N., & Weindling, M. (2007). Perceptions of parent–staff communication in neonatal intensive care: The findings from a rating scale. *Journal of Neonatal Nursing*, *13*(2), 64–74.

Robichaux, C. M., & Clark, A. P. (2006). Practice of expert critical care nurses in situations of prognostic conflict at the end of life. *American Journal of Critical Care*, *15*(5), 480–491.

Roué, J. M., Kuhn, P., Maestro, M. L., Maastrup, R. A., Mitanchez, D., Westrup, B., & Sizun, J. (2017). Eight principles for patient-centred and family-centred care for newborns in the neonatal intensive care unit. *Archives of Disease in Childhood: Fetal and Neonatal Edition*, *102*(4), F364–F368.

Royal College of Nursing. (2015). *Career, education and competence framework for neonatal nursing in the UK.* London: Royal College of Nursing.

Royal College of Paediatrics and Child Health. (2017). *Your baby's care: A guide to the National Neonatal Audit programme.* London: Royal College of Paediatrics and Child Health.

Segers, E., Ockhuijsen, H., Baarendse, P., van Eerden, I., & van den Hoogen, A. (2018). The impact of family centred care interventions in a neonatal or paediatric intensive care unit on parents' satisfaction and length of stay: A systematic review. *Intensive and Critical Care Nursing. 50*, 63–70.

Shaw, R. J., Deblois, T., Ikuta, L., Ginzburg, K., Fleisher, B., & Koopman, C. (2006). Acute stress disorder among parents of infants in the neonatal intensive care nursery. *Psychosomatics, 47*(3), 206–212.

Shin, H., & White-Traut, R. (2007). The conceptual structure of transition to motherhood in the neonatal intensive care unit. *Journal of Advanced Nursing, 58*(1), 90–98.

Skene, C., Franck, L., Curtis, P., & Gerrish, K. (2012). Parental involvement in neonatal comfort care. *Journal of Obstetric, Gynecologic & Neonatal Nursing, 41*(6), 786–797.

Skene, C., Gerrish, K., Price, F., Pilling, E., Bayliss, P., & Gillespie, S. (2019). Developing family-centred care in a neonatal intensive care unit: An action research study. *Intensive and Critical Care Nursing, 50*, 54–62.

Stefana, A., Padovani, E. M., Biban, P., & Lavelli, M. (2018). Fathers' experiences with their preterm babies admitted to neonatal intensive care unit: A multi-method study. *Journal of Advanced Nursing, 74*(5), 1090–1098.

Thomas, L. (2008). The changing role of parents in neonatal care: a historical review. *Neonatal Network, 27*(2), 91–100.

Thomson-Salo, F., Kuschel, C. A., Kamlin, O. F., & Cuzzilla, R. (2017). A fathers' group in NICU: Recognising and responding to paternal stress, utilising peer support. *Journal of Neonatal Nursing, 23*(6), 294–298.

Turrill, S. (1999). Interpreting family-centred care within neonatal nursing. *Paediatric Nursing, 11*(4), 22–24.

Warren, B. (2000). The premature infant in the mind of the mother. In Tracey, N. (Ed.) *Parents of preterm infants: Their emotional world*. Philadelphia: Whurr Publishers.

Warren, I. (2017). Family and Infant Neurodevelopmental Education: An innovative, educational pathway for neonatal healthcare professionals. *Infant, 13*(5), 200–203.

Whyte, D. (Ed.). (1997). *Explorations in family nursing*. London and New York: Routledge.

Wigert, H., Johansson, R., Berg, M., & Hellström, A. L. (2006). Mothers' experiences of having their new-born child in a neonatal intensive care unit. *Scandinavian Journal of Caring Sciences, 20*(1), 35–41.

Wigert, H., Blom, M. D., & Bry, K. (2014). Parents' experiences of communication with neonatal intensive-care unit staff: an interview study. *BMC Pediatrics, 14*(1), 304.

Williams, K., Patel, K., Stausmire, J., Bridges, C., Mathis, M., & Barkin, J. (2018). The neonatal intensive care unit: Environmental stressors and supports. *International Journal of Environmental Research and Public Health, 15*(1), 60. doi:10.3390/ijerph15010060.

5 DEVELOPMENTALLY FOCUSED NURSING CARE

Alison O'Doherty

CONTENTS

INTRODUCTION AND BACKGROUND

The term 'developmental care' is used to describe broadly those interventions which support and facilitate the stabilisation, recovery and development of infants and families undergoing intensive care and beyond, to promote optimal outcomes. This chapter will discuss key issues in relation to this vitally important area of care, including fundamental theory and principles underpinning the practice and interventions that healthcare professionals and parents should implement together to optimise infant developmental outcomes. Importantly, the preceding chapter on families and the key messages of family integration and inclusion apply also to this chapter.

THEORETICAL APPROACHES TO DEVELOPMENTAL CARE

The theoretical basis for our current understanding of developmental care stems from both animal and clinical studies. Animal models demonstrate that the brain has critical stages in development which require optimal environmental exposure to enhance brain development (Als et al., 2004). Over the last 30 years, advancement in the field of neonatology has improved survival and decreased the incidence of major long-term disabilities among the preterm population. However, the increasing survival of low birth weight infants, particularly those at the limits of viability, has created new challenges and neurodevelopmental outcomes for preterm infants and remains a significant concern for health professionals (Baron et al., 2011; Lavallée et al., 2018). There remains, therefore, a genuine need to explore strategies which support outcomes in the neonatal unit (NNU) so that these are optimised during and after transition to home (Dusing et al., 2018) to ensure the best future for our vulnerable patients.

Although it is accepted that foetal development and *in utero* experience may not be the appropriate theoretical model for our understanding of the newborn environment and the delivery of care, it seems appropriate to mimic the uterine environment where practically possible in infants born preterm. Premature birth disrupts the process of foetal maturation; preterm infants are developmentally unprepared for the sensory input that they are exposed to, particularly in the neonatal intensive care unit. While illness and treatments may have adverse effects on the rapidly developing brain, it is the environment of care which is often intensive, stressful and sometimes traumatic (Altimier and Phillips, 2013) to both preterm infants and their families (see figure 5.1). From birth, the premature infant is subjected to fluctuations in temperature, touch, noxious sounds, bright lights, interrupted and inadequate sleep, parental separation and a multitude of painful procedures, along with repetitive, non-nurturing handling. The preterm infant's rapidly developing but immature brain is particularly vulnerable within this stressful environment (Bröring et al., 2017).

Delivering critical care in such circumstances is complex, and it is important to acknowledge the difficulties of integrating the 'art' and 'science', the technological treatments and the humanitarian acts of nurture, considering how they can be combined to best effect. As discussed in chapter 4, apart from the management of the infant, psychosocial support of the parents and extended family/friends is essential in the delivery of true family-centred care. It is worth reiterating this important point. In addition, it is known that various degrees of parental involvement in care activities have been reported in the literature through the decades (Maree and Downes, 2016). However, as we have already seen, there is increasing recognition of the importance of viewing parents as partners in care and allowing parents to take on roles and responsibilities as primary caregivers (Lee and O'Brien, 2014). To enable parents to be involved in their baby's care, many units are developing family support programs to improve education and psychosocial support for parents (Jiang et al., 2014) within a family integrated care (FIC) philosophy (Lee and O'Brien, 2018).

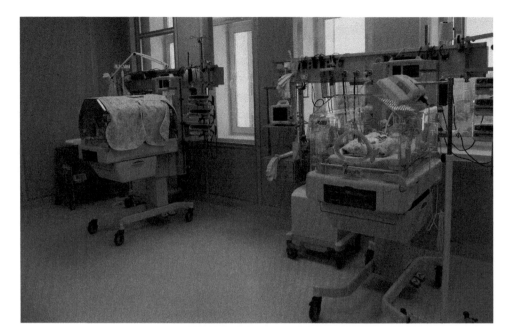

Figure 5.1 The neonatal intensive care environment

Preterm infants may spend months in the NNU during a critically important developmental period. The importance of environmental exposures on long-term physical, psychological and neurodevelopmental outcomes is now recognised (Santos et al., 2015). Preterm infants experience multiple noxious stimuli such as toxic light and sound, social deprivation and chemical exposure, all of which can have a negative impact on neurodevelopment. Optimising the neonatal environment could improve neurobehavioural outcomes for infants born preterm (Santos et al., 2015). This has implications for investment in training, environmental modification and other resources. Developmental care is thus viewed as an expansion of neonatology in which evolving family and family systems interface with the biological, environmental and psycho-emotional risks of preterm birth.

With increased understanding of developmental theory and systematic behavioural assessment, the emphasis of developmental care moves towards a more individualised and holistic approach, rather than the general introduction of developmentally supportive initiatives, such as modifying the environment or the provision of positioning aids. Nevertheless, both approaches are important; there are many initiatives of a general nature which will facilitate developmental stability, but individualised assessment will highlight the emerging agenda for the infant and enable care to be delivered according to infant cues. Advocacy is a fundamental principle of nursing care, and the ability to communicate effectively with parents, the extended family and friends is an essential component.

PRINCIPLES OF DEVELOPMENTALLY FOCUSED CARE

Developmental support programmes/interventions have been guided by different theoretical models and approaches have varied from single interventions to a collation of individualised developmentally focused care strategies aiming to minimize the negative effects of neonatal intensive care and to maximise infant and family outcomes (Altimier and Phillips, 2016; Burke, 2018). They have generally aimed to address one or more of the following areas which will be discussed in turn:

- *Managing sensory overload and/or deprivation:* Interventions which counteract sensory overload or deprivation, for example, reducing stress responses or promoting positive sensory experiences.
- *Promoting parent–infant attachment:* Interventions which aim to help parents to resolve the emotional crisis of preterm birth and promote maternal-infant attachment.
- *Behaviour and behavioural assessment*: Interventions that help parents to be more sensitive and responsive to their baby's behaviour and improve social interactions, practical caregiving or confidence.
- *Behavioural and development interventions:* Interventions aimed at managing the environment and preventing long-term developmental effects of being born early and admitted to neonatal care.

Managing sensory overload/deprivation

One approach views the infant as an 'extrauterine foetus' with the assumption that after birth, development is likely to progress as it would prior to birth. From this perspective, the NNU is seen as being overly stimulating compared to the natural uterine environment. The infant can easily become stressed, displayed by a variety of signals or cues (see figure 5.2 and table 5.2). The theory is that preterm infants' brain development may be further compromised by sensory overstimulation by bright lights, noise, handling and pain caused by NNU care processes such as heel lancing, venepuncture and suctioning (Mento and Bisiacchi, 2012; Roofthooft et al., 2014).

Therefore, to limit the effects of the NNU, proponents of this approach advocate minimal handling and reduced sensory input. This protection from potential hazards is thought to reduce the stress response and thus promote greater stability and increased tolerance of handling. An alternative approach is that the infant's developmental trajectory varies considerably after birth and progress is inherently and inevitably different, regardless of gestation. As the infant is deprived of appropriate *in utero* sensory input, additional stimuli are provided to improve outcome. Some studies have used a single intervention such as maternal voice indicating positive outcomes for preterm infants (Krueger, 2010). A review of the literature indicated that maternal voice had beneficial effects on preterm infants' stability both physiologically and behaviourally (Filippa et al., 2017). Other stimuli cited in the

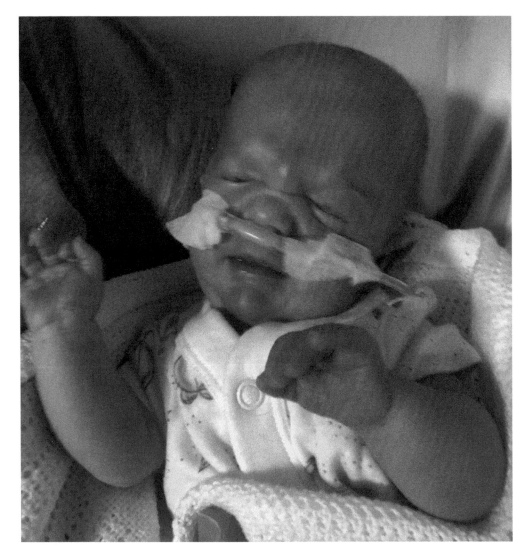

Figure 5.2 The stressed and the calm infant (continued opposite)

literature are heart sounds, providing rhythmic stimuli that simulate low frequency sounds and the cyclic nature of womb sounds resulting in decreased heart rates, improved sleep patterns and increased sucking/feeding behaviour (Loewy et al., 2013), tactile (massage, stroking), visual (mobiles, facial presentation), while others have used a combination of strategies (Kanagasabai et al., 2013).

Many NNUs are experiencing changes in their approaches to developmental care as they consider and incorporate the philosophy of individualised developmental care. A systematic review found evidence supporting individualised programmes of developmental care

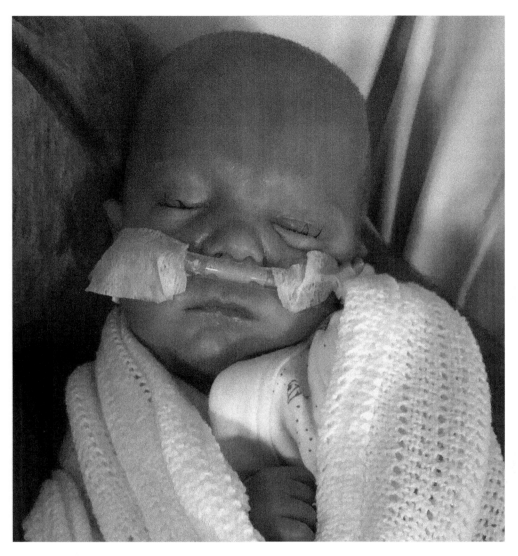

Figure 5.2 (continued)

but recommended further research examining the outcomes for preterm infants receiving developmental care and/or individualised developmental care programmes (Lengendre et al., 2011).

The developmental needs of preterm infants are complex, as they attempt to balance their lack of foetal experiences with the hazards of treatments necessary for survival. Current understanding would suggest that both approaches have merit depending upon the individual infant's medical condition, age and developmental stage and the environ-ment of care.

Parent-infant attachment

The foeto-maternal and maternal-infant relationship is also in deficit and requires consideration from a developmental perspective. The stress, uncertainty and anxiety that many parents of preterm infants experience can significantly affect development of parent-child bond and parental mental health (Alkozei et al., 2014), having a permanent detrimental impact on the successful establishment of the parenting role. The importance of early social interactions between infants and their parents, such as holding, touching and eye contact have been well researched in relation to attachment (Flacking et al., 2012). There is a plethora of literature advocating the importance of involving mothers in caregiving activities such as kangaroo care, breastfeeding, and other caregiving activities with the aim of improving maternal-infant bonding, attachment and outcomes (Pineda et al., 2018). However, as discussed in chapter 4, there is limited information about the experiences of preterm infants' fathers during the NNU stay; fathers often represent themselves as an observer of care, frequently left out from primary caregiving (Provenzi and Santoro, 2015). It is important that neonatal staff actively and effectively engage with fathers as well as mothers when implementing developmental care.

We have seen how family-centred models of care have considerably improved the situation of parents, whereby healthcare professionals aim to support families to be more involved in their infant's care (Gooding et al., 2011). Although family-centred care has now become an accepted care philosophy adopted by NNUs, some caregiving activities may continue to be performed by nurses and other health professionals, with parental involvement often being restrictive (Gooding et al., 2011). However, with the more recent advent of FIC, a comprehensive family-integrated care programme for parents of preterm infants (Broom et al., 2017) described earlier, it is vital that developmental care is an interconnected component of this – in other words, viewing and treating parents as active participants in care provision including developmental care interventions involving parent and staff education and psychosocial support (Lee and O'Brien, 2014). Indeed, where families were fully integrated into the neonatal team and actively provided much of their baby's care, this showed many benefits to both parents and infants. Mothers had lower stress scores and felt more knowledgeable and confident, while babies had improved weight gain and a higher rate of breastfeeding exclusively at discharge (O'Brien et al., 2013). To link this to developmental care, parental education on how to support their baby's emerging developmental needs is increasingly regarded as an essential component of optimal care (Bracht et al., 2013). By understanding infant behaviour, parents can observe more closely the individuality of their infant, become able to 'reset' their own expectations of infant behaviour and development and thus offer more infant-led support. This involvement helps parents feel more empowered to make decisions about their baby's care.

Brazelton (1973) was among the first to note the highly organised term infant's abilities to be active participants and social partners who affect caregiving behaviours. Als (1982) observed that preterm infants, although less organised, were similarly competent for their stage of development. She proposed a dynamic model for preterm infant behavioural organisation, known as synactive theory of development, which identified subsystems (auto-nomic, motor, state, attention-interactional and regulatory) of functioning which interact with each other and are influenced by the infant's internal and external environment. This model provides a basis with which to understand preterm infant behaviour, assess subsystems functioning and thus identify the emerging developmental goals. Using the synactive theory improves the scope for facilitative parent teaching, as parents learn to understand the indi-viduality of their infant and ways in which they can offer support which promotes stability and development.

In order to incorporate developmentally focused care, healthcare professionals must have knowledge and understanding of preterm infant developmental theory, be able to assess behaviours and interpret their meaning in the context of internal and external factors. In addition, it is essential that practitioners can determine and deliver an appropriate plan of care, have the resources to deliver the required strategy and ability to evaluate its effectiveness.

Behaviour and behavioural assessment

Advances in neuroimaging and research have provided a broader insight into third trimester brain development, and what has previously been viewed as simply developmentally sup-portive care is now recognised to be also neuroprotective care (McGrath et al., 2011; Discenza, 2015). To better understand the developmental problems associated with pre-maturity, it is important to understand the basics of neurosensory development of the pre-term infant. The neurological and sensory systems do not exist as separate entities, but are interdependent and comprise the neurobehavioural and neurosensory development of the infant. Every sensory experience is recorded in the brain leading to a behavioural response, thereby leading to a further sensory experience. This reaction is the basis for neurobehavioural and neurosensory development (Altimier and Phillips, 2016).

The preterm infant has a unique repertoire of behaviours that caregivers can observe and these behaviours are a window for understanding the developing brain (Vittner and McGrath, 2019). Parental ability to interpret the infant's behavioural cues has been shown to strengthen parent–infant interaction during the first year of life (Flacking et al., 2012). The following themes identified from the literature and various practical initiatives are likely to support the goal of improved medical and developmental outcomes for infants under-going intensive care, or enhance parent–infant interaction and subsequent psychosocial relationships:

■   Behavioural assessment
■   Recognition and appropriate management of distress and pain
■   Reduction of environmental hazard
■   Promotion of contingent handling
■   Postural support
■   Family-centred, developmentally focused models of care.

Well term newborns have stable autonomic and motor systems function and rapidly acquire distinct state system organisation. State refers to the level of consciousness displayed by the infant. This is determined by the level of arousal and the ability to respond to stimuli. Sleep and drowsy states predominate, but term infants can achieve quiet and active alert states as well as fussy, irritable and lusty cry states. They can be readily consoled and satisfied and are able to 'shut out' stimulation for rest and sleep. The emerging task of the term newborn is for increasing time in alert states with growing differentiation and responsiveness. An active and responsive social partner is essential to support this development which should be rewarding and stimulating for both participants and supportive of an increasing interest in the external world. The capacity of the infant for active participation in developing and maintaining a relationship with others and thus affecting his or her social environment and emerging developmental agenda is described by Brazelton (1973; 1984; Brazelton and Nugent, 1995).

Als (1982) was among the first to assert that preterm infants also had distinct behavioural patterns and that it was possible to assess and interpret them. These behaviours are grouped according to five physiological and behavioural subsystems of functioning and include an integrated set of autonomic (respirations, colour, tremors/startles), motor (tone, movement and postures), state (ranges of state and patterns of transitional states), and interaction attention (range and transition into and out of alertness) behaviours (Als, 1986). Preterm infants, while driven by the similar goals of stability and organisation, are at a stage of development which is more concerned with their internal world. They have immature systems organisation and their behaviours are consequently more diffuse and less stable. The autonomic subsystem, demonstrable through respiratory, cardiovascular and digestive function, often requires support to enable stable functioning, and this stability is likely to be under duress when challenged by handling, environmental disturbance, pain and illness. Stability and organisation in all other subsystems depend upon autonomic stability and within this model, can be viewed as the basis for more complex, hierarchical developmental tasks. The motor system, demonstrable through muscle tone, posture and movements, is the second emerging subsystem. Preterm infants have reduced muscle bulk and power and an immature central nervous system which inhibits smoothness and purposefulness of movement and may result in a flattened and extended posture.

One major component in preterm infants' growth and development is adequate sleep (Brummelte et al. 2012; van den Hoogen et al., 2017). Sleep plays an important role in preterm infants' illness recovery, brain development and energy utilisation (Mahmoodi et al., 2016). Preterm infants with unstable sleep/wake states are at high risk of later neurological problems (Serenius et al., 2013). Inpatients in the NNU are exposed to repeated environmental stimuli causing frequent disruptions to the infant's sleep/wake cycles. Recognising the importance of sleep to the developing preterm infant it is essential that health professionals providing care in the NNU environment incorporate developmentally supportive care strategies into their caregiving routine.

Sleeping and waking states represent a level of maturity of the central nervous system, the infant's relationship with the external environment and the ability to regulate and stabilise underlying internal systems. The organisation of sleep and wake states relates closely to brain maturation and reflects the central wellbeing of the nervous system (Holditch-Davis, 2010). Sleep and wake cycles begin at around 26 to 28 weeks' gestational age. Sleep states of preterm infants were originally recognised by observing infant behaviours. This observation of behaviours and changes in physiology has now added electroencephalography (EEG) and continuous electroencephalography (aEEG) to the studies of sleep and sleep cycles (Graven and Browne, 2008a). Prior to 36 weeks' gestation, there is poor coordination between states and with decreasing gestation, behaviours which demonstrate particular states are increasingly difficult to identify, even by trained observers. State transitions are diffuse, erratic and more easily influenced by internal and external stressors. Preterm newborns spend greater amounts of time in light sleep or drowsy states and have difficulty in achieving deep sleep. Deep sleep and quiet alertness, when infants are socially responsive, are rarely observed in NNU conditions and require facilitation from contingent handling and environmental manipulation. The active alert state which is usually generated by caregiving regimens may result in hyper-alertness and arousal followed by system collapse/compromise.

Two additional subsystems, the attention-interactional and the regulatory subsystems, are the final components of the synactive theory of development (Als, 1982). Attention and interaction are assessed when the infant is in an alert state and regulation is an assessment of the infant's success in achieving a balance in the subsystems. Each subsystem can be described independently but it is the processes of subsystems' interaction or synaction combined with the infant's interaction with their environment which completes the developmental theory. With experience and reflection, practitioners can begin to assess the attention-interactional and regulatory abilities of infants, but careful assessment of the autonomic, motor and state subsystems can provide sufficient knowledge of an individual's developmental agenda to determine appropriate interventions in most practical situations.

There are several sleep–wake scoring systems, based on careful observations of term and preterm infants (see table 5.1). The Neonatal Behavioural Assessment Scale (NBAS; Brazelton, 1973) catalogues detailed definitions of infants' behavioural states. The scores are used to determine predominant states, transitions between states and the quality of alertness. It has the advantage of being widely used in research and clinical practice and is relatively easy to use due to the distinct definitions (Brazelton and Nugent, 1995). However, due to the small number of states described, it fails to capture the indeterminate and transitory qualities of preterm infant behavioural states.

Thoman's revised state scoring system (1990) is more sensitive and has inter-rater and test-retest reliability with preterm infants (Holditch-Davis, 1990). There are ten states which differentiate state-related behaviours in preterm infants and those with perinatal complications. This system is more difficult to learn, and training is not readily available, but it has been shown to have predictive validity with later developmental out-come. Anderson's state scoring system (ABSS) was devised following earlier work with preterm infants and was used to demonstrate a relationship between heart rate, energy consumption and behavioural state (Ludington, 1990). There are few published studies using this scale, so its reliability and validity are not well established; however, it was constructed specifically for preterm infants and was based on extensive observations of their behaviours. Although similar to other scales, it is more complex, as it takes into account physiological parameters and thus is derived from a different theoretical base (Holditch-Davis, 1990). It is likely to be a useful instrument for quantitative studies into the relationships between interventions and infant state, but its use as a clinical instrument is not yet clearly defined.

Als (1982) defines behavioural state in greater detail in the Assessment of Preterm Infant Behaviour (APIB) which is a modification of the NBAS (Brazelton 1973; 1984). This scale more closely describes the state-related behaviours of preterm infants' responses to their internal and external environments and can be used with infants of very low gestational ages. The scale has been expanded to account for the immature and diffuse nature of emer-ging preterm state-related behaviours. As the scale is based on the NBAS, it is more familiar to researchers and clinicians, but training and supervision in its use are essential. The advan-tage of the system is its use as part of a holistic assessment and care planning programme, where state functioning is an important consideration. According to the synactive theory of development (Als, 1982), stability and organisation in autonomic and motor function can support and facilitate state system stability, thus enabling the infant to engage with the external world or settle into better quality sleep states. Sleep–wake state is more difficult to assess because of the subtle definitions described; nevertheless, it is essential to rec-ognise the current functioning of this subsystem to protect the infant from stressors and to facilitate and support emerging competencies.

A modified sleep–wake assessment which has practical validity and 95% inter-rater reliability with experienced nurses has been developed by Reid (2000). Although it is less sensitive than other preterm sleep–wake assessments, it can be readily utilised in general practice with minimal training and supervision.

Behaviours fall into two categories: stress or avoidance signals, where the stimula-tion is beyond the infant's capacity to assimilate and approach, or stability signals, where the behaviours demonstrate organisation or self-regulatory activity (table 5.2). Approach signals inform the observer of the infant's current stable functioning and point to the next level of developmental goals.

Behaviours should be assessed before, during and following handling activity. It is important to take note of the context of the intervention, including the responses of the infant to caregiving and the influences of the environment. A developmental review should therefore consist of observations of infant behaviour, an assessment of the current level of functioning and recommendations which support stability within the infant's immediate

TABLE 5.1 SLEEP–WAKE SCORING

Brazelton (1973)	Thoman (1990)	Anderson	Als (1982)	Reid (2000)
1 Deep sleep	1 Quiet sleep	1 Quiet sleep, regular respiration	1B Very still deep sleep	1 Very quiet sleep, regular respiration
2 Light sleep	2 Active-quiet transitional sleep	2 Quiet sleep, irregular respiration, slight movement	1A Deep sleep	2 Quiet sleep, irregular respirations, slight movement
3 Drowsy	3 Active sleep		2B Light sleep	
4 Alert	4 Sleep–wake transition	3 Active sleep, irregular respiration, movement	2A Noisy light sleep	3 Restless sleep, unsettled, some movement
5 Considerable motor activity	5 Drowsy		3A Drowsy with activity	
6 Crying	6 Daze		3B Drowsy	4 Drowsy, inattentive, some movement
	7 Alert	4 Very active sleep, whole body movement	4A Quiet awake or hyperalert	
	8 Non-alert waking		4B Bright alert	5 Quiet, awake, calm, focused attention
	9 Fuss	5 Drowsy	5A Active	
	10 Crying	6 Alert, slight movement, fixated eyes	5B Considerable activity	6 Restless awake, irregular respirations, suck-searching, some movement
		7 Quiet awake, no movement	6A Crying	
		8 Awake, some movement	6B Lusty crying	
		9 Awake, whole body movement		7 Fussing, grunting, increased movement
		10 Fussing, prolonged exhalation		
		11 Crying		8 Crying, facial grimace, tongue or jaw tremor
		12 Hard crying, clenched fists		

environment of care. Wider developmental issues such as modifications to the environment at large, education of staff and parents, and institutional awareness, all have an impact on the ability to integrate developmentally focused care, but careful, systematic observation is pivotal to its success.

TABLE 5.2 STRESS AND STABILITY SIGNALS

Stress signals	Stability and organisation signals
Autonomic system	
Respiratory pause, tachypnoea, gagging, gasping or sighing	Stable heart rate, respiratory rate, oxygenation and colour
Colour, vascular and visceral changes	Tolerance of enteral feeds
Tremor, twitch or startle	
Posset, vomit or hiccough	
Bowel strain	
Cough, sneeze or yawn	
Motor system	
Hyperflexion – trunk, limbs, fists, feet, neck	Smooth, well-modulated movements
Protective manoeuvres – hand on face, salute, high guard arm position	Relaxed postures and tone, with increasing flexion towards midline
Frantic, diffuse activity	Mobility and efficient self-regulatory activity, e.g.
Fixed, stereotypical postures	■ hand and foot clasping
	■ hand-to-mouth activity
	■ grasping and handholding
	■ suck-searching and sucking
State system	Clear, robust sleep states
Diffuse, oscillating sleep–wake state, whimper or high-pitched cry	Clear, robust, rhythmic cry
Strained or irritable fussiness or cry, lack of consolability	Ability to self-quiet or to be consoled
Eye floating or staring, lack of facial expression, strained or panicked alertness	Alert, intent or animated facial expression
Active averting	Focused wide-eyed alertness

BEHAVIOURAL AND DEVELOPMENTAL INTERVENTIONS

Managing the neonatal environment

The birth of any infant presents a dramatic change in environment. The well full term infant is ready for the transition to extrauterine life and quickly adapts with increasing interest in it. In contrast, the immaturity of physiological systems in the preterm infant makes this transition difficult and consequently the complex environment of the NNU becomes overly stimulating, creating a state of sensory overload in the baby. While there are several sources of stress, of particular concern are non-contingent or aversive handling events and the effect of sound and light on the sensory modalities of hearing and vision which are particularly immature in the preterm infant. Preterm babies have to adapt to extrauterine environment with immature body systems which include musculoskeletal, neuromuscular, cardiovascular, pulmonary and integumentary systems (Kanagasabai et al., 2013). The goal of nursing care then is to create a physical environment and approach to caregiving interventions that support the infant's physiological and neurodevelopmental needs.

There are recommendations for NNU design, including the structure, lighting, noise control, infection control, family space and other considerations (White et al., 2013). In general, these suggest that there are many practical ways in which subdued calmness and appropriate caregiving can be achieved without making structural changes. The literature describes numerous methods that have been shown to reduce noise levels within the NNU but, despite this, noise levels remain above the recommended level (Casavant et al., 2017). Noise reduction strategies described in the literature include implementation of 'quiet time'; however, evidence suggests that a 'culture of silence' is needed throughout the day and night to enhance infant neurodevelopment and growth (Swathi et al., 2014).

Sound hazard: Sound is heard in two dimensions: pitch (frequency) and loudness (decibels). Early auditory development involves the structural parts of the ears that develop in the first 20 weeks of gestation, and the neurosensory part of the auditory system that reaches the critical stage of development from 25 weeks' gestation to approximately 5–6 months post-term (Graven and Browne, 2008b). *In utero* sounds are muted through a fluid-filled environment. In contrast, on NNU infants are frequently exposed to noise that is often undesirable, which is predominately mechanical rather than social (Hunter et al., 2014). The auditory experience is therefore very different, and greater care is needed to protect babies.

Concerns in the preterm infant relating to sound exposure are repeated arousal causing significant physiologic effects such as increased heart rate, blood pressure and respiratory rate, decreased oxygen saturations, apnoea and bradycardia, increased intracranial pressure (Wachman and Lahav, 2011) as well as an inability to achieve relaxed sleep and alertness (Kuhn et al., 2012). Excessive noise levels in the NNU can cause damage to the cilia of the developing cochlea with an increasing susceptibility to hearing loss, and arousal in infants exposed to continuous loud sound (Moon, 2011).

Much of the literature focuses on immediate and medium-term effects of sound; there is little evidence on the consequences of sound on long-term development. Further controlled trials are needed to determine the effects of more extensive exposure to NNU noise on early brain maturation and long-term developmental outcomes (Wachman and Lahav, 2011).

The American Academy of Pediatrics recommends that sound levels in the NNU should not exceed the maximum acceptable level of 45 decibels (Almadhoob and Ohlsson, 2015) and with the cooperation of the whole team it is possible to modify sound bursts over this level. However, careful monitoring and audit are needed as well as a commitment to amend the physical environment where required. Optimising the acoustic environment is crucial; the challenge is for the NNU to be quiet enough to avoid physiological instability but to simultaneously provide optimal stimuli to support cognitive development of the preterm infant (Chow and Shellhaas, 2016). Supporting early vocal contact between mothers and preterm infants can impact the functional development of auditory brain development (Filippa et al., 2015). Therefore, the provision of auditory stimulation in the form of a softly modulated voice when the infant is receptive can help to promote alertness. Parents have described seeing their baby respond to their voice by turning, eye opening, calming or becoming animated as a powerful emotional event, which helps them to feel closer to their infant.

Light hazard: Light is measured in two ways: illuminance (the amount of light measured in lux), and irradiance (the kind of light measured in $\mu W/cm^2/nm$). In NNUs, lighting levels are variable with some units providing continuous high-intensity light and others reduced levels with diurnal patterning. Infants may also be exposed to additional amounts of light from their proximity to windows and the use of medical equipment and procedural lamps.

While there are no studies showing adverse long-term effects of exposure to variable levels of lighting, it is generally accepted that preterm infants need protection from light exposure. The visual system of the preterm infant is functionally and structurally incomplete and infants require dimness and sleep to support development (Graven and Browne, 2008c). The visual system is not developmentally ready for external visual stimuli. The visual system *in utero* develops in the absence of light stimulation, therefore the bright lighting conditions in the NNU appear to affect brain cell activity, sleep–wake state and intense light exposure producing stress-like responses in the infant (Graven, 2011). Reduced lighting has been found to stabilise the baby's heart rate, respiratory rate, blood pressure and motor activity. Preterm infants are unable to shut out stimulation for rest and sleep and are unable to achieve wide-eyed alertness unless environmental conditions are modified. If sleep–wake state is carefully observed under dimmed lighting conditions, it becomes apparent that this environment can improve the quality of sleep and promote alert states. Under bright and constant lighting, infants' autonomic and motor systems are likely to be aroused and they may remain in transitional states with closed eyes, neither deeply asleep nor available for social contact.

The lighting of clinical areas is an important environmental consideration. Practitioners need to balance the need for soft lighting to promote rest and sleep and support alertness with the need for close observation of the infant. Bright, overhead lighting is inappropriate for the needs of fragile preterm infants who are unable to shut out the stimulation if they remain unprotected. Dimmer switches should be fitted to overhead lights to modify lighting conditions. Spotlights or angle poise lighting can be utilised to illuminate a particular cot space, which prevents other infants in the nursery from being exposed. Wall-mounted up-lighters can provide ambient lighting while improving the clinical atmosphere and appearance of the nursery.

There are inevitable limits to the extent of environmental modification, particularly if it is not possible to make structural changes. It is possible, however, to focus on the immediate cot space to reduce the impact of the clinical environment in vulnerable infants. Incubator hoods or blankets can be used to absorb noise and attenuate lighting conditions. Thick, soft blankets and quilts around the mattress have a dual purpose of promoting comfort and absorbing incubator and tubing noise. Exposure to extreme lighting and abrupt fluctuations in lighting can disrupt the sleep of the premature infant; an important consideration as sensory system and brain development occur during sleep (Graven and Browne, 2008c). Lighting should be adjusted according to the infant's stage of development and strategies should be employed to individualise lighting to accommodate the needs of the caregiver and the infant. The provision of quiet time where activity, sound and lighting are reduced can enable infants to rest and sleep. A gradual lengthening of this period may be possible if infant behaviour is noted to improve because of the reduced activity. The quality of sleep and alert states should be monitored, as well as physiological parameters which suggest more stable autonomic functioning. Improved motor system stability may also be observed; tremor, startle, frantic diffuse or extensor activity should be replaced by more relaxed postures, tone and movements with self-regulatory activity.

Handling

Handling is the most direct source of stress for infants on the NNU; it is a well-known hazard to which experienced nurses are well attuned. The majority of handling episodes are inevitably unpleasant, stressful or painful, and for the most vulnerable infants these experiences dominate. More robust infants make efforts to regulate themselves by grasping, sucking and boundary searching, but more fragile infants are unable to mount the resources needed to stabilise and organise their behaviour. A systematic review by Valeri et al. (2015) found evidence for an association between painful experiences in preterm infants and adverse developmental outcomes, including cognitive and motor development. Chapter 6 has a detailed focus on pain and stress management in neonatal care.

Contingent care: Handling can also be the most effective source of comfort and pleasure. Human contact, particularly parental contact, can be both stimulating and stabilising, provided that it is appropriate, and the surrounding environment is conducive. The introduction of positive handling experiences is important at every stage of the infant's progress, but it is important to monitor their tolerance. Even low-key, gentle handling can cause distress if not delivered in the context of the environment or with consideration to the schedule of care. For example, it may be unreasonable to expect an infant to respond to parental contact following practical caregiving such as nappy change or feeding, when resources are depleted. Yet between the caregiving schedule, the infant may be lying quietly alert and socially available. Parents' expectations of social contact generally revolve around practical caregiving, but this may not be the most appropriate time for promoting alert and animated interaction. Lighting, sound and activity levels as well as infant preparedness must be taken into consideration prior to social handling if parent–infant interaction is to be optimised. Parents should be encouraged to spend time observing their babies, to become accustomed to their individuality, as an important first step towards contingent interaction.

With guidance, many parents could develop observational skills which would support practical caregiving, and similarly, parents who are unable to provide direct care can still have an important role to play, being better equipped to advocate for their babies. Parents may be more sensitive to their baby's needs, which is a sound basis for better quality interaction, and may help to improve parental self-esteem.

Handling stress can be reduced by incorporating measures to stabilise the infant's status and minimising the risk of overloading their capacity to assimilate events. Babies frequently demonstrate reduced stress responses in contained, flexed postures as motor stability is achieved and underlying physiological stress responses are minimised. Autonomic and motor stability can be supported by hands-on containment, concave nests with deep boundaries or swaddling, and by maintaining flexed, midline postures and head support while performing cares. These techniques provide greater opportunity for the baby to tolerate the intervention without aversion, stress or total systems collapse. In the most fragile infants undergoing hazardous care activities, it may be necessary for two people to perform the intervention: one to maintain flexed containment, and one to deliver the treatment or care. This approach to handling can have a marked effect on systems stability, and reflecting on the comparative outcomes of different handling techniques is a worthwhile exercise.

Autonomic stability can be supported by gently introducing the handling episode through voice and soft touch, in order to prevent immediate stress responses; this may also help to prevent the baby from remaining in a constant state of partial arousal or exhaustion. The environment and schedule of care are also important for the more mature and robust infants; consider, for example, oral feeding. The organisation and energy required for feeding success are considerable, and infant efforts can be significantly supported by ensuring that they are in optimal readiness. Any source of stress, for example vigorous handling or background activity, can provoke failure as behavioural organisation fails to cope with the additional demands.

To support the infant's responsiveness to social handling, it is essential that care is scheduled in a way which is realistic for the baby's abilities and which supports the parents' needs. This will often require teaching parents to adjust their expectations and to understand their baby's need for low-key, unimodal interaction.

Postural support

Developmentally supportive positioning is important in the NNU for several reasons: to promote comfort and respiratory function, maintain skin integrity, and facilitate infant alertness. Preterm infants are deprived of intrauterine development during the third trimester of pregnancy. This trimester encourages the development of physiologic flexion, including shoulder flexion, scapular protraction, hip and knee flexion and posterior pelvic tilt (Zarem et al., 2013). The late stages of pregnancy also encourage midline orientation (Waitzman, 2007). A flexed midline body alignment promotes healthy musculoskeletal development (Hunter et al., 2014), supports neurodevelopment and promotes self-soothing (Waitzman, 2007).

As preterm infants are deprived of this critical stage of development, they often lack muscle tone, and this causes their body to maintain an extended posture. Preterm infants left in unsupported extended positions can exhibit increased stress and agitation with worsened physiological instability.

Preterm infants are unable to counteract the effects of gravity and without support will develop imbalance between active and passive muscle tone, stereotypical head, shoulder and hip flattening which in turn, leads to problems with mobility (Hunter, 2010). Therefore, support with positioning is critical for the short- and long-term development of the premature infant. However, the long-term benefits of these developmental interventions with the aim of improving functional outcomes for preterm infants remains unclear (Spittle et al., 2015)

Appropriate positioning promotes self-regulation and facilitates the infant's participation in normal sensorimotor experiences, such as bringing the hand to mouth and face, whereas inappropriate positioning may contribute to physiological distress and behavioural disorganisation (Vergara and Bigsby, 2004). This results in an inability to engage in self-regulatory behaviours such as exploration of the face and mouth, hand and foot clasping, boundary searching, and flexion and extension of the limbs.

Furthermore, infants who are unable to maintain flexed postures or summon protective manoeuvres may remain in autonomic arousal at a cost to their energy and oxygen expenditure and systems stability. The goals of postural support are therefore multidimensional:

- support of physiological stability
- prevention of **abduction** or rotated postures of shoulders and hips and flattening of the head
- prevention of pressure damage from persistent stereotypical or favoured positions
- promotion of mobility and motor systems stability and development
- facilitation of protective manoeuvres and self-regulatory behaviours.

It is essential to support the baby in a range of positions to promote optimum outcome. To facilitate flexion patterns, there are numerous position recommendations that caregivers can utilise, such as side-lying, prone when awake, **supine** with external supports to mimic the curled, flexed position in the womb (Nightlinger, 2011), and some form of hip and shoulder elevation in prone positions to help reduce flattening. Various commercial products are available for swaddling, nesting and stabilising positions, but 'home-made' resources can be equally effective (see figure 5.3).

Overall, physiological stability is the prime goal of nursing the acute or chronically ill infant and any postural intervention should be considered not only for its intrinsic value but also for optimising this subsystem stability.

Cranial moulding: The incidence of positional plagiocephaly has increased over recent decades. Cranial moulding has a negative effect on the physical development of preterm infants (Collett et al., 2005). Infants with head flattening tend to position themselves preferentially on the flattened side, which can lead to contractures of the neck muscles and torticollis (Hunter, 2010). Preventative measures such as developmentally appropriate positioning can minimise the risk of positional plagiocephaly, with a reduction in bilateral head flattening in infants who receive regular repositioning, compared to infants who do not receive the intervention (Wielenga et al., 2011). In addition to repositioning, many infants also benefit from a soft head boundary. When in supine postures, the head can be supported to enable occipital lying, the only position which aims to reduce the incidence and severity of head flattening. This can be achieved using a soft roll or small sheet closely contouring the head, but loose enough to ensure some mobility. The use of neck rolls should be avoided as they may cause neck extension and thus, through damage, the delicate vessels at the back of the neck may alter cerebral blood flow. The sheet can be fixed in position by gently tucking it under the shoulders. This elevation will help the shoulders to fall naturally into midline and support mobility of the upper limbs. Cushioned mattresses or gel pillows will provide a 'nesting' effect; the gentle indentation supports flexion and containment and reduces the gravity effect on pressure areas. However, more research is required to establish the efficacy of interventions described above to prevent head moulding (Wielenga et al., 2011).

Prone position: Prone positions are frequently utilised in the NNU when infants are undergoing respiratory support or recovering from respiratory illness as oxygenation and lung expansion are thereby optimised. A systematic review by Gillies et al. (2012) concluded that prone positioning was significantly more beneficial than other positions in terms of improving ventilation, oxygenation and chest wall stability for ventilated preterm infants hospitalised with acute respiratory distress. As infants recover, prone positions are normally replaced in accordance with the recommendations for reducing the risk of sudden infant death syndrome by supine or side-lying postures. In prone postures, gravity has its greatest effect. The head is always on one side or the other, and hips are forced into abduction and rotation as the infant cannot maintain elevation or lower limb flexion under the pelvis. Shoulders are forced into the mattress, particularly if there is any pelvic elevation and the mattress is flat. Although the lower parts of the limbs can mobilise, mobility is considerably reduced without postural support in the prone position. If the mattress is elevated to aid respiratory function, it can reduce the pressure effects on the shoulders, neck and head. However, it also forces the infant to slide down the cot where lower limbs are cramped against the fixed cot boundary. Support around the buttocks can help to fix the infant in a stable prone position.

Pelvic elevation has been advocated by Downs et al. (1991) to prevent hip abduction and rotation and promote lower limb flexion. However, care must be taken to ensure that the infant's weight is not transferred to the femur and knee, as this may cause other problems with hip development (Monterosso et al., 2003). Hip slings have been used to fix the lower body in position and provide some degree of pelvic elevation, but they do not prevent hip abduction. Small pillows or rolls can be placed under the infant's pelvis and trunk to elevate the hips and thus enable some protraction of the lower limbs. It is important to ensure that the elevation does not cause respiratory impairment, the infant appears relaxed and comfortable, the weight of the body is evenly distributed, and limbs are mobile. Small pillows or gel mattresses can also be used to elevate the upper trunk to allow for some shoulder and hip protraction around it. Similarly, simply elevating the shoulders from the mattress gives some scope for supporting the head and neck at an oblique angle to prevent persistent side-lying.

Supine position: Although supine lying with midline occipital support is the position which best promotes mobility, it is associated with decreased ventilation and increased energy expenditure in some early studies, and therefore more frequently utilised in the mature and stable infant (Martin et al., 1979; Masterson et al., 1987). These studies should be interpreted with some caution as supine positions were frequently unsupported; that is, infants were not necessarily supported in centralised flexed postures as would be the case today. This position requires some degree of 'nesting' around the infant to maintain head, shoulders, pelvis and limbs in midline flexion. A small degree of hip and shoulder elevation from the boundary will promote limb mobility, support midline alignment and facilitate self-regulatory behaviours such as hand-to-mouth activity. This can be achieved by a combination of nesting into soft bedding, and the use of close, flexible boundaries around the infant's entire body. The lower limbs should be supported in flexed postures, but as limb mobility is facilitated in this position, opportunities for stretching and exten-sion should be provided. Often limbs can be found draped over the boundary, but this does not mean they no longer need boundary support. They are, in fact, being supported well enough to flex and extend at will while utilising some degree of shoulder and pelvic support. The effects of gravitational pressure are more evenly distributed in the supine midline position, and the pressure on the occipital region should ensure a more rounded head shape.

Side-lying position: Side-lying postures tend to minimise hip and shoulder rota-tion and abduction. Limbs should be flexed towards the midline axis (**adduction**). This posture can be maintained by swaddling in soft, flannelette sheeting. The infant's back should be rounded and may require some boundary support from a small rolled sheet or towel.

It is essential that boundaries are flexible to closely follow the contours of the body. Anteriorly, the infant may benefit from the placement of a soft toy or filled silicone glove within reach of the hands but away from the face. This will provide an opportunity for grasping and tactile stimulation and may encourage flexion towards the object. Side-lying can also be used to treat unilateral lung disease with better oxygenation being achieved by positioning the unaffected lung uppermost (Heaf et al., 1983).

Overall for postural care, attention to detail is crucial to the dual goals of prevention of postural deformity and the facilitation of self-regulation and mobility. It is important to ensure that side-lying and supine postures are utilised, and position changes are planned to incorp-orate a varied range of positions (see figure 5.3 (a) to (e)). It is also essential to assess the effectiveness of the intervention by ensuring that the infant tolerates the new position and that it supports both mobility and comfort.

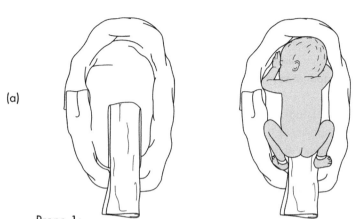

(a)

Prone 1:
Softly rolled sheet or blanket positioned in a complete circle. One smaller softly rolled sheet placed over the sheet circle and cover sheet, folded to support pelvic and thoracic lift. Arms and shoulders can be elevated to improve lung function, or fixed and tucked under the thorax. An additional cover may be needed to tuck under the nesting sheet. This serves to draw the nest closer into the infant, supporting flexed containment.

(b)

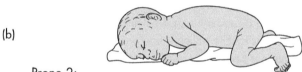

Prone 2:
Nappy roll length-wise under the body from head to hips. This may require additional rolls or blankets across the baby. The head can be supported at an oblique angle, if tolerated.

(c)

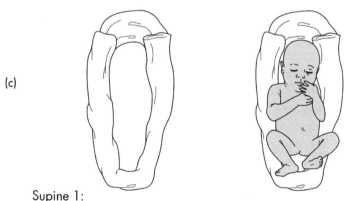

Supine 1:
Soft blanket or sheet rolled into a nest encourages flexion of lower limbs, brings shoulders forward and keeps the head in mid-line. If this continues round the contours of the head it may promote comfort. A small degree of neck flexion, if tolerated, can provide greater stability.

Figure 5.3 Postural support for infants in the NNU (adapted from Edinburgh Sick Children's NHS Trust, Maureen Grant, Superintendent Physiotherapist)

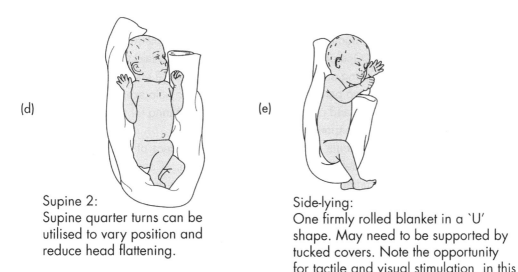

(d)

Supine 2:
Supine quarter turns can be
utilised to vary position and
reduce head flattening.

(e)

Side-lying:
One firmly rolled blanket in a 'U'
shape. May need to be supported by
tucked covers. Note the opportunity
for tactile and visual stimulation in this
position.

Figure 5.3 (continued)

DEVELOPMENTAL MODELS OF CARE

To fully utilise developmental knowledge, it is essential to incorporate theoretical concepts and practical skills into the model of care. This will ensure that experienced practitioners convey their values to less experienced team members and developmental practice is regarded as an essential component of neonatal nursing care. Effective documentation will ensure that care planning decisions are based on careful assessment, and implementation is continued over shift changes. Issues such as mobility, sensory stimulation, comfort and communication needs are thus considered to be as important as physiological needs, and developmental considerations become fundamental to neonatal care. As these issues are incorporated into practice, it is important to evaluate the outcomes, for both individuals and populations. Documentary evidence of the effects of the implementation of a particular strategy, such as reference to more stable functioning, provides the justification for its continuation in a plan of care. Audit of longer-term outcomes such as ventilator days, days on oxygen, days to full feeds and days to discharge, may provide the evidence which will support further investment and practice development in a wide range of strategies and interventions.

The support of parent–infant relationships is perhaps the most important developmental intervention of all, as it is this relationship which will have the greatest impact on long-term developmental outcome. Developmental models of care must therefore place the emotional and educational needs of parents at the centre of practice. This means going beyond the practical caregiving approach and providing structured support for behavioural observation and contingent handling skills development. Parents should be encouraged to actively contribute to care planning decisions and be fully informed and supported as partners in care. Parents with babies requiring intensive care are at increased risk of psycho-emotional difficulties such as depression and emotional distress (Lefkowitz et al., 2010; Gönülal et al., 2014). One of the main factors that may be linked to increased anxiety and depression is lack of coping strategies and parental support (Lefkowitz et al., 2010). It is important that NNUs develop parent support programmes to help express these feelings in order for parents to recover and proceed with the tasks of caring for their baby, while at the same time resuming daily responsibilities.

Communicating with parents is clearly an important aspect of nursing care and a developmentally focused model should ensure minimal levels of communication are routinely incorporated and documented, for example, teaching plans, interaction support, crisis interviews, practical and social problems and discharge planning. Semi-formal interviews with parents can reveal many underlying difficulties, but these are unlikely to be revealed if communication consists of opportunistic conversation at the cot side, with the multitude of distractions and lack of privacy. This model of care therefore advocates a prearranged meeting with parents on a regular basis, where information-giving, decision-making and evaluation can take place with nurses who are familiar with the baby and family.

It can be seen that baby and family are at the centre of this model (figure 5.4). However, some of the considerations apply to the infant and educational issues clearly apply only to parents. Sensory and comfort needs, and emotional and communication needs can apply to both. All should be assessed to see if they require intervention which is then planned, implemented and evaluated according to individual requirements. The model does not have to differentiate between a need, problem or potential problem if they are regarded as systematic considerations. All aspects must be assessed, and the appropriate

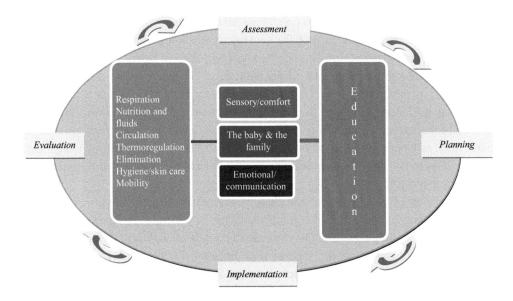

Figure 5.4 Family-centred developmental model of care

strategy devised to meet the need, deal with the problem or prevent a potential problem from developing.

Documentation to support the developmental aspects of the model can be devised in the same way that clinical assessments and plans are devised. Charts can record sleep–wake state, postural support, parent interaction and teaching plans. Care plans can record behavioural assessment, interventions and evaluations. Developmental progress can thus be submitted for audit to evaluate the effectiveness of developmentally focused care over time and make resource decisions which will influence the future direction of practice development.

CONCLUSION

Developmental care has emerged as a neuroprotective care concept aimed at preventing long-term consequences associated with the environment of care, promoting the optimal organisation and neurodevelopment of preterm infants, as well as involving parents as partners in care (Kenner and McGrath, 2014; Altimier et al., 2015). Developmental interventions have the potential to enhance the effectiveness of neonatal services by supporting traditional medical and nursing care. Neonatal nurses are the primary caregivers in the neonatal environment; they are in a key position to influence the environment of the developing neonate, as well as therapeutic interventions (Altimier et al., 2015).

Finally, although research has demonstrated the potential to improve outcome and reduce healthcare expenditure, there is no prescriptive approach and there are few conclusive solutions which apply in general, although modification to the environment is likely to benefit all infants and parents experiencing intensive care. An understanding of developmental theory and knowledge of behavioural assessment will serve to promote a creative approach to individualised holistic family-centred care which reflects the fundamental values and beliefs of neonatal nursing.

CASE STUDIES

Case study 1: Two-day old premature baby

Jacob is a 2-day-old baby boy born at 24 weeks' gestation. Following a traumatic delivery requiring resuscitation, he is fully ventilated within a humidified incubator and is also being monitored by ECG, pulse oximetry and arterial line blood gas analysis. He also has an intravenous long line in situ for nutrition and drugs.

Q.1. Firstly, consider the foetal environment: the consistent temperature, gravitational support and containment, attenuated light and sound, and nutritional, hormonal and psychological influences. Now consider the

C
A
S
E

S
T
U
D
Y

postnatal environment that Jacob was born into and his early care in the first few hours. How has this affected him and how would you manage the neonatal environment?

As someone who is looking after Jacob and his parent, you watch him for a while and note the following:

You note an infant in light sleep who, upon handling, immediately becomes hyperalert and agitated with extensor postures and 'panicked' facial expression. You also note the difficulty in achieving a quiet, alert state with responsive and animated facial expression. You have the additional problem of being unable to detect distinct states due to the infant's immature behaviours and the environment in which the infant is nursed. With reference to the key points within the chapter, consider the following questions:

Q.2.   What do you notice about Jacob's behaviour?

Q.3.   How would you explain this to the parents and how would you work with the parents to address the behaviours?

Q.4.   What developmental care strategies could parents employ with your support, in this case, and why?

Case study 2: Three-week-old premature twin boys

Sebastian and Paulo are 3-week-old twins who were born at 25 weeks' gestation to Italian parents, visiting the UK on holiday. Sebastian has suffered a grade 2 bleed (IVH) on his left side but regardless of this, he has progressed well and has been taken off all forms of ventilatory support just requiring some low flow oxygen in the special care unit. Paulo however, has not progressed so well, had become septic and was re-ventilated after being on high flow oxygen therapy, currently being nursed in the intensive care unit. He has been diagnosed with a grade 2 and 3 bleed on the right and left sides respectively.

With reference to the key points within the chapter, consider the following questions:

Q.1.   How would you work with the parents to manage this situation?

Q.2.   What strategies are required for both infants to optimise their wellbeing and prevent any longer-term development problems?

Q.3.   What members of the neonatal multidisciplinary team should you involve to also work with the parents?

Case study 3: An eight-week-old premature baby on a developmental care programme

Baby Callum was born at 23 weeks and is now 8 weeks old. After a very unstable few weeks, he is starting to show progress in all areas but remains oxygen-dependent with difficulty tolerating his feeds. He has been reviewed by a developmental care specialist who is trained in 'NIDCAP'. Along with the parents, they explain to you about the importance of observing the reactions of Callum in different environmental conditions. They also note the circumstance which supports his efforts to quieten and relax or reach alertness. They observe his behaviour during periods of high activity and note the stress responses as well as comparing state system stability in relation to the environment of care.

With reference to the key points within the chapter, consider the following questions:

Q.1. What do these observations and explanations mean to you and why are they important for the infant and family?

Q.2. How can you support the family during this current time in line with these types of observations?

Q.3. What interventions are required, working towards discharge home, to minimise adverse outcomes?

For suggested answer guides to the questions posed in these case studies, please refer to the web-based companion site specific to this chapter (see URL below).

WEB-BASED RESOURCES

For further information, online resources and greater detail on the case studies featured in this chapter go to www.routledge.com/cw/nicnursing

References

Alkozei, A., McMahon, E., & Lahav, A. (2014). Stress levels and depressive symptoms in NICU mothers in the early postpartum period. *The Journal of Maternal-Fetal & Neonatal Medicine*, 27(17), 1738–1743.

Almadhoob A, Ohlsson A. (2015). Sound reduction management in the neonatal intensive care unit for preterm or very low birth weight infants. *Cochrane Database of Systematic Reviews*, Issue 1. Art. No.: CD010333. DOI: 10.1002/14651858.CD010333.pub2

Als, H. (1982). Toward a synactive theory of development: Promise for the assessment and support of infant individuality. *Infant Mental Health Journal*, 3(4), 229–243.

Als, H. (1986). A synactive model of neonatal behavioural organisation: Framework for the assessment of neurobehavioural development in the premature infant and for support of parents in the intensive care environment. In Sweeney, J. K. (Ed.) *The High-Risk Neonate: Developmental Therapy Perspectives* (pp. 3–53). London: The Haworth Press.

Als, H., Duffy, F. H., McAnulty, G. B., Rivkin, M. J., Vajapeyam, S., Mulkern, R. V., ... & Fischer, C. (2004). Early experience alters brain function and structure. *Pediatrics, 113*(4), 846–857.

Altimier, L., & Phillips, R. M. (2013). The neonatal integrative developmental care model: Seven neuroprotective core measures for family-centered developmental care. *Newborn and Infant Nursing Reviews, 13*(1), 9–22.

Altimier, L., & Phillips, R. (2016). The neonatal integrative developmental care model: Advanced clinical applications of the seven core measures for neuroprotective family-centered developmental care. *Newborn and Infant Nursing Reviews, 16*(4), 230–244.

Altimier, L., Kenner, C., & Damus, K. (2015). The wee care neuroprotective NICU program (Wee Care): The effect of a comprehensive developmental care training program on seven neuroprotective core measures for family-centered developmental care of premature neonates. *Newborn and Infant Nursing Reviews, 15*(1), 6–16.

Baron, I. S., Erickson, K., Ahronovich, M. D., Baker, R., & Litman, F. R. (2011). Neuropsychological and behavioral outcomes of extremely low birth weight at age three. *Developmental Neuropsychology, 36*(1), 5–21.

Bracht, M., O'Leary, L., Lee, S. K., & O'Brien, K. (2013). Implementing family-integrated care in the NICU: A parent education and support program. *Advances in Neonatal Care, 13*(2), 115–126.

Brazelton, T. B. (1973). *Neonatal Behavioural Assessment Scale: Clinics in Developmental Medicine. No. 50.* https://nidcap.org/wp-content/uploads/2013/12/Brazelton-1973-BNBAS.pdf

Brazelton, T. B. (1984). *Neonatal Behavioural Assessment Scale* (2nd Edition). Philadelphia: Lippincott.

Brazelton, T. B. and Nugent, J. K. (1995). *Neonatal Behavioral Assessment Scale* (3rd Edition). London: MacKeith Press.

Broom, M., Parsons, G., Carlisle, H., Kecskes, Z., Dowling, D., & Thibeau, S. (2017). Exploring Parental and Staff Perceptions of the Family-Integrated Care Model. *Advances in Neonatal Care, 17*(6), E12–E19.

Bröring, T., Oostrom, K. J., Lafeber, H. N., Jansma, E. P., & Oosterlaan, J. (2017). Sensory modulation in preterm children: Theoretical perspective and systematic review. *PloS One, 12*(2), e0170828.

Brummelte, S., Grunau, R. E., Chau, V., Poskitt, K. J., Brant, R., Vinall, J., ... & Miller, S. P. (2012). Procedural pain and brain development in premature newborns. *Annals of Neurology, 71*(3), 385–396.

Burke, S. (2018). Systematic review of developmental care interventions in the neonatal intensive care unit since 2006. *Journal of Child Health Care, 22*(2), 269–286.

Casavant, S. G., Bernier, K., Andrews, S., & Bourgoin, A. (2017). Noise in the Neonatal Intensive Care Unit: What Does the Evidence Tell Us? *Advances in Neonatal Care, 17*(4), 265–273.

Chow, V. Y., & Shellhaas, R. A. (2016). Acoustic environment profile of the neonatal intensive care unit: High ambient noise and limited language exposure. *Journal of Neonatal Nursing, 22*(4), 159–162.

Collett, B., Breiger, D., King, D., Cunningham, M., & Speltz, M. (2005). Neurodevelopmental implications of 'deformational' plagiocephaly. *Journal of Developmental and Behavioral Pediatrics, 26*(5), 379.

Discenza, D. (2015). Neuro-NICUs: Nurturing the tiniest of brains. *Neonatal Network, 34*(5), 291–293.

Downs, J. A., Edwards, A. D., McCormick, D. C., Roth, S. C., & Stewart, A. L. (1991). Effect of intervention on development of hip posture in very preterm babies. *Archives of Disease in Childhood, 66*(7), 797–801.

Dusing, S. C., Tripathi, T., Marcinowski, E. C., Thacker, L. R., Brown, L. F., & Hendricks-Muñoz, K. D. (2018). Supporting play exploration and early developmental intervention versus usual care to enhance development outcomes during the transition from the neonatal intensive care unit to home: A pilot randomized controlled trial. *BMC Pediatrics, 18*(1), 46.

Filippa, M., Frassoldati, R., Talucci, G., & Ferrari, F. (2015). Mothers singing and speaking to preterm infants in NICU. *Journal of Pediatric and Neonatal Individualized Medicine, 4*(2):e040238.

Filippa, M., Panza, C., Ferrari, F., Frassoldati, R., Kuhn, P., Balduzzi, S., & D'amico, R. (2017). Systematic review of maternal voice interventions demonstrates increased stability in preterm infants. *Acta Paediatrica*, *106*(8), 1220–1229.

Flacking, R., Lehtonen, L., Thomson, G., Axelin, A., Ahlqvist, S., Moran, V. H., ... & SCENE group. (2012). Closeness and separation in neonatal intensive care. *Acta Paediatrica*, *101*(10), 1032–1037.

Gillies D., Wells D., Bhandari A.P. (2012). Positioning for acute respiratory distress in hospitalised infants and children. *Cochrane Database of Systematic Reviews*, Issue 7. Art. No.: CD003645. DOI: 10.1002/14651858.CD003645.pub3

Gönülal, D., Yalaz, M., Altun-Köroğlu, Ö., & Kültürsay, N. (2014). Both parents of neonatal intensive care unit patients are at risk of depression. *Turkish Journal of Pediatrics*, *56*(2), 171–176.

Gooding, J. S., Cooper, L. G., Blaine, A. I., Franck, L. S., Howse, J. L., & Berns, S. D. (2011). Family support and family-centered care in the neonatal intensive care unit: origins, advances, impact. In *Seminars in Perinatology*, *35*(1), 20–28.

Graven, S. N., & Browne, J. V. (2008a). Sleep and brain development: The critical role of sleep in fetal and early neonatal brain development. *Newborn and Infant Nursing Reviews*, *8*(4), 173–179.

Graven, S. N., & Browne, J. V. (2008b). Auditory development in the fetus and infant. *Newborn and Infant Nursing Reviews*, *8*(4), 187–193.

Graven, S. N., & Browne, J. V. (2008c). Sensory development in the fetus, neonate, and infant: introduction and overview. *Newborn and Infant Nursing Reviews*, *8*(4), 169–172.

Graven, S. N. (2011). Early visual development: implications for the neonatal intensive care unit and care. *Clinics in Perinatology*, *38*(4), 671–683.

Heaf, D. P., Helms, P., Gordon, I., & Turner, H. M. (1983). Postural effects on gas exchange in infants. *New England Journal of Medicine*, *308*(25), 1505–1508.

Holditch-Davis, D. (1990). The development of sleeping and waking states in high-risk preterm infants. *Infant Behavior and Development*, *13*(4), 513–531.

Holditch-Davis, D. (2010). Development of sleep and sleep problems in preterm infants. *Encyclopedia on Early Childhood Development*. Centre of Excellence for Early Childhood Development, Montreal, Quebec, Canada, 1–8.

Hunter, J. (2010). Therapeutic positioning: neuromotor, physiologic and sleep implications. In McGrath, C. K. J. (Ed.) *Developmental Care of Newborns and Infants. A guide for health professionals* (2nd Edition). Glenview: NANN.

Hunter, J., Lee, A., & Altimier, L. (2014). Neonatal Intensive Care Unit. In Case-Smith, J., & O'Brien, J. C. (Eds.) *Occupational Therapy for Children and Adolescents* (7th Edition). St Louis: Mosby.

Jiang, S., Warre, R., Qiu, X., O'Brien, K., & Lee, S. K. (2014). Parents as practitioners in preterm care. *Early Human Development*, *90*(11), 781–785.

Kanagasabai, P. S., Mohan, D., Lewis, L. E., Kamath, A., & Rao, B. K. (2013). Effect of multisensory stimulation on neuromotor development in preterm infants. *The Indian Journal of Pediatrics*, *80*(6), 460–464.

Kenner, C., & McGrath, J. M. (Eds.) (2014). *Developmental care of newborns & infants. A guide for health professionals*. St Louis: Mosby.

Krueger, C. (2010). Exposure to maternal voice in preterm infants: A review. *Advances in Neonatal Care*, *10*(1), 13–20.

Kuhn, P., Zores, C., Pebayle, T., Hoeft, A., Langlet, C., Escande, B., ... & Dufour, A. (2012). Infants born very preterm react to variations of the acoustic environment in their incubator from a minimum signal-to-noise ratio threshold of 5 to 10 dBA. *Pediatric Research*, *71*(4–1), 386–392.

Lavallée, A., De Clifford-Faugère, G., Garcia, C., Oviedo, A. N. F., Héon, M., & Aita, M. (2018). Part 1: Narrative overview of developmental care interventions for the preterm newborn. *Journal of Neonatal Nursing*. *25*(1), 3–8.

Lee, S. K., & O'Brien, K. (2014). Parents as primary caregivers in the neonatal intensive care unit. *CMAJ*, *186*(11), 845–847.

Lee, S. K., & O'Brien, K. (2018). Family integrated care: Changing the NICU culture to improve whole-family health. *Journal of Neonatal Nursing, 24*(1), 1–3.

Lefkowitz, D. S., Baxt, C., & Evans, J. R. (2010). Prevalence and correlates of posttraumatic stress and postpartum depression in parents of infants in the Neonatal Intensive Care Unit (NICU). *Journal of Clinical Psychology in Medical Settings, 17*(3), 230–237.

Legendre, V., Burtner, P. A., Martinez, K. L., & Crowe, T. K. (2011). The evolving practice of developmental care in the neonatal unit: A systematic review. *Physical & Occupational Therapy in Pediatrics, 31*(3), 315–338.

Loewy, J., Stewart, K., Dassler, A. M., Telsey, A., & Homel, P. (2013). The effects of music therapy on vital signs, feeding, and sleep in premature infants. *Pediatrics, 131*(5), 902–918.

Ludington, S. M. (1990). Energy conservation during skin-to-skin contact between premature infants and their mothers. *Heart & Lung: The Journal of Critical Care, 19*(5 Pt 1), 445–451.

McGrath, J. M., Cone, S., & Samra, H. A. (2011). Neuroprotection in the preterm infant: further understanding of the short-and long-term implications for brain development. *Newborn and Infant Nursing Reviews, 11*(3), 109–112.

Mahmoodi, N., Arbabisarjou, A., Rezaeipoor, M., & Mofrad, Z. P. (2016). Nurses' awareness of preterm neonates' sleep in the NICU. *Global Journal of Health Science, 8*(6), 226–233.

Maree, C., & Downes, F. (2016). Trends in family-centered care in neonatal intensive care. *The Journal of Perinatal & Neonatal Nursing, 30*(3), 265–269.

Martin, R. J., Herrell, N., Rubin, D., & Fanaroff, A. (1979). Effect of supine and prone positions on arterial oxygen tension in the preterm infant. *Pediatrics, 63*(4), 528–531.

Masterson, J., Zucker, C., & Schulze, K. (1987). Prone and supine positioning effects on energy expenditure and behavior of low birth weight neonates. *Pediatrics, 80*(5), 689–692.

Mento, G., & Bisiacchi, P. S. (2012). Neurocognitive development in preterm infants: insights from different approaches. *Neuroscience & Biobehavioral Reviews, 36*(1), 536–555.

Monterosso, L., Kristjanson, L., Cole, J., & Evans, S. F. (2003). Effect of postural supports on neuromotor function in very preterm infants to term equivalent age. *Journal of Paediatrics and Child Health, 39*(3), 197–205.

Moon, C. (2011). The role of early auditory development in attachment and communication. *Clinics in Perinatology, 38*(4), 657–669.

Nightlinger, K. (2011). Developmentally supportive care in the neonatal intensive care unit: An occupational therapist's role. *Neonatal Network, 30*(4), 243–248.

O'Brien, K., Bracht, M., Macdonell, K., McBride, T., Robson, K., O'Leary, L., ... & Lee, S. K. (2013). A pilot cohort analytic study of Family Integrated Care in a Canadian neonatal intensive care unit. *BMC Pregnancy and Childbirth, 13*(1), S12.

Pineda, R., Bender, J., Hall, B., Shabosky, L., Annecca, A., & Smith, J. (2018). Parent participation in the neo-natal intensive care unit: Predictors and relationships to neurobehavior and developmental outcomes. *Early Human Development, 117*, 32–38.

Provenzi, L., & Santoro, E. (2015). The lived experience of fathers of preterm infants in the Neonatal Intensive Care Unit: a systematic review of qualitative studies. *Journal of Clinical Nursing, 24*(13–14), 1784–1794.

Reid, T. (2000). Maternal identity in preterm birth. *Journal of Child Health Care, 4*(1), 23–29.

Roofthooft, D. W., Simons, S. H., Anand, K. J., Tibboel, D., & van Dijk, M. (2014). Eight years later, are we still hurting newborn infants? *Neonatology, 105*(3), 218–226.

Santos, J., Pearce, S. E., & Stroustrup, A. (2015). Impact of hospital-based environmental exposures on neurodevelopmental outcomes of preterm infants. *Current Opinion in Pediatrics, 27*(2), 254–260.

Serenius, F., Källén, K., Blennow, M., Ewald, U., Fellman, V., Holmström, G., ... & Olhager, E. (2013). Neurodevelopmental outcome in extremely preterm infants at 2.5 years after active perinatal care in Sweden. *Jama, 309*(17), 1810–1820.

Spittle, A, Orton, J., Anderson, P. J., Boyd, R., & Doyle L. W. (2015). Early developmental intervention programmes provided post hospital discharge to prevent motor and cognitive impairment in preterm infants. *Cochrane Database of Systematic Reviews*, Issue 11. Art. No.: CD005495. DOI: 10.1002/14651858.CD005495.pub4

Swathi, S., Ramesh, A., Nagapoornima, M., Fernandes, L. M., Jisina, C., Suman Rao, P. N., & Swarnarekha, A. (2014). Sustaining a 'culture of silence' in the neonatal intensive care unit during nonemergency situations: A grounded theory on ensuring adherence to behavioral modification to reduce noise levels. *International Journal of Qualitative Studies on Health and Well-being*, *9*(1), 22523. doi:10.3402/qhw.v9.22523.

Thoman, E. B. (1990). Sleeping and waking states in infants: A functional perspective. *Neuroscience & Biobehavioral Reviews*, *14*(1), 93–107.

Valeri, B. O., Holsti, L., & Linhares, M. B. (2015). Neonatal pain and developmental outcomes in children born preterm: A systematic review. *The Clinical Journal of Pain*, *31*(4), 355–362.

van den Hoogen, A., Teunis, C. J., Shellhaas, R. A., Pillen, S., Benders, M., & Dudink, J. (2017). How to improve sleep in a neonatal intensive care unit: a systematic review. *Early Human Development*, *113*, 78–86.

Vergara, E., & Bigsby, R. (2004). *Developmental and Therapeutic Interventions in the NICU*. Brookes Pub.

Vittner, D., & McGrath, J. M. (2019). Behavioral Assessment. In Tappero, E. P., & Honeyfield, M. E. (Eds.) *Physical Assessment of the Newborn: A Comprehensive Approach to the Art of Physical Examination* (6th Edition). New York: Springer Publishing Company.

Wachman, E. M., & Lahav, A. (2011). The effects of noise on preterm infants in the NICU. *Archives of Disease in Childhood: Fetal and Neonatal Edition*, *96*(4), F305–F309.

Waitzman, K. A. (2007). The importance of positioning the near-term infant for sleep, play, and development. *Newborn and Infant Nursing Reviews*, 7(2), 76–81.

White, R. D., Smith, J. A., & Shepley, M. M. (2013). Recommended standards for newborn ICU design. *Journal of Perinatology*, *33*(S1), S2–16.

Wielenga, J., Mansvelt, P., & van den Hoogen, A. (2011). Is cranial molding preventable in preterm infants? A systematic literature review of the effectiveness of interventions. *Pediatric Intensive Care Nursing*, *12*(1–2), 3–10.

Zarem, C., Crapnell, T., Tiltges, L., Madlinger, L., Reynolds, L., Lukas, K., & Pineda, R. (2013). Neonatal nurses' and therapists' perceptions of positioning for preterm infants in the neonatal intensive care unit. *Neonatal Network*, *32*(2), 110–116.

6 MANAGEMENT OF PAIN AND STRESS IN THE NEONATAL UNIT

Kaye Spence

CONTENTS

GUIDANCE ON HOW TO ENHANCE PERSONAL LEARNING FROM THIS CHAPTER

Key points covered in this chapter

- The pathophysiology of pain in neonates.
- Stress and pain in the neonatal unit – nursing and medical interventions that cause pain, preventative measures, assessment tools and management strategies.
- Parental perceptions of pain in the neonatal unit.

Reflection

Reading through the chapter, you are encouraged to engage with the key points and related literature in an enquiring way. Ask these questions:

- Why is the recognition and management of neonatal stress and pain so important?
- What is the wider impact of stress and pain in the neonatal unit – consider short- and long-term outcomes, and how it may affect families?
- What measures for pain management are in place in your work environment? Do you need to address this subject?

Implications for nursing care

- Finally: how will this chapter enable you to consider and implement pain management strategies and support parents concerning this aspect?

INTRODUCTION AND BACKGROUND

There have been major changes in the attitudes and practices of clinicians in recognising and managing pain in neonates over the past 40 years. With a proliferation of groundbreaking research, there has been a change in the way pain is assessed and managed as the focus is on the understanding of short-term and long-term consequences of pain. Unfortunately, pain remains an emotive issue for clinicians and the infant's inability to express pain can still result in under- or overtreatment of pain. The identification of prolonged, persistent or chronic pain continues to be a challenge as we seek the evidence for these types of pain in neonates (Anand, 2017).

Pain assessment and management are controversial in small and sick neonates. There are many assessment tools available for acute pain; however, these remain underused in the neonatal unit (NNU) and special care units (SCU). Choosing a suitable tool that can be standardised across all neonatal settings remains a challenge, and guideline statements now recommend that procedural pain is covered with some analgesia. This chapter aims to provide the evidence for best practice for the assessment and management of pain in neonates. Nurses prevail on the front line in ensuring that neonates and their families receive the best care for managing painful interventions. Despite an overwhelming volume of research, an evidence-practice gap for the assessment and management of pain in neonates persists (Spence et al., 2010).

DEVELOPMENT OF THE PAIN PATHWAYS

Pain pathways consist of a network that communicates unpleasant sensations of noxious stimuli throughout the body. At birth, neonates have a developing and incomplete **myelinated** nervous system; however, all the components of the **nociceptive** (pain) pathways are present. Thus, a newborn infant's nervous system is fully capable of transmitting, perceiving, responding to and remembering noxious stimuli even though it is not yet fully developed (Verriotis et al., 2016).

Nociception (the detection of noxious stimuli) occurs when harmful impulses are transferred to the spinal cord through thinly myelinated and unmyelinated nerve fibres (see figure 6.1). These neuronal connections to the cortex are essential for the experience of pain

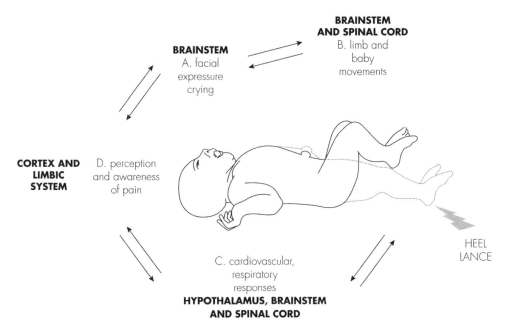

Figure 6.1 Pain pathways in the neonate (adapted from Slater et al., 2007, with permission from Elsevier)

and these occur late in gestation (ibid.). Physiological and behavioural response to noxious stimulation may occur early in development, as the connections to the cortex, where pain perception is mediated, are immature (Slater et al., 2007). Responses to noxious stimuli, such as limb withdrawal and increased heart rate, do not require the involvement of higher (cortical) brain structures; they are reflexes mediated at the level of the brainstem or spinal cord. As a result, these responses are measures of nociception rather than the perception of pain (ibid.).

Three key aspects of sensory processing in the spinal cord underlie responses to pain in the neonate. First, an infant's spinal sensory nerve cells are more excitable than an adult's. This makes their spinal reflex response to a harmful stimulus much greater and more prolonged. Second, individual sensory nerve cells in neonates have a much larger area of skin – or receptive fields – than in adults. This means reflex responses can be triggered from a larger body area. Receptive fields combine to form a 'map' or image of our body surface in our brain and enable us to locate a stimulus in a particular part of our body. In neonates, the larger receptive fields result in a less precise or 'smeared' body map where the newborn responds less selectively and produces the same reflex to a light touch (Fitzgerald, 2015).

EARLY PAIN EXPERIENCES

The plasticity of the developing brain contributes to its vulnerability to the stressors that cause long-term developmental changes, ultimately leading to adverse neurological outcomes. Observational studies have highlighted the impact of early pain experience upon later pain behaviour (Schwaller and Fitzgerald 2014).

Neonatal unit environmental influences

Brummelte et al. (2012) found that a reduction of white matter and subcortical grey matter maturation occurred when there were a higher number of skin breaks, which are markers for early neonatal pain-related stress. Very preterm infants, who have a greater number of invasive procedures during their hospital stay, when adjusted for clinical confounders, have been shown to have an altered brain microstructure and poorer cognitive outcome at 18 months' corrected age (Vinall et al., 2014). Procedures commonly carried out in the NNU have been found to be painful, such as suprapubic aspiration (Kozer et al., 2006), eye examination (Mitchell et al., 2004), nappy change (Holsti et al., 2005) and central line placement (Taddio et al., 2006). Developmental care practices were found to decrease the pain response to routine nursing procedures in medically stable preterm infants (Cignacco et al., 2012; Warren et al., 2016). It is important to consider these influences and the context of the infant experiencing painful procedures during caregiving.

Surgery

Infants who undergo a surgical procedure in the neonatal period are vulnerable to pain in the postoperative period as a result of surgery itself as well as from continuing post-operative interventions, which can be numerous and repeated. Postoperative analgesia should be planned and organised prior to surgery (Howard et al., 2012) as well as appropriate to developmental age, surgical procedure, and clinical setting to provide safe, sufficiently potent, and flexible pain relief. Neonatal surgery has been associated with changes in pain responses later in life. Infants who had surgery in the newborn period had increased perioperative analgesic requirements for subsequent surgery (Peters et al., 2005). More persistent changes in sensory processing were found in children of 8–12 years following neonatal intensive care and the degree of change was more marked in those who also required surgery during the neonatal period (Walker et al., 2009).

Chronic pain

Inadequate pain management has been identified as a risk factor for chronic pain, indicating that newborns subjected to neonatal intensive care may be at risk of developing a chronic pain state (Anand et al., 2014). Anand (2017) suggests that the importance of investigating behavioural and environmental interventions for infant chronic pain may be safer than drug therapies. The message for the neonatal nurse is that being aware of the consequences of pain, no matter how harmless it may appear, is to know that it has the potential to cause harm. Modifications of practice to meet the individualised needs of each infant should be part of every nurse's practice.

TYPES OF NEONATAL PAIN

Defining an infant's pain can aid clinicians' level of concern, focus their attention towards specific assessment methods, and allow them to weigh the risks/benefits of appropriate interventions (Anand, 2017). Pain definitions can assist in understanding the causes of pain in neonates, developmental considerations, genetic, epigenetic or other factors that contribute to poor outcomes or long-term complications, and to help in choosing appropriate management for both acute and non-acute pain (Anand, 2017). Consideration of the various types of pain are shown in table 6.1.

PAIN AND STRESS

The terms 'neonatal pain' and 'neonatal stress' are often used interchangeably. Stress responses can be specific to a particular source, or non-specific and more generalised. Yet pain is always stressful while stress is not necessarily painful. It remains very difficult

TABLE 6.1 TYPES OF NEONATAL PAIN

Pain term	Onset	Duration	Character[a]	Primary hyperalgesia
Acute episodic	Immediate	0–120[b] minutes	Sharp, well-localised	Present, mild, short-lasting
Acute recurrent	Immediate	Variable	Sharp, well-localised	Present, moderate or severe
Prolonged[c]	Rapid, may be gradual	One hour to 24 hours[b]	Sharp, diffusely localised	Present, moderate or severe
Persistent[c]	Rapid or gradual	Cumulative one to seven days	Dull/sharp, diffusely localised	Present, moderate or severe
Chronic	Usually gradual	Eight days or longer	Dull, diffusely localised	May be present or absent, mild if present

(adapted from Anand, 2017)

a Based on descriptions in adult patients, but may be discerned by a careful physical examination.

b Some infants with increased sensitivity to pain may have a slower decay of the acute pain following an invasive procedure, thus justifying some overlap in the durations of acute episodic pain and prolonged pain.

c Continuous pain may be characterised as either 'prolonged' or 'persistent'.

to distinguish where stress ends and the painful experience begins (Raeside, 2013; Provenzi et al., 2015). When pain is provoked through activation of nociceptors, noticeable signs such as crying, or heart rate variability can be detected. Crying and increased heart rate can both show a high sensitivity for pain, though neither crying nor heart rate are specific to pain. The sudden appearance of these signs after a potentially painful stimulus can give reliable information on the presence of pain (Bellieni et al., 2015, 2018). From the perspective of the neonatal nurse, the Neonatal Infant Stressor Scale can aid with formulating a management plan of accumulated stress in preterm neonates (Newnham et al., 2009). Figure 6.2 outlines the context of pain or stress when assessing pain in neonates.

ASSESSMENT OF PAIN

The neonatal nurse plays a crucial role in the assessment of pain, which should form part of his or her routine observations. The physiological and behavioural responses to acute pain are well characterised in newborns and used for assessments. There is a difference between scoring pain and detecting pain: using a pain score enables assessment on the level of pain, detection identifies the presence or absence of pain. The ideal goal is the avoidance of pain, with at least the detection of arising pain, to enable a change in the procedure or behaviour, as no amount of pain can be called 'tolerable' in a baby (Bellieni et al., 2015; 2018).

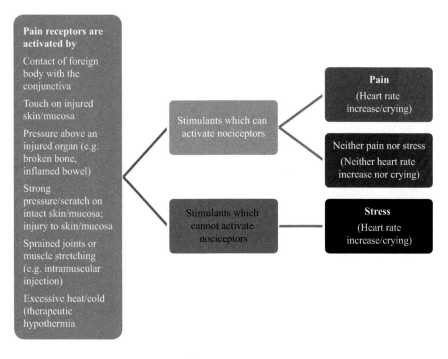

Figure 6.2 Contextual assessment of pain (adapted from Bellieni et al., 2015)

Pain tools can only be used as a guide for practice and decisions. By undertaking a pain assessment, it opens up the dialogue between clinicians and often leads to joint decisions in the management of an infant's pain and/or discomfort. One cannot choose a single tool as this choice will depend on gestational age, type of painful stimulus and the infant's environment (de Melo et al., 2014). Multidimensional or one-dimensional scales are suggested; however, they must be reliable and validated. Harrison et al. (2015) recommend the use of a pain assessment method which is already developed and tested in the clinical area, suitable for the specific unit/setting/population, feasible to use, acceptable to staff, used consistently, used in ward rounds, handovers, and in clinical care to make decisions about pain management.

Table 6.2 describes some of the assessment tools in current use.

MANAGEMENT OF PAIN, STRESS AND DISCOMFORT

Comfort/non-pharmacological interventions

The first line of pain management is to ensure basic comfort measures are instituted. These include positioning the infant in a non-stressful way and ensuring there are boundaries to assist in self-regulation as a method of relieving stress. In addition, the use of a pacifier

TABLE 6.2 OVERVIEW OF PAIN ASSESSMENT TOOLS

Tool	Variables	Type of pain	Population	Clinical use
BIIP (Behavioural Indicators of Infant Pain) (Holsti and Grunau, 2007)	Sleep/wake states, five facial actions and two hand actions.	Procedural	Preterm	Reliability, moderate concurrent validity with a multidimensional pain scale (NIPS)
CHEOPS (Children's Hospital of Eastern Ontario Pain Scale)	Calmness, physical movement, facial tension, alertness, respiratory response heart rate, blood pressure.	Procedural and postoperative	Preterm, term neonates and older infants	Reliability and validitiy
COMFORT Scale (Van Dijk et al., 2005)	Movement, calmness, facial tension, alertness, respiration rate, muscle tone, heart rate, blood pressure.	Postoperative	0 to 3-year-old infant Ventilated and non-ventilated	Reliability, validity, clinical utility
CRIES (Crying, requires O2 for saturations above 95%, increased vital signs, expression and sleeplessness)	Cry, saturations, expression, sleep, heart rate and blood pressure.	Procedural and Postoperative	Preterm and term	Reliability and validity
N-PASS (Neonatal Pain, Agitation, and Sedation Scale)	Crying, irritability, behavioural state, facial expression, extremity tone, vital signs.	Postoperative, procedural	Ventilated	Reliability, validity, includes sedation end of scale, does not distinguish pain from agitation
NFCS (Neonatal Facial Coding System) (Peters et al., 2003)	Facial expressions, eyes squeezed, bulging brow, open lips, taut tongue, and deepening of nasolabial folds.	Procedural		Reliability, validity, clinical utility, high degree of sensitivity to analgesia

TABLE 6.2 (Cont.)

Tool	Variables	Type of pain	Population	Clinical use
NIPS (Neonatal Infant Pain Score) (Lawrence et al., 1993)	Facial expression, crying, breathing patterns, arm and leg movements, arousal.	Procedural	Preterm and full term	Reliability, validity
PAT (Pain Assessment Tool) (Spence et al., 2005)	Physiological, behavioural, nurse's, perception.	Postoperative, ventilated	Term and preterm	Reliability and validity, comfort measures part of use, clinical utility
PIPP-R (Premature Infant Pain Profile – Revised) (Stevens et al., 2014)	Heart rate, oxygen saturation, facial actions; takes state and gestational age into account.	Procedural, postoperative (minor)	Preterm and term neonates	Reliability, validity, clinical utility well established

adapted from Bellieni et al., 2015)

to encourage non-nutritive sucking, ensuring the nappy is dry and comfortable, and environmental modification to ensure lights are dimmed, and the noise and activity kept to a minimum. Handling infants has been found to increase the pain response after procedures (Cameron et al., 2007).

To protect the neurodevelopment of preterm and sick term infants and to provide best practice in neonatal intensive care, emphasis has been put on humane neonatal care, individualised developmentally supportive care, and family-centred care (Marfurt-Russenberger et al., 2016); these are discussed in detail in chapters 4 and 5. There are many non-pharmacological interventions that can be implemented either singularly or in conjunction with each other. Box 6.1 lists each of these, as well as the actions and evidence for reducing pain and/or stress during acute pain interventions (see figure 6.3).

Pharmacological interventions

Pharmacological agents may be required to alleviate pain in neonates in intensive care who are subjected to numerous invasive procedures, or in the postoperative period. There is considerable clinical and experimental evidence to support the practice of providing adequate analgesia for newborns undergoing invasive medical, surgical, diagnostic or therapeutic procedures, or who develop conditions associated with considerable pain, such as necrotising enterocolitis. Long-term follow-up of infants who have received morphine in the NNU has shown favourable outcomes (De Graaf et al., 2013). Despite an overwhelming volume of evidence, analgesia remains under-utilised (Carbajal et al., 2015; Prestes et al., 2016).

BOX 6.1 NON-PHARMACOLOGICAL PAIN MANAGEMENT IN NEONATES

Non-nutritive sucking

- Reduced physiological response
- Reduced behavioural response
- 4 RCT and meta-analysis

Breastfeeding

- First-line intervention
- Depends on the sweetness of the milk
- Used in conjunction with other interventions

Sucrose therapy

- Considered to be the role of endogenous opioids
- 30+ RCT on single dose for procedures

Swaddling

- Stimulation of proprioceptive system
- Reduced physiological response, i.e. heart rate, saturated oxygen
- Few studies in to efficacy of this procedure

Facilitated tucking

- Reduced pain during ETT suctioning
- Increased quietening, reduction in crying
- Used in conjunction with sucrose
- 3 RCT

Skin-to-skin contact

- Stimulation of proprioceptive system
- Reduced physiological response, i.e. heart rate
- 24+ RCT on single dose for procedures

Kangaroo care

- Stimulation of proprioceptive system
- Reduced physiological response, i.e. heart rate

- Crossover RCTs, consists of preterm neonates not ventilated
- Result in reduced heart rate, crying and pain score

Massage

- Suggested to provide tactile and kinesthetic stimuli
- Modulates behaviour to pain response
- Few studies into efficacy of this procedure

Auditory

- Affects descending pain modulation mechanism
- No RCTs, few observation studies
- Limited proven efficacy, needs more research

Environment

- Lighting, day, clustering procedures and night cycles
- Reduce physiological stress response
- 42 clinical trials, varied levels of evidence.

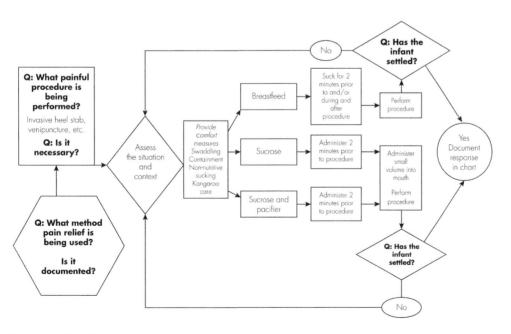

Figure 6.3 Algorithm for the management of procedural pain

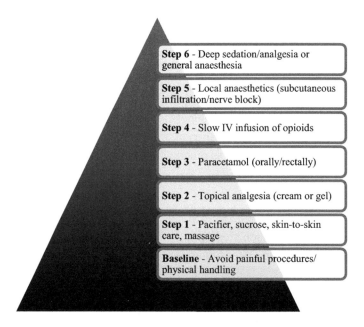

Figure 6.4 Stepwise approach to neonatal analgesia (adapted from Durrmeyer, et al., 2010)

Figure 6.4 depicts a suggestion of escalating analgesia in neonates. It is recommended that all NNUs have a plan for the use of analgesia, and this should include regular identification and assessment of pain. Fundamentally, however, as indicated in figure 6.4, the aim should be the prevention of unnecessary pain. Pharmacological agents used in the NNU are described in box 6.2.

FAMILIES

Parents of infants in the NNU may worry that their baby is experiencing pain, and this concern may contribute to increased parental stress. Franck et al. (2011) identified six conceptual categories which parents found distressing about their baby's pain. These were: (1) causes of infant pain; (2) parent concerns about infant pain and pain management; (3) parent information needs; (4) parent involvement; (5) differing views among parents and healthcare professionals about the care of infant pain; and (6) parent views on how healthcare professionals can improve infant pain care. Nurses can assist parents by being aware of these issues and address them as they talk about the baby's pain or potential pain.

Nurses cannot care for neonates without considering the parents and their involvement in their baby's care. Communication regarding neonatal pain is a challenge and may be difficult, leading to frustration for both parents and nurses (Elias et al., 2014) and

BOX 6.2 PHARMACOLOGICAL INTERVENTIONS FOR PAIN MANAGEMENT IN THE NNU

Opioids – intravenous

- The gold standard for relief of moderate to severe pain in neonates.
- Potential adverse effects of opioids include the slowing of gastric and intestinal motility, feeding intolerance, and adverse neurological effects.
- Prolonged use may lead to opioid dependance and tolerance.

MORPHINE

- Most widely used and studied opioid in critically ill infants.
- Side effects include marked respiratory depression, bradycardia and hypotension.
- Has a long half-life (6 to 14 hours in preterm, 2 to 11 hours in term infants).
- Continuous infusion of 10 micrograms/kg/hour does not harm general outcomes.
- Tolerance may develop after prolonged use (3–4 days in preterm infants).
- Slow weaning is recomended.
- No adverse effects on long-term outcomes in preterm infants.

FENTANYL

- A potent synthetic opioid.
- It penetrates the central nervous system (CNS) rapidly and the serum half-life is 1 to 15 hours.
- Infants receiving a fentanyl infusion should be observed closely for chest wall rigidity, urine retention and laryngospasm.
- Infusions of fentanyl for >5 days have shown significant withdrawal symptoms.

Paracetamol

- Infants who receive intravenous paracetamol as primary analgesic after major surgery require significantly less morphine than those who receive a continuous morphine infusion.
- Multiple intravenous administrations of paracetamol in the very preterm infant results in a predictable pharmacokinetic profile (van Ganzewinkel et al., 2014).
- Prolonged administration of paracetamol 7.5mg/kg/day every six hours was not associated with impaired hepatic conjugation or glutathione depletion.

- Caution is warranted, as safety data on the prolonged administration of paracetamol exceeding five doses in very preterm infants is still lacking.

Epidural analgesia

- **Caudal** catheters were found to account for 50% of neonatal epidural catheters.
- The commonest drugs are bupivacaine, lidocaine and ropivacaine.

Local wound analgesia

- Bupivacaine is an amide local anaesthetic with a slow onset and a long duration of action, which may be prolonged by the addition of a vasoconstrictor.
- The wound catheter is placed during surgery to provide postoperative pain relief.

Topical agents

- Topical local anaesthetics can be used for venepuncture pain.
- Topical local anaesthetics alone are insufficient for heel lance pain.
- Topical tetracaine plus morphine is superior to topical analgesia alone for central venous catheter insertion pain in ventilated infants.
- When using a topical local anaesthetic, it must be applied correctly, and sufficient time allowed for it to become effective.
- EMLA contains lidocaine 2.5% and prilocaine 2.5%, which can produce local anaesthesia when applied to intact skin as a cream. It is applied to the centre of the area to be anaesthetised and covered with an occlusive dressing. Cream and dressing are removed after 30 minutes for venepuncture and 45 min for venous cannulation.

Sweet-tasting solutions

- Sucrose may contribute to pain response reduction in examination for retinopathy of prematurity.

an undercurrent of anxiety. Parents may be apprehensive about actively participating in their baby's pain care, in case they are labelled as 'demanding'. Good communication and support are paramount, as witnessing their baby's pain can be very distressing for parents. Box 6.3 contains suggestions for effective parent communication around the subject of pain.

BOX 6.3 EXAMPLE OF A PARENT INFORMATION BROCHURE ABOUT SUPPORTING THEIR BABY DURING A PAINFUL PROCEDURE

Identifying your baby's responses You can assist the nurses and doctors by describing your baby's responses to them. The nurses may assess your baby's signals by using a standard chart.

How to comfort your baby If a procedure is required that is likely to cause your baby pain, you can comfort the baby by holding or supporting them during the procedure. If you are breastfeeding, it can be helpful to give your baby a breastfeed a couple of minutes before the procedure. If you are not breastfeeding, then ask the nurses to provide some sucrose for your baby prior to the procedure.

Being present during procedures Holding your baby during a procedure may comfort your baby; however, you may decide that this is too uncomfortable for you to do.

CLINICAL PRACTICE

Clinical guidelines

Position statement and clinical practice recommendations for pain assessment in the non-verbal patient have been developed and issued in many countries by professional groups, project teams and individual institutions (Bennett et al., 2009; Spence et al., 2010; The Hospital for Sick Children, 2017). Guidelines are a useful way of putting the evidence for pain assessment and management into practice. However, it is the responsibility of practicing clinicians to be aware of the guidelines supporting their own practice and to adhere to these recommendations. The use of evidence-based guidelines has led to a significant reduction in opioid exposure, and in the number of infants requiring methadone for iatrogenic narcotic dependence (Rana, 2017). Harrison et al. (2015) have called for a consistent and coordinated approach to improving neonatal pain management by implementing recommendations included in nationally and internationally endorsed guidelines.

Caregiver knowledge and response to infant pain

Gaps in knowledge can be attributed to the lack of basic knowledge about pain behaviour, over-reliance on an invasive short-term pain model, pain measurement issues, and lack of knowledge about contributing factors to the painful experience (Cong et al., 2014). How nurses respond to the infant's pain is often influenced by their personal perception of pain and their work with others in the care team (Elias et al., 2014).

Studies have shown that similar ratings on a pain scale may have different meanings for various caregiver groups, which can result in different management strategies (Pillai Riddell and Craig, 2006). Nurses were found to appropriately identify pain display indicators such as crying, vital sign changes and body movement; however, having this specific pain assessment knowledge did not translate to their care practices (Campbell-Yeo, 2008). When caring for a neonate in pain, nurses can have emotional reactions or an empathetic response (Campbell-Yeo, 2008), both of which play a central role in the recognition and treatment of pain. However, Guedj et al. (2014) found there was a variation in pain management practices between day and night, with less analgesia being used at night, and less attention to weaning analgesia. The presence of parents and written protocols could contribute to the variation of practices and quality of care around the clock. Constant efforts to improve care quality should thus include standardisation of care across 24 hours, and pain management guidelines should be followed (Guedj et al., 2014). Elias et al. (2014) established that adults found identifying pain in neonates difficult, but the reasons for this require further investigation.

Part of the nurse's role is advocacy for best practice by ensuring guidelines are in place and used to inform practice. Effectiveness of practice is measured by way of clinical audits monitoring whether pain management is individualised, and practice based on evidence.

Ethical aspects of neonatal pain

Pain assessment and management can raise ethical issues for neonatal staff with the infant's best interests being of primary concern. When neonates are subjected to painful procedures, it can be argued that this is not in the infant's best interest (see chapter 9, ethical issues) to withhold pain relief (Spence, 2000). If pain relief is withheld on the assumption that the medicine may be harmful to the infant, then this raises the issue of the boundaries of preserving life and health. The ethical issues associated with the treatment for neonatal pain are complex. The long-term consequences of continued exposure to pain experienced by neonates are unknown. Therefore, the focus for this dilemma should be to try and reduce the exposure to pain. Consideration of each potentially painful procedure needs to be a priority for each caregiver. The number of painful procedures carried out in the NNU needs to be reduced, and the indiscriminate use of routines without a clear rationale reviewed by the multidisciplinary team.

CONCLUSION

Neonatal pain is an emotive issue. Neonatal nurses can help alleviate pain and suffering through careful assessment and ensuring appropriate interventions are provided. By understanding the mechanisms of neonatal pain pathways, nurses should be able to demonstrate effective assessment skills, which in turn contribute to best practice. Despite a large amount of evidence regarding painful procedures and effective management, clinical practice is still variable and not always in keeping with this evidence. Nurses with an awareness of pain in the newborn will be empowered to provide interventions to ensure that neonates in NNU and SCU will receive adequate relief not only from procedural pain, but also from chronic pain associated with ventilation and surgery, as well as exposure to stress.

CASE STUDIES

Case study 1: Neonatal stress

Naomi has been in the NNU for four weeks now. She was delivered by caesarean section at 28 weeks' gestation because her mother went into labour with ruptured membranes. Naomi was on mechanical ventilation for two weeks and is now on non-invasive respiratory support (CPAP). She is receiving small volumes of expressed breast milk via her gastric tube. You have been assigned to care for Naomi on your shift.

Q.1. On receiving handover from your colleague how would you determine if Naomi is comfortable?

Q.2. What signs of stress would you be looking for when you are undertaking care activities for Naomi?

Q.3. How might you determine if Naomi has been experiencing stressful events either on the past shift or during your shift?

Q.4. What are some of the detrimental effects of stress for neonates in the NNU?

Case Study 2: Pain assessment

Angus was born at 34 weeks' gestation and he is now five days of age. On his mother's antenatal ultrasound scan he was diagnosed with a congenital heart defect. He had surgery on the second day of life for a narrowing of his aortic arch. He was ventilated in the postoperative period for three days and was receiving a fentanyl infusion for his pain. On the medical ward round the team asked for the rate of his fentanyl infusion to be reduced in preparation for extubation.

Q.1. How would you assess Angus' readiness for a reduction in his analgesia?

Q.2. You have been asked what the trends in his pain score are prior to reducing the analgesia. Using a suitable pain assessment scale check the algorithm to gauge the scores that would be suitable for weaning the analgesia.

C
A
S
E

S
T
U
D
Y

Q.3. You have been assigned a new staff member to work with you in caring for Angus. As part of your mentorship you decide to teach them about how to assess a baby's pain. What do you need to consider in explaining how to assess a baby's pain using a pain scale?

Case study 3: Pain management

George is a 26-week gestation infant weighing 875 grams. He was delivered by emergency caesarean section following maternal antepartum haemorrhage. His mother did not receive antenatal corticosteroids. He was born in fair condition and was intubated and given surfactant immediately after delivery. Following stabilisation, he is transferred to the NNU, where he continues to require mechanical ventilation. Umbilical arterial and venous lines are sited for monitoring and intravenous therapy and medication.

Q.1. Does George need any pain relief given that he is so premature? Please qualify your answer.
Q.2. Which drugs could be used in this situation?
Q.3. Are there any non-pharmacological strategies you could employ to keep George comfortable?
Q.4. How would you assess whether the pain-relieving strategies were effective?
Q.5. Can you think of any pharmacological interventions appropriate for procedural pain?

For suggested answer guides to the questions posed in these case studies, please refer to the web-based companion site specific to this chapter (see URL below).

WEB-BASED RESOURCES

For further information, online resources and greater detail on the case studies featured in this chapter go to www.routledge.com/cw/nicnursing

References

Anand, K. J., Kramer, B. W., & Andriessen, P. (2014). Chronic pain in the newborn: toward a definition. *The Clinical Journal of Pain, 30*(11), 970–977.
Anand, K. J. (2017). Defining pain in newborns: Need for a uniform taxonomy? *Acta Paediatrica, 106*(9), 1438–1444.
Bellieni, C. V., Tei, M., & Buonocore, G. (2015). Should we assess pain in newborn infants using a scoring system or just a detection method? *Acta Paediatrica, 104*(3), 221–224.

Bellieni, C. V., Tei, M., Cornacchione, S., Di Lucia, S., Nardi, V., Verrotti, A., & Buonocore, G. (2018). Pain perception in NICU: A pilot questionnaire. *The Journal of Maternal-Fetal & Neonatal Medicine*, *31*(14), 1921–1923.

Bennett, M., Carter, B., Dooley, F., Goddard, J., Gordon, J., Hartley, J., ... & Monahan, N. (2009). *The Recognition and Assessment of Acute Pain in Children. Update of Full Guideline*. London: Royal College of Nursing.

Brummelte, S., Grunau, R. E., Chau, V., Poskitt, K. J., Brant, R., Vinall, J., ... & Miller, S. P. (2012). Procedural pain and brain development in premature newborns. *Annals of Neurology*, *71*(3), 385–396.

Cameron, E. C., Raingangar, V., & Khoori, N. (2007). Effects of handling procedures on pain responses of very low birth weight infants. *Pediatric Physical Therapy*, *19*(1), 40–47.

Campbell-Yeo, M., Latimer, M., & Johnston, C. (2008). The empathetic response in nurses who treat pain: Concept analysis. *Journal of Advanced Nursing*, *61*(6), 711–719.

Carbajal, R., Eriksson, M., Courtois, E., Boyle, E., Avila-Alvarez, A., Andersen, R. D., ... & Papadouri, T. (2015). Sedation and analgesia practices in neonatal intensive care units (EUROPAIN): Results from a prospective cohort study. *The Lancet Respiratory Medicine*, *3*(10), 796–812.

Cignacco, E., Sellam, G., Stoffel, L., Gerull, R., Nelle, M., Anand, K. J. S., Engberg, S. (2012). Oral Sucrose and 'Facilitated Tucking' for Repeated Pain Relief in Preterms: A Randomized Controlled Trial. *Pediatrics* 129, 2.

Cong, X., McGrath, J. M., Delaney, C., Chen, H., Liang, S., Vazquez, V., ... & Dejong, A. (2014). Neonatal nurses' perceptions of pain management: Survey of the United States and China. *Pain Management Nursing*, *15*(4), 834–844.

De Graaf, J., van Lingen, R. A., Valkenburg, A. J., Weisglas-Kuperus, N., Jebbink, L. G., Wijnberg-Williams, B., ... & Van Dijk, M. (2013). Does neonatal morphine use affect neuropsychological outcomes at 8 to 9 years of age? *PAIN*, *154*(3), 449–458.

de Melo, G. M. D., Lélis, A. L. P. D. A., Moura, A. F. D., Cardoso, M. V. L. M. L., & Silva, V. M. D. (2014). Pain assessment scales in newborns: Integrative review. *Revista Paulista de Pediatria*, *32*(4), 395–402.

Durrmeyer, X., Vutskits, L., Anand, K. J. S., Rimensberger, P. (2010). Use of Analgesic and Sedative Drugs in the NNU: Integrating Clinical Trials and Laboratory Data. *Pediatric Research*. *67*(2), 117–127.

Elias, L. S. D. T., dos Santos, A. M. N., & Guinsburg, R. (2014). Perception of pain and distress in intubated and mechanically ventilated newborn infants by parents and health professionals. *BMC Pediatrics*, *14*(1), 44.

Fitzgerald, M. (2015). What do we really know about newborn infant pain? *Experimental Physiology*, *100*(12), 1451–1457.

Franck, L. S., Oulton, K., Nderitu, S., Lim, M., Fang, S., & Kaiser, A. (2011). Parent involvement in pain management for NICU infants: A randomized controlled trial. *Pediatrics*, *128*(3), 510–518.

Guedj, R., Danan, C., Daoud, P., Zupan, V., Renolleau, S., Zana, E., ... & Durand, P. (2014). Does neonatal pain management in intensive care units differ between night and day? An observational study. *BMJ Open*, *4*(2), e004086.

Harrison, D., Bueno, M., & Reszel, J. (2015). Prevention and management of pain and stress in the neonate. *Research Reports in Neonatology*, *5*, 9–16.

Holsti, L., Grunau, R. E., Oberlander, T. F., & Whitfield, M. F. (2005). Prior pain induces heightened motor responses during clustered care in preterm infants in the NICU. *Early Human Development*, *81*(3), 293–302.

Holsti, L., & Grunau, R. E. (2007). Initial validation of the behavioral indicators of infant pain (BIIP). *Pain*, *132*(3), 264–272.

Howard, R., Carter, B., Curry, J., Jain, A., Liossi, C., Morton, N., ... & Williams, G. (2012). Good practice in postoperative and procedural pain management. *Paediatric Anaesthesia*, *22*(July Sup), 1–79.

Kozer, E., Rosenbloom, E., Goldman, D., Lavy, G., Rosenfeld, N., & Goldman, M. (2006). Pain in infants who are younger than 2 months during suprapubic aspiration and transurethral bladder catheterization: A randomized, controlled study. *Pediatrics*, *118*(1), e51–e56.

Lawrence, J., Alcock, D., McGrath, P., Kay, J., MacMurray, S. B., & Dulberg, C. (1993). The development of a tool to assess neonatal pain. *Neonatal Network, 12*(6), 59–66.

Marfurt-Russenberger, K., Axelin, A., Kesselring, A., Franck, L. S., & Cignacco, E. (2016). The experiences of professionals regarding involvement of parents in neonatal pain management. *Journal of Obstetric, Gynecologic & Neonatal Nursing, 45*(5), 671–683.

Mitchell, A., Stevens, B., Mungan, N., Johnson, W., Lobert, S., & Boss, B. (2004). Analgesic effects of oral sucrose and pacifier during eye examinations for retinopathy of prematurity. *Pain Management Nursing, 5*(4), 160–168.

Newnham, C. A., Inder, T. E., & Milgrom, J. (2009). Measuring preterm cumulative stressors within the NICU: the Neonatal Infant Stressor Scale. *Early Human Development, 85*(9), 549–555.

Peters, J. W., Koot, H. M., Grunau, R. E., de Boer, J., van Druenen, M. J., Tibboel, D., & Duivenvoorden, H. J. (2003). Neonatal Facial Coding System for assessing postoperative pain in infants: item reduction is valid and feasible. *The Clinical Journal of Pain, 19*(6), 353–363.

Peters, J. W., Schouw, R., Anand, K. J., van Dijk, M., Duivenvoorden, H. J., & Tibboel, D. (2005). Does neonatal surgery lead to increased pain sensitivity in later childhood? *Pain, 114*(3), 444–454.

Pillai Riddell, R. R., & Craig, K. D. (2006). Judgments of infant pain: The impact of caregiver identity and infant age. *Journal of Pediatric Psychology, 32*(5), 501–511.

Prestes, A. C. Y., Balda, R. D. C. X., dos Santos, G. M. S., de Souza Rugolo, L. M. S., Bentlin, M. R., Magalhães, M., ... & Guinsburg, R. (2016). Painful procedures and analgesia in the NNU: What has changed in the medical perception and practice in a ten-year period? *Jornal de Pediatria (Versão em Português), 92*(1), 88–95.

Provenzi, L., Fumagalli, M., Sirgiovanni, I., Giorda, R., Pozzoli, U., Morandi, F., ... & Montirosso, R. (2015). Pain-related stress during the Neonatal Intensive Care Unit stay and SLC6A4 methylation in very preterm infants. *Frontiers in Behavioral Neuroscience, 9*, 99.

Raeside, L. (2013). Neonatal pain: Theory and concepts. *Working Papers in Health Sciences, 1*(4), 1–6.

Rana, D. (2017). Reduced narcotic and sedative utilization in a NNU after implementation of pain management guidelines. *Journal of Perinatology 37*(9), 1038.

Schwaller, F., & Fitzgerald, M. (2014). The consequences of pain in early life: Injury-induced plasticity in developing pain pathways. *European Journal of Neuroscience, 39*(3), 344–352.

Slater, R., Fitzgerald, M., & Meek, J. (2007). Can cortical responses following noxious stimulation inform us about pain processing in neonates? *Seminars in Perinatology, 31*(5), 298–302.

Spence, K. (2000). The best interest principle as a standard for decision making in the care of neonates. *Journal of Advanced Nursing, 31*(6), 1286–1292.

Spence, K., Gillies, D., Harrison, D., Johnston, L., & Nagy, S. (2005). A reliable pain assessment tool for clinical assessment in the neonatal intensive care unit. *Journal of Obstetric, Gynecologic, & Neonatal Nursing, 34*(1), 80–86.

Spence, K., Henderson-Smart, D., New, K., Evans, C., Whitelaw, J., Woolnough, R., & Australian and New Zealand Neonatal Network. (2010). Evidencd-based clinical practice guideline for management of newborn pain. *Journal of Paediatrics and Child Health, 46*(4), 184–192.

Stevens, B. J., Gibbins, S., Yamada, J., Dionne, K., Lee, G., Johnston, C., & Taddio, A. (2014). The premature infant pain profile-revised (PIPP-R): initial validation and feasibility. *The Clinical Journal of Pain, 30*(3), 238–243.

Taddio, A., Lee, C., Yip, A., Parvez, B., McNamara, P. J., & Shah, V. (2006). Intravenous morphine and topical tetracaine for treatment of pain in preterm neonates undergoing central line placement. *Journal of the American Medical Association, 295*(7), 793–800.

The Hospital for Sick Children ('SickKids'). (2017) *Guidelines for Pain Assessment and Management for Neonates*. Toronto: SickKids.

Van Dijk, M., Peters, J. W., Van Deventer, P., & Tibboel, D. (2005). The COMFORT Behavior Scale: a tool for assessing pain and sedation in infants. *The American Journal of Nursing, 105*(1), 33–36.

Van Ganzewinkel, C., Derijks, L., Anand, K. J. S., Van Lingen, R. A., Neef, C., Kramer, B. W., & Andriessen, P. (2014). Multiple intravenous doses of paracetamol result in a predictable pharmacokinetic profile in very preterm infants. *Acta Paediatrica*, *103*(6), 612–617.

Verriotis, M., Chang, P., Fitzgerald, M., & Fabrizi, L. (2016). The development of the nociceptive brain. *Neuroscience*, *338*, 207–219.

Vinall, J., Miller, S. P., Bjornson, B. H., Fitzpatrick, K. P., Poskitt, K. J., Brant, R., … & Grunau, R. E. (2014). Invasive procedures in preterm children: Brain and cognitive development at school age. *Pediatrics*, *133*(3), 412.

Walker, S. M., Franck, L. S., Fitzgerald, M., Myles, J., Stocks, J., & Marlow, N. (2009). Long-term impact of neonatal intensive care and surgery on somatosensory perception in children born extremely preterm. *PAIN*, *141*(1–2), 79–87.

Warren, I., Hicks, B., Kleberg, A., Eliahoo, J., Anand, K. J., & Hickson, M. (2016). The validity and reliability of the EV aluation of IN tervention Scale: Preliminary report. *Acta Paediatrica*, *105*(6), 618–622.

7 NEONATAL PALLIATIVE CARE

Sharon Nurse

CONTENTS

GUIDANCE ON HOW TO ENHANCE PERSONAL LEARNING FROM THIS CHAPTER

Key points covered in this chapter

- The principles of neonatal palliative care.
- Decision-making and assessment of the family needs in relation to neonatal palliative care including a consideration of the barriers.
- Family and staff support strategies for neonatal palliative care.

Reflection

Reading through the chapter, you are encouraged to engage with the key points and related literature in an enquiring way. Ask these questions:

- What important aspects of care would you consider when dealing with an baby and family who require palliative care?
- How does this chapter closely link with chapters 8 and 9 on bereavement care and ethical issues in the neonatal unit?
- What guidance is available to provide key information about this area of practice?

Implications for nursing care

- Finally: how will this chapter enable you to understand the principles of best practice for neonatal palliative care? Consider the implications of what you learn for your nursing care relating to this area.

INTRODUCTION AND BACKGROUND

Perinatal palliative care refers to the provision of services for expectant parents who receive a diagnosis of a life-limiting foetal condition which might result in the baby living for only hours or days, although some may live for much longer. The charity Together for Short Lives defines it as follows: '*Palliative care for a foetus, neonate, or infant with a life-limiting condition is an active and total approach to care, from the point of diagnosis or recognition, throughout the child's life, at the time of death and beyond*' (Dickson, 2017, p. 13). Before the invention of ventilators and synthetic drugs, neonatologists could do little else for premature babies but keep them warm, feed them breast milk and isolate them from other individuals – essentially this was palliative care (Marc-Aurele and English, 2017). However, neonatology has made significant advances in the last 30 years and despite the developments in treatments, some infants do not have good outcomes. Therefore, a palliative care model is required within the neonatal context (Kilcullen and Ireland, 2017). While improvements have occurred in family-centred care, communication, pain management and bereavement care, there remains a need to integrate palliative care with intensive care rather than wait until the terminal phase of a baby's life when they are imminently dying (Carter, 2018). Many deaths in this context occur in the acute setting of the neonatal unit (NNU) Twamley et al., 2012. Currently, the prolonged lifespan of babies who are extremely premature or have more complex health needs is mostly due to early diagnosis and intervention during pregnancy as well as improved medical and surgical treatments. Overall, not every baby can survive their condition and associated neonatal care, and indeed many will have life-limiting conditions which require expert care for the duration of their short lives.

This chapter will examine the options for care available to families of babies with life-limiting conditions as well as principles of palliative care considering cultural, spiritual and emotional dimensions. The barriers to implementation of family-centred palliative care, education and support for staff will also be included. This chapter should be read in conjunction with chapters 8 and 9 which cover bereavement care and ethical issues respectively, as the principles and issues are closely linked.

PRINCIPLES OF NEONATAL PALLIATIVE CARE

Midwives play a vital role in foetal assessment and diagnosis of life-limiting conditions in pregnancy, but also in bereavement counselling following diagnosis, as well as supporting parents in the planning and preparation of the birth and immediate postnatal care (Peacock et al., 2015). Throughout the pregnancy there should be parallel planning whereby a palliative care approach is initiated while ongoing support and antenatal care is provided by midwives, obstetricians and children's hospices staff where appropriate. It has become apparent that the involvement of children's hospice should be integral to palliative care provision in order to deliver holistic care for babies and their families. Research has indicated that although expert neonatal nursing care is vital for babies in their final hours of life, where a palliative care consultation was sought during pregnancy, fewer medical procedures were carried out on the baby and increased support services were already in place ready to assist following the baby's birth (Twamley et al., 2012).

The British Association of Perinatal Medicine (BAPM) produced national guidance in the form of a framework for clinical practice (2011) which sets out the principles of palliative care for infants in the perinatal setting (see figure 7.1). Mancini et al. (2014) published specific guidance to neonatal nurses delivering palliative care in the acute neonatal setting.

Principles of care should embrace physical, emotional, social and spiritual elements and focus on enhancement of quality of life for the infant and support for the family. It

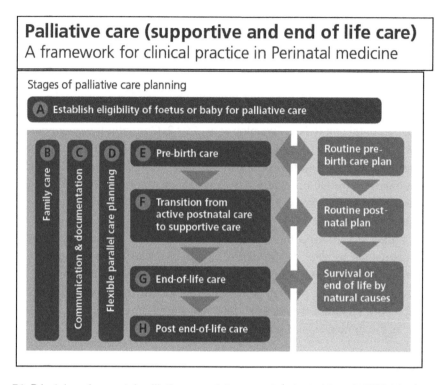

Palliative care (supportive and end of life care)
A framework for clinical practice in Perinatal medicine

Stages of palliative care planning

(A) Establish eligibility of foetus or baby for palliative care

(B) Family care (C) Communication & documentation (D) Flexible parallel care planning

(E) Pre-birth care → Routine pre-birth care plan

(F) Transition from active postnatal care to supportive care → Routine post-natal plan

(G) End-of-life care → Survival or end of life by natural causes

(H) Post end-of-life care

Figure 7.1 Principles of neonatal palliative care: A framework (adapted from BAPM, 2011)

includes the management of distressing symptoms, the provision of short breaks and care through death and bereavement (Dickson, 2017).

DECISION-MAKING IN PALLIATIVE CARE IN NEONATOLOGY

Not all babies will be suitable for palliative care, as sadly some babies' conditions may deteriorate rapidly, preventing a plan of care or choices for parents who have been given the diagnosis of a life-limiting condition early in pregnancy. An overview of the types of conditions that are deemed appropriate for palliative care are outlined in table 7.1. Protocols for end-of-life care must be in place for any pregnancy or newborn baby where complex needs are likely to present, so that they are managed effectively but sensitively. Decisions should be made as to which babies are suitable for palliative care and consideration given as to the impact that kind of care will have on the whole family. It is also important to consider the setting in which palliative care will be offered; if this includes hospice or homecare then support and collaboration with hospice and community staff is required urgently to plan appropriate but realistic care.

TABLE 7.1 CONDITIONS FOR PERINATAL PALLIATIVE CARE

Category 1	An antenatal or postnatal diagnosis of a condition which is not compatible with long-term survival, e.g. bilateral renal agenesis or anencephaly.
Category 2	An antenatal or postnatal diagnosis of a condition which carries a high risk of significant morbidity or death, e.g. severe bilateral hydronephrosis and impaired renal function.
Category 3	Babies born at the margins of viability, where intensive care has been deemed inappropriate.
Category 4	Postnatal clinical conditions with a high risk of severe impairment of quality of life and when the baby is receiving life support or may at some point require life support, e.g. severe hypoxic-ischaemic encephalopathy.
Category 5	Postnatal conditions which result in the baby experiencing 'unbearable suffering' during their illness or treatment, e.g. severe necrotising enterocolitis, where palliative care is in the baby's best interests.

(adapted from BAPM, 2011)

Palliative care might be described as short term or long term. Short term refers to cases where there is withdrawal of life-sustaining treatment like ventilation, after which the baby might be expected to live only a few hours or days. Long-term palliative care will apply in cases when baby is likely to live for a longer period of time or it is anticipated that there is more time for family involvement and participation in the care of the baby, thereby impacting on quality of life.

Ethical dilemmas are inherent in making difficult decisions regarding withdrawal of treatment in the NNU, sometimes resulting in conflict between parents and staff, or indeed between staff members. Moreover, the multidisciplinary team may face new ethical considerations when parents continue pregnancies after receiving life-limiting foetal diagnoses and desire palliative care (Mendes et al., 2017). In this milieu of rapid advancements in diagnostics and interventions, continued risk for significant morbidity and mortality, and uncertainty regarding outcomes, ethical challenges are ever-present (Marty and Carter, 2018). Obviously, discussions will take place between the multidisciplinary team using all current clinical evidence pertaining to the baby's condition before and after consulting parents. Conversations with parents must be honest and respectful, avoiding inconsistent communication and in clear language, so that multiple interpretations do not affect parental responses and decisions impacting on palliative interventions for the baby (Mendes et al., 2017). Stories in the press of 'miracle babies' often portray cures, but do not expand on the morbidity rates and long-term challenges for children and their families later. Every hospital Trust in the UK has a clinical ethics committee which can be helpful when opinions differ and a consensus between staff and/or parents cannot be reached. (Ethical issues are discussed in greater detail in chapter 9). It is vital throughout the decision-making process that parents are reassured that withdrawal of treatment does not mean withdrawal of care, but merely a shift in the focus of care.

MULTI-AGENCY ASSESSMENT OF THE FAMILY'S NEEDS

Designing a care plan that is holistic but realistic is a challenge in itself; involvement of all stakeholders is essential and effective communication between members of the multidisciplinary team is vital if the care is to be provided in a seamless, cohesive manner (Parravicini, 2017).

With reference to Together for Short Lives guidance the following points should be considered:

- Multi-agency planning should commence as soon as possible after diagnosis of a life-limiting condition during pregnancy; this might involve neonatal staff, obstetrician, General Practitioner (GP), health visitor, social worker, community children's nurses, children's hospice, community palliative care nurses, nutritionists and others.
- There should be a holistic approach to planning and implementation of care.
- The baby should always be central to the process and the family a part of the team caring for their baby.
- Family integrated care should be practised always.
- The family's religious, spiritual, cultural and personal beliefs should be respected.
- Jargon-free language should be used and written information provided where possible. Interpreters should be employed where necessary.
- Assessment information and care plans should be freely accessible to the family.
- There should be clarity in who is taking the lead role in the baby's care.
- Contact details of all relevant staff should be made available to parents (Dickson, 2017).

The children's palliative care team should be involved from the antenatal diagnosis where possible, so that advice and guidance can be offered well in advance of their involvement after the baby's birth. The earlier palliative care nurse contact is initiated, the sooner this enables the development of relationships and the building of trust between parents and staff who will provide support later. A visit to the children's hospice might be beneficial, allowing parents to meet the staff and familiarise themselves with the facilities available to them as a family.

PALLIATIVE CARE SETTING

Choices available to parents of babies requiring palliative care:

- Remain in NNU (preferably in a side room)
- Antenatal or postnatal ward (side room) with neonatal nurse's support
- Transfer to children's hospice
- Home to family with support from palliative care community staff, GP and hospital contact.

The 'place of care' may not always be the preferred 'place of death' and should be decided by the family with appropriate support and guidance (Craig and Mancini, 2013). Parents need information to assist them in making the right decision for their family and working together with the healthcare team in providing quality care. To facilitate changes in the baby's condition and how this impacts on care goals, it is vital that there is good communication between parents and staff. Timing of information is crucial to allow parents to plan transfers and familiarise themselves with new surroundings such as the hospice and staff. Some parents may need to make appropriate adaptations to their home to facilitate the equipment necessary in caring for the baby.

Detailed, clear information is required regarding potential changes in their baby's condition, feeding, medications required and the management in response to ongoing symptoms. Homecare, while suitable for some families, will require greater support from community staff, and this may not always be feasible. Installation of equipment and administration of medicines may raise additional barriers to implementing a homecare plan – this must be realistic. Neonatal units may not have access to neonatal community teams, meaning that many babies will receive care from generic children's nursing teams who may not have specialised palliative care experience.

Home or hospice care

This type of care often provides a more family-centred environment where siblings and grandparents can become more involved. A step-down approach to palliative care can be challenging for some parents after the high-tech NICU environment. Currently, neonatal services across the UK are striving to develop stronger links between children's hospice services and palliative care teams in the community to provide quality homecare. Ideally, these children's services should work closely with neonatal staff to provide neonatal palliative care in the home, resulting in the optimum model of care (Engelder et al., 2012). Local models of homecare will differ, but they must be family-centred, allowing flexibility so that issues such as location, professional expertise and nursing care are all facilitated (National Health Service (NHS) England, 2018). Together for Short Lives highlight the need for multi-agency care planning and go so far as to provide guidance for extubation at home within a children's palliative care framework (Dickson, 2017).

Palliative care in the neonatal unit

This entails managing the baby's care once the decision has been made to withdraw life-sustaining treatment. Mancini et al. (2014) suggest the following themes for consideration when planning care:

■　　Discussion with parents regarding matters such as location of care delivery, which family members will be present, special requests regarding involvement in care.

photographs, films, memory-making such as footprints, handprints and artwork. If appropriate, discussions around the possibility of a post-mortem may be required and assistance with arranging the funeral.

- Pain relief: The intravenous (IV) route is preferable for rapid symptom management, non-pharmacological interventions such as non-nutritive sucking, reduced noise and light, music, comfort positioning, cuddling baby and breastfeeding if appropriate.

- Physiological monitoring – monitors should be disconnected with visual monitoring by nurses and auscultation when necessary.

- Fluids and nutrition are only to be administered if the baby is expected to survive for more than a few hours, but the baby's cues need to be responded to in order to avoid distress or suffering. If possible avoid insertion of central lines or peripheral IV lines. Hospice or homecare feeding will require parental training and support by community staff.

- Ventilation and oxygen – explanations for parents regarding extubation, the procedure itself and the effects on the baby (death may not follow extubation immediately). Parents may wish to hold the baby throughout the procedure with nursing support.

- Location of care: privacy in the NNU, preferably a side room. Transfer to hospice if baby is expected to survive for a prolonged period (previously discussed with parents and the hospice place booked in advance). Liaison between hospice and senior medical/nursing staff in the NNU is essential. Homecare requires a good community palliative care team, GP support, and liaison with local hospital and ambulance service.

SUPPORT FOR FAMILIES

Following delivery of the baby, the parents should be cared for with the utmost sensitivity and compassion and all staff should be aware of the situation before entering the room. Kenner et al. (2015) provided a series of considerations in supporting grieving parents:

- Psychological and emotional support: Nursing and medical staff will be the primary providers of immediate emotional and psychological support to families offering suitable choices tailored to their needs (Mancini et al., 2014; Hall et al., 2015).

- Professionals should be aware of the stages of grieving and recognise distress in families, finding ways of engaging and exploring their feelings and emotions. Psychosocial support should be offered to grandparents and siblings also.

- Where necessary, translation should be available, so that every parent is treated equally with cultural and religious needs being addressed.

- Parents may require support if they have another sick baby in the NNU or siblings at home. Social services may be of help in arranging support and financial advice where required.

- Support and guidance might be required around decisions on post-mortem examination and organ donation to validate the family's loss.

- Contact details of staff members/support groups both within the hospital and outside should be made available to families.
- Formal appointments with consultants and bereavement counsellors may be arranged if parents wish to avail themselves of the services. A follow-up appointment around 6 to 8 weeks following the baby's death should be arranged with the lead consultant and named nurse to address any unanswered questions or concerns and to discuss the autopsy report if applicable.

Spiritual support for parents

'*Facing neonatal loss is frequently experienced as traumatic assault on parents' spiritual and existential world of meaning*' (Rosenbaum et al., 2011, p. 84). Families may have made decisions which have left them feeling guilty and bereft from a cultural and spiritual perspective. It is vital for parents to feel that the decision to withhold life-sustaining treatment is a shared one, or that hospital staff suggested the plan of action thereby relinquishing any fears or guilt on their part. Each family's experience of grief will be unique, but it is imperative that health professionals respect and support spiritual practices during and following the baby's death. Nurses should contact the family's religious advisor, or in the absence of this person, the hospital chaplain will be on call for emergencies. Being experienced in supporting families through death in bereavement, chaplains can be very helpful in supporting families while navigating the NNU experience. Nurses may feel inadequate or helpless to relieve the sadness and loss that parents are experiencing while their baby is dying, but Rosenbaum et al. (2011, p. 67) argue that '*the power of presence is profound*' and that just being there for them and acknowledging their loss can mean so much to families. Being respectful of the family's faith and providing a private and peaceful environment enabling them to carry out their religious practices is extremely important as it hopefully will help them achieve spiritual peace.

KEY POINTS WHEN PLANNING DISCHARGE FROM THE NEONATAL UNIT

Together for Short Lives suggest that the discharge planning team should consist of the parents, family GP, neonatologist, neonatal nursing and community staff (palliative care and children's nurses) (Dickson, 2017). Table 7.2 outlines issues which need to be addressed to make the transition or 'step-down' from neonatal care to home or hospice as smooth as possible.

CARE OF THE BABY AND FAMILY AT THE POINT OF DEATH

Care of the dying baby is discussed in chapter 8 and so only specific palliative care issues relating to the death of the baby at home or in hospice care will be summarised in this section.

TABLE 7.2 ISSUES FOR CONSIDERATION WHEN PLANNING DISCHARGE FROM THE NNU

Environment	Does the home environment have sufficient space for the baby, equipment and the rest of the family?
Equipment	■ Shape and size may make transportation and installation difficult. ■ Oxygen and suction may need to be installed. ■ Parents must be trained in using some equipment. ■ Maintenance and safety in the home must be considered.
Nursing needs	■ Level of professional nursing care required? ■ What percentage of care will be carried out by parents? ■ Are there any potential gaps in the service provision? ■ Will there always be provision of expert palliative care nurses?
Routine medication	Only essential medicines will be continued via an easily accessible route.
Symptom management	Written symptom management plans and education of parents regarding these is vital.
Feeding plan	Is enteral feeding alone appropriate? Comfort rather than nutritional goals may become a priority. Parents need to be taught how to feed their baby.
Ongoing/flexible care plans	The baby may not die within the anticipated timeframe, so frequent care plan reviews are essential. Consider the use of checklists to ensure nothing is missed (Taylor et al., 2018).
24-hour access to parental support and advice	Identify individuals/groups and their contact details to ensure timely responses to requests for help.
Hospital readmission	Agree thresholds and arrangements for readmission prior to discharge.
Care team	Multidisciplinary team involvement – all teams should have relevant information on care plans, symptom management and ongoing care.
Care after death	■ Who is contacted? ■ Confirmation and certification of baby's death. ■ Transfer to funeral home and burial advice.
Parental education	Goals of care, carrying out baby's care needs, expectations, medicines administration and who to call for help in the emergency.

Hopefully a plan of care has already been agreed between parents and professionals about how they would like their baby's care to be carried out in the final moments. It is important that the parents have the care and support of nurses with whom they have developed a trusting relationship, so that a family-centred approach to care is used, particularly when siblings and other family members are present.

The following suggestions might enhance the quality of care and the overall experience of the family at this emotional time (Dickson, 2017):

■ The environment should be quiet and peaceful with appropriate light and comfort measures available to baby and family, utilising home furnishings such as cushions, blankets etc.

■ The family may need someone to take any phone calls and engage with visitors, ensuring that the parents have undisturbed, private time with their baby.

■ Nursing staff should make themselves available but remain unobtrusive, only attending to the baby's needs when necessary.

■ Pain relief should be managed as before, but used judiciously at this point in time. Comfort measures such as cuddling, kangaroo care, non-nutritive sucking, or lying together with parents and siblings could be employed.

■ Parents may wish to move to a specific place, a room, a garden or somewhere that holds significance for them as a family. Nurses should assist them with transferring the baby or any equipment needed.

■ Hospice community nurses often spend time with siblings if parents feel they need to be alone with their baby at the end, or perhaps have anxieties about siblings' possible reactions to death. This is a good time to engage brothers and sisters in memory-making activities or storytelling.

Cultural needs should also be met. The family may have expressed a wish to engage in practices relative to their faith and this should be facilitated if the baby is being cared for in a hospice environment. Some suggestions for consideration:

■ Using simple terms and phrases with help from a translator if necessary.

■ Providing written material in the family's primary language where possible.

■ Awareness of culturally appropriate behaviour, e.g. eye contact or touch is sometimes considered inappropriate.

■ Extra sensitivity may be required if the baby has a congenital malformation as in some cultures the mother may be blamed.

■ An autopsy may be refused possibly leading to the need for a court order.

■ Some cultures do not encourage holding or touching a dead or dying baby or the use of pain-relieving measures; this can be challenging for some healthcare professionals.

■ Fear of the unknown and basic distrust of authority figures could make communication and trust quite difficult so having someone from the same religion or ethnicity would be helpful (Catlin and Carter, 2002).

■ Culturally sensitive grief counselling or contact with parents from a similar cultural ethnicity may be beneficial to grieving parents.

SUPPORT FOR NEONATAL STAFF IN THE PROVISION OF PALLIATIVE CARE

Emotional support

Providing care for dying babies and support for the parents is very intense. Ideally all staff involved should have access to clinical psychologists, counsellors or at least 'time out' with senior staff to engage in discussions and debriefing where necessary. Care-related grief may be magnified in the neonatal nurse who has developed a relationship with the family over a period of time. An ongoing source of stress and anxiety, particularly for junior neonatal nurses, is that of lacking confidence and perceived lack of competence in caring for babies and their families at the end of life (Nurse and Price, 2017). A large percentage of nurses in the study by Peng et al. (2013) expressed a lack of knowledge in pain control management or recognition of symptoms of pain and distress. Calls for increased education in pre- and post-registration programmes on end-of-life and palliative care is evident in literature owing to the low percentages of staff having palliative care experience (Contros et al., 2004; Thompson and Hall, 2007). Professionals in the NNU often feel compelled to balance the ethical principles of beneficence and non-maleficence in order to provide morally focused care and a 'good death' for the baby (Mendel, 2014).

These simple suggestions might go some way in providing psychological and emotional support for nurses affected by bereavement in the NNU:

■ Peer support or a 'buddying' scheme for more junior members of staff.
■ Acknowledge your colleague's pain with a chat or a hug.
■ A telephone call when off duty from the manager.
■ Staff meetings where outward displays of emotion can be acknowledged in a more private setting and appropriate support offered (Welborn, 2017).
■ Sessions on self-care to reduce the risk of burn-out from compassion fatigue.
■ Multidisciplinary meetings where specific cases are discussed, and everyone's perspective is respected, creating an environment conducive to learning and healing.

Education of staff

Research identifies that continuing education in palliative care and bereavement is essential to enhancing nurses' confidence and competence (Mancini et al., 2013; Kain, 2013; 2017). However, it has also been identified that there is a lack of specific training in palliative care (Gilmour et al., 2017). Unfortunately, end-of-life care in NNUs is frequently delivered in an inconsistent manner, particularly when clear practice guidelines are absent (Marchuk, 2016). A neonatal palliative care education programme (Mancini, 2011) within the North West London Perinatal Network, accessed by 183 health professionals in the first year, resulted in improved palliative care in the region.

Education in end-of-life/palliative care should include:

■ Communicating appropriately/supporting parents and families (culturally and spiritually).
■ Practical care of the baby including pain management and other comfort measures.
■ Liaison with the multidisciplinary team and hospital staff.
■ Care of the baby and family at the point of death (family-centred care).
■ Making memories.
■ Bereavement support mechanisms in hospital and community.

Education can be offered in the form of conferences, study days, short study sessions, simulation-based scenarios, interactive workshops on communication as well as online education programmes.

With staff shortages and increasing difficulty in releasing staff for study, it is important to consider a more blended learning approach utilising online resources alongside shorter face-to-face teaching sessions, enabling education to be more accessible for learners. Integration of education into everyday practice requires mentorship of more inexperienced staff by senior practitioners, practice educators, advanced neonatal nurse practitioners and medical staff in order to create an environment conducive to learning and increasing confidence (Nurse and Price, 2017). Training and education in neonatal palliative care should become a mandatory requirement in all neonatal curricula and meet agreed national standards to ensure equity of quality care across the region. Table 7.3 outlines suggestions as to the way forward in neonatal palliative care education.

BARRIERS TO THE PROVISION OF NEONATAL PALLIATIVE CARE

Barriers have been identified as those including nurses' values and moral dilemmas, beneficence and non-maleficence, nurses' exposure to death, emotional control and protection, stress, grief, lack of optimal environment, and lack of education in palliative care principles (Kilcullen and Ireland, 2017). Kain (2006) identified common themes in barriers due to nurses' past traumatic experiences relating to death, difficulties in communication with parents, conflicting opinions when making decisions, the NNU environment, lack of peer support and again, no formal training. Nurse education still lacks the appropriate content, leaving nurses feeling unsure and unable to provide competent, high-quality palliative care (Kain, 2006; Martin, 2013).

One interesting suggestion is the difficulty for some staff to change from a curative to palliative model of care and the baby's impending death engendering a sense of failure for them. Other barriers can be attributed to inadequate environmental conditions in the NNU,

TABLE 7.3 GOALS OF NEONATAL PALLIATIVE CARE EDUCATION

- Time-out sessions where staff explore their own beliefs and perceptions about death debating ethical dilemmas and legal issues which might impact on delivery of care in the NNU.
- Information on attitudes and behaviours used alongside specific skills and knowledge provided as formal education sessions but also incorporated into clinical practice through mentorship.
- A bespoke education pack in each NNU with information on practice guidelines, bereavement follow-up information, memory-making and other information for more junior staff and students.
- Mentorship or 'buddying' for junior staff by senior nurses in NNU enabling them to learn in practice.
- Teaching at the cot side by experienced staff.
- Increased collaboration with children's palliative care nurses; intra-disciplinary learning.
- Working alongside palliative care staff, either through secondment programmes or post-graduate training programmes.
- Specific neonatal palliative care modules offered as online, interactive learning making education more accessible to busy staff.
- Clear learning objectives set out for practitioners.
- Competencies clearly set out and once achieved should be signed off by senior/ education staff.
- Delivery of education using 'in-house' sessions enabling better attendance.
- Regular and sustained skills sessions as part of internal training programmes within hospitals.
- Nurses' teaching ward rounds or problem-based learning sessions.
- Simulation teaching both in the hospital and universities for educating staff in clinical and communication skills as well as team-working and leadership skills.

such as lack of space, lack of comfortable chairs, lack of privacy, and minimal parental and family facilities.

Barriers also may exist in offering choices with regard to the place of care, and how care is delivered. Timing and initiation of palliative care can be problematic when decisions are still pending on diagnosis and prognosis. Hospice care is still not considered an option for some neonatal staff, partly due to lack of awareness of the services available and the expertise therein. With a consideration of homecare, funding for vital equipment and its servicing remain problematic (Noyes, 2002). Communication between hospital and community services can result in a reduction in choice for parents at an already stressful time in their life.

The timing of when to start advance care planning conversations remains an issue for healthcare professionals. The value of doing this in stages and considering the environment where the conversations are held is important. Timely planning is vital to avoid difficult conversations at a crisis point and for coordination of care. Good advance care planning is to provide the best person-centred care for the child and experience for the family (Jack et al., 2018).

Training programmes for staff covering the tenets of palliative care, including symptom management, analgesic use and communication skills, as well as regular multidisciplinary forums and debriefs, are necessary to improve the care provided to all babies with life-limiting and life-threatening conditions and their families (Martin, 2013).

CONCLUSION

To summarise, when a baby is affected by a life-limiting or life-threatening condition and prolongation of survival is no longer feasible or appropriate, a plan of palliative care focusing on the infant's comfort and family support is essential. Moreover, there is a need to guide and standardise practices with the provision of guidelines that address babies' basic needs, to achieve a state of comfort during the course of illness while including and supporting the family throughout. Barriers to provision of effective and compassionate palliative care must be addressed and minimised or eliminated. A multidisciplinary team approach addressing both the infants' medical and non-medical needs, parental grieving process, and healthcare professionals' distress should be embraced.

CASE STUDIES

For each of these cases below:

Q.1. What are the key issues and care considerations for these infants and families?
Q.2. Can you write these out in relation to a plan of palliative care for each one?
Q.3. What are the reasons for your answers?
Q.4. What potential situations may occur that might mean you will need to revise your plan?

Case study 1: The infant with a congenital syndrome

Jacob was born at term and has Edwards Syndrome, which was diagnosed postnatally. His parents are Polish and have lived in the UK for the past two years. They have two other children; Marcos who is four and Katrina who is eight years old. Jacob is now a week old and, following discussion with the neonatal multidisciplinary team (MDT), the decision is made for Jacob to be discharged home for palliative care. The family live in a two-bedroom, third-floor flat.

Case study 2: The infant with severe hypoxia at birth

Devindar is a post-term baby, now 4 days old, who suffered severe hypoxia at birth during a prolonged and difficult labour and has a diagnosis of severe hypoxic-ischaemic encephalopathy. Therapeutic cooling has been undertaken but this did not result in any

C
A
S
E

S
T
U
D
Y

improvement in his condition and he has no spontaneous effort to breath. Devinder's parents are Sikhs and have three older children aged 2, 5 and 14 years old respectively. The nursing team has discussed the situation with the parents and they understand that a plan of palliative care is now the next step in their son's care.

Case study 3: The preterm infant with devastating necrotising enterocolitis

Eve was born at 24 weeks' gestation to parents, Brigit and Patrick, after a sudden delivery 20 minutes after presenting in the labour ward. After an unstable period of ventilation, she had stabilised at age 10 days and was on bi-level continuous positive airway pressure. Early feeding had started via a nasogastric tube and this was being increased slowly. However, Eve developed necrotising enterocolitis on day 11 of life which showed no improvement after medical management. She went to theatre but unfortunately, her bowel was so damaged that none of it was viable, requiring the difficult decision to return her to the neonatal unit for palliative care. Parents are Irish Catholic and have one other boy, Daniel who is 18 months old.

For suggested answer guides to the questions posed in these case studies, please refer to the web-based companion site specific to this chapter (see URL below).

WEB-BASED RESOURCES

For further information, online resources and greater detail on the case studies featured in this chapter go to www.routledge.com/cw/nicnursing

References

British Association of Perinatal Medicine (2011). *Palliative Care: A framework for clinical practice in peri-natal medicine.* London: British Association of Perinatal Medicine.

Carter, B. (2018). Pediatric Palliative Care in Infants and Neonates. *Children, 5*(2), 21.

Catlin, A., & Carter, B. (2002). Creation of a neonatal end-of-life palliative care protocol. *Journal of Perinatology, 22*(3), 184–195.

Contro, N. A., Larson, J., Scofield, S., Sourkes, B., & Cohen, H. J. (2004). Hospital staff and family perspectives regarding quality of pediatric palliative care. *Pediatrics, 114*(1), 1248–1252.

Craig, F., & Mancini, A. (2013). Can we truly offer a choice of place of death in neonatal palliative care? *Seminars in Fetal and Neonatal Medicine, 18*(2): 93–98.

Dickson, G. (2017). A perinatal pathway for babies with palliative care needs. Bristol: Together for Short Lives.

Engelder, S., Davies, K., Zeilinger, T., & Rutledge, D. (2012). A model program for perinatal palliative services. *Advances in Neonatal Care, 12*(1), 28–36.

Gilmour, D., Davies, M. W., & Herbert, A. R. (2017). Adequacy of palliative care in a single tertiary neonatal unit. *Journal of Paediatrics and Child Health, 53*(2), 136–144.

Hall, S. L., Cross, J., Selix, N. W., Patterson, C., Segre, L., Chuffo-Siewert, R., ... & Martin, M. L. (2015). Recommendations for enhancing psychosocial support of NICU parents through staff education and support. *Journal of Perinatology, 35*(S1), S29–S36.

Jack, B. A., Mitchell, T. K., O'Brien, M. R., Silverio, S. A., & Knighting, K. (2018). A qualitative study of health care professionals' views and experiences of paediatric advance care planning. *BMC Palliative Care, 17*(1), 93.

Kain, V. (2006). Palliative care delivery in the NICU: What barriers do neonatal nurses face? *Neonatal Network, 25*(6), 387–392.

Kain, V. J. (2013). An exploration of the grief experiences of neonatal nurses: A focus group study. *Journal of Neonatal Nursing, 19*(2), 80–88.

Kain, V. J. (2017). The Praecox Program: Pilot testing of an online educational program to improve neonatal palliative care practice. *Journal of Neonatal Nursing, 23*(4), 188–192.

Kenner, C., Press, J., & Ryan, D. (2015). Recommendations for palliative and bereavement care in the NICU: a family-centered integrative approach. *Journal of Perinatology, 35*(S1), S19–S23.

Kilcullen, M., & Ireland, S. (2017). Palliative care in the neonatal unit: neonatal nursing staff perceptions of facilitators and barriers in a regional tertiary nursery. *BMC Palliative Care, 16*(1), 32.

Mancini, A. (2011). Developing a neonatal palliative care education programme within the North West London Perinatal Network. *Journal of Neonatal Nursing, 17*(4), 146–149.

Mancini, A., Kelly P., & Bluebond-Lanner, M. (2013). Training staff for the future in neonatal palliative care. *Seminars in Fetal and Neonatal Medicine, 18*; 111–115.

Mancini, A., Uthaya, S., Beardsley, C., Wood, D., & Modi, N. (2014). Practical guidance for the management of palliative care on neonatal units. *London: Royal College of Paediatrics and Child Health*.

Marc-Aurele, K. L., & English, N. K. (2017). Primary palliative care in neonatal intensive care. In *Seminars in Perinatology, 41*(2), 133–139.

Marchuk, A. (2016). End-of-life care in the neonatal intensive care unit: applying comfort theory. *International Journal of Palliative Nursing, 22*(7), 317–323.

Martin, M. (2013). Missed opportunities: a case study of barriers to the delivery of palliative care on neonatal intensive care units. *International Journal of Palliative Nursing, 19*(5), 251–256.

Marty, C. M., & Carter, B. S. (2018). Ethics and palliative care in the perinatal world. In *Seminars in Fetal and Neonatal Medicine, 23*(1), 35–38.

Mendel, T. R. (2014). The use of neonatal palliative care: Reducing moral distress in NICU nurses. *Journal of Neonatal Nursing, 20*(6), 290–293.

Mendes, J., Wool, J., & Wool, C. (2017). Ethical Considerations in Perinatal Palliative Care. *Journal of Obstetric, Gynecologic & Neonatal Nursing, 46*(3), 367–377.

National Health Service (NHS) England (2018). *Increasing neonatal palliative care support*. NHS England.

Noyes, J. (2002). Barriers that delay children and young people who are dependent on mechanical ventilators from being discharged from hospital. *Journal of Clinical Nursing, 11*(1), 2–11.

Nurse, S., & Price, J. (2017). 'No second chance'–Junior neonatal nurses experiences of caring for an infant at the end-of-life and their family. *Journal of Neonatal Nursing, 23*(2), 50–57.

Parravicini, E. (2017). Neonatal palliative care. *Current Opinion in Pediatrics, 29*(2), 135–140.

Peacock, V., Price, J., & Nurse, S. (2015). From pregnancy to palliative care: Advancing professional midwifery practice? *The Practising Midwife, 18*(10), 18–20.

Peng, N. H., Chen, C. H., Huang, L. C., Liu, H. L., Lee, M. C., & Sheng, C. C. (2013). The educational needs of neonatal nurses regarding neonatal palliative care. *Nurse Education Today, 33*(12), 1506–1510.

Rosenbaum, J. L., Smith, J. R., & Zollfrank, R. (2011). Neonatal end-of-life spiritual support care. *The Journal of Perinatal & Neonatal Nursing, 25*(1), 61–69.

Taylor, N., Liang, Y. F., & Tinnion, R. (2018). Neonatal palliative care: A practical checklist approach. *BMJ Supportive & Palliative Care*, bmjspcare-2018.

Thompson, L., & Hall, C. (2007). Exploring student nurses educational needs in relation to end-of-life care in children. *Journal of Children's and Young People's Nursing, 1*(6), 281–286.

Twamley, K., Kelly, P., Moss, R., Mancini, A., Craig, F., Koh, M., ... & Bluebond-Langner, M. (2013). Palliative care education in neonatal units: impact on knowledge and attitudes. *BMJ Supportive & Palliative Care, 3*(2), 213–220.

Welborn, A. C. (2017). Supporting the neonatal nurse in the role of final comforter. *Journal of Neonatal Nursing, 23*(2), 58–64.

8 NEONATAL BEREAVEMENT CARE

Jo Cookson

CONTENTS

GUIDANCE ON HOW TO ENHANCE PERSONAL LEARNING FROM THIS CHAPTER

Key points covered in this chapter

- Definitions of loss and grief, and the nature of the grieving process.
- How to care for families experiencing a bereavement on the NNU.
- The wider impact of the perinatal loss of a baby.

Reflection

Reading through the chapter, you are encouraged to engage with the key points and related literature in an enquiring way. Ask these questions:

- What reactions and behaviours can you expect from grieving parents, and how can you in turn respond to them in a supportive manner?
- How can you effectively approach bereavement care in accordance with the parents' wishes, with the aim that they may reflect in a positive light on this later on?
- What are your considerations following the death of a baby with regard to the wider family and ongoing support for the parents following discharge home?

Implications for nursing care

- Finally: this chapter should facilitate your understanding of perinatal loss, and how to care for affected families. How might your nursing care be impacted by what you have learned?

INTRODUCTION AND BACKGROUND

The death of a neonate is a comparatively rare event in the western world and remains one of the greatest challenges in the neonatal unit (NNU). For parents, the profound and often unexpected loss results in a complex process of grieving and attempts to find strategies of coping with bereavement. Perinatal loss needs to be recognised as a unique type of bereavement in which parents often experience an intense response that will cause changes in several domains of their lives, including emotional, physical, financial, spiritual and social aspects.

Experiencing the death of a baby affects families and professionals, creating both challenges and opportunities for best practices. The aim is to ensure quality care provision, imperative in such circumstances. All parents will recall the care provided in their pregnancy and at the time of birth. When a baby dies, the quality of this care becomes even more crucial, as it can have profound short- and long-term effects on their wellbeing, their ability to care for others and their contact with health services in the future (Cacciatore, 2010; Downe et al., 2013). This chapter aims to identify the unique impact of grief in relation to neonatal death. The individual needs of families who experience the death of a baby will be considered, and best practice matters discussed. The need for effective communication in this situation is essential. An understanding of how to sensitively and effectively communicate with bereaved families will be explored and considered.

BEREAVEMENT, MOURNING AND GRIEF

Terms such as grief, mourning and bereavement are often used interchangeably, but an understanding of the discreet differences of these concepts is vital. It is important to acknowledge that loss and grief may not be solely linked to the actual death of a neonate. Such feelings may be experienced when reality clashes with an expected future. For many parents of preterm and sick newborns, there is often a sense of loss and grief, even if their baby does not die. Frequently, there is a sense of lost opportunity, especially where longer-term morbidity issues present when mortality is evaded (Steele and Mancini, 2013).

Bereavement

Bereavement is an objective fact. It is the state of having lost someone. Neonatal nurses may come across parents wondering if the loss of their baby – especially if it is their only child – means that they are no longer considered parents in the eyes of society. This change in status may be especially painful because it minimises or denies their loss. Parental bereavement following infant death is unique, due to the limited amount of time parents spend with their baby, resulting in few memories for parents to maintain a connection to the infant after death (Currie et al., 2018).

Mourning

Mourning is a sign of distress caused by loss. Most societies have rituals which are followed as part of the mourning process. This may include wearing specific clothes, withdrawing from everyday life, and adopting forms of behaviour to indicate that they have experienced a loss. Mourning in the UK may be difficult for parents who have experienced neonatal death, as family and friends may struggle to recognise the fact that the parents experience the loss of a baby as profoundly as they would that of an adult.

Grief

Grief is a painful biological manifestation that can reveal itself in many different ways. It can affect a person in a physical, psychosocial, emotional or behavioural way (Worden, 2009). A varied emotional response is to be expected, causing complexities that professionals working within NNUs need to be aware of. Although the experience of loss is similar across different cultures, it is imperative to remember that the way it is expressed may not be. Some cultures value stoicism, others may be verbally expressive, while others may prefer privacy at this difficult time (England and Morgan, 2012). The role of the neonatal nurse at such a time is to remain non-judgemental and responsive to parents' wishes.

MODELS OF GRIEF AND LOSS

The grieving process has been repeatedly explored over the years. Some early theories have focused on stages of grief, where emotional responses such as denial, confusion or anger, bargaining, depression and acceptance were recognised (Kübler-Ross, 2014). Health professionals need to have an awareness that parents may not proceed through and experience all stages of this cycle and will definitely not proceed through them in a particular order. Therefore, while to be able to consider some of the emotions that may be displayed is extremely useful, they should not be applied in a prescriptive manner. More recent theorists have emphasised the social and cultural context of bereavement and grief, with the consideration of such dimensions leading to the dual process model (Stroebe & Schut, 1999; 2010). This theory recognises the individuality of the grief response and the journey through the grief process. It suggests that bereaved parents often move between confrontation and avoidance, rather than experiencing grief as a series of stages (see figure 8.1). It is acknowledged that there may be a tendency to oscillate and hesitate through these stages (Papa et al., 2014; Currie et al., 2016). The oscillation is seen as movement between the more passive styles of grief to a more active approach, without the presence of a time limit. Thus, bereaved individuals will fluctuate between confronting their grief, while at other times dealing with everyday tasks required for living, or a welcome distraction from their intense emotions (Stroebe et al., 2007).

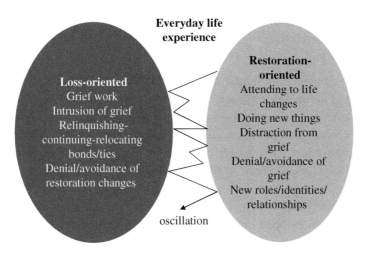

Figure 8.1 A dual process model of coping with loss (adapted from Stroebe and Schut, 1999)

RESPONDING TO LOSS

Grief is often fluid and a labile emotional state (Worden, 2009). Some parents may be experiencing loss and bereavement for the first time in their lives, unprepared for the emotional chaos that will ensue. Bereaved parents need to be made aware that grief is a very individual experience, with a wide range of feelings and physical responses (see box 8.1). Grief is intensely personal, and there is no right or wrong way to perceive this. There is, however, some evidence to suggest that grieving parents find it helpful to have information about the range of feelings they may experience (Schott et al., 2007). This helps them cope by 'normalising' the copious emotions they may encounter, and realising that they are not alone in their suffering.

Traditional models of grief assume that after a period of time this will become resolved. It is now acknowledged that bereaved people will continue to feel a bond with a person who has died, and that this person will continue to be part of their lives (Walter and McCoyd, 2009). Experience indicates that parents do not want to forget their baby who has passed away (Davies, 2004). Parents may find their grief overwhelming, and this may isolate them from family and friends. Within Western societies, people are generally given a few weeks to make the transition from bereavement to normal everyday life (Behrman and Field, 2003). When an infant has spent all his or her life in a NNU, their existence may not be acknowledged by the wider society. Parents have reported that friends and family often suggest the loss may have 'been for the best', or that the optimum way to come to terms with the loss is to have another baby as soon as possible. Their experience of caring for a baby in a NNU is negated, because there is no visible proof of the baby's life to the outside world. This lack of recognising the baby as an individual in their own right may impact on

> ## BOX 8.1 A MOTHER'S REFLECTION ON THE COMPLEX NATURE OF GRIEF IN THE PERINATAL PERIOD
>
> *Bereaved parents, no matter how long ago our loss, we carry on, we might smile and we might laugh and we might be genuinely happy – but what we never, ever do – is forget. You can help us make our memories rich and meaningful. I wish I had photographs of my son naked. It might seem strange but years later, I feel guilty as his mother that I never saw him properly. I know he was in poor condition, so the nurse very kindly wrapped him up and took him away to dress him. She meant well, but I regret not dressing him myself, I would have been so proud of myself for doing that. I could have really been a Mum to him in those brief moments, and photographs that took me back to that special time would have been amazing!*
>
> Mother of Rowan
>
> ### Reflection point
>
> Consider how this bereaved mother's story will affect your own professional practice? Think of how you could adapt practice in your own clinical area to improve the memories of bereaved parents?

how parents mourn and grieve for their loss, which can significantly affect parents' health and functioning (Youngblut et al., 2017).

DEATH IN THE NEONATAL UNIT – PROVIDING HOLISTIC AND INCLUSIVE CARE

Following the death of a neonate, parents and families need to be provided with holistic care sensitive to their individual needs, and specific interventions offered to help them (Banerjee et al., 2016). Professionals should apply a person-centred attitude to care, listening to parents' wishes. There is a need to ensure a standardised approach to care with provision of written policies and standards (Kenner et al., 2015). The parents need to be given time to articulate their individual requirements, with support and guidance from healthcare professionals. Parents' personal, cultural, spiritual and religious needs must be considered to facilitate this (Youngblut et al., 2017). Research suggests parents value clear communication, education about grieving and demonstrated emotional support by staff but at the same time there are deficiencies in staff knowledge and education in this area (Robertson et al., 2011). Moreover, 20–30% of affected parents expressed feelings that such considerations were lacking (Redshaw et al., 2014).

> **BOX 8.2 THE IMPORTANCE OF COMMUNICATION BETWEEN NEONATAL AND MATERNITY SERVICES**
>
> *While my husband had left to arrange overnight accommodation at the hospital, I asked the doctor if I should express milk, as the midwives had suggested I should do so. I was told, 'Let's see if he survives first.' These words were like a bullet through my heart. The doctor was shocked I didn't know how serious his condition was, but all day we had been told he was stable and not given the full details, even the midwives that had been with us were shocked by this news.*
>
> Mother of Isaac

A holistic approach to care should be adopted by the wider healthcare teams involved in the family's care. This necessitates clear communication and cooperation between teams, with appropriate referrals to relevant organisations for ongoing support. Collaboration with maternity services is particularly crucial, so parents are well supported during the immediate postnatal period (see box 8.2).

CULTURAL ELEMENTS OF LOSS

While professionals should have an understanding of how parents' personal, cultural, spiritual and religious needs may affect their choices and decisions, assumptions should never be made (Sadeghi, et al., 2016). It is important that professionals do not presume anything regarding parents' wishes based on their socioeconomic status, religion or personal circumstances. Such considerations may well influence decision-making with regard to funerals and post-mortem consent, yet these factors will not necessarily dictate decisions. Individuals supporting parents affected by infant loss should listen with a non-judgemental approach.

COMMUNICATION

When caring for bereaved parents, it is essential that healthcare professionals have the necessary communication skills to effectively and sensitively interact. Even where excellent clinical care is delivered, the use of poor communication skills can overshadow the parents' experience (Downe et al., 2013). As well as professional expertise, parents value the use of empathy and kindness. Often bereaved parents will recall the staff who acknowledged their immense loss while treating their baby with the utmost respect and dignity (Henley and Schott, 2008). The offer of empathetic support is fraught with difficulties for several reasons. What is well received with one bereaved family may not be fitting under different circumstances. Listening is an essential skill and a form of support imperative to bereaved families. Appropriate silences should be utilised as much as possible. Finding time to truly listen can be difficult for staff who are working under clinical pressure, so that it may be tempting to do or say something, rather than just to listen. However, this skill should never be underestimated. Parents will value the presence of a professional to listen as they talk about their experience and deliver appropriate information or suggestions. Parents value staff who accept what they say without judgement, remain calm as they express strong emotions, and avoid giving platitudes or empty reassurance (Henley and Schott, 2008). When parents are offered supportive listening from healthcare professionals, it can have a profound effect on short- and long-term wellbeing (Kenworthy and Kirkham, 2011; Crawley et al., 2013).

Verbal communication

Words need to be chosen extremely carefully when communicating with parents. Bereaved families have expressed that they want honest and frank information about their child's health, even if this means receiving bad news (Harvey et al., 2008). Unfortunately, a lack of training means that parents do not always feel information is delivered sensitively (Siassakos, 2018).

Medical terminology should be avoided where possible, with health professionals taking a lead from the bereaved parents and the terminology they use when discussing their loss. For example, if parents refer to their baby by their chosen name, it is best practice to also use their name. It is also important to appreciate the effect traumatic news can have on people's ability to retain information they receive. It may be necessary to repeat facts on several occasions, perhaps rephrasing them (Woodroffe, 2013). Parents should be encouraged to ask questions and to clarify aspects they struggle to comprehend. In between discussions, parents should have access to members of staff who are able to answer their questions (Henley and Schott, 2008). In general, parents appreciate staff who demonstrate the significance of the information being given. Health professionals should remain truthful, be honest about uncertainties where they exist, and acknowledge how difficult this must be for parents. Provision of sensitive, therapeutic communication with parents is a vital part of quality bereavement care (Currie et al., 2016).

Nonverbal communication

Nonverbal cues are extremely powerful and should therefore be considered in any communication situation. Aspects such as posture, facial expressions, gestures, proximity and tone of voice all send out profound messages. Bereaved parents are extremely sensitive to such communication, often realising something is wrong before the verbal message has been imparted, purely from interpreting nonverbal cues of professionals (Siassakos, 2018).

> ## BOX 8.3 COMMUNICATION WITH BEREAVED PARENTS
>
> - *Use sensitive communication when informing parents of the expected sequence of events*
> - *Discuss the current situation and ensure parents are fully informed about what is happening, including them in decisions related to their care and the care of their baby*
> - *Give the parents time to absorb information and allocate time to ask questions*
> - *Listen to the parents; their views and wishes should be acknowledged and respected*
> - *Offer support and listen to the parents as they talk about their feelings and concerns.*
>
> (adapted from SANDS, 2016)

Similarly, nonverbal communication signals from parents can usually provide good insight, particularly where there is a lack of congruency. Parents are extremely intuitive in such situations and will often guess the nature of the news. This will generate considerable anxiety and additional distress for the parents, while reducing their trust of the health professionals caring for their baby (Stillbirth and Neonatal Death Society (SANDS), 2016). An awareness regarding cultural differences in nonverbal communication is crucial: facial expressions and the appropriateness of eye contact vary across cultures. Healthcare professionals should therefore not make assumptions about someone's meaning or level of understanding purely from nonverbal signals. Where parents do not use English as their first language, access to trained interpreters should be standard practice. An interpreter will be able to translate information provided by the health professional but will also be able to explain to both staff and parents any cultural or other issues that may be hindering mutual understanding. Box 8.3 summarises important aspects of communication in bereavement.

CARING FOR THE DYING BABY

An infant dying on a NNU is likely to have gone through a period of intensive care provision. The parents will have witnessed their baby attached to a variety of machines and tubes, surrounded by technology and protected by the plastic incubator. Some parents can begin to withdraw emotionally and physically from the baby in anticipation of their loss (Hindmarch, 2016). Professionals supporting parents who are displaying such withdrawal should do their utmost to encourage them to participate in the personal care of their child. Disengagement can lead to feelings of immense guilt following the death.

Additionally, consideration needs to be attributed to the environment at the point of death. This has already been discussed in chapter 7, where salient points for contemplation are identified.

An individualised approach to the immediate time surrounding death needs to be established. Some parents will want to be alone with their baby before, during or after the death, while others will take comfort from having professionals present to support them and answer any questions they may have. Some parents will want to hold their child as he or she is dying, while others may find little comfort in doing so. Seeing and holding babies after death has become common practice in many NNUs. Some parents may benefit from this, but others may not wish to hold their baby and 'encouraging' them to do so in the belief that it will facilitate the grieving process is unhelpful. It is imperative that health professionals supporting parents at this time sensitively discuss and offer options that are possible while taking a clear lead from the requests of parents. This should be done tentatively and gently, as it can be difficult for distressed parents to refuse if these suggestions are perceived as instructions. Evidence from a systematic review of studies that explored support for mothers, fathers and families after perinatal death concluded that the proposed benefits of interventions such as seeing and holding the baby remain inconclusive. (Koopmans et al., 2013). However, they also conclude that, under the right circumstances and guided by compassionate, sensitive and experienced staff, parents' experiences of seeing and holding their deceased baby is often very positive.

Spiritual and religious considerations

Some parents may take comfort from being able to hold spiritual and religious ceremonies or rituals to celebrate their child's life. Again, assumptions should not be made that this will be wanted or accepted, but the possibility should be sensitively introduced and discussed. Once the baby has died, some cultures observe certain rituals relating to the care of the dead. This may include specification as to who should handle them and how they may be washed and dressed. Parents of babies dealing with death for the first time may be unsure of rituals relating to their social customs and may look to staff in the NNU to help inform them of the requirements. Having links with a range of faith and social communities can be helpful at this time and should usually already be established by the unit in readiness of need relating to sound cultural care (Butler and Neimeyer, 2012).

Memory-making

A perinatal loss poses numerous challenges. While many parents have established a bond with their child, often there are few or no tangible memories that can be shared with other people. Parents may welcome suggestions and ideas from experienced staff, such as encouraging parents to talk to and touch their baby. The offer of skin-to-skin contact with their baby can provide important memories to recall and provide comfort in the future.

Parents should be encouraged to create keepsakes and take photographs and videos of their child as concrete memories to share with others. Parents who were not offered or who declined the memory-making process often regretted this subsequently (Harvey et al., 2008). Most NNUs are now benefiting from charities such as 4Louis (see figures 8.2 and 8.3) and SANDS who are providing free memory boxes to support this process, supplying a special place for the storage of significant keepsakes (see box 8.4).

Tangible mementoes connected to the baby will help to confirm their existence and provide comfort to the parents in the long term (see box 8.5).

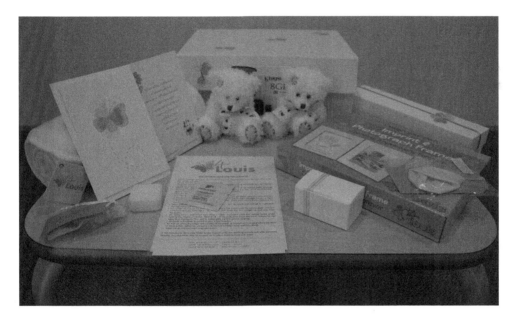

Figure 8.2 4Louis memory box

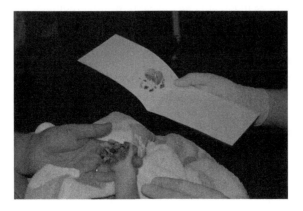

Figure 8.3 Memory-making

BOX 8.4 KEEPSAKES

- Hand and foot prints
- Lock of hair
- Clay models of the baby's hands or feet if possible
- A record of baby's weight and length
- Clinical items used when caring for the baby
- Any blankets or toys used by the baby
- Baby's cord clamp
- Identification bracelet
- Cot card
- Photographs

BOX 8.5 THE IMPORTANCE OF MEMORY BOXES

When we made the decision to turn his life support off, we realised that he didn't have a teddy. I made the decision to buy him one but had no idea where I could get one from. I asked the staff member who told me not to worry and that she would sort it; she came back a short time later with a memory box which included a change of clothes and two teddy bears. This meant that the last few precious moments could be spent with our baby.

Father of Isaac

Wherever possible, parents should be supported to consider the transference of their baby's care to an appropriate children's hospice. This is an environment less clinical, and here parents may spend as much time as possible, without restrictions, with their baby. This can also reduce the pressure on clinical staff working in busy NNUs, who often find the time to spend with bereaved families is limited. Please see chapter 7 for more details on palliative care planning.

Choices should be offered with an assurance that staff will respect parental wishes where possible. In most situations, it is feasible for parents to change their minds. For example, they may decide not to hold their dead baby initially but decide later that they wish to do this. Staff need to be aware of the changes that take place in bodies after they die and alert parents to these, otherwise this can cause distress (McHaffie et al., 2001). Where the environmental temperature is high, changes in the baby's appearance take place more rapidly. Advice should be sought from a mortuary technician about how long the baby's body can remain out of the mortuary before noticeable changes take place. This is particularly important if the parents want to take their baby home. Ideally, bereaved families should have access to a cool cot to allow for the maximum amount of time to be spent with their baby. If parents request to take their baby home for a period of time, there is no reason why this cannot be facilitated. No explicit documentation needs to accompany the baby, but it may be good practice to issue a letter to avoid any misunderstandings. In this particular instance, a cool cot is necessary to keep the baby's body protected against the degenerative process following death.

Photographs

Photography can be an important way for families to remember their baby, although this may not be acceptable across all cultures. Having photographs of their baby can provide visual proof of the reality of their baby's life (Kenner et al., 2015). Evidence suggests that parents value photographs, but where possible professionals need to minimise the invasive nature of the clinical environment, as images of babies with numerous wires and tubes can be difficult for parents (Harvey et al., 2008). Specialised bereavement photography courses are now being developed for health professionals involved in this sensitive area, to ensure that long-lasting sensitive images are obtained (see figure 8.4 for an example). It is important to consider other family members at this time: it can be comforting for siblings to have photographs taken with the baby. Families should never feel pressurised to take photographs, yet if they are unsure, it may be helpful to inform them that parents have often

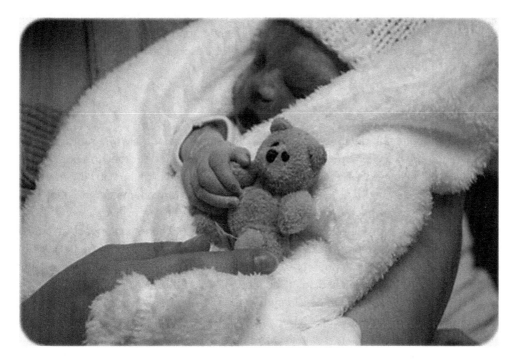

Figure 8.4 Minimising the presence of invasive medical devices

cited regret over this decision or are unhappy with the quality or number of photographs they have taken (Blood and Cacciatore, 2014).

POSTNATAL CARE FOLLOWING A LOSS

The psychological impact of stillbirth and neonatal death on parents is profound. Both practical and psychological support is needed from close family members, friends, health professionals and others. Ongoing support is often a lacking element of the parents' care pathway. Around 21% of parents are not given information about counselling services when discharged home for hospital services (Redshaw et al., 2014). Therefore, professionals on the NNU should ensure that all parents have contact details for further support facilities upon discharge, as well as closely communicating with maternity and community services following a baby's death.

MULTIPLE PREGNANCIES

Where one baby from a set of multiples is dying, the situation can be complex and emotionally charged. Parents should be encouraged to spend time with their healthy baby as well as the one who is unlikely to survive. It is important that where multiple births are involved, the babies should be held and photographed together. Neonatal nurses supporting parents should continue to provide the usual bereavement support while acknowledging the conflicting emotions of both joy and grief parents will be experiencing (Kenner et al., 2015).

FATHERS AND SAME-SEX PARTNERS

The effect of perinatal death on fathers and partners is not always recognised or acknowledged. Men are often expected to suppress their grief in order to support their partner who, it is assumed, will suffer more intensely from the loss of the baby (Murray et al., 2000). Men may also find that the need for them to return to work means that they have to suppress feelings of grief in order to resume their place in the everyday world. Some research suggests the possibility of asynchronous grieving – where men appear to recover from the loss of the baby more quickly than their partner (Oliver, 1999; Murray et al., 2000). However, most studies involving men have small samples and high drop-out rates, so it is impossible to generalise these findings (Badenhorst et al., 2006).

It is furthermore important to consider the evolving paternity role within society, which is likely to impact on the intensity of grief as fathers become more involved during the pregnancy. Fathers need to be allowed to grieve in their own time, without having expectations imposed on them (Koopmans et al., 2013). Neonatal death results in a unique type of grief in that it affects both parents equally and simultaneously. Parents need to be guided in understanding this complexity to respect and accept each other's response to the grieving process. Couples also need to be aware of the challenge of supporting the other partner when both are grieving. Neonatal nurses should encourage parents to take time to listen to each other and to seek outside, specialist counselling support if required (Albuquerque et al., 2016).

EXTENDED FAMILY

From the beginning of a neonatal journey, siblings need to be as closely involved as possible, and not infrequently parents may need advice on how to facilitate this in the NNU environment. The quality of communication they experience will have a lasting influence on how well siblings will cope with the evolving situation. Historically it was believed that if children were not involved and told about illness and death, it would not affect them. This has been demonstrated to be inaccurate (Woodroffe, 2013). The work of the organisation Child Bereavement UK has clearly shown the psychological dangers of children who are left to their imagination where death is concerned, leading to often dysfunctional thinking and behaviour in later life. Information (available via their website) may enable parents to have appropriate and sensitive discussions with their other children (Child Bereavement UK, 2018).

Parents should also be encouraged to involve other family members if they wish. Consideration needs to be given to other siblings (figure 8.5) and grandparents who may

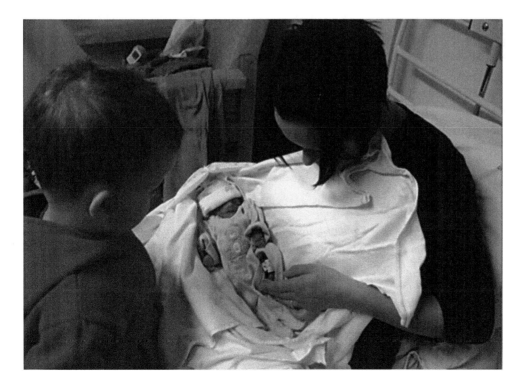

Figure 8.5 Involving siblings in bereavement care

want the opportunity to see and hold the baby and say their own goodbyes. In the long term, this may assist in their ability to support the parents if others too, have memories to share. All visiting restrictions should be removed where possible, to ensure the family's needs are met.

CHALLENGING ISSUES TO CONSIDER

Perinatal autopsy

All parents whose baby dies should be offered the opportunity to have a post-mortem examination. In England this practice is governed by the Human Tissue Act 2004 and the Human Tissue Authority (HTA, 2011). Specific training for health professionals is required to discuss this sensitive issue. Although often a doctor will discuss autopsy with parents, nursing and midwifery staff need to be prepared if information and clarification are needed. Such discussions may be particularly problematic if parents who both have parental responsibility disagree about whether a post-mortem examination should take place, necessitating NNU staff to be familiar with the legislation (see box 8.6).

Organ donation

Newborn organ donation is still relatively uncommon practice within the UK. While overall increase in rates across the general population continues to rise, this has not been replicated in the neonatal population. However, following the release of guidelines from the Royal College of Paediatrics and Child Health (RCPCH) on diagnosing brainstem death in neonates between 37 weeks' gestation to 2 months of age, there is a potential to increase the number of successful neonatal donations (RCPCH, 2015). Often a paternalistic approach to bereavement care results in professionals not discussing the option of

---

BOX 8.6 CONSENT FOR POST-MORTEM EXAMINATION

Where there is a conflict between those accorded equal ranking, this should be discussed sensitively with all parties, whilst explaining clearly that so far as the HT Act is concerned, the consent of one of those ranked equally in the hierarchy is sufficient for the procedure to go ahead. This does not mean that the consent of one person must be acted on, and a decision not to proceed may be made on the basis of the emotional impact that this would have on family and friends.

(HTA 2017, p. 10)

organ donation as part of palliative care conversations, believing it may cause more emotional distress for the family. This, however, is an evolving concept of neonatal bereavement care with successful cases cited in the literature that allude to the positive experience for the bereaved family (Atreja et al., 2014).

To assist in improving current neonatal donation rates, a strategic plan has been released in 2019 by the National Health Service (NHS) blood and transplant team which aims to ensure that a framework is developed that will embed organ donation as a routine end-of-life choice for all families facing the death of their child, where organ donation may be possible (NHS Blood and Transplant, 2019). It is crucial that, where neonatal organ donation is being considered, any initial discussions involve the transplant team (Mancini et al., 2014). This should include notifying the Specialist Nurse in Organ Donation (SNOD). All NHS Trusts will have a SNOD who will not only be able to offer advice to professionals regarding the suitability of organ donation in individual cases, but will also, where possible, attend as preliminary discussions with parents are raised. This topic needs to be broached with parents at a suitable time, in a sensitive manner, with appropriate professionals involved. Where a SNOD is part of such discussions, the rate of consent is higher (Hawkins et al., 2018). As well as being trained to open the discussion sensitively, they will be able to support and guide clinical staff through the process and will ensure parents are given all information relating to the end-of-life care, post-mortem examination, and how memory-making will be facilitated.

Parents need to be reassured that if they do or do not opt to donate their baby's organs it will not affect the baby's care (SANDS, 2016). Where parents refuse to consider organ donation, their wishes should always be respected. The offer of organ donation is an important development for bereaved families, as where organ donation has been possible parents have cited that they have been able to take comfort knowing that something remarkable has transpired from their own loss (Bliss, 2010).

STAFF SUPPORT AND TRAINING

Death, as well as the beginning of life, has an impact upon the lives of those it touches. The nature of this impact is often socially constructed (Kenworthy and Kirkham, 2011). The repercussions on healthcare professionals of supporting parents through a neonatal death must therefore also be considered. While there is a growing body of evidence regarding best practice points for delivering effective care for bereaved families on a NNU, little is known regarding the grief nurses experience when a newborn in their care dies. Neonatal nurses, support staff and doctors require an appreciation of the emotional burden of a patient's death on their own wellbeing. Caring for neonates at the end of life as well as supporting the family can be extremely intense and cause significant moral distress. An acknowledgement of this should be ingrained in a unit's culture, with the possibility to support staff during such times. This is often provided on an ad hoc basis with little opportunity for staff to learn how to develop effective grief management skills (Kain, 2013). Creating a platform of appropriate clinical supervision where staff are able to discuss issues will ultimately assist in alleviating some of the distress often cited by nurses working in this complex area of practice (Mendel, 2014).

Staff who support parents through a bereavement as part of their role may also find the national bereavement care network helpful (https://bereavement-network.rcm.org.uk/). This is an online resource which aims to enhance the knowledge, insight and understanding of professionals surrounding bereavement and bereavement care in the perinatal period. It furthermore offers a forum to enable professionals to share best practice, as well as informing users of relevant recent developments within this field, with valuable resources to enhance practice.

CONCLUSION

The complexity of bereavement care often causes anxiety for neonatal nurses involved. The emphasis with this must be on the main principles of supportive practice, good communication and an individualised approach to care provision. As parents will continue to live with the memories generated at this difficult time, how these are constructed is of the highest importance and must therefore be parent-led. To facilitate this, neonatal nurses need to be able to provide information regarding all available options and achieve a balance of being guided by parents with regard to their wishes, while simultaneously supporting them in caring for their dying baby.

CASE STUDY

CASE STUDIES

First, looking back at boxes 8.1 and 8.2, consider how these bereaved mothers' stories will affect your own professional practice? Think of how you could adapt practice in your own clinical area to improve the memories of bereaved parents.

Case study 1 – Organ donation

Dale and Chloe have given birth to a daughter, Ellie, at 39 weeks' gestation. Chloe presented to the maternity services with a heavy vaginal bleed and was immediately taken for an emergency caesarean section because of placental abruption. Ellie was born in a poor condition and no heart rate was noted at birth. She had advanced resuscitation by the attending neonatal team including intubation, cardiac compressions and resuscitation drugs. A heart rate was first heard at 10 minutes of age. Ellie fulfilled the criteria for therapeutic hypothermia. After a period of 3 days of cooling, she remained neurologically compromised and did not demonstrate any spontaneous respiratory effort. On examination, she had fixed dilated pupils and absent gag and deep tendon reflexes.

Magnetic resonance imaging (MRI) was undertaken on day 5 and demonstrated extensive changes in the white matter and basal ganglia, suggestive of severe hypoxic-ischaemic brain damage. The neonatal team agree that further intensive care is futile and are considering re-orienting Sophie's care to palliation. Throughout Ellie's stay on the NNU, Dale and Chloe have been made aware of how critical her status was and have 'prepared themselves for the worst' prior to her MRI. Once the results are discussed with the parents, they express a wish to donate Ellie's organs following her death.

Would Ellie be eligible for organ donation?

Case study 2 – Planning holistic bereavement care

Tyler was born at 24 weeks and doing well initially, but sadly deteriorated with fulminant necrotising enterocolitis at 10 days of age. He is too unstable for an operation, and within a few hours it becomes evident that Tyler will not survive for much longer. His parents, Matilda and Jamil, have two other children, Daisy aged 7, and Jackson aged 4 years. Jamil was raised in the Muslim faith but is not practicing this as part of his adult life or raising his children in accordance with it.

Q.1. What are your immediate considerations with regard to planning Tyler's care around his death?
Q.2. Given that Jamil is not a practicing Muslim, would you address religious aspects as part of the family's bereavement care?
Q.3. Which points would you like to discuss with Matilda and Jamil with regard to their other children?

For suggested answer guides to the questions posed in these case studies, please refer to the web-based companion site specific to this chapter (see URL below).

WEB-BASED RESOURCES

For further information, online resources and greater detail on the case studies featured in this chapter go to www.routledge.com/cw/nicnursing

References

Albuquerque, S., Pereira, M., & Narciso, I. (2016). Couple's relationship after the death of a child: A systematic review. *Journal of Child and Family Studies, 25*(1), 30–53.

Atreja, G., Zhu, F., & Godambe, S. (2014). Neonatal organ donation: Thinking ahead. *Pediatrics, 133*, e82–87.

Badenhorst, W., Riches, S., Turton, P., & Hughes, P. (2006). The psychological effects of stillbirth and neonatal death on fathers: Systematic review. *Journal of Psychosomatic Obstetrics & Gynecology, 27*(4), 245–256.

Banerjee, J., Kaur, C., Ramaiah, S., Roy, R., & Aladangady, N. (2016). Factors influencing the uptake of neonatal bereavement support services: Findings from two tertiary neonatal centres in the UK. *BMC Palliative Care, 15*(1), 54.

Behrman, R. E., & Field, M. J. (Eds.) (2003). *When children die: Improving palliative and end-of-life care for children and their families*. Washington: National Academies Press.

Bliss. (2010). *Making Critical Decisions for your Baby*. London: Bliss.

Blood, C., & Cacciatore, J. (2014). Best practice in bereavement photography after perinatal death: Qualitative analysis with 104 parents. *BMC Psychology, 2*(1), 15.

Butler, R. J., & Neimeyer, R. A. (2012). Constructions of death and loss: A personal and professional evolution. *Reflections in Personal Construct Theory*. Wiley online library.

Cacciatore, J. (2010). The unique experiences of women and their families after the death of a baby. *Social Work in Health Care, 49*(2), 134–148.

Child Bereavement UK (2018). *Explaining Miscarriage, Stillbirth or the Death of a Newborn Baby to Young Children*. Retrieved from https://childbereavementuk.org/wp-content/uploads/2018/06/Explaining-miscarriage-stillbirth-or-the-death-of-a-newborn-baby-to-young-children-June-2018.pdf

Crawley, R., Lomax, S., & Ayers, S. (2013). Recovering from stillbirth: the effects of making and sharing memories on maternal mental health. *Journal of Reproductive and Infant Psychology, 31*(2), 195–207.

Currie, E. R., Christian, B. J., Hinds, P. S., Perna, S. J., Robinson, C., Day, S., & Meneses, K. (2016). Parent perspectives of neonatal intensive care at the end-of-life. *Journal of Pediatric Nursing, 31*(5), 478–489.

Currie, E. R., Christian, B. J., Hinds, P. S., Perna, S. J., Robinson, C., Day, S., … & Meneses, K. (2018). Life after loss: Parent bereavement and coping experiences after infant death in the neonatal intensive care unit. *Death Studies*, 1–10.

Davies, R. (2004). New understandings of parental grief: Literature review. *Journal of Advanced Nursing, 46*(5), 506–513.

Downe, S., Schmidt, E., Kingdon, C., & Heazell, A. E. (2013). Bereaved parents' experience of stillbirth in UK hospitals: A qualitative interview study. *BMJ Open, 3*(2), e002237.

England, C. & Morgan, R., (2012). *Communication Skills for Midwives: Challenges in Everyday Practice*. London: McGraw-Hill Education (UK).

Harvey, S., Snowdon, C., & Elbourne, D. (2008). Effectiveness of bereavement interventions in neonatal intensive care: A review of the evidence. In *Seminars in Fetal and Neonatal Medicine, 13*(5), 341–356.

Hawkins, K. C., Scales, A., Murphy, P., Madden, S., & Brierley, J. (2018). Current status of paediatric and neonatal organ donation in the UK. *Archives of Disease in Childhood, 103*(3), 210–215.

Henley, A., and Schott, J. (2008). The death of a baby before, during or shortly after birth: Good practice from the parents' perspective. *Seminars in Fetal and Neonatal Medicine, 13*(5), 325–328.

Hindmarch, C. (2016). *On the Death of a Child*. Oxford & New York: Taylor & Francis.

Human Tissue Authority (HTA). (2011). *Human Tissue Act 2004*. Human Tissue Authority.

Human Tissue Authority (HTA). (2017). *Code A: Guiding principles and the fundamental principle of consent*. Human Tissue Authority.

Kain, V. J. (2013). An exploration of the grief experiences of neonatal nurses: A focus group study. *Journal of Neonatal Nursing*, 19(2), 80–88.

Kenner, C., Press, J., & Ryan, D. (2015). Recommendations for palliative and bereavement care in the NICU: A family-centered integrative approach. *Journal of Perinatology*, 35(S1), S19–S23.

Kenworthy, D., & Kirkham, M. (2011). *Midwives coping with loss and grief: Stillbirth, professional and personal losses.* London & New York: Radcliffe Publishing.

Koopmans, L., Wilson, T., Cacciatore, J., & Flenady, V. (2013). Support for mothers, fathers and families after perinatal death. *Cochrane Database of Systematic Reviews*, Issue 6. Art. No.: CD000452. DOI: 10.1002/14651858.CD000452.pub3

Kübler-Ross, E. (2014). *On death and dying.* (Reprint edition). London and New York: Routledge.

McHaffie, H., Fowlie, P. W., Hume, R., Laing, I., Lloyd, D., & Lyon, A. (2001). *Crucial decisions at the beginning of life: Parents' experiences of treatment withdrawal from infants.* Oxford: Radcliffe Medical Press.

Mancini, A., Uthaya, S., Beardsley, C., Wood, D., & Modi, N. (2014). Practical guidance for the management of palliative care on neonatal units. London: Royal College of Paediatrics and Child Health.

Mendel, T. R. (2014). The use of neonatal palliative care: Reducing moral distress in NICU nurses. *Journal of Neonatal Nursing*, 20(6), 290–293.

Murray, J. A., Terry, D. J., Vance, J. C., Battistutta, D., & Connolly, Y. (2000). Effects of a program of intervention on parental distress following infant death. *Death Studies*, 24(4), 275–305.

NHS Blood and Transplant. (2019). *Paediatric and Neonatal Deceased Donation. A Strategic Plan. NHS Blood and Transplant.* Retrieved from www.odt.nhs.uk/odt-structures-and-standards/key-strategies/paediatric-and-neonatal-donation-strategy/

Oliver, L. E. (1999). Effects of a child's death on the marital relationship: A review. *Omega-Journal of Death And Dying*, 39(3), 197–227.

Papa, A., Lancaster, N. G., & Kahler, J. (2014). Commonalities in grief responding across bereavement and non-bereavement losses. *Journal of Affective Disorders*, 161, 136–143.

Redshaw, M., Rowe, R., & Henderson, J. (2014). Listening to Parents after stillbirth or the death of their baby after birth. *University of Oxford: National Perinatal Epidemiology Unit.*

Robertson, M. J., Aldridge, A., & Curley, A. E. (2011). Provision of bereavement care in neonatal units in the United Kingdom. *Pediatric Critical Care Medicine*, 12(3), e111–e115.

Royal College of Paediatric and Child Health. (2015). *The Diagnosis of Death by Neurological Criteria in Infants Less Than Two Months Old.* London: RCPCH.

Sadeghi, N., Hasanpour, M., Heidarzadeh, M., Alamolhoda, A., & Waldman, E. (2016). Spiritual needs of families with bereavement and loss of an infant in neonatal intensive care unit: A qualitative study. *Journal of Pain and Symptom Management*, 52(1), 35–42.

Schott, J., Henley, A., & Kohner, N. (2007). *Pregnancy loss and the death of a baby: guidelines for professionals.* London: Bosun Press.

Siassakos, D., Jackson, S., Gleeson, K., Chebsey, C., Ellis, A., Storey, C. … & Hillman, J. (2018). All bereaved parents are entitled to good care after stillbirth: A mixed-methods multicentre study (INSIGHT). *BJOG: An International Journal of Obstetrics & Gynaecology*, 125(2), 160–170.

Steele, P., & Mancini, A. (2013). The neonatal experience–loss and grief without a bereavement. *Infant*, 9(3), 92–93.

Stillbirth and Neonatal Death Society (2016). *Pregnancy Loss and the Death of a Baby: Guidelines for Professionals. 4th Edition.* London: SANDS

Stroebe, M., & Schut, H. (2010). The dual process model of coping with bereavement: A decade on. *OMEGA-Journal of Death and Dying*, 61(4), 273–289.

Stroebe, M., & Schut, H. (1999). The dual process model of coping with bereavement: Rationale and description. *Death Studies*, 23(3), 197–224.

Stroebe, M., Schut, H., & Stroebe, W. (2007). Health outcomes of bereavement. *The Lancet.* 370: 1960–73.

Walter, C. A., & McCoyd, J. L. M. (2009). *Grief and loss across the lifespan: A biopsychosocial perspective.* New York: Springer Publishing Company.

Woodroffe, I. (2013). Supporting bereaved families through neonatal death and beyond. *Seminars in Fetal and Neonatal Medicine, 18*(2), 99–104.

Worden, J. W. (2009). *Grief Counselling and Grief Therapy. 4th Edition.* London: Routledge.

Youngblut, J. M., Brooten, D., Glaze, J., Promise, T., & Yoo, C. (2017). Parent grief 1–13 months after death in neonatal and pediatric intensive care units. *Journal of Loss and Trauma, 22*(1), 77–96.

9 LEGAL AND ETHICAL ISSUES IN NEONATAL CARE

Debra Nicholson and Katherine Noble

CONTENTS

GUIDANCE ON HOW TO ENHANCE PERSONAL LEARNING FROM THIS CHAPTER

Key points covered in this chapter

■ Legal issues as applicable to neonatal care including foetal and neonatal rights, limits of viability, consent and duty of care.

■ Ethical theories and principles as they apply to neonatal care in line with the 'best interests' of the infant and family.

■ An overview of decision-making in the neonatal unit within a legal and ethical perspective.

Reflection

Reading through the chapter, you are encouraged to engage with the key points and related literature in an enquiring way. Ask these questions:

■ How do you ensure you uphold sound legal and ethical principles in the best interests of the infant and family?

■ Who is involved in legal and ethical decision-making in neonatal care?

■ Can you apply the content of this chapter to any situation(s) you have encountered in practice?

Implications for nursing care

■ Finally: how will this chapter enable you to consider and understand legal and ethical principles of neonatal care? Consider the implications of what you learn for your nursing care relating to both these important, interrelated areas.

INTRODUCTION AND BACKGROUND

Major improvements in technology and clinical care mean that extremely premature and very ill babies have better chances of survival and making a good recovery, as touched on in earlier chapters. However, it can be difficult to predict whether an individual infant will have a limited lifespan and the extent to which he or she will recover from any health problems or develop disabilities. This means that families and health professionals sometimes must make complex and emotionally demanding decisions about an infant's treatment and care (Nuffield Council on Bioethics, 2014; Green et al., 2017). An understanding therefore of these complexities is essential for the multidisciplinary team (MDT) to make sense of situations that present legal and/or ethical dilemmas. Although ethical dilemmas occur across all specialties, they are particularly common in modern neonatal practice. This chapter will explore some of the key legal principles, ethical frameworks and theories including the best interest principle in relation to decision-making for these babies and families. While legal and ethical issues are covered in separate sections, there are many overlaps and commonalities between both. The chapter will consider related issues that present in modern neonatal practice such as the importance of family inclusion, consent, shared decision-making and, less commonly, tissue and organ donation. Nurses are in a focal position to be fully engaged in neonatal bioethical discussions and decisions about care, in conjunction with the parents and the MDT. The Nursing and Midwifery Council (NMC, 2018) states that nurses must be able to recognise ethical challenges in their role and to practice in accordance with legal, professional and ethical frameworks to overcome these challenges.

LEGAL AND ETHICAL CONSIDERATIONS IN NEONATAL INTENSIVE CARE

Legal principles

Law affects almost everything we do and can be defined as a rule enacted and recognised as commanding or forbidding certain actions, or a body of such rules (Griffith and Tengnah, 2016). Rules can both guide and serve as standards for behaviour. But all rules, whether they are legal, moral, ethical or social, have the same basic characteristics: they set standards of how things ought or ought not to be, and lay down a standard of behaviour which must be complied with if the rule affects us (Hendrick, 2000). Nurses should therefore be aware of relevant legislation and health and social care policies to be able to apply them in their practice. A vital role of nurses in these cases is to advocate for the infant or child and the family, and to ensure that their legal rights are upheld and respected (Hagger et al., 2016). Knowledge of specific legal principles and laws relevant to neonatology is essential in modern healthcare (DeTora and Cummings, 2015). Table 9.1 outlines some key legal principles that should be understood by nurses and the MDT to protect both themselves and the infant and family at a usually vulnerable time.

These important legal considerations, highlighted above, should not be addressed in isolation and they all interlink in some way. For example, obtaining valid, informed consent to medical treatment is a fundamental principle of modern medical practice (Williams and Perkins, 2011). The law pertaining to who does and who does not have parental responsibility is complicated and often poorly understood. Parental responsibility is a concept of having the rights, duties, powers and responsibilities which a parent has in relation to the child and his or her property. It was introduced by the Children Act 1989 and contains a list of key roles; the guiding principle being that of the child's best interests (Williams and Perkins, 2011).

Other specific legal areas will now be addressed that are pertinent to the area of neonatal care specifically, as distinct from other areas of healthcare; namely, foetal rights and

TABLE 9.1 LEGAL PRINCIPLES IN NEONATAL CARE: THE NURSE'S ROLE

Legal issue	Application to neonatal care
Safeguarding / child protection	Nurses should use their experience and clinical judgement to make informed decisions in relation to the safety of infants in the neonatal unit and identify factors for concern in families.
	Through continued education and professional development, nurses can increase their knowledge on potential indicators for infant abuse and preventative measures.
	An environment must be created in which not only the infant feels secure but also the parents so that they can promote a healthy start to their relationship (Care Quality Commission (CQC), 2016; Rogers & Nurse, 2018).
Minimising risk and litigation	To protect the vulnerable infant, all nursing care practices should be delivered with safety as a central consideration including adherence to local/national policies and practice guidelines relating to clinical tasks and staffing levels (National Quality Board, 2018). Governance processes should also be followed (CQC, 2016).
Accountability	Neonatal nurses, whether at the bedside or in advanced practice, are morally, ethically and legally accountable for their nursing judgements and actions and must comply with The Code (NMC, 2018) to ensure their practice meets the standards required not only by the NMC, but also by patients (infants and families) and the general public. Compliance with *'the professional standards that registered nurses and midwives must uphold [is] not negotiable or discretionary'* (NMC, 2018, p. 3).
Consent	Nurses in conjunction with the MDT, have both a legal and a professional obligation to ensure that parents are informed about the proposed treatment and care of their infant and that this consent is sought before starting treatment. Consent will only be valid if full information has been given (Shenoy et al., 2003; BAPM, 2014; Vasu, 2017; Taylor, 2018). Consent principles in line with the above-mentioned governance processes must also be applied to parental consent for their involvement in research.
Confidentiality	Neonatal nurses must ensure that personal and sensitive information about the infant and family is protected and not shared openly with others (Sudia-Robinson, 2013) avoiding any breach of data protection rules and laws that are in place.
Duty of care	This refers to obligations placed on people to act towards others in a certain way (Royal College of Nursing (RCN), 2019). Nurses have a moral or legal obligation to ensure the safety or wellbeing of others. Neonatal nurses specifically have a duty to act in the infant's best interests (Mancini et al., 2014), both legally and professionally. They can use the guidance and frameworks outlined in this chapter to assist with knowledge about decision-making to uphold this essential principle.
Parental responsibility	This refers to legal rights and responsibilities as a parent. Neonatal nurses must be aware of the Children Act 2004 (Workingwithkids.co.uk, 2017) in relation to an understanding of this term and how it applies to their practice when dealing with parents.

the concept of personhood, before turning to a discussion of ethical principles and application to neonatal practice.

Foetal rights, personhood, age of viability

Under English law, foetuses have no independent legal status. Once born, babies have the same rights to life as other people (Nuffield Council on Bioethics, 2014). The law's main concern with gestational age lies in the concept of viability. This is not only a matter of UK jurisprudence; viability is universally regarded as an important milestone (Laurie et al., 2016). In an era of fast improving neonatal care, ethical care of infants born at the threshold of viability is increasingly complex (Boyle et al., 2004). Indeed, outcome of these infants is marked by the potential for complications that can impact on the quality of life for children and families (Einaudi et al., 2015). Ethical frameworks should be used to approach ethical dilemmas in patient care and assist in the decision-making process. Wherever possible, practitioners and parents should mutually decide on the most appropriate treatment; however, when conflict arises, legal frameworks can be applied. The fundamental legal perspective in relation to children and young people is that the best interests of the child must be paramount (Hagger et al., 2016).

There are varied positions on when a foetus is afforded the status of personhood. These positions have foundations in law, morality, religion and biomedical science. In some instances, the foetus is considered a person from the point of conception, but there are many thresholds during embryonic development that differing perspectives consider attainment of moral status. For many, however, birth is considered to be a highly significant moment in the foetus becoming a person with full moral status. The Nuffield Council could not reach a unanimous conclusion as to the point in time at which moral status should be afforded to the foetus; however, they regard the moment of birth, which is straightforward to identify, and usually represents a significant threshold in potential viability, as the significant point of transition not just for legal judgments about preserving life but also for moral ones (Nuffield Council on Bioethics, 2014). In neonatal care, personhood is not the only consideration regarding moral, legal and ethical thinking. Age of viability is tremendously relevant to determine whether life of the foetus is sustainable. Embryonic development of the lungs is highly significant in relation to survival and outcome of the preterm infant, as it is during the period of 22 to 24 weeks that the basic structure of the area of the lung where gaseous exchange occurs is formed and vascularised (Glass et al., 2015) and surfactant production begins; both are paramount to enable life. There is international consensus that at 22 weeks of gestation there is no hope of survival, and that up to 22^{+6} weeks is considered to be the 'cut-off' or threshold for human viability. From week 25^{+0} onwards there is general agreement that active management should be offered. Delivery between these two gestational age limits is the most challenging (Royal College of Obstetricians and Gynaecologists (RCOG), 2014). The Nuffield Council have developed criteria to guide clinicians when considering whether to resuscitate babies born at the limits of viability. A link to this document can be found in the web-based companion (see link at the end of this chapter).

In brief, the criteria provide useful information on how to manage resuscitation of infants born at varying gestations from 22 weeks' gestation and above, with recommendations changing at each week as gestation progresses through to 25 weeks and above. The discussion about the age of foetal viability involves two quite separate issues. One is the increase in survival rates for babies born extremely prematurely; the second is abortion – which, in the UK, is available up to 24 weeks' gestation. From a legal perspective it is clear that international human rights law deems human rights to apply prior to birth, but by reducing the 'normal' limit for abortion to 24 weeks, UK law seems to recognise that a foetus has acquired some additional human rights at this stage of its gestation that it did not have prior to this (British Medical Association, 2007). Quite often due to this notion 24 weeks' gestation is often referred to as the age of viability. Chapter 3 has details on the updated guidance published by the British Association of Perinatal Medicine (BAPM, 2019).

Closely linked to legal considerations are ethical principles which will now be discussed, in line with the specific application to the neonatal setting.

Ethical principles

Foetal and neonatal medicine raises several ethical issues including: the value of human life, the concept of 'best interests', deliberately ending life and decision-making (Nuffield Council on Bioethics, 2014). Much has been said about the ethics of delivery room resuscitation; however most neonatal deaths now occur after intensive care is reoriented or following limitation or non-escalation of treatment orders. Due to a combination of factors including technological advances, improved service delivery and greater parental involvement, it seems that ethical dilemmas are ever more challenging to resolve (Kirkbride, 2013; Sacco and Virata, 2017).

Although a preterm baby is one born before 37 weeks, there is a wide variation in that group, from extremely preterm to late preterm (Paterson and Redpath, 2013). Advances in this area have been remarkable, leading to a substantial reduction in mortality. Nevertheless, ethical questions remain, about resources, about whether the outcomes for some babies are too burdensome, about criteria and authority for decision-making, and on stress and burn-out for adults involved, both professionals and parents. Of these, the most challenging is the issue of over-burdensome outcomes of treatment to achieve survival. Parents too may feel '*overwhelmed by the demands of having to care for a preterm infant while at the same time coming to terms with a pregnancy that did not meet their expectations*' (Paterson and Redpath, 2013, p. 19). Where an infant appears to have poor prognosis, it may be argued that it is best either not to begin or to withdraw treatment. The difficulty of a decision to act is that, while resuscitation may be successful, the result may be a severely handicapped survivor; and this is not even to mention the resource implications of such a decision (Laurie et al., 2016).

Neonatal ethical standards seem to have lagged behind delivery of neonatal intensive care. Potential reasons for this include: agreement of how to manage care varies among physicians, nurses, and families, all who have different values, beliefs, and priorities; advances in neonatal technology have determined that those caring for neonates have not been afforded with sufficient training and time to resolve difficult end-of-life dilemmas; both of these factors therefore contribute to an overall lack of capability of providers to discuss ethical care (Pasarón, 2013). Although there is no scope within this chapter to explore different ethical theories and principles in great detail, some areas of concern and practical neonatal intensive care-related dilemmas based on principles of ethics will follow. For more detailed information, reference should be made to the work of Beauchamp and Childress (2009).

The main focus will now turn to an overview of the four main ethical theories and then a discussion of the basic bioethical principles of autonomy, beneficence and non-maleficence, and justice. Central to any of the following discussion is the notion of upholding what is in the best interest of the baby and the vital inclusion and involvement of the family.

ETHICAL THEORIES

Utilitarianism or consequentialism

This first theory adopts the belief that actions are right or wrong according to the balance of their good and bad consequences. The right act is therefore considered to be the one that produces the best overall result and is determined from an impersonal perspective considering that all parties are equally considered. A major criticism of utilitarianism is this impersonal approach. It would in the most part be seemingly impossible to apply this theory to neonatal nursing, at the foundation of which is to ensure that every infant should be treated as an individual, considering the needs of the baby and family at the centre of care. There are, of course, limited occasions when a utilitarian-based decision may be the appropriate one to implement. An example of this would be where the maximum safety of all persons within the neonatal unit (NNU) had to be ensured such as a fire evacuation.

Deontology/Kantianism

Deontology results from the work of Immanuel Kant (1724–1804) and is obligation- or duty-based. The overarching theme is that the duty is performed, irrespective of the consequences (Chadwick and Gallagher, 2016). An example of this, which could be applied to neonatal care, is the duty to preserve life. If this duty were upheld in the truest sense, it would exclude any decisions regarding withholding or withdrawing life-sustaining treatments and prevent the application of the best interest standard.

Virtue-based theory

Virtue ethics are concerned with the moral character or the virtues of the decision-maker, rather than what is right, the duty of the decision-maker or the consequences of their decision. The idea underpinning virtue ethics is that when people are faced with complex moral dilemmas or situations, they will select the right decision because doing the right thing is fundamental to a virtuous person's character (Butts and Rich, 2015). Although virtue ethics may influence one's perception of another, even virtuous people are fallible, thus highlighting an elementary flaw when applying this theory to practice in isolation.

Rights-based theory

Generally speaking, rights are moral and legal claims that entitle us to demand that we are treated in a just and equitable way (Benatar, 2006). As individuals' rights can conflict with each other, this indicates no right can be considered absolute. However, most rights can be deemed obligatory if not overridden by competing rights. Rights usually arise from legal and moral sources and from pertinent documents such as the Human Rights Act (1998). Related to human rights and related topics, there are key articles of reference for neonatal nurses (a weblink can be found within the web-based companion, see URL at the end of this chapter). Within neonatal nursing, rights-based theory poses conflicting perspectives, as the infant's rights and parents' rights may be directly infringing upon each other, placing the healthcare providers in a difficult position. It seems prudent, therefore, to have an awareness of all these ethical theories to help shape decision-making within the neonatal intensive care unit, however caution should be sought when using one theory in isolation.

ETHICAL FRAMEWORKS

As we have seen, technological advances have altered the boundary relating to what is defined as 'viability', and there is an increased need to consider quality of life in intervention decisions (Lantos, 2018). An approach to decision-making that accounts for the complexity of both the MDT and family values is essential. Beauchamp and Childress (2009) 'Four Principles' is one of the most widely used frameworks and offers a broad consideration of medical ethics issues generally. The Four Principles are general guides that leave considerable room for judgement on specific cases.

Bioethical framework

The four bioethical principles, now discussed in turn, are depicted in figure 9.1.

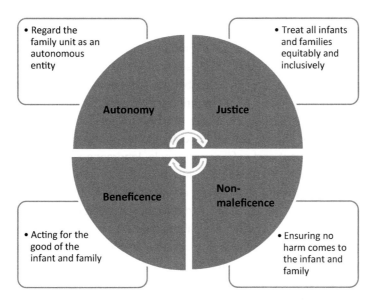

Figure 9.1 The four bioethical principles

AUTONOMY

When considering making decisions within neonatal care, it is important to remember the infant is not an autonomous being. To be considered autonomous it is widely thought that a person must be able to perceive themselves as a rational individual who has the capacity to make informed choices through uncoerced decisions. Where the patient is considered incompetent or non-autonomous, decisions are made by a proxy or surrogate decision-maker. This would usually be the baby's parents; under the terms of the Mental Capacity Act 2005, they must be presumed to be competent to do so unless otherwise proven. In some cases, the courts will be forced to act in the capacity of surrogate decision-maker to ensure the rights of the infant are protected and care is delivered considering their best interest (Wilkinson, 2006). The decision-making process within neonatal care is unique in nature, as it considers an infant who has never been autonomous, and the natural focus of neonatal care tends to be the infant's interests opposed to their rights (Spence, 2000). The best interest standard is disputed in this principle and is meant to be protective of a person unable to make decisions of his or her own by transferring the assessment of risks and benefits of treatment options and their alternatives to a surrogate. The baby's parents may not be best placed to make decisions in isolation as they may not possess the appropriate knowledge or perspective to do so. It is the responsibility of healthcare providers to ensure that every reasonable effort has been made to enable parents to understand the information presented. An example of this is the use of interpreters or relevant communication aids.

BENEFICENCE AND NON-MALEFICENCE

Beneficence can be defined as an action of charity, mercy or kindness with a strong intention to do good to others (Kinsinger, 2009), so relating to benevolence. Beneficence also strives to reach an outcome that provides benefit for the recipient (Baumrucker et al., 2008). In contrast, non-maleficence is the principle of doing no harm. The Code is very clear when identifying that fulfilling the duties of both principles is a core responsibility for all nurses (NMC, 2018). Nurses are and should be held accountable for their practice, ensuring they are competent and safe professionals. Ignorance is not accepted as a justification when harm occurs, as nurses are duty bound to ensure that they act within the level of their competence (NMC, 2018). If faced with a situation they are not competent to manage, they should recognise their limits and refer the situation to another member of the team. Harm incidents that occur within clinical practice are usually caused by human error or iatrogenesis, harm caused by initiating treatment/care. When such incidents do occur, the staff involved are assessed using the Bolam principle, in which staff are measured by the standard of practice deemed acceptable and reasonable by a responsible group of practitioners from the same specialty (Tingle and Cribb,2013). This ensures a fair and just review of the incident as to whether it was avoidable and managed appropriately.

As principles, non-maleficence and beneficence are usually in tension with one another, primarily because beneficence considers burden versus benefit of treatment within the best interest standard, whereas non-maleficence could be considered as continuing futile treatment by not causing death (Stone, 2018). It is important to acknowledge that the purpose of intensive care is not to prolong life with futile treatment, but to restore the health of the person (Stone, 2018). From this perspective, continuation of futile intensive care could even be considered as a technological form of harm, as it is not going to achieve the desired outcome (Wyatt, 1985). It is difficult to balance these two principles when applying them to specific dilemmas in neonatal intensive care such as withholding and withdrawing life-sustaining treatment, again highlighting the need for a pragmatic approach when approaching ethical principles in isolation.

JUSTICE

The fourth ethical principle, justice, refers to ensuring each person is given what they are due. It can be considered in terms of fairness, equality, need or any other criterion that is material to the justice decision. In healthcare, justice often focuses on equitable access to care resource allocation and protection of the patient's rights (Pasarón, 2013). It would therefore seem obvious that the cost of neonatal care, while just for the patients that receive it, may not be considered so in a struggling healthcare economy. When resources are already limited, it could be considered unjust to fund an expensive area of healthcare when this funding could be used elsewhere for patients that may have better outcomes and survival rates. Pasarón (2013) objects to this perspective, highlighting that there is insufficient data to support these claims. It is clear that there are no easy answers as to how justice can

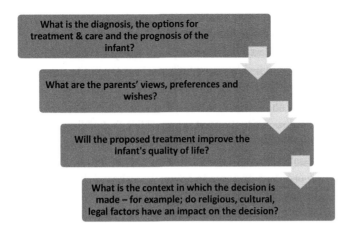

Figure 9.2 The four-quadrant approach to ethical decision-making in the neonatal unit (adapted from Jonsen et al., 2008)

be truly implemented within an imperfect society (Beauchamp and Childress, 2009). The application of ethics and moral decision-making to practice is not just about life and death decisions or the provision of resources on a national scale. It is present in everyday life, and neonatal nurses, as autonomous practitioners, should be encouraged to develop their awareness of the subject. When in context, it is easy to determine how these ethical considerations can be seen in everyday practice. An example of this is allocating staff to infants, when considering the needs of the babies are matched against the skills of the staff and the overall needs of the unit. This can be seen as an unconscious use of the ethical principles to ensure that care is provided safely and effectively.

The four-quadrant approach

Another framework for ethical decision-making is the four-quadrant approach – see figure 9.2. This provides a set of questions to follow when exploring particular cases.

WITHHOLDING AND WITHDRAWING TREATMENT

Due to the advancements in both perinatal and neonatal care, there are more frequent instances where infants of borderline viability are resuscitated at birth. These situations call for medical and nursing teams in collaboration with parents to make some very difficult decisions regarding withholding or withdrawing life-sustaining treatments (McHaffie et al., 2001; Royal College of Paediatrics and Child Health (RCPCH), 2004; Bhatia, 2015). Professionals should not only be fully aware of the ethical and legal issues but also about how to manage such difficult decisions to the satisfaction of parents, the judiciary, and the public (Avery, 2016). There are also instances where infants have been born and developed past the age of viability but have conditions that are incompatible with life, such as congenital abnormalities, for example anencephaly or Trisomy 18 (Edwards syndrome). In other situations, ongoing treatment has become futile and continuing to provide care is no longer considered to be in the best interest of the baby; examples of this are infants that have received therapeutic hypothermia and when the treatment is completed they have no cerebral function present. In these situations, it is imperative that all the ethical and legal considerations have been addressed to ensure the most appropriate outcome. Clinicians are duty bound to act in the best interest of the infant and should use all available guidance to do so. Internationally, the literature appears to advocate a shared decision-making approach, in which clinicians (members of medical and nursing teams in the UK) and parents work collaboratively to recognise the infant's best interests. The guidance provided by the RCPCH (2004); which has foundations in UK law and strives for best ethical practice, agrees that parental agreement is essential when considering withholding or withdrawing treatment for neonates (Larcher et al., 2015). The dynamics of complex decision-making between all parties will be explored further later in this chapter. The RCPCH provides an essential framework that echoes the voice of law, and although it is a clinical guideline, it assumes much of the same language as a legal ruling (Bhatia, 2015). It is common and accepted practice to withdraw life-sustaining treatment where parents and the neonatal MDT believe that the distress caused by such intervention outweighs the benefits. This 'weighing-up' of risks versus benefits is part of the decision-making process and must always be viewed within the context of the 'best interest' principle to which the chapter will now turn.

DECISION-MAKING AND THE 'BEST INTERESTS' PRINCIPLE

Admission of a baby to a NNU is anxiety-provoking for parents and information about interventions may not be understood or retained (Carter et al., 2005). Nonetheless, parents may be asked to sanction proposed interventions based on medical 'best interests' (Vasu, 2017). The principle of 'best interests' is central to medical practice and UK law. It states that in all matters affecting any child, his or her best interest should be the paramount consideration. Parents, doctors and others involved in the decision-making process may have different ideas about what is in the best interest of the baby (Nuffield Council on Bioethics, 2014). Gillam et al. (2017) present differences in viewpoint in the case of deciding whether to resuscitate an infant born at 24 weeks whose parents did not want any active resuscitation, but who went on to survive without complications with an uncertain outcome. They concluded that there must be shared decisions made with both parents and unbiased information from expert health professionals. It is important to recognise that there may be some situations where the plan upholds the rights and best interest of the baby, but the result is in discord between the parents and care providers (Bhatia, 2015). Conflict in decision-making and suggested strategies are summarised in table 9.2.

TABLE 9.2 CONFLICT IN DECISION-MAKING IN THE NEONATAL UNIT

Challenges and conflicts	Strategies
Conflict within the family	Give honest and timely information. Involve key members of the family
	Involve religious figure according to the values and background of the family.
Conflict between parents and the neonatal MDT	Regular meetings and communication between the MDT and the parents/family.
Communication challenges and barriers	Involve advocacy services to bridge any communication barriers.
	Consider language/information needs, both verbal and written in line with cultural and ethnic background of the family.
Parents with limited competence to make decisions (due to age, capacity, illness)	Involve other members of the MDT – e.g. social worker, family support workers, family advocates and support services.

Regardless of the presence of conflict, what must always be upheld is what is deemed in the 'best interest' of the infant. The 'best interest' principle has its foundation in the Children Act 1989. The overriding principle of the Children Act 1989 is that the baby's or child's welfare and best interests must be of the highest regard in all decisions concerning their upbringing. The way the 'best interest' of the very premature newborn is determined needs to keep time with the evolving importance of shared decision-making and family-centred care (Jefferies et al., 2012). This evolution requires that the very concept of 'best interest' as well as the modalities to clinically determine it, be transformed to transcend the traditional basis in the principles of bioethics and the definition of ethical dilemmas as 'conflicts between principles' (Daboval and Shidler, 2014). Daboval and Shidler (2014) also state, however, that there is no single, unequivocal definition of the 'best interest' of a seriously compromised newborn. The General Medical Council (GMC, 2018) states that authoritative clinical guidance must be used to determine what treatment may be in a neonate's best interests. The RCPCH (2004) describes five situations in which it is considered ethical, legal and in the child's best interest to withhold life-sustaining treatment, one of which is the 'no chance' situation. This situation is described as '*such severe disease that life-sustaining treatment simply delays death without significant alleviation of suffering*' (RCPCH, 2004, p. 10).

Although clinical practices are evolving toward shared decision-making, a significant proportion of neonatologists believe they provide the 'best' answers in the quest for the best interest of sick infants, not recognising the fact that the interpretation of research data predicting prognosis may vary even among themselves (Haward et al., 2011; 2017). Thus a collaborative approach is paramount, meaning that all persons with relevant advocacy for the baby, having taken into account long- and short-term issues, partake in the decision-making process (Kohsman, 2016).

Parents are generally considered to have the moral authority to make decisions in their child's best interests in all the circumstances of life, though not as if they owned them. Doctors have a responsibility to promote the best interests of the newborn baby and will be able to give a prediction on the outcome for the baby based on their knowledge and experience. Nurses spend a great deal of time with the parents and their baby, and are therefore well placed to provide additional insights into the best interest of both the child and his or her family (Nuffield Council on Bioethics, 2014).

TISSUE AND ORGAN DONATION

Finally, when a decision has been reached to withdraw treatment, parents are approached in appropriate situations to determine whether they would consider their baby to become a tissue or organ donor. Immediate focus should be applied to consent rates and supporting family decision-making in the most effective way possible (Hawkins et al., 2018). In the past, neonates have not been eligible for organ donation owing to the technical difficulties and the high risk for graft complication involved with transplant of their small organs. At present, less than 1% of all organ and tissue donations come from donors younger than 1 year (Stiers et al., 2015). Neonatal organ and tissue donation has only come into existence in the latter part of the twentieth century and is still an uncommon procedure following death in the NNU (Godfrey and Kish, 2014). Organ transplantation involves a potentially lifesaving gift from the donor to the recipient. However, numerous ethical considerations exist, especially in paediatrics and neonates. Practitioners involved in paediatric and neonatal organ transplantation should apply the four principles of biomedical ethics, namely autonomy, non-maleficence, beneficence and justice (Sarnaik, 2015).

The decision to donate a newborn's organs is most often a parental responsibility. The legal standard is that parents consent for their child with the understanding that they are making decisions in the best interest of the child. Unfortunately, because of the inability to use organ donations from many of the deceased infants belonging to the NNU population of donors, there remain many cases of death where parents are not informed about organ donation. In addition, sometimes medical professionals find it difficult to discuss organ donation with families who are experiencing the intense grief associated with loss of an infant. Organ donation in the NNU rarely occurs; criteria exist that are based on what is considered technically feasible for transplantation of donated organ and tissue. These criteria often include weight and gestational age limitations, and absence of infection or malignancy, as well as constraints related to optimal timing following circulatory death and hospital geography (Godfrey and Kish, 2014). Neonates with birth defects likely to be lethal immediately after birth represent another potential group of organ donors. Anencephaly is a severe neural tube defect in which the cerebral hemispheres including the neocortex, part of the meninges, skull and scalp are missing. Infants born with this condition are blind, deaf, unconscious and unable to perceive pain (Sarnaik, 2015).

The loss of a loved one is a devastating time, particularly for the parents of a newborn baby. Despite the intense emotions that accompany loss, many parents want to make sense of the tragedy by being able to keep another family from experiencing the same tragedy through organ donation. The option for organ, tissue and cell donation and transplantation provides a second chance at life for thousands of people each year, and is often seen by families as a way to help others while facilitating their own healing. By allowing their child to be a source of organ donation, parents are giving the gift of hope to many other families whose lives could be enhanced through transplantation or vital transplantation research (Godfrey and Kish, 2014).

Finally, the chapter pays attention to both the family's and the nurse's roles to emphasise the key part that both play in delivery of safe and ethically sound care in the NNU.

FAMILY-CENTRED PRINCIPLES OF INCLUSIVE, ETHICAL CARE

By changing the paradigm of neonatal care and integrating parents into the care team, the family integrated care (FIC) model, as discussed in chapter 4, ensures that babies receive care within a holistic framework and that parents are a core part of any decision-making. In addition, within the often difficult and complex ethical decision-making that takes place as discussed earlier, it is also vital that the family's individualised cultural needs and values are considered. The holistic perspective is depicted in figure 9.3.

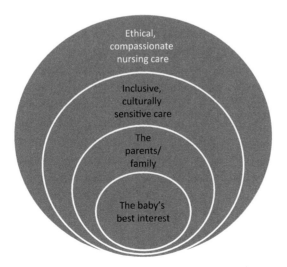

Figure 9.3 Family-centred, inclusive and ethical care of the infant in the neonatal unit

THE NURSE'S ROLE IN LEGAL AND ETHICAL ISSUES IN THE NEONATAL UNIT

The nurse's role as a key component of the neonatal MDT has been touched on throughout this chapter. However, it is worth concluding the chapter with a few final points about the nursing context. It is essential that nurses are able to recognise legal and ethical challenges and practise in line with national guidance and frameworks. Neonatal nurses are in a unique position to be advocates for the babies and families they care for. They understand the beliefs and values of families including the individualised wishes they may have within their ethnic, cultural and religious backgrounds. Cultural competence is vital in line with respecting the cultural, ethnic, and socioeconomic diversity of all families in the NNU and ensuring their best interests are upheld. In line with this, culturally inclusive care should be considered and implemented by the whole MDT (Hendson et al., 2015) and nurses as a key player in the team should continue to work towards greater cultural competence (Heitzler, 2017) to ensure family's' diverse and holistic needs are met. This important topic is given further coverage in chapters 7 and 8, palliative and bereavement care respectively.

Finally, the link between law and ethics requires further emphasis. Nurses should have knowledge and skills to practise safe acts in line with regulations that will ultimately guide and influence them to provide holistic, ethical and compassionate care; this is the essence of good nursing practice for the best interests of the neonatal population and their families (Al-Breiki, 2017).

CONCLUSION

Nurses, the MDT and parents ought to be able to meet the challenges and complexities of modern neonatal care including advanced technology, uncertain outcomes and the legal and ethical issues that may arise, free of any coercion, fear or guilt, and equipped with the knowledge of appropriate frameworks to guide them. Only in this type of environment can they truly embrace advocacy and practise soundly in consideration of the four key biomedical ethical principles discussed (Pasarón, 2013) and the 'best interest' principle. While there is no single strategy that should be used, collaboration is the preferred approach, since this requires the MDT to recognise areas of controversy and identify a solution incorporating the perspectives of all parties (Vivar, 2006, cited in Hagger et al., 2016), including the family at all times through the entire decision-making process. Ultimately, the best interests of the infant must be paramount in any ethical and legal decision-making that takes place within the NNU.

CASE STUDIES

For each of these cases below:

Q.1. What are the key legal and ethical issues in these three cases?
Q.2. What would you consider in line with the 'best interest' principle?
Q.3. What are vital considerations for supporting the parents/family in these cases?
Q.4. Can you identify the areas of conflict in decision-making in these cases and possible ways to resolve them?
Q.5. What are the reasons for your answers?

Case study 1: An ethical dilemma in the delivery suite

Faye was born very prematurely and because her mum, Freda, had not had any antenatal care, the exact estimated date of delivery was uncertain. An assessment by the neonatal team came to the decision that she presented like a baby born at 22–23 weeks. Faye required prolonged resuscitation after delivery and her heart rate remained low with very little spontaneous breathing. Freda wanted full resuscitation to continue and for Faye to be admitted to the neonatal unit for full intensive care. She was estranged from her partner, Faye's father Pete, and they had separated when she was in the early stages of pregnancy. They were unmarried with no other children. Pete did not wish Faye to receive full intensive care as he felt it was not in her best interest.

Case study 2: A child protection dilemma

Tim is a very growth-restricted baby boy, born at 37 weeks' gestation to Linda, a known drug user (heroin). Linda lives in a hostel run by a local charity and has been on a methadone programme although the compliance with this is erratic. Her two other children are in temporary foster care. There is also a history of domestic abuse from Linda's ex-partner and he is aware that Tim has been born although he is not permitted to visit the neonatal unit. Following birth, Tim shows withdrawal signs and is very irritable, inconsolable with an episode of fitting. He is placed onto methadone.

Case study 3: Ethical and legal issues in the older infant

Rosemary was born at term and spent a period of 10 weeks being very unstable requiring respiratory support and displaying symptoms of hypotonia, muscle weakness, pneumonia, and swallowing and feeding difficulties. After a recent extubation, she required re-ventilation and a diagnosis returned of spinal muscular atrophy. Her

C
A
S
E

S
T
U
D
Y

respiratory drive continued to worsen, eventually diminishing completely and she was unable to tolerate any enteral feeding. Her parents Precious and Zane, who had four other children all healthy, wanted full ventilation support to continue. The consultant had spoken to them about Rosemary's poor prognosis and the fact that she would be unable to breathe without this support.

For suggested answer guides to the questions posed in these case studies, please refer to the web-based companion site specific to this chapter (see URL below).

WEB-BASED RESOURCES

For further information, online resources and greater detail on the case studies featured in this chapter go to www.routledge.com/cw/nicnursing

References

Al-Breiki, M. (2017). What Influence Nurses Practice More: Law or Ethics. *JOJ Nurse Healthcare*. 5(3), 103.

Avery, G. (2016). *Law and ethics in nursing and healthcare: An introduction*. London: Sage.

Baumrucker, S. J., Sheldon, J. E., Stolick, M., Morris, G. M., VandeKieft, G., & Harrington, D. (2008). The ethical concept of 'best interest'. *American Journal of Hospice and Palliative Medicine*, 25(1), 56–62.

Beauchamp, T. L., & Childress, J. F. (2009). *Principles of Biomedical Ethics* (6th Edition). Oxford: Oxford University Press.

Benatar, D. (2006). Bioethics and health and human rights: A critical view. *Journal of Medical Ethics*, 32(1), 17–20.

Bhatia, N. (2015). *Critically Impaired Infants and End of Life Decision Making: Resource Allocation and Difficult Decisions*. Oxford: Routledge.

Boyle, R. J., Salter, R., & Amander, M. W. (2004). Ethics of refusing parental requests to withhold or withdraw treatment from their premature baby. *Journal of Medical Ethics*, 30(4), 402–405.

British Association of Perinatal Medicine (BAPM). (2014). *Consent for common neonatal investigations, interventions and treatments*. London: British Association of Perinatal Medicine.

British Association of Perinatal Medicine. (2019). *Perinatal Management at less than 27 weeks' Gestation. A Framework for Practice*. London: British Association of Perinatal Medicine.

British Medical Association. (2007). *The law and ethics of abortion*. London: British Medical Association.

Butts, J.B., & Rich, K.L. (2015). *Nursing Ethics* (4th edition). Burlington, MA: Jones and Bartlett.

Care Quality Commission. (2016). *Inspection Framework: NHS Acute (specialist children's hospitals. Core Service: Neonatal Services*. www.cqc.org.uk/sites/default/files/20160713_NHS_specialist_core_service_inspection_framework_neonatal_services.pdf

Carter, J. D., Mulder, R. T., Bartram, A. F., & Darlow, B. A. (2005). Infants in a neonatal intensive care unit: parental response. *Archives of Disease in Childhood: Fetal and Neonatal Edition*, 90(2), F109–F113.

Chadwick, R., & Gallagher, A. (Eds.) (2016). *Ethics and Nursing Practice: A Case Study Approach. 2nd Edition*. London: Palgrave.

Children Act. (1989). www.legislation.gov.uk/ukpga/1989/41.

Daboval, T., & Shidler, S. (2014). Ethical framework for shared decision making in the neonatal intensive care unit: Communicative ethics. *Paediatrics & Child Health, 19*(6), 302–304.

DeTora, A. W., & Cummings, C. L. (2015). Ethics and the law: Practical applications in the neonatal intensive care unit. *NeoReviews, 16*(7), e384–e392.

Einaudi, M. A., Gire, C., Auquier, P., & Le Coz, P. (2015). How do physicians perceive quality of life? Ethical questioning in neonatology. *BMC Medical Ethics, 16*(1), 50.

General Medical Council. (2018). *Ethical guidance*. General Medical Council.

Gillam, L., Wilkinson, D., Xafis, V., & Isaacs, D. (2017). Decision-making at the borderline of viability: Who should decide and on what basis? *Journal of Paediatrics and Child Health, 53*(2), 105–111.

Glass, H. C., Costarino, A. T., Stayer, S. A., Brett, C. M., Cladis, F., & Davis, P. J. (2015). Outcomes for extremely premature infants. *Anesthesia and Analgesia, 120*(6), 1337–1351.

Godfrey, K., & Kish, M. Z. (2014). Neonatal Liver Cell Donation: A Case Report. *Neonatal Network, 33*(6), 315–321.

Green, J., Darbyshire, P., Adams, A., & Jackson, D. (2017). Quality versus quantity: The complexities of quality of life determinations for neonatal nurses. *Nursing Ethics, 24*(7), 802–820.

Griffith, R. & Tengnah, C. (2016). *Law and professional issues in Nursing. 4th Edition*. Sage Publications Ltd.

Hagger, V., Ellis, C., & Strumidlo, L. (2016). Legal and ethical issues in neonatal nursing: A case study. *Nursing Standard, 30*(44), 48–53.

Haward, M. F., Kirshenbaum, N. W., & Campbell, D. E. (2011). Care at the edge of viability: Medical and ethical issues. *Clinics in perinatology, 38*(3), 471–492.

Haward, M. F., Gaucher, N., Payot, A., Robson, K., & Janvier, A. (2017). Personalized decision making: Practical recommendations for antenatal counseling for fragile neonates. *Clinics in Perinatology, 44*(2), 429–445.

Hawkins, K. C., Scales, A., Murphy, P., Madden, S., & Brierley, J. (2018). Current status of paediatric and neonatal organ donation in the UK. *Archives of Disease in Childhood, 103*(3), 210–215.

Heitzler, E. T. (2017). Cultural competence of obstetric and neonatal nurses. *Journal of Obstetric, Gynecologic & Neonatal Nursing, 46*(3), 423–433.

Hendrick, J. (2000). *Law and ethics in nursing and health care*. Cheltenham: Nelson Thornes.

Hendson, L., Reis, M. D., & Nicholas, D. B. (2015). Health care providers' perspectives of providing culturally competent care in the NICU. *Journal of Obstetric, Gynecologic & Neonatal Nursing, 44*(1), 17–27.

Human Rights Act. (1998). Great Britain. Human Rights Act 1998: Elizabeth ll. (1998). London: The Stationery Office.

Jefferies, A. L., Kirpalani, H. M., Canadian Paediatric Society, & Fetus and Newborn Committee. (2012). Counselling and management for anticipated extremely preterm birth. *Paediatrics & Child Health, 17*(8), 443–443.

Jonsen, A. R., Siegler, M., & Winslade, W. J. (2008). *Clinical ethics: A practical approach to ethical decisions in clinical medicine. 3rd Edition*. London: McGraw-Hill.

Kinsinger, F. S., (2009). Beneficence and the professional's moral imperative. *Journal of Chiropractic Humanities, 16*(1), 44–46.

Kirkbride, V. (2013). Managing complex ethical problems on the neonatal unit. *Infant, 9*(2), 66–70.

Kohsman, M. G. (2016). Ethical considerations for perinatal toxicology screening. *Neonatal Network, 35*(5), 268–276.

Lantos, J. D. (2018). Ethical problems in decision making in the neonatal ICU. *New England Journal of Medicine, 379*(19), 1851–1860.

Larcher, V., Craig, F., Bhogal, K., Wilkinson, D., & Brierley, J. (2015). Making decisions to limit treatment in life-limiting and life-threatening conditions in children: a framework for practice. *Archives of Disease in Childhood, 100* (Suppl 2), s1–s23.

Laurie, G. T. Harmon, SHE. & Porter, G. (2016). *Law and medical ethics.* (10th Edition). Oxford: Oxford University Press.

Mancini, A., Uthaya, S., Beardsley, C., Wood, D., & Modi, N. (2014). *Practical guidance for the management of palliative care on neonatal units*. London: Royal College of Paediatrics and Child Health.

McHaffie, H. E., Laing, I. A., Parker, M., & McMillan, J. (2001). Deciding for imperilled newborns: Medical authority or parental autonomy? *Journal of Medical Ethics*, *27*(2), 104–109.

Mental Capacity Act. (2005). www.legislation.gov.uk/ukpga/2005/9.

National Quality Board (2018) Safe, Sustainable and Productive Staffing. An improvement resource for neonatal care. https://improvement.nhs.uk/documents/2978/Safe_Staffing_Neonatal_FINAL_PROOF_27_June_2018.pdf.

Nuffield Council On Bioethics. (2014). *Critical care decisions in fetal and neonatal medicine: Ethical issues. A guide to the Report.* Nuffield Council on Bioethics.

Nursing and Midwifery Council (NMC). (2018). *Professional standards of practice and behaviour for nurses, midwives and nursing associates.* London: NMC. www.nmc.org.uk/standards/code/

Pasarón, R. (2013). Neonatal bioethical perspectives: practice considerations. *Neonatal Network*, *32*(3), 184–192.

Paterson, L., & Redpath, I. (2013). Preterm infant care. *Nursing Standard*, *27*(49).

Rogers, A., & Nurse, S. (2018). Child protection in the neonatal unit. *Journal of Neonatal Nursing*, *25*(2), 99–101.

Royal College of Nursing. (2019). *Duty of Care.* www.rcn.org.uk/get-help/rcn-advice/duty-of-care

Royal College of Obstetricians & Gynaecologists. (2014). Perinatal management of pregnant women at the threshold of infant viability (the obstetric perspective) scientific impact paper no. 41. *UK: RCOG.*

Royal College of Paediatrics and Child Health. (2004). *Witholding or Withdrawing Life Sustaining Treatment in Children: A Framework for Practice.* Royal College of Paediatrics and Child Health.

Sacco, J., & Virata, R. (2017). Baby O and the withdrawal of life-sustaining medical treatment in the devastated neonate: A review of clinical, ethical, and legal issues. *The American Journal of Hospice & Palliative Care*, *34*(10), 925–930.

Sarnaik, A. A. (2015). Neonatal and paediatric organ donation: Ethical perspectives and implications for policy. *Frontiers in Pediatrics.* 100(3): 1–7.

Shenoy, S., Archdeacon, C., Kotecha, S., & Elias-Jones, A. C. (2003). Current practice for obtaining consent in UK neonatal units. *Bulletin of Medical Ethics*, (188), 17–19.

Spence, K. (2000). The best interest principle as a standard for decision making in the care of neonates. *Journal of Advanced Nursing*, *31*(6), 1286–1292.

Stiers, J., Aguayo, C., Siatta, A., Presson, A. P., Perez, R., & DiGeronimo, R. (2015). Potential and actual neonatal organ and tissue donation after circulatory determination of death. *JAMA Pediatrics*, *169*(7), 639–645.

Sudia-Robinson, T. (2013). Legal and Ethical Issues in Neonatal Care. In Kenner, C., & Wright Lott, J. (Eds.) *Comprehensive Neonatal Nursing care* 5th Edition (pp. 863–867). New York: Springer Publishing Company.

Stone E. G. (2018). Evidence-Based Medicine and Bioethics: Implications for Health Care Organizations, Clinicians, and Patients. The Permanente Journal, 22, 18–30.

Taylor, H. (2018). Informed consent 1: Legal basis and implications for practice. *Nursing Times*, *114*(6), 25–28.

Tingle, J., & Cribb, A. (Eds.) (2013). Nursing law and ethics (3rd Edition). Chichester: John Wiley & Sons.

Vasu, V. (2017). Pilot evaluation of parental and professional views regarding consent in neonatal medicine by telephone interviews and questionnaires. *BMJ Paediatrics Open*, *1*(1).

Wilkinson, D. (2006). Is it in the best interests of an intellectually disabled infant to die? Journal of Medical Ethics, 32(8), 454–459.

Williams, C. A., & Perkins, R. (2011). Consent issues for children: A law unto themselves? *Continuing Education in Anaesthesia, Critical Care & Pain*, *11*(3), 99–103.

Workingwithkids.co.uk. (2017). *Children Act 2004.* www.workingwithkids.co.uk/childrens-act.html

Wyatt, J. S. (2009). *Matters of Life and Death* (2nd Edition). Westmont, Illinois: InterVarsity Press.

PART 3
CLINICAL ASPECTS OF NEONATAL CARE

Clinical aspects of neonatal care: The parent voice

He was very sick, and it was 'touch and go' if he would survive. He needed so much support for his breathing and his heart and was attached to all sorts of machines and tubes to keep him alive. I remember the noises, the bleeps and flashing lights … Relentless. The technology was daunting and scary, but it saved his life.

The care he had from the whole team was amazing … everything was explained to us and we came to finally understand what everything meant.

Even the smallest things we could do were important- expressing my milk and holding his hand … Even through the incubator walls and the mist.

One step at a time … gradually he got better but it seemed endless and like it was never going to happen. The sight of him without any machines and wires was quite a day … A relief to know that we could finally go home and start some normality.

Voice of a mother of a 25-week gestation baby, Luca (pseudonym) who spent 17 weeks in neonatal care.

Adapted from Petty et al., 2019a; 2019b

See chapter 4 reference list for full citations.

10 EARLY CARE OF THE NEWBORN

Sarah Fitchett

CONTENTS

GUIDANCE ON HOW TO ENHANCE PERSONAL LEARNING FROM THIS CHAPTER

Key points covered in this chapter

- Preparation for caring for the newborn infant in the first hour of life, including antenatal and perinatal considerations.
- Principles of neonatal resuscitation and the newborn life support algorithm.
- Care considerations after successful resuscitation.

Reflection

Reading through the chapter, you are encouraged to engage with the key points and related literature in an enquiring way. Ask these questions:

- How can you improve outcomes by optimising care in the Golden Hour?
- Would you feel confident and competent to participate in neonatal resuscitation, and are you familiar with the algorithm?
- How can you support families in caring for their baby after he or she has required resuscitation at birth?

Implications for nursing care

- Finally: consider how this new information will impact on your nursing care in relation to antenatal preparation for neonatal care, interventions during the Golden Hour and post-resuscitation care.

INTRODUCTION AND BACKGROUND

Resuscitation at birth is a relatively frequent occurrence. Approximately 10% of newborns will require help to establish breathing at birth, with 1% requiring more extensive resuscitation (Dempsey et al., 2015; Wyllie et al., 2015). These numbers suggest that most infants will respond to good airway and respiratory management, but that a small proportion will go on to require further interventions of chest compressions and resuscitative drugs.

Neonatal nurses, as either the lead practitioner or assistant, are often involved in the resuscitation of high-risk infants in the delivery room and infants in their care on the neonatal unit (NNU). In order to comply with The Code (Nursing and Midwifery Council (NMC), 2018), it is imperative that they deliver care based upon best evidence and practice available, and that associated knowledge and skills are kept up to date. This chapter examines the literature currently available with regard to effective practices in the early care of the newborn baby requiring neonatal care; starting with antenatal and perinatal care, then leading on to a discussion of the first sixty minutes of postnatal life known as the 'The Golden Hour' (Sharma, 2017a). The chapter will then discuss resuscitation of the newborn in line with current evidence-based practice.

ANTENATAL AND PERINATAL INTERVENTIONS

Referral and transfer to tertiary facilities in the case of threatening preterm birth substantially improve infant outcomes. It is required for all women at risk of preterm birth that antenatal care includes administration of antenatal corticosteroids, treatment of infections, prevention of preterm labour, and counselling and planning for the best and safest mode of delivery. If safe and feasible for both mother and baby, any woman presenting at a non-tertiary centre with inevitable delivery of a very low birth weight (VLBW) infant should be transferred to a tertiary centre (Vintzileos et al., 2002; Doyle et al., 2009; American College of Obstetricians and Gynecologists, 2011; Roberts et al., 2017; National Institute for Health and Care Excellence (NICE), 2019a). *In utero* transfers have better clinical outcomes than transfers following birth (Fowlie et al., 2008).

Tocolytics

The aim of tocolytics is to prolong the pregnancy for up to 48 hours allowing for the administration of antenatal corticosteroids and transfer to a tertiary centre for ongoing care, thus improving the neonatal outcome (Voltolini et al., 2013). Nifedipine is a calcium channel blocker, and one of the main tocolytics used. The inhibition of the return of calcium ions across cell membranes decreases smooth muscle tone. Nifedipine is given orally, and doses are adjusted in line with the observed response of uterine activity.

Antibiotics

Preterm birth has been associated with infection; commonly a transvaginally ascending infection. The routine prescribing of maternal antibiotics where membranes are intact is not recommended due to potential masking of a subclinical infection and prolonging a hostile intrauterine environment with its increased risks of cerebral palsy (Kenyon et al., 2001). A Cochrane review recommends prescribing antibiotics where specific clinical indications arise, such as preterm pre-labour rupture of the membranes (PPROM), Group B Streptococcus colonisation, or chorioamnionitis (Kenyon et al., 2013).

Antenatal corticosteroids

Antenatal corticosteroids are administered to the mother at risk of preterm labour between 24 and 35^{+6} weeks' gestation to improve infant outcomes (Roberts et al., 2017; Travers et al., 2017). They enhance foetal surfactant production by maturing type II pneumocytes and accelerating foetal lung maturity, increasing the volume of terminal air sacs, allowing closer alignment to the blood vessels for gaseous exchange. In addition, corticosteroids activate epithelial sodium channels and commence the process of removing fluid from the lungs. Further documented benefits include decreased risk of a patent ductus arteriosus (PDA), intraventricular haemorrhage (IVH) and necrotising enterocolitis (NEC), reduced need for respiratory support, reduced systemic infections in the first 48 hours of life and reduction in neonatal mortality. Timing is critical to maximise the benefits, with the optimum timeframe between administration and delivery to be between 24 hours to 7 days. A repeat course may be considered depending on the timing of the first course and if delivery is likely within 48 hours. (NICE, 2019). In this case, antenatal corticosteroid administration is beneficial in reducing respiratory distress syndrome although may potentially reduce foetal growth and subsequently birth weight. The corticosteroids used are betamethasone or dexamethasone.

Magnesium sulphate

Magnesium sulphate is widely used for seizure prophylaxis in pre-eclampsia and as a treatment for eclampsia. It is not used as a tocolytic agent, although there is evidence it is neuroprotective to the foetus when administered shortly before preterm birth. It reduces the risk of cerebral palsy by a third (Doyle et al., 2009).

Antenatal counselling and team briefing

Antenatal counselling is essential, as one of its main goals is to assist parents in informed decision-making relating to the initiation of resuscitation or the provision of comfort care only. A senior neonatologist should be present at these discussions if extremely preterm delivery is expected and thus ensure that the parents have good understanding of the possible outcomes (Jefferies and Kirpalani, 2012). Statistics and information given should be in a format that can be understood by parents, should be personalised and address the needs of the family including the impact on later life (Janvier and Mercurio, 2013). Discussions may remain open, and wishes can be further discussed and renegotiated when needed. Where possible, all this information should be supported in a written format, to allow parents to revisit it whenever required.

NICE (2015) emphasises an individual's rights to be involved in decisions about their care; an opinion echoed within the POPPY study (Staniszewska et al., 2012) which suggests parents should be with their baby at the centre of neonatal care. Therefore, shared decision-making and family-centred care should be the goals of antenatal counselling. Effective counselling comprises the assessment of risks, communication of those risks, and ongoing support for the parents. When undertaken before a preterm delivery it has demonstrated many benefits for parents, such as the reduction of parental anxiety, increased knowledge, facilitation of informed decision-making and connecting with the neonatal clinicians, and having a rapport with them prior to the delivery (Brett et al., 2011; Cummings, 2015). The neonatal team should always be prepared for parental questions and anxiety. Part of this role is to ensure that questions are answered openly, factually and honestly, taking care not to generalise and to avoid assumptions being made. Knowing the impact of the information being shared can then determine the approach, with an aim to limit distress where possible. There needs to be an awareness that some parents may react in a manner which communicates anger or aggression. This is secondary to a physiological response to the fears brought on by the delivery of bad news. Such situations need to be managed sensitively, responding to parents with a calm demeanour and non-threatening body language, while assessing the situation for a need to withdraw to ensure personal safety. Chapter 3 has more information on perinatal decision-making in the face of pending preterm delivery.

THE GOLDEN HOUR

The concept of The Golden Hour incorporates evidence-based interventions for term and preterm neonates in the first sixty minutes of postnatal life which can improve long-term outcomes. It reinforces the philosophy of communication and collaboration ensuring a standardised approach by all healthcare professionals involved (Reynolds et al., 2009). The Golden Hour interventions (see box 10.1) include neonatal resuscitation, post-resuscitation care, transportation of the sick newborn to the NNU, respiratory and cardiovascular support, and initial care in the nursery environment. Doyle and Bradshaw (2012) list the key areas of the Golden Hour as: resuscitation, thermoregulation, rapid treatment of sepsis, timely parenteral nutrition administration, euglycaemia and completed admission within sixty minutes of delivery.

Studies evaluating the Golden Hour concept in preterm neonates demonstrated a reduction in detrimental short-term outcomes such as hypothermia, hypoglycaemia, and subsequently the decrease in IVH, bronchopulmonary dysplasia (BPD), and retinopathy of

---

> ## BOX 10.1 COMPONENTS OF THE GOLDEN HOUR
>
> 1   Antenatal counselling and team briefing
> 2   Delayed cord clamping
> 3   Prevention of hypothermia/temperature maintenance
> 4   Support to respiratory system
> 5   Support to cardiovascular system
> 6   Early nutritional care
> 7   Prevention of hypoglycaemia
> 8   Initiation of breastfeeding
> 9   Infection prevention
> 10 Starting of therapeutic hypothermia for birth asphyxia
> 11 Laboratory investigation
> 12 Monitoring/record
> 13 Communication with family.
>
> (adapted from Sharma, 2017a and 2017b; Sharma et al., 2017)

prematurity (ROP) when a policy, guideline or protocol is followed (Bissinger and Annibale, 2010; Soll and Pfister, 2011; Sharma, 2017). Ensuring that all practitioners follow the 5 moments of hand hygiene during all aspects of care is also essential. Hand hygiene is the single most important activity that can be undertaken by everyone in contact with the infant to minimise the likelihood of the transmission of infection in every setting.

The first four areas from this list of care interventions above (1: attendance at delivery, 2: delayed cord clamping (DCC), 3: prevention of hypothermia/temperature maintenance, and 4: supporting the respiratory system) will now be discussed. Further detail on these areas along with the remaining nine topics (5–13) are covered in the relevant sections elsewhere in the book.

Attendance at delivery

Decisions about resuscitation should be made by an experienced neonatologist or paediatrician to whom this responsibility has been designated. Experienced neonatal staff need to be present at delivery (commonly two doctors/Advanced Neonatal Nurse Practitioners (ANNPs) and a neonatal nurse) and ensure that introductions have been made to the parents with explanations as to their presence. The team should be aware of any treatment plans agreed with parents during antenatal counselling, also ensuring familiarity with obstetric history. A significant amount of preparation is required not only for the pending delivery, but the baby's care during the first hour of life. The team attending the birth of a high-risk neonate should decide on a team leader and allocate roles prior to the delivery of the baby. This role allocation can avoid confusion over interventions, thus streamlining the process of resuscitation. It can be beneficial if staff present state their responsibilities prior to the resuscitation. A 'hands-off' leadership role at resuscitation allows an objective view of events to occur.

Delayed cord clamping

This area of practice has recently changed. The Royal College of Obstetricians and Gynaecologists (RCOG), The International Federation of Gynaecology and Obstetrics and the World Health Organization (WHO) no longer recommend immediate cord clamping (WHO, 2014; RCOG, 2015). WHO state that delayed cord clamping (DCC) (1 to 3 minutes after birth) is recommended for all infants (preterm and term). Early clamping (at less than 1 minute) is not recommended unless the neonate is significantly compromised and needs to be moved for resuscitation immediately. NICE (2019b) suggests that for healthy infants at term the cord is not clamped in the first 60 seconds and that it should be clamped before 5 minutes, although women should be supported if they wish this to be delayed further. Delaying cord clamping by at least a minute is more representative of a physiological process and has been shown to improve iron storage in infancy. DCC for 1 minute has demonstrated a reduction in hospital mortality for preterm infants by 32%, improved blood pressure, reduced the need for blood transfusions by 10%, reduced IVH and NEC, and can reduce infection (Mercer et al., 2006; Fogarty et al., 2018). In Baby-Directed Umbilical Cord Clamping (Baby-DUCC), the umbilical cord remains patent until the infant's lungs are exchanging gases. This has been shown to be feasible even in situations where resuscitative measures were required (Blank et al., 2018).

Supporting the respiratory system: preventing hypoxia

Hypoxia before, during or after birth is an important cause of neonatal mortality and morbidity (Seikku et al., 2016). Hypoxia is defined as a condition in which an extreme decrease in the concentration of oxygen in the body leads to loss of consciousness or death. In the perinatal period, this hypoxia with concurrent hypercapnia and acidosis leading to circulatory compromise is usually secondary to impaired placental gas exchange (Wyllie et al., 2016). Early detection is essential to minimise any potential irreparable damage. Assessment of hypoxia at the moment of birth is undertaken by cord blood gas analysis, where blood is sampled from the umbilical artery and umbilical vein and analysed on a blood gas machine.

Hypoxia is the stimulus for the onset of breathing at birth, therefore relative oxygen depletion is part of the normal process of labour, with the healthy foetus being equipped with several protective mechanisms to prevent hypoxic damage to vital organs. The high affinity for oxygen of foetal haemoglobin supports the delivery of oxygen to the tissues. This mechanism allows oxygen extraction at tissue level to increase by almost 100% during hypoxaemic events, delaying hypoxic damage (Bocking et al., 1992; Talner et al., 1992). The foetal heart rate is a major determinant of **cardiac output**. It is four times greater than that of an adult per kilogram body weight, as it is the combined output of right and left ventricles, with 50% of the output directed to the placenta (Cohn et al., 1974). The combination of these mechanisms allows a wide safety margin of adequate oxygen delivery during labour.

In short-duration hypoxaemic events, the heart rate of the mature foetus will fall, but myocardial contractility is increased, and cardiac output is maintained due to an associated increase in arterial blood pressure (Cohn et al., 1974). This autoregulatory process is modulated at cellular level via metabolic feedback regulation of the calibre of the arterioles and capillary sphincters (Talner et al., 1992). The heart and brain are efficient at **autoregulation** and can maintain their blood flow over a wide range of perfusion pressures and oxygen contents. Hypoxaemic events of this type are intermittent during labour, and the ability of the foetus to quickly redistribute oxygenated blood is very important.

When there is no stress, the foetal and newborn heart is working at close to capacity merely to satisfy normal demands of tissues and growth (Talner et al., 1992); therefore, any increased output requirement to satisfy suboptimal tissue oxygen demand cannot be sustained for long and myocardial contractility will fail. So, while the foetus can make circulatory adjustments to compensate for the rigours of labour, under severe conditions these adaptive mechanisms will be overwhelmed, the shunting of blood towards vital organs and cerebral oxygen delivery will reduce, as blood pressure and cardiac output fall.

The ability of an organ to maintain aerobic metabolism is dependent on the amount of energy needed to maintain functional activity, the amount of oxygen delivered to the tissue and the amount of oxygen extracted by the tissue. The variation in response during labour is related to maturity, with immature foetal tissue being generally more robust. The smaller body mass to placental size gives a larger oxygen reserve to the premature foetus (Greene and Rosen, 1995). As ventricular pressure falls there is a corresponding decrease in cerebral blood flow (CBF). During severe asphyxia, CBF is directed to the brain stem rather than the cerebrum, which increases the likelihood of damage to the cerebrum and cortex (Bennet et al., 2003). When organ blood flow and oxygen delivery are severely compromised, increased tissue extraction of oxygen will not be able to compensate fully for the decrease in oxygen delivery.

Hypoxia is the most common cause of perinatally acquired severe brain injury in the full-term infant (Vasudevan and Levene, 2013). Practitioners working within the field of neonatal care need to be able to ameliorate its potentially devastating effects by prompt and skilled resuscitation. This is true also in management of the preterm infant who, if neglected in the first few minutes of life, is more likely to succumb to hypoxic and thermal stresses that will undoubtedly adversely affect that infant's outcome.

Prevention of hypothermia/temperature maintenance

Hypothermia remains a worldwide problem, especially for small infants and those born preterm. Across all gestations, admission temperature is a strong predictor of mortality and morbidity (Perlman et al., 2015). Effective thermal management is crucial to successful extrauterine transition. Interventions and measures to minimise heat loss are integral to the Golden Hour management: maintaining a draught-free, warm delivery room at a set room temperature (26°C) to prevent convective heat losses; using pre-warmed towels (to prevent conductive heat loss); use of a plastic wrap/bag (to prevent evaporative losses in preterm infants); pre-heated radiant heat sources; and the availability of thermal adjuncts such as a mattress.

The use of exothermic sodium acetate gel mattresses (TransWarmer©) during newborn resuscitation and stabilisation of preterm infants is effective in preventing heat loss (Almeida, 2009; Ibrahim and Yoxall, 2010; Chawla et al., 2011). These mattresses emit latent heat of crystallisation when activated (Carmichael, 2007). The thermal mattress must be activated prior to use to prevent any unnecessary heat losses that may occur as a consequence of placing an infant on a non-activated mattress (McCarthy et al., 2012). The use of plastic coverings/bags is also effective in the reduction of heat loss, mortality, and morbidity in preterm infants (Li et al., 2016; Oatley et al., 2016). These are used without drying the baby except for the head and applying a hat. They do not interfere with the ongoing management and monitoring of the infant (McCarthy et al., 2013).

All the above measures can prevent hypothermia and hypothermia-associated morbidity and mortality risks (McCall et al., 2018).

These fundamental aspects of neonatal care initiated at the delivery of the infant aim to ensure that a core temperature of 36.5–37.5°C (Royal College of Paediatrics and Child Health, 2018) is maintained, and as a result minimal oxygen consumption and energy expenditure occurs. The intrauterine environment is approximately 38°C, and the temperature of the foetus is between 0.5°C and 1.5°C greater than the maternal temperature. As soon as the baby is delivered, heat losses by convection, radiation and evaporation are high. VLBW infants are at an even greater risk of cold stress due to their unfavourable surface to mass ratio. The core temperature of a newborn baby can drop by as much as 5°C in the first 10–20 minutes of life, if measures to prevent heat loss are not initiated (Champlain Maternal Newborn Regional Program (CMNRP), 2013). Cold stress is associated with hypoxia and acidosis, factors which inhibit surfactant production in the newborn and should be avoided. Mild hypothermia previously thought to be inevitable carries an unacceptable risk.

RESUSCITATION

The aims of resuscitation are to establish and maintain a clear airway by ventilation and oxygenation, ensure effective circulation, correct acidosis, prevent hypothermia, hypoglycaemia, and haemorrhage. Successful resuscitation requires the coordinated efforts of a professional team. Infants who require resuscitation at birth fall into two broad categories: those who have undergone a period of hypoxic stress *in utero*, and those who are prone to hypoxaemia in the immediate postnatal period due to inadequate pulmonary development, airway obstruction or congenital malformations. Significant hypoxia will lead to irreparable hypoxic tissue damage, so anticipation of the need for resuscitation prior to delivery is crucial.

It is important to have an appreciation for the events that may lead to acute hypoxia. An interruption to placental oxygen supply causes the foetus to make breathing attempts. If these fail to inflate the lungs with air, the baby loses consciousness. A continuation of hypoxia of the respiratory centre within the brain results in the cessation of breathing – usually within two to three minutes; this is termed primary apnoea. After the baby has been in a state of primary apnoea for one to two minutes, the result is a period of gasping, which is followed by terminal apnoea. If no intervention occurs at this point, the baby will die.

Anticipation

The likelihood of neonatal resuscitation is increased by certain several known maternal, foetal and intrapartum factors. These include maternal disease, such as pre-eclampsia, maternal infection/chorioamnionitis, substance misuse in pregnancy or maternal sedation, foetal abnormality, intrauterine growth restriction, antepartum or intrapartum haemorrhage, prolonged rupture of membranes, foetal compromise indicated by decelerations of the heart rate or meconium-stained amniotic fluid, preterm labour, induction of labour, prolonged labour, instrumental and operative delivery, and obstetric emergencies such as a cord prolapse or shoulder dystocia. However, unexpected situations where resuscitation is required will also arise. Therefore, on arriving in the delivery room, details with regard to the gestation of the infant and any known problems should be elicited prior to the baby being born. If time permits, a more detailed history can be taken; but the above will enable a plan to be formulated quickly as to whether the infant may need intervention, or whether more help may be needed in the case of multiple births.

Preparation of environment and equipment

Preparation prior to the birth is the key to success. Before every delivery, the room should routinely be prepared as a warm, draught-free environment so heat loss is minimised. The working condition of any equipment should be checked and prepared, so that everything that may be required is close to hand. Staff should check there is adequate equipment supply on each resuscitaire or in the resuscitation trolley, if twins, triplets or higher multiples are being expected. The use of a pre-resuscitation check list can make the process of equipment checking quick and easy.

While it may appear obvious that equipment is checked, and be sufficient for the task in hand, failure of this simple procedure has been previously implicated in a proportion of neonatal deaths reported annually in the UK (National Patient Safety Agency (NPSA), 2010). Equipment for resuscitation may vary depending on the place of birth, e.g. community

BOX 10.2 BASIC RESUSCITATION EQUIPMENT IN HOSPITAL

- Radiant warmer – flat surface, heat source, light source, timer/clock
- Stethoscope
- Warm towels
- Suction unit with tubing, yankauer and various sizes of suction catheters
- Blended air/oxygen supply with flow regulation and adjustable pressures
- Pulse oximetry
- T-piece system, e.g. neopuff™
- Self-inflating bag
- Assorted face mask sizes
- Oropharyngeal airways – various sizes for preterm and term babies
- Plastic Bags/wraps for preterm babies.

Delivery rooms should have equipment available for more advanced resuscitation

- Laryngoscope handles (disposable options are now available)
- Various blades (disposable options are now available)
- Endotracheal tubes (ETT) – various sizes and introducers
- ETT fixation equipment according to local procedures
- End-tidal CO_2 detectors
- Resuscitation drugs
- Syringes, needles
- Umbilical artery catheter (UAC)/umbilical venous catheter (UVC) insertion pack
- Intraosseous needle
- Nasogastric tube and fixation source
- Surfactant administration / instillation kit.

or hospital setting, yet all staff must be familiar with what is available for use, including the decontamination procedure following equipment use (box 10.2).

Correct personal protective equipment should be available and worn to protect the baby and the attending professional.

The ABC (D and E) of resuscitation

The Resuscitation Council UK suggests the use of an algorithm which incorporates an ABCD approach to neonatal resuscitation, based on continuous assessment of the baby (see figure 10.1 and box 10.3). As this forms the basis for education of midwives, nurses

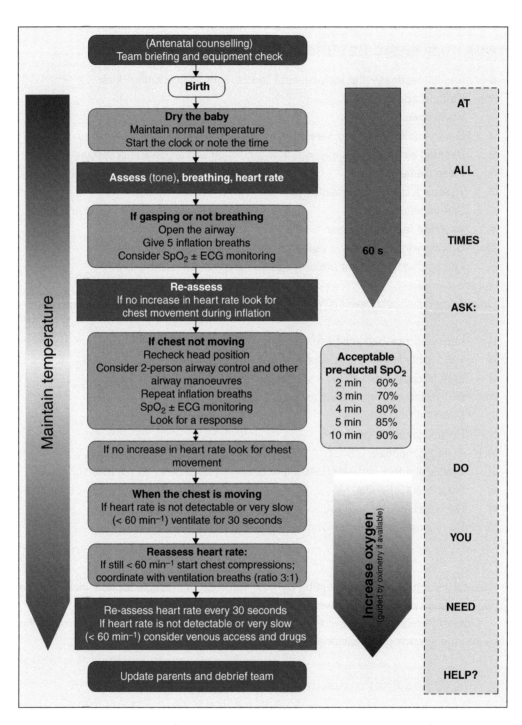

Figure 10.1 The NLS Algorithm (with permission from the Resuscitation Council UK)

BOX 10.3 A, B, C

- ■ The heart rate remains <60bpm after 5 inflation breaths (chest wall movement seen).
- ■ Give 30 seconds of ventilation breaths (rate of 30 breaths per minute).
- ■ Reassess the heart rate.
- ■ If still no improvement, start chest compressions at a ratio of 3:1 (3 compressions: 1 breath).

---

and medical staff during Neonatal Life Support (NLS) courses, aiming to standardise the approach to resuscitation at birth, neonatal nurses should be familiar with this. Each aspect of the algorithm will be discussed in the following sections.

APGAR SCORING AND ASSESSMENT AT BIRTH

Every baby should be assessed immediately after birth. The concept of Apgar scoring is discussed in chapter 2, assessment of the neonate.

AIRWAY

After ensuring thermal control, airway management is the next consideration if the infant has a slow heart rate or is not breathing. The goal of providing support to the respiratory system is to help in the smooth transition of the gas exchanging organ from placenta to lung. The key points in successful airway management are:

- ■ *Open airway* Particularly in compromised/floppy infants, the airway can be occluded as the prominent occiput forces the head into a flexed position. The relatively large tongue can also cause obstruction.
- ■ *Head in neutral position* This should provide an open airway by counteracting the problems described above. Neutral head position (see figure 10.2) can be achieved by a simple chin lift, or by placing a 2cm thick roll under the baby's shoulder. With either manoeuvre, care must be taken not to over-extend the head, as this in itself can cause airway obstruction.

BREATHING

The spontaneously gasping infant who has central cyanosis and/or a heart rate around 100 beats per minute (bpm) is likely to respond quickly to airway opening and minimal resuscitative measures such as facial oxygen. Apnoea, pallor or a heart rate less than 100bpm

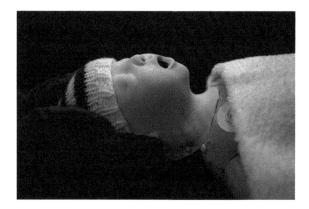

Figure 10.2 Neutral Head Position (Source: Fitchett's Photography)

indicates the necessity for positive-pressure ventilation (PPV) via a mask. When an infant is born in less than optimal condition, it is resuscitation that mimics the adaptation to extra-uterine life. A healthy baby born in good condition can clear approximately 100mL of lung fluid spontaneously within minutes of birth (Bland, 1988). It is this airway-liquid clearance and lung aeration, which allows for the establishment of a functional residual capacity (FRC) and the delivery of tidal volumes, which are essential for gaseous exchange. Table 10.1 explores the key aspects of 'breathing' during neonatal resuscitation.

The face mask With both the T-piece and self-inflating bag, an appropriate-sized mask is required, which should fit over the nose and mouth, without occluding the orbital ridges (see figure 10.3). When applying the face mask, remember the '3 P's':

■ *Position* To obtain a good seal, the mask should be rolled on from the cleft of the chin to the bridge of the nose.
■ *Pressure* Applying gentle, well-balanced pressure to the non-deformable top portion of the mask with thumb and forefinger held in a 'C' shape aids in achieving a good seal without leaks.
■ *Pull* The remaining three fingers are placed to form an 'E' on the jaw line with the ring finger on the angle of the jaw. Drawing the mandibular ridge upwards lifts the jaw into the mask, thus applying a single-handed jaw thrust.

Troubleshooting If no chest wall movement is observed during PPV, the most likely reason is the absence of an open airway. Thus, the first steps should be to revisit the fundamental basics, such as head positioning and mask fit, with an attempt to repeat inflation breaths. The baby's condition will not change and resuscitation cannot progress until an airway is established and chest movement is seen.

TABLE 10.1 THE 'B' OF NEONATAL RESUSCITATION

Equipment check	■ Safety check of a 500mL self-inflating bag-valve mask system *or*
	■ (preferably) a T-piece resuscitator
	   ■ Peak Inspiratory Pressure (PIP) set at **30cmH₂O for the term baby and 20–25cmH₂O for the preterm baby**
	   ■ Positive end-expiratory Pressure (PEEP) set at 5cmH₂O
	      ■ Gas blender set to **air (21%) for term babies** or **21–30% for preterm babies <30 weeks' gestation**
	■ Selection of mask sizes (see below)

5 inflation breaths	■ Give 5 inflation breaths, sustained for 2–3 seconds each ■ Observe for chest wall movement (the chest may not rise with the first few inflation breaths as the fluid is being moved out from the lungs, but it should be seen of the fourth or fifth inflation breath if the technique is correct and the airway is open ■ Reassess the heart rate
Ventilation breaths	Ventilation breaths are delivered at a rate of 30 breaths per minute if ■ Chest wall movement was observed during inflation breaths ■ The heart rate has improved but the baby remains apnoeic/is still breathing irregularly ■ The heart rate remains slow but chest wall movement was seen during inflation breaths. Continue to observe for consistent chest wall movement, and reassess the baby after 30 seconds.

(adapted from Wyllie et al., 2016)

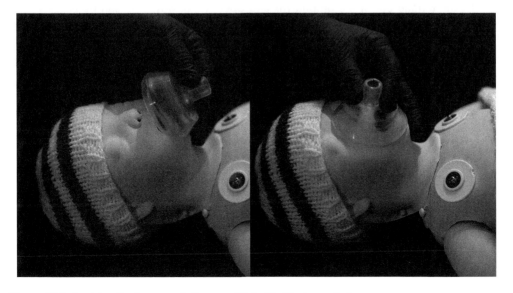

Figure 10.3 Applying the face mask (Source: Fitchett's Photography)

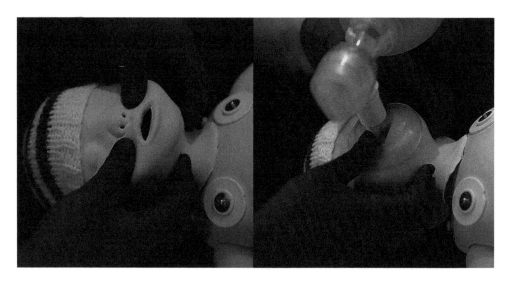

Figure 10.4 Jaw thrust (Source: Fitchett's Photography)

There are, however, two other airway manoeuvres that can be used if this is not successful:

■ *Two-person jaw thrust* Jaw thrust will lift the tongue out of the oropharynx and open the airway. The first person applies jaw thrust and maintains a good seal with the mask, while five inflation breaths are delivered by the second person (see figure 10.4).

■ *Oropharyngeal airway* Insertion of a correctly sized oropharyngeal airway (OPA) will lift the tongue out of the oropharynx and open the airway. This can be an excellent method of maintaining the airway if alone. Insertion of the OPA should be under direct vision with the aid of a laryngoscope to depress the tongue. Prior to insertion of the OPA, inspect the mouth and oropharynx for any particulate matter that may need removing by suction under direct vision. Suction should never be performed blindly or stimulate the posterior larynx or pharynx as this may induce adduction of the vocal cords or a profound vagal bradycardia.

REMEMBER

■ After any airway-opening manoeuvre, give 5 inflation breaths if the chest wall has not previously been seen to move.

■ Observe for chest wall movement during PPV.

■ Reassess the baby's heart rate after you have repeated your inflation breaths.

Most infants will respond favourably to mask ventilation (Ersdal et al., 2012), but a pro-portion will require endotracheal intubation, due to extreme prematurity, severe asphyxia, altered anatomy or poor response to PPV. If this is anticipated or found to be required, a practitioner skilled in endotracheal intubation should be in attendance as unsuccessful intubation attempts are counterproductive and make subsequent attempts more difficult.

Positive end-expiratory pressure The application of positive end-expiratory pressure (PEEP) at resuscitation may have several benefits for the premature infant. It is thought to not only optimise alveolar expansion and conserve and prolong the effectiveness of surfactant (Wyszogrodski et al., 1975; Froese et al., 1993), but also attenuate the potential damaging effects of high inspiratory pressures (Carlton et al., 1990).

If the use of a bag-valve mask system is required due to the absence of a T-piece or gas supply, practitioners need to be aware that this does not provide PEEP.

Oxygen Current evidence available suggests that resuscitation in air is as effective as receiving 100% oxygen. Supplementation of this can be considered if there is a failure of the heart rate to respond to successful lung inflation or in response to pulse oximetry readings (Davis et al., 2004). High oxygen concentrations, leading to oxygen toxicity, can damage hypoxic cells and tissues. This is caused by the production of free radicals and antioxidants and contributes to brain injury in the baby who has suffered a hypoxic-ischaemic event. The antioxidant defense system develops towards the end of pregnancy and neutralises free radicals and antioxidants. Due to this system not being established, preterm babies below 30 weeks' gestation are at greater risk from oxidative stress and the inflammatory cycle. This can damage the heart, lungs, brain and kidneys, contributing to the pathogenesis of morbidities such as ROP, BPD, NEC and PDA in the premature population (Ozsurekci and Aykac, 2016).

Hyperoxia reduces cerebral blood flow in both term and preterm infants. Persistent cerebral vasoconstriction when high oxygen levels are used may make the brain more sus-ceptible to hypoxic episodes or ischaemia, which may increase the risk of cerebral damage in the newborn period, delay the onset of spontaneous respirations, and increase the risk of short-term mortality. In the term hypoxic population, high oxygen concentrations may also be damaging due to hypoxic reperfusion injury. Research suggests that restoration of blood supply containing a high concentration of oxygen is more detrimental than restoration of the circulation alone, as it appears to create radical oxygen metabolites that lead to further pathological changes.

While the prevention of hypoxia must remain a high priority during neonatal resuscita-tion, the indiscriminate use of oxygen needs careful consideration in order to prevent poten-tial long-term adverse sequelae. Oxygen should be increased and decreased according to the response of the heart rate and oxygen saturation levels observed using pulse oxim-etry. As air is the initial gas chosen, oxygen should be readily available for infants who do not respond adequately. It is now recommended that all infants should be monitored with pulse oximetry at delivery as a real-time measurement. Pulse oximetry is a non-invasive monitoring method which measures the arterial haemoglobin saturation. The application of a pulse oximeter on the right hand, in the early stages of a resuscitation allows for the monitoring of pre-ductal oxygen saturations and hence cerebral oxygen saturations are also recorded. Accuracy may be affected if cardiac output and perfusion of the infant are very poor. Acceptable pre-ductal saturations can be found in chapter 3, table 3.3.

CIRCULATION

The heart rate should be assessed by auscultation over the apex beat using a stethoscope. Palpation of the apex or the umbilical stump is not recommended, as it has been found that slow pulsation does not always accurately reflect the true heart rate (Owen and Wyllie, 2004). More recently, electrocardiography has been advocated as a quick and accurate way of determining heart rate in the delivery room (Dawson et al., 2018). The most frequent cause of an inadequate heart rate is ineffective ventilation, and once this is established, most heart rates will increase. It is rare for a baby to require cardiac compressions: 0.1% term or near-term infants and between 2 and 10% of preterm infants.

The aim of cardiac compressions is to re-establish effective heart pumping through the movement of the oxygenated blood from the pulmonary veins to the coronary arteries. As breaths are being delivered, ensure that the chest is inflating with each breath. At this stage, it is appropriate to increase the oxygen concentration. Help should have been requested and if it has not already been applied, a pulse oximeter will be beneficial in assessing how effective the process is. The quality of compressions cannot be overemphasised – too rapid a rate will not allow for the relaxation phase of the chest compressions, which will hinder its effectiveness. The 3:1 ratio will give 120 cycles per minute, for example, 90 cardiac compressions to 30 breaths. However, the quality is more important than the quantity. Reassessment should take place every 30 seconds. Once the infant's heart rate is above 60bpm and rising, chest compressions can be discontinued. Ventilation breaths need to continue until spontaneous respiration occurs – reassess the heart rate every 30 seconds to ensure it remains above 100bpm or use a pulse oximeter (figure 10.5).

DRUGS

Neonatal cardiopulmonary resuscitation (CPR) in the delivery room is rare, as less than 0.1% of newborns fail to respond to effective lung inflation and require extensive resuscitation in the form of chest compressions with or without the use of epinephrine (Kapadia and Wyckoff, 2012). In the unlikely event that the infant's heart rate is still not improving – remaining below 60bpm – or is not detectable despite adequate ventilation and good-quality compressions, drug therapy (see table 10.2) needs to be considered. Drugs are not a first-line action in neonatal resuscitation.

TABLE 10.2 DRUGS IN NEONATAL RESUSCITATION

Drug	Dose	Mechanism of action
Adrenaline (epinephrine)	0.1mL/kg of 1:10,000 0.3mL/kg of 1:10,000 (repeat dose)	■ Endogenous **catecholamine** with α- and β-adrenergic effects ■ α-mediated vasoconstriction results in improved coronary perfusion pressure and myocardial blood flow ■ Administration is intravenous (IV) or intraosseous; may consider endotracheal instillation (Halling et al., 2017) ■ Risk of arrhythmias when multiple doses administered
Sodium bicarbonate	2–4mL/kg of 4.2%	■ Reversal of acidosis within the heart may facilitate the action of adrenaline (Preziosi et al., 1993) ■ Administration is IV or intraosseous ■ Cautious use in preterm infants – associated with hypernatraemia and IVH (Howell 1987; Ginsberg and Goldsmith 1998)
Glucose	2.5mL/kg of 10%	■ Intracardiac **glycogen** stores are likely to become depleted during acidosis ■ Glucose may be helpful where there has been no response to adrenaline and sodium bicarbonate ■ Administration is IV or intraosseous
Volume	10mL/kg 0.9% sodium chloride	■ To correct hypovolaemia where this is suspected as the underlying cause for perinatal compromise ■ Avoid excessive volume replacement ■ Administration is IV or intraosseous.

(adapted from Wyllie et al., 2016)

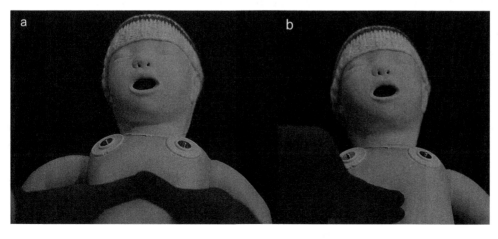

Figure 10.5 Chest Compressions (Source: Fitchett's Photography)

The administration of drugs needs to be achieved as close as possible to the heart, so best via an umbilical venous catheter (UVC). Administration into a peripheral vein is unlikely to reach the heart in the event of a complete circulatory arrest, even with effective ventilation and chest compressions. Umbilical catheterisation is also quicker and easier in a baby that is peripherally poorly perfused. An alternative route is the intraosseous route. After the administration of each drug a small flush, usually of 0.9% sodium chloride, must be given. The continuation of good-quality ventilation and cardiac compressions is imperative; drugs will otherwise not be effective.

Drug therapy during resuscitation remains a controversial area in relation to the most appropriate and most effective agents, dosages, routes of administration and speed of delivery. These controversies are, in part, due to many of the drug dosages being extrapolated from adult data. Also, once anatomical and physiological differences in the neonate are considered, for example, the presence of lung fluid, right-to-left shunts, and the susceptibility of the neonatal brain to haemorrhage, these extrapolations may be inappropriate (Perlman et al., 2012). Indeed, the use of drugs at all in certain groups of infants may in itself be inappropriate, as their necessity seems to be associated with an extremely poor outcome (Perondi et al., 2004).

WHEN TO STOP RESUSCITATION

There is little existing guidance on when resuscitation should be discontinued. Everybody with a responsibility of attending high-risk deliveries needs to have an awareness of their local NNU/maternity unit guidance in relation to this. What is known is that the decision should be made in the best interest of the baby. Prior to discontinuation of resuscitation, the person leading the situation should invite all other team members to suggest or contribute to further treatment options. Everybody involved should participate in the discussions whether resuscitation ought to be continued. This process should also include conversations with the obstetric team and a review of the obstetric history, and at this point the parents also need to be spoken to about potential plans to cease resuscitative measures.

A retrospective study exploring this suggests that resuscitation beyond 10 minutes is not justified if there is no spontaneous cardiac output following effective resuscitation. If the baby has a spontaneous heart rate but is making no respiratory effort, assisted ventilation should continue. More recently, however, it has been suggested that an Apgar score of 0 at 10 minutes does not determine a universally poor outcome and should therefore be used cautiously to aid decision-making (Kasdorf et al., 2015; Shah et al., 2015).

This is in keeping with other evidence advocating that resuscitation at birth should continue until 20 minutes in the absence of a clinically detectable heartbeat. In the case of uncertainty with regard to the discontinuation of resuscitation, clinicians should continue to provide resuscitation for longer, to allow consideration of withdrawal of life-sustaining treatment later if the clinical condition then indicates that the prognosis is poor (Wilkinson and Stenson, 2015).

If the decision is made to discontinue resuscitation, there needs to be ethical justification for stopping. This will need to be that a poor outcome is highly likely, a high risk of mortality and that survival will be with severe disability. Parents' views are critical to the decision-making process, especially in the marginally viable gestation neonates.

MECONIUM-STAINED AMNIOTIC FLUID

Antenatal or intrapartum meconium release is referred to as meconium staining of amniotic fluid (MSAF). This is an important sign of deteriorating foetal wellbeing and adverse outcomes in terms of morbidity and mortality (Desai et al., 2017). Risk factors for the *in utero* passage of meconium include post-maturity (>41 weeks' gestational age), small size for gestational age, and conditions that compromise foetal wellbeing, such as placental insufficiency and cord compression (Crowley, 2015). Continuous foetal heart rate monitoring is recommended where there is evidence of MSAF, to detect possible foetal compromise in case this indicates acute or chronic hypoxia.

MSAF is present in approximately 13% of all live births and reported rates documented are between 8 and 20%. It has been demonstrated to be as high as 23–52% at 42 weeks' gestation and 27.1% at 41 weeks' gestation (Argyridis and Arulkumaran, 2016). Preterm births are not frequently associated with MSAF. The majority of neonates born with MSAF are healthy, but in about 2–10% meconium aspiration syndrome develops, presenting with severe respiratory compromise (Desai et al., 2017).

COMMUNICATION WITH PARENTS

Communicating with the parents is a vital aspect of neonatal care and should always be a priority of care and not an afterthought. Clinicians should ensure that the parents understand about their baby's health at the time of delivery, during and after resuscitation. Complete, direct and honest individualised information from nurses and physicians is helpful and seen as the cornerstone of Family-Centred Care (FCC). Wherever possible, the parents should be spoken to together regarding what is likely to happen following the delivery (for example, immediate removal of the infant to the resuscitation area), so that they are aware of the situation and prepared as to why these interventions may be necessary. This is not always possible when a baby is born unexpectedly compromised. Neonatal resuscitation events are unique in that there are usually other persons in the immediate vicinity who are not directly (practically) involved with the situation.

During delivery room resuscitation, parents are most certainly present and witnessing events as they occur. Their role as bystanders in the emergency situation can be traumatic

---

BOX 10.4 POINTS TO DOCUMENT FOLLOWING BIRTH

- Apgar score
- Interventions required during resuscitation
- Time respirations were established
- Birth weight
- Axillary temperature at time of admission to the NNU
- Timing of surfactant instillation
- Time of umbilical catheterisation
- Time of commencement of ventilation or non-invasive respiratory support
- Time of commencement of therapeutic hypothermia
- Time of administration of first feed
- Time of commencement of intravenous fluids and parenteral nutrition
- Time of administration of the first dose of antibiotics
- Complications secondary to any neonatal procedure
- Size and depth of endotracheal tube (ETT), umbilical catheters and depth of feeding tube fixation.

---

for both parents. This has implications for the professionals' demeanor and parental support both during and after the resuscitation. Parent presence during any lifesaving procedure can aid and support the bereavement process in the event that their infant dies. If the baby requires admission to the NNU post-resuscitation, this needs to be explained to the parents in a sensitive manner. Chapter 4 discusses FCC in more depth.

RECORD KEEPING

Accurate and contemporaneous record keeping of the resuscitation and documentation of interventions undertaken during the Golden Hour alongside their timing is essential (box 10.4). It allows the team to review this and identify a potential need for improvement. Having one member of the team allocated and solely dedicated to recording the events and interventions as they occur during resuscitation facilitates accurate and contemporaneous documentation. Prior to leaving the delivery room for transfer to the NNU, identification of the baby must be established in the form of name bands (National Patient Safety Agency (NPSA), 2005).

POST-RESUSCITATION CARE

Continuing observation is necessary for any infant who has required resuscitation and has any need for ongoing support. This includes heart rate, oxygen saturations and temperature.

Determined on an individual basis, this may include cord gases, placental histology, screening for sepsis, cardiovascular and respiratory management including the correction of any metabolic acidosis. The main aim of post-resuscitation care is the early identification of the unwell or deteriorating neonate, as timely recognition will ensure appropriate referral, diagnosis and management.

The signs and symptoms of a deteriorating neonate can be either obvious or initially non-specific. Nurses and midwives must have the required knowledge to recognise any deviations from the norm or the normal for each individual baby. Tools exist to assist healthcare professionals to identify signs and symptoms of deterioration. One such tool is the Newborn Early Warning Score (NEWS). Any concerns with observations made should be escalated to the appropriate personnel – this may vary from unit to unit. Utilising a recognised tool is a good indicator of physiological trends and a sensitive indicator of any abnormal physiology. Identifying problems prompts earlier review in those babies that are showing deterioration and using a standardised escalation system can aid in reducing sudden collapse or unexpected death.

Infants who have required resuscitation or are preterm and meet the criteria for admission to the NNU will need to be transferred safely from the delivery room. During the transfer they will need to have their temperature maintained, airway secured and have heart rate and oxygen saturations monitored throughout. Occasionally, IV access is gained prior to transfer. Transfer to the NNU will need a coordinated approach and should be undertaken on either a resuscitaire or in a transport incubator, depending on the unit's available equipment and location in relation to the delivery room.

RESUSCITATION TRAINING AND EDUCATION

The presence of a practitioner experienced in neonatal resuscitation is crucial at high-risk deliveries. It is therefore essential that skills and competence are maintained, and refresher sessions are attended to ensure there is no deterioration in psychomotor skills following training. Three months after an educational session has been attended, skills have been shown to deteriorate (Cusack and Fawke, 2012). Simulation-based training is the gold standard in both graduate and postgraduate education. When skills are acquired within a simulated setting, they are transferable into the clinical environment, with a resultant improvement in patient outcomes. Simulation should not replace exposure and experience of real-time clinical practice, but utilising this expansion of resuscitation training and dedicated airway management training can ensure that exposure to skills continues despite reduced bedside practice opportunities.

CONCLUSION

Management in the perinatal and early postnatal period including the first hour of care can directly affect long-term outcomes, necessitating a careful, structured approach. This chapter has highlighted the importance of sound antenatal and perinatal care as well as the anticipation of the need for resuscitation, enabling good preparation prior to delivery. Any practitioner attending high-risk deliveries needs to be familiar with the fundamental principles of neonatal resuscitation and be skilled in delivering this, for which ongoing training is required. Post-resuscitation care needs to include conversations with the parents of perinatal events, and the implementation of safety measures for the newborn infant, which may constitute NNU admission or close observation. The neonatal nurse's role in this is central, ensuring that the needs of both parents and baby are met during this crucial time.

CASE STUDIES

Case study 1: Delivery of an extremely preterm infant

Ava is 24^{+3} weeks' gestation and was delivered by Claire, a primi-gravida mother, after early onset of labour.

Q.1.   How would you prepare the equipment and environment prior to the birth of Ava?

Q.2.   Which members of the multidisciplinary team need to be informed of the impending delivery?

Q.3.   How could Ava's parents Claire and Richard best be prepared for her birth? At birth Ava's colour is pink with gasping breaths, no cry, hypotonic, heart rate is 100bpm and rising.

Q.4.   Explain how you would use the Apgar score to assess Ava's condition at birth.

Q.5.   What are your initial management priorities following delivery? Discuss the care for Ava in relation to the components of the Golden Hour.

Case study 2: Term baby compromised at delivery

Amy gave birth to her first baby Jack in the delivery suite. When Jack was born his colour was blue, heart rate was slow, he had reduced tone and after stimulation he grimaced and gasped but made no further attempts to breathe.

Q.1. What are the initial actions that you would take to resuscitate Jack?

Q.2. How would you size a face mask for Jack?

Q.3. What are the ongoing observations following resuscitation? What assessment tool would be used on the postnatal ward?

For suggested answer guides to the questions posed in these case studies, please refer to the web-based companion site specific to this chapter (see URL below).

WEB-BASED RESOURCES

For further information, online resources and greater detail on the case studies featured in this chapter go to www.routledge.com/cw/nicnursing

References

Almeida, P. G., Chandley, J., Davis, J., & Harrigan, R. C. (2009). Use of the heated gel mattress and its impact on admission temperature of very low birth-weight infants. *Advances in Neonatal Care*, 9(1), 34–39.

American College of Obstetricians and Gynecologists. (2011). ACOG Practice Bulletin No. 120: Use of prophylactic antibiotics in labor and delivery. *Obstetrics and Gynecology*, 117(6), 1472.

Argyridis, S., & Arulkumaran, S. (2016). Meconium stained amniotic fluid. *Obstetrics, Gynaecology & Reproductive Medicine*, 26(8), 227–230.

Bennet, L., Westgate, J. A., Gluckman, P. D., & Gunn, A. J. (2003). Fetal Responses to Asphyxia. In Stevenson, D. K., Sunshine, P., & Benitz, W. E. (Eds) *Fetal and neonatal brain injury: mechanisms, management, and the risks of practice* (pp. 83–110), Cambridge: Cambridge University Press.

Bissinger, R. L., & Annibale, D. J. (2010). Thermoregulation in very low-birth-weight infants during the golden hour: results and implications. *Advances in Neonatal Care*, 10(5), 230–238.

Bland, R.D. (1988). Lung liquid clearance before and after birth, *Seminars in Perinatology*, 12: 124–33.

Blank, D. A., Badurdeen, S., Kamlin, C. O. F., Jacobs, S. E., Thio, M., Dawson, J. A., … & Davis, P. G. (2018). Baby-directed umbilical cord clamping: A feasibility study. *Resuscitation*, 131, 1–7.

Bocking, A. D., White, S. E., Homan, J., & Richardson, B. S. (1992). Oxygen consumption is maintained in fetal sheep during prolonged hypoxaemia. *Journal of Developmental Physiology*, 17(4), 169–174.

Brett, J., Staniszewska, S., Newburn, M., Jones, N., & Taylor, L. (2011). A systematic mapping review of effective interventions for communicating with, supporting and providing information to parents of preterm infants. *BMJ Open*, 1(1), e000023.

Carlton, D. P., Cummings, J. J., Scheerer, R. G., Poulain, F. R., & Bland, R. D. (1990). Lung overexpansion increases pulmonary microvascular protein permeability in young lambs. *Journal of Applied Physiology*, 69(2): 577–583.

Carmichael, A., McCullough, S., & Kempley, S. T. (2007). Critical dependence of acetate thermal mattress on gel activation temperature. *Archives of Disease in Childhood: Fetal and Neonatal Edition*, 92(1), F44–F45.

Champlain Maternal Newborn Regional Program (CMNRP). (2013). Newborn Thermoregulation. www.cmnrp.ca/uploads/documents/Newborn_Thermoregulation_SLM_2013_06.pdf

Chawla, S., Amaram, A., Gopal, S. P., & Natarajan, G. (2011). Safety and efficacy of Trans-warmer mattress for preterm neonates: Results of a randomized controlled trial. *Journal of Perinatology, 31*(12), 780.

Cohn, H. E., Sacks, E. J., Heymann, M. A., & Rudolph, A. M. (1974). Cardiovascular responses to hypoxemia and acidemia in fetal lambs. *American Journal of Obstetrics & Gynecology, 120*(6), 817–824.

Crowley, M. A. (2015). Neonatal Respiratory Disorder. In Martin, R. J., Fanaroff, A. N., & Walsh, M. C. (Eds.) *Fanaroff and Martins Neonatal-Perinatal Medicine. Disease of the Fetus and Infant* (10th Edition) (pp. 1113–1136). Philadelphia PA: WB Saunders.

Cummings, J. (2015). Antenatal counseling regarding resuscitation and intensive care before 25 weeks of gestation. *Pediatrics, 136*(3), 588–595.

Cusack, J., & Fawke, J. (2012). Neonatal resuscitation: are your trainees performing as you think they are? A retrospective review of a structured resuscitation assessment for neonatal medical trainees over an 8-year period. *Archives of Disease in Childhood: Fetal and Neonatal Edition, 97*(4), F246–F248.

Davis, P. G., Tan, A., O'Donnell, C. P., & Schulze, A. (2004). Resuscitation of newborn infants with 100% oxygen or air: A systematic review and meta-analysis. *The Lancet, 364*(9442), 1329–1333.

Dawson, J. A., Schmölzer, G. M., & Wyllie, J. (2018). Monitoring heart rate in the delivery room. *Seminars in Fetal and Neonatal Medicine.* 23(5): 327–332.

Dempsey, E., Pammi, M., Ryan, A. C., & Barrington, K. J. (2015). Standardised formal resuscitation training programmes for reducing mortality and morbidity in newborn infants. *Cochrane Database of Systematic Reviews.* Issue 9. Art. No.: CD009106. DOI:10.1002/14651858.CD009106.pub2

Desai, D., Maitra, N., & Patel, P. (2017). Fetal heart rate patterns in patients with thick meconium staining of amniotic fluid and its association with perinatal outcome. *International Journal of Reproduction, Contraception, Obstetrics and Gynecology, 6*(3), 1030–1035.

Doyle, L. W., Crowther, C. A., Middleton, P., Marret, S., & Rouse, D. (2009). Magnesium sulphate for women at risk of preterm birth for neuroprotection of the fetus. *Cochrane Database of Systematic Reviews,* Issue 1. Art. No.: CD004661. DOI: 10.1002/14651858.CD004661.pub3

Doyle, K. J., & Bradshaw, W. T. (2012). Sixty golden minutes. *Neonatal Network, 31*(5), 289–294.

Ersdal, H. L., Mduma, E., Svensen, E., & Perlman, J. M. (2012). Early initiation of basic resuscitation interventions including face mask ventilation may reduce birth asphyxia related mortality in low-income countries: A prospective descriptive observational study. *Resuscitation, 83*(7), 869–873.

Fogarty, M., Osborn, D. A., Askie, L., Seidler, A. L., Hunter, K., Lui, K., ... & Tarnow-Mordi, W. (2018). Delayed vs early umbilical cord clamping for preterm infants: a systematic review and meta-analysis. *American Journal of Obstetrics and Gynecology, 218*(1), 1–18.

Fowlie, P., Booth, P., & Skeoch, C. (2008). Moving the preterm infant. In McGuire, W., & Fowlie, P. (Eds.) *ABC of Preterm Birth (ABC Series).* London: Blackwell Publishing.

Froese, A. B., Mcculloch, P. R., Sugiura, M., Vaclavik, S., Possmayer, F., & Moller, F. (1993). Optimizing alveolar expansion prolongs the effectiveness of exogenous surfactant therapy in the adult rabbit. *American Review of Respiratory Disease, 148*(3), 569–577.

Ginsberg, H. G., & Goldsmith, J. P. (1998). Controversies in neonatal resuscitation. *Clinics in Perinatology, 25*(1), 1–15.

Greene, K. R. , & Rosen, K. G. (1995). Intrapartum asphyxia. In Levene, M. I., & Lilford, R. J. (Eds.) *Fetal and Neonatal Neurology and Neurosurgery,* 2nd Edition (ppcvfv). Edinburgh: Churchill Livingstone.

Halling, C., Sparks, J. E., Christie, L., & Wyckoff, M. H. (2017). Efficacy of intravenous and endotracheal epinephrine during neonatal cardiopulmonary resuscitation in the delivery room. *The Journal of Pediatrics, 185,* 232–236.

Howell, J. H. (1987). Sodium Bicarbonate in the Perinatal Setting–Revisited. *Clinics in Perinatology, 14*(4), 807–816.

Ibrahim, C. P., & Yoxall, C. W. (2010). Use of self-heating gel mattresses eliminates admission hypothermia in infants born below 28 weeks gestation. *European Journal of Pediatrics, 169*(7), 795–799.

Janvier, A., & Mercurio, M. R. (2013). Saving vs creating: perceptions of intensive care at different ages and the potential for injustice. *Journal of Perinatology, 33*(5), 333–335.

Jefferies, A. L., & Kirpalani, H. M. (2012). Counselling and management for anticipated extremely preterm birth. *Paediatrics & Child Health*, *17*(8), 443–446.

Kapadia, V., & Wyckoff, M. H. (2012). Chest compressions for bradycardia or asystole in neonates. *Clinics in Perinatology*, *39*(4), 833–842.

Kasdorf, E., Laptook, A., Azzopardi, D., Jacobs, S., & Perlman, J. M. (2015). Improving infant outcome with a 10 min Apgar of 0. *Archives of Disease in Childhood: Fetal and Neonatal Edition*, *100*(2), F102–F105.

Kenyon, S. L., Taylor, D. J., & Tarnow-Mordi, W. F. (2001). Broad-spectrum antibiotics for spontaneous preterm labour: the ORACLE II randomised trial. *The Lancet*, *357*(9261), 989–994.

Kenyon, S., Boulvain, M., & Neilson, J.P. (2013). Antibiotics for preterm rupture of membranes. *Cochrane Database of Systematic Reviews*, Issue 12. Art. No.: CD001058. DOI: 10.1002/14651858. CD001058.pub3

Li, S., Guo, P., Zou, Q., He, F., Xu, F., & Tan, L. (2016). Efficacy and safety of plastic wrap for prevention of hypothermia after birth and during NICU in preterm infants: A systematic review and meta-analysis. *PloS One*, *11*(6), e0156960.

McCall, E. M., Alderdice, F., Halliday, H. L., Vohra, S., & Johnston, L. (2018). Interventions to prevent hypothermia at birth in preterm and/or low birth weight infants. *Cochrane Database of Systematic Reviews*, Issue 2. Art. No.: CD004210. DOI: 10.1002/14651858.CD004210.pub5

McCarthy, L. K., Hensey, C. C., & O'Donnell, C. P. (2012). In vitro effect of exothermic mattresses on temperature in the delivery room. *Resuscitation*, *83*(10), e201–e202.

McCarthy, L. K., Molloy, E. J., Twomey, A. R., Murphy, J. F., & O'Donnell, C. P. (2013). A randomized trial of exothermic mattresses for preterm newborns in polyethylene bags. *132*(1), e135–141.

Mercer, J. S., Vohr, B. R., McGrath, M. M., Padbury, J. F., Wallach, M., & Oh, W. (2006). Delayed cord clamping in very preterm infants reduces the incidence of intraventricular hemorrhage and late-onset sepsis: a randomized, controlled trial. *Pediatrics*, *117*(4), 1235–1242.

National Institute for Health and Care Excellence. (2015). *Intrapartum Care (QS105)* London: National Institute for Health and Care Excellence.

National Institute for Health and Care Excellence. (2019a). *Preterm labour and birth.* London: National Institute for Health and Care Excellence.

National Institute for Health and Care Excellence. (2019b). *Antenatal Care for Uncomplicated Pregnancies (CG62).* London: National Institute for Health and Care Excellence.

National Neonatal Audit Programme (NNAP) (2018). *Royal College of Paediatrics and Child Health. NNAP* Online https://nnap.rcpch.ac.uk/.

National Patient Safety Agency. (2005). *Safer Practice Notice – Wristbands for hospital inpatients improves safety.* http://dim.ch-saintonge.fr/Dim/Web/Dossiers%20th%C3%A9matiques/0%20Identito-Vigilance/0%20Wristbands%20for%20hospital%20%20inpatients%20improve%20safety.pdf.

National Patient Safety Agency. (2010). *Neonatal Resuscitation – Signal.* National Patient Safety Agency.

Nursing and Midwifery Council. (2018). *The Code: Professional standards of practice and behaviour for nurses, midwives* and nursing associates. NMC.

Oatley, H. K., Blencowe, H., & Lawn, J. E. (2016). The effect of coverings, including plastic bags and wraps, on mortality and morbidity in preterm and full-term neonates. *Journal of Perinatology*, *36*(S1), S83–S89.

Owen, C. J., & Wyllie, J. P. (2004). Determination of heart rate in the baby at birth. *Resuscitation*, *60*(2), 213–217.

Ozsurekci, Y., & Aykac, K. (2016). Oxidative stress related diseases in newborns. *Oxidative Medicine and Cellular Longevity*, *2016*. 2768365.

Perlman, J., Kattwinkel, J., Wyllie, J., Guinsburg, R., Velaphi, S., & Nalini Singhal for the Neonatal ILCOR Task Force Group. (2012). Neonatal resuscitation: In pursuit of evidence gaps in knowledge. *Resuscitation*, *83*(5), 545–550.

Perlman, J. M., Wyllie, J., Kattwinkel, J., Wyckoff, M. H., Aziz, K., Guinsburg, R., ... & Szyld, E. (2015). Part 7: Neonatal resuscitation: 2015 international consensus on cardiopulmonary resuscitation and emergency cardiovascular care science with treatment recommendations. *Circulation*, *132*(16_ suppl_1), S204–S241.

Perondi, M. B. M., Reis, A. G., Paiva, E. F., Nadkarni, V. M., & Berg, R. A. (2004). A comparison of high-dose and standard-dose epinephrine in children with cardiac arrest. *New England Journal of Medicine*, *350*(17), 1722–1730.

Preziosi, M. P., Roig, J. C., Hargrove, N., & Burchfield, D. J. (1993). Metabolic acidemia with hypoxia attenuates the hemodynamic responses to epinephrine during resuscitation in lambs. *Critical Care Medicine*, *21*(12), 1901–1907.

Reynolds, R., Pilcher, J., Ring, A., Johnson, R., & McKinley, P. (2009). The Golden Hour: Care of the LBW infant during the first hour of life one unit's experience. *Neonatal Network*, *28*(4), 211–219.

Roberts, D., Brown, J., Medley, N., & Dalziel, S. R. (2017). Antenatal corticosteroids for accelerating fetal lung maturation for women at risk of preterm birth. *Cochrane Database of Systematic Reviews*, Issue 3. Art. No.: CD004454. DOI: 10.1002/14651858.CD004454.pub3

Royal College of Obstetricians and Gynaecologists. (2015). *Clamping of the Umbilical Cord and Placental Transfusion* London: Royal College of Obstetricians and Gynaecologists.

Royal College of Paediatrics and Child Health & Healthcare Quality Improvement Partnership (2018). *National Neonatal Audit Programme 2018 Annual Report on 2017 data*. Royal College of Paediatrics and Child Health.

Seikku, L., Gissler, M., Andersson, S., Rahkonen, P., Stefanovic, V., Tikkanen, M., ... & Rahkonen, L. (2016). Asphyxia, neurologic morbidity, and perinatal mortality in early-term and postterm birth. *Pediatrics*, e20153334.

Shah, P., Anvekar, A., McMichael, J., & Rao, S. (2015). Outcomes of infants with Apgar score of zero at 10 min: The West Australian experience. *Archives of Disease in Childhood: Fetal and Neonatal Edition*, *100*(6), F492–F494.

Sharma, D. (2017a). Golden hour of neonatal life: Need of the hour. *Maternal Health, Neonatology and Perinatology*, *3*(1), 16.

Sharma, D. (2017b). Golden 60 minutes of newborn's life: Part 1: Preterm neonate. *The Journal of Maternal-Fetal & Neonatal Medicine*, *30*(22), 2716–2727.

Sharma, D., Sharma, P., & Shastri, S. (2017). Golden 60 minutes of newborn's life: Part 2: Term neonate. *The Journal of Maternal-Fetal & Neonatal Medicine*, *30*(22), 2728–2733.

Soll, R. F., & Pfister, R. H. (2011). Evidence-based delivery room care of the very low birth weight infant. *Neonatology*, *99*(4), 349–354.

Staniszewska, S., Brett, J., Redshaw, M., Hamilton, K., Newburn, M., Jones, N., & Taylor, L. (2012). The POPPY study: developing a model of family-centred care for neonatal units. *Worldviews on Evidence-Based Nursing*, *9*(4), 243–255.

Talner, N. S., Lister, G., & Fahey, J. T. (1992). Effects of asphyxia on the myocardium of the fetus and newborn. In Polin, R. A., & Fox, W. W. (Eds) *Fetal and Neonatal Physiology. Philadelphia, Saunders*, 759–768.

Travers, C. P., Clark, R. H., Spitzer, A. R., Das, A., Garite, T. J., & Carlo, W. A. (2017). Exposure to any antenatal corticosteroids and outcomes in preterm infants by gestational age: Prospective cohort study. *BMJ*, *356*, j1039.

Vasudevan, C., & Levene, M. (2013). Epidemiology and aetiology of neonatal seizures. In *Seminars in Fetal and Neonatal Medicine*, *18*(4), 185–191.

Vintzileos, A. M., Ananth, C. V., Smulian, J. C., Scorza, W. E., & Knuppel, R. A. (2002). The impact of prenatal care in the United States on preterm births in the presence and absence of antenatal high-risk conditions. *American Journal of Obstetrics and Gynecology*, *187*(5), 1254–1257.

Voltolini, C., Torricelli, M., Conti, N., Vellucci, F. L., Severi, F. M., & Petraglia, F. (2013). Understanding spontaneous preterm birth: From underlying mechanisms to predictive and preventive interventions. *Reproductive Sciences, 20*(11), 1274–1292.

Wilkinson, D. J., & Stenson, B. (2015). Don't stop now? How long should resuscitation continue at birth in the absence of a detectable heartbeat? *Archives of Disease in Childhood: Fetal and Neonatal Edition, 100*(6), F476–F478.

World Health Organisation. (2014). *Guideline: Delayed Cord Clamping for improved maternal and infant health and nutrition outcomes.* Geneva: WHO.

Wyllie, J., Bruinenberg, J., Roehr, C. C., Rüdiger, M., Trevisanuto, D., & Urlesberger, B. (2015). European Resuscitation Council Guidelines for Resuscitation 2015: Section 7. Resuscitation and support of transition of babies at birth. *Resuscitation, 95,* 249–263.

Wyllie, J., Ainsworth, S., Tinnion, R., & Hampshire, S. (2016). *Newborn Life Support. (4th Edition).* London: Resuscitation Council UK.

Wyszogrodski, I., Kyei-Aboagye, K., Taeusch Jr, H. W., & Avery, M. E. (1975). Surfactant inactivation by hyperventilation: conservation by end-expiratory pressure. *Journal of Applied Physiology, 38*(3), 461–466.

11 MANAGEMENT OF THERMAL STABILITY

Tracey Jones

CONTENTS

GUIDANCE ON HOW TO ENHANCE PERSONAL LEARNING FROM THIS CHAPTER

Key points covered in this chapter

- The physiological basis of neonatal thermoregulation.
- Mechanisms of neonatal heat gain and heat loss.
- Thermal management in the neonatal unit.

Reflection

Reading through the chapter, you are encouraged to engage with the key points and related literature in an enquiring way. Ask these questions:

- Have you observed infants who are hypothermic or hyperthermic and what were the potential adverse outcomes because of this?
- How did these infants present?
- How were these infants managed?

Implications for nursing care

■ Finally: how will this chapter enable you to consider best practice in thermal care of the high-risk infant in neonatal care? Consider the implications of what you learn for your nursing care relating to this area.

INTRODUCTION AND BACKGROUND

Thermal management has been integral to neonatal nursing care since studies published in the early 1990s evidenced the consequence of thermal injury (Fastman et al., 2014). Normal thermal control for the term infant requires some assistance by the midwife attending delivery, and the neonatal nurse and multidisciplinary team (MDT) thereafter. Hypothermia (body temperature below normal) on admission to neonatal units (NNUs) is a problem worldwide, across all climates, particularly for small infants and those born too early (McCall et al., 2014; Yip et al., 2017; McCall et al., 2018). Data from the National Neonatal Audit Programme (NNAP; Royal College of Paediatrics and Child Health (RCPCH), 2018) and recent results of the ATAIN (Avoiding Term Admissions Into NNUs) study (National Health Service (NHS) Improvement, 2017) demonstrated the impact of poor thermal management in relation to term infant admissions to NNUs throughout the UK. Other countries have either reported similar issues or acknowledged the importance of managing neonatal thermoregulation (Yip et al., 2017; Frazer et al., 2018; Laptook et al., 2018). This chapter provides an overview of physiology and mechanisms of neonatal thermoregulation, heat loss and heat gain, and the management strategies required to ensure sound thermal control.

PHYSIOLOGICAL BASIS OF NEONATAL THERMOREGULATION

Thermal control must be initiated by the infant at birth. Temperature is regulated by balancing heat production against heat loss, a balance that is continually being disturbed by changes in metabolic rate or external factors (Knobel, 2014). Newborns lose heat rapidly and the body temperature begins to fall immediately following birth; this can drop 2–3°C in the first 30 minutes (Fastman et al., 2014). Particular issues for newborn infants are immaturity of the hypothalamus, the thermoregulatory control centre in the mid-brain, and large surface area to body weight ratio, leading to immature thermal control. When born early, the physiological pathways necessary to commence heat production are struggling to meet thermoregulatory demands even more; there is limited adipose tissue (brown fat), reduced subcutaneous (insulating) fat and thin, unkeratinised skin prone to transdermal heat and water losses in the preterm infant. Overall, there are insufficient reserves to maintain thermal stability without compromising other body systems.

Whatever the situation, to manage hypothermia successfully, the neonatal nurse must have knowledge of the systems involved in initiating and maintaining thermal stability, as well as understanding how to assist the infant in the vital transition time after birth. The role of the neonatal nurse is crucial in limiting heat loss at birth and in establishing a suitable environment in which the infant is cared for. In the NNU, expertise is essential in choosing the right thermal environment for the infant whatever the gestation.

MECHANISMS OF HEAT GAIN

Non-shivering thermogenesis

The newborn infant has limited capabilities to produce heat by shivering, and when a baby is born prematurely, poor muscular development means the neonate has no means of changing position to preserve heat. Infants have more sweat glands than adults, but the ability to use them as a form of heat reduction is limited, as they are regulated by the hypothalamus via the nervous system, which is poorly myelinated. In the premature neonate, the sweat glands have not completely formed, and the secretory coils of the glandular segment and the sweating response to external stimuli are reduced (Oranges et al., 2015). The primary source of heat in the newborn is **non-shivering thermogenesis**, which involves the use of **brown adipose tissue** (BAT) to produce heat (Asakura, 2004).

Thermogenesis is initiated by three different mechanisms: (1) cutaneous cooling; (2) oxygenation; and (3) separation from the placenta. An increase in oxygen content of blood with increased flow is needed for the initiation of the system. Separation from the placenta when the cord is cut plays a vital role in maximising non-shivering thermogenesis (Asakura, 2004). The mechanisms of non-shivering thermogenesis include the metabolism of BAT, the secretion of noradrenaline and the release of thyroxin (see figure 11.1).

BROWN ADIPOSE TISSUE

The majority of brown fat is located around the neck, between the scapulae, across the clavicular line and around the sternum. It also surrounds the major thoracic vessels and kidneys. Brown fat cells contain a nucleus, glycogen and **mitochondria**. The mitochondria are numerous and provide energy for metabolic conversion (Enerbäck, 2010). Brown fat has a high concentration of stored triglycerides, and the presence of thermogenin means that when fat is oxidised, heat is produced rather than energy. Glucose is the main energy substrate in the very low birth weight (LBW) infant, providing it has entered the cells. Glucose cannot enter the cells if there are low amounts of amino acids, and where these are reduced, insulin production is also lowered, leading ultimately to glucose intolerance and intracellular failure.

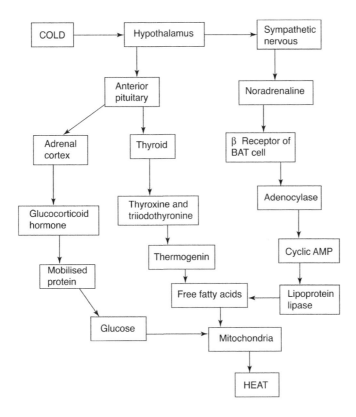

Figure 11.1 The mechanisms of non-shivering thermogenesis

GLUCONEOGENESIS

Non-shivering thermogenesis is dependent on a source of energy from glucose and fatty acids; therefore, if the body is unable to generate new glucose, this source of heat production will be affected. Gluconeogenesis is the process that converts proteins and lipids into glucose to meet requirements. Corticotrophin released from the anterior pituitary gland stimulates the release of glucocorticoid hormone from the adrenal cortex, to free proteins within the cells to be metabolised into glucose. In the preterm or small for gestational age (SGA) infant, the stores may be depleted, thus inhibiting gluconeogenesis. Hormonal levels may also be inadequate, such as thyroid-stimulating hormone (TSH) and adrenocorticotropic hormone (ACTH), which influence thyroxine and the adrenal cortex and assist in gluconeogenesis (Aylott, 2006a).

INSULIN

Insulin acts in the liver and muscles to increase glycogen synthesis, and in the adipose cells it increases glucose uptake and the conversion of carbohydrate to fat. It decreases lipolysis and raises the uptake of free fatty acids. There is rapid **glycogenolysis** after birth, subsequent to falling levels of insulin. There is a response from glucagon stimulating the sensory nervous system to release catecholamine which frees hepatic cyclic adenosine monophosphate (cAMP). Surges of glucagon and cAMP help to change the activity of the liver from glycogen to glucose production (Knobel, 2014; Knobel-Dail, 2014).

NORADRENALINE

Non-shivering thermogenesis is controlled by the release of noradrenaline. Infants born before term have a substantially reduced adrenal medulla, potentially causing adrenal insufficiency. Cord blood catecholamines are low and the infant's ability to withstand cold stress is reduced. Noradrenaline binds to β_1-receptors increasing cAMP by releasing **adenosine triphosphate** (ATP) from adenocyclase. This increase in cAMP causes the release of kinase which, in turn, leads to a breakdown of the triglycerides in BAT, which releases fatty acids to be combusted by the mitochondria. The fatty acids are readily available on the outer membrane of the mitochondria. Premature infants have inefficient heat production by non-shivering thermogenesis and have an inability to exhibit peripheral vasoconstriction either due to immaturity or poor vasomotor tone (Knobel et al., 2009).

THE THYROID GLAND

TSH, which stimulates thermogenesis (Endo and Kobayashi, 2008) is released by the anterior pituitary gland. Free fatty acids and thermogenin accelerate heat production. Thermogenin increases with gestation, so although there may be sufficient thyroxine (T_4) at 25 weeks, the thermogenin available to convert it is low. Serum concentrations of TSH increase rapidly for 10 minutes after delivery, then gradually fall over 48 hours, which is thought to indicate the acute use of stored pituitary TSH. The levels of T_4, free T_4 and triiodothyronine (T_3) are significantly low in sick infants. Where thyroid efficacy is lacking, more energy is expended in thermogenesis, it is less fuel-efficient, and more fat is burned so the preterm infant, already with a limited ability to produce heat, is further challenged by the extra energy demands (Clemente et al., 2007; Carrascosa et al., 2008).

THERMAL RECEPTORS

In the infant, the hypothalamus reacts to cold stimulus by causing vasoconstriction of the cutaneous blood vessels via the sympathetic nervous system (though this is limited) and increases the metabolic rate by releasing noradrenaline and enhancing T_4 release (Marieb and Hoehn, 2015).

Vasoconstriction

Where there is a layer of subcutaneous fat, peripheral vasoconstriction can result in some reduction in heat loss, especially in full-term infants. However, in the very preterm baby, this layer of fat is very thin and therefore there is little or no reduction in heat loss through vaso-constriction, exacerbated by the fact that the ability to vasoconstrict is significantly reduced (Knobel et al., 2009; Petty, 2010).

MECHANISMS OF HEAT LOSS

It is important to not only understand the physiology of heat production, but also to be aware of the means external to the infant by which heat is gained or lost. Insulation will reduce any transfer of heat. There are two forms of insulation – internal and external. Internal insulation is provided by the layer of subcutaneous fat, which starts developing from 26 to 29 weeks' gestation. Fat is a poor conductor of heat, and its depth will contribute to its effectiveness. The smaller infant has had less chance to develop this layer of insulation. Transfer of heat between the environment and the infant occurs by evaporation, radiation, convection and conduction. These are outlined now along with associated strategies to prevent heat loss.

Evaporation

Evaporation is the insensible water loss from the skin's surface and the respiratory mucosa dependent on air speed and relative humidity (Asakura, 2004). Evaporative losses account for a large proportion of total heat loss immediately after delivery or during bathing. Under normal conditions in a term infant, evaporative heat loss is about a quarter of the resting heat production. However, the preterm infant has much higher evaporative losses as a consequence of transepidermal water loss, which is up to six times higher per unit surface area in an infant of 26 weeks' gestation. In very preterm infants, a diminished capacity for metabolic heat production coupled with a high surface area to volume ratio and an imma-ture epidermal barrier leads to extraordinarily high evaporative heat losses (Doglioni, 2014). Evaporative losses can be minimised by drying immediately after delivery of term infants. For infants born at ≤30 weeks, wrapping in polyethylene at delivery and humidifying the incu-bator will eliminate/reduce evaporative losses (McCall et al., 2018).

Radiation

Radiation involves transfer of radiant energy from the surface of the body to surrounding surfaces that are not in contact with the infant; this is in the form of electromagnetic waves (Hall, 2011). Up to 60% of heat can be lost this way. More heat is transferred if the surrounding surfaces are cold. This process is reversed where a radiant heat source is used to warm the infant, although only in the short term. Loss through radiation can be limited by ensuring that the delivery room is at least 25°C, and, when necessary, admitting infants into a pre-warmed, double-walled incubator and not placing them near cold exterior walls or windows. Overheating should be avoided by careful monitoring of the infant's temperature if under a radiant heat source.

Convection

Convection involves heat loss due to the movement of air on the skin surface. Therefore, it is important to protect the infant from draughts, wrapping them to reduce exposure of the skin surface. Low birth weight infants should be nursed in incubators with warm air circulating. Delivery of oxygen – if used for more than a short period – should have added warmth because the cool gas is exchanged for warm expired carbon dioxide (Meyer et al., 2015).

Conduction

Conduction involves the transfer of heat from one object to another when they are in contact with each other, such as the infant being placed on a cool surface (Knobel, 2014; Knobel-Dail, 2014). It can also refer to heat conducted from the core of the body to the cooler skin surface. Losses by conduction (approximately 3%) can be minimised by use of warmed blankets, pre-warmed clothing, pre-warmed incubators and resuscitaires, warm coverings for scales and X-ray plates.

Heat exchanged through the respiratory tract

Expired air is more humid than inspired air. This results in an evaporative loss of water and heat from the respiratory tract. There is also a small amount of convective heat transfer. As a result of the alternate inspiratory warming and expiratory cooling of the air, the convective heat exchange depends on the temperature of the inspired air (Sweet et al., 2017).

Surface area

The newborn infant has a large surface area compared to his or her mass. There is an imbalance in the smaller neonate between the heat-producing ability (mass) and the heat-loss potential (surface area; Petty, 2010; Turnbull and Petty, 2013a; 2013b). This large surface area to body mass ratio requires a high calorific intake to support temperature balance and this should be taken into account when prescribing fluid. Modi (2004) recommends that a judgement should be made of the likely magnitude of insensible water loss, taking into account sources of radiant heat, ambient humidity, and gestational and postnatal age. Experiments have shown that heat loss increases with an increase in the ratio of body surface area to body mass (Elabassi et al., 2004); therefore, the very LBW infant will have greater potential for heat loss.

Immature skin

Skin maturation in preterm infants, unlike the maturation of renal function, is not accelerated by antenatal steroid exposure, but is accelerated by birth (Modi, 2004). It is thought that transfer from the intrauterine aquatic environment to the external atmospheric environment stimulates and accelerates the maturation of skin (Oranges et al., 2015). Histological analysis has shown that epidermal development is complete *in utero* at 34 weeks' gestation, and infants of 30–32 weeks have a barrier function comparable to that of adults. Preterm skin is also more gelatinous and transparent than at term. The stratum corneum, the outer horny layer of the epidermal barrier, conserves the body contents, resists noxious agents and protects against trauma. The immaturity of this layer means that the risk of percutaneous absorption of drugs or chemicals is increased. Immaturity also means that the skin is permeable to gases, allowing for the passive diffusion of oxygen in and carbon dioxide out along a concentration gradient. The skin of a preterm infant comprises up to 13% of his or her body weight compared to 3% in an adult. The infant of 26 weeks has developed a keratinised stratum corneum, but the epidermis is only two or three cells thick leading to more significant transepidermal water and heat loss via evaporation described earlier (Chiou and Blume-Peytavi, 2004).

Transepidermal water loss

Transepidermal water loss (TEWL) is a physical process dependent on the epidermal barrier, temperature, air speed and humidity. In infants born at 24–25 weeks' gestation, TEWL is about 60g/m^2/hour (about 140 mL/kg/day in a 1000g baby) at a relative humidity of 50% in the first two days after birth (approximately five times higher than in term infants; see figure 11.2); this decreases significantly by day 3, to around 45g/m^2/hour and to 24g/m^2/hour by 28 days. In babies born at lesser degrees of prematurity, by 2–3 weeks of age, skin maturity is similar to that of full-term infants. By 32 weeks' gestation, TEWL has fallen to the same order of magnitude as in term infants at 6–8g/m^2/hour (about 12 mL/kg/day; Modi, 2004; Ågren et al., 2006). When 100% humidity is added to the incubator, TEWL does not occur (Waldron and MacKinnon, 2007). However, this addition of humidity to reduce TEWL may actually delay the maturation of the epidermis, as it has been shown that there is more rapid maturation of skin barrier function at lower humidity (Ågren et al., 2006).

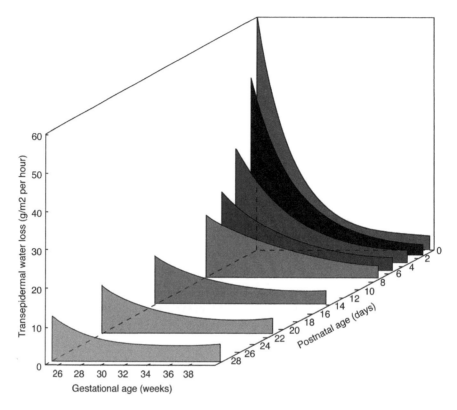

Figure 11.2 The regression of transepidermal water loss at different postnatal ages (adapted from Hammarlund et al., 1983, with permission from Wiley Blackwell Publishers)

THERMAL INSTABILITY

Hypothermia

The sick newborn infant is more prone to hypothermia, especially where respiratory disease is a problem. Non-shivering thermogenesis requires the presence of oxygen to metabolise BAT. If the infant suffers a degree of hypoxia, the limited ability to produce heat is further diminished (Aylott, 2006b; Turnbull and Petty, 2013b). Preterm and SGA infants are at increased risk from hypothermia (Yip et al., 2017) and nursing interventions and excessive handling have been associated with temperature instability (Deguines et al., 2013). The cardiovascular responsiveness of growth-restricted infants is absent in the first few days of life, which impairs their ability to mount a thermal response. Evidence continues to link hypothermia after birth with neonatal morbidity and mortality (Waldron and MacKinnon, 2007; Frazer et al., 2018; Laptook et al., 2018). Laptook et al. (2007) examined 5,277 infants born between 2002 and 2003 weighing 401–1,499g. Hypothermia was prevalent in this group, with 14.3% of the infants having an admission temperature less than 35°C, and 32.6% having a temperature between 35°C and 35.9°C. Even though figures have improved, an inverse association between temperature and mortality risk persists (Laptook et al., 2018).

Since hypothermia is known to be linked to both morbidity and mortality in preterm infants, it is very important to address their temperature requirements as a priority (Laptook et al., 2007). The admission temperature of infants admitted to neonatal units has become one of the key indicators in the UK NNAP highlighted earlier. Monitoring the standard of care provided by specialist NNUs is essential to inform efforts to give all babies the best possible chance of surviving and reaching their full potential. The most recent NNAP data indicates that in 2017, more babies born at <32 weeks' gestation were admitted with a temperature within the recommended range of 36.5–37.5°C than in 2016 (61% in 2016; 64% in 2017). This improvement in normothermia is seen in most units, suggesting changes in clinical practices. However, the report states that there remains room for further improvement in the promotion of normothermia on admission to NNUs for very preterm infants, and recommends putting a care bundle in place, developed with MDT input, which mandates the use of evidence-based strategies to encourage admission normothermia of very preterm babies. These will be discussed later.

Cold stress

Neonatal hypothermia limits have been defined by various researchers and organisations over the years. Given the normal temperature of an infant being 36.5° to 37.5°C (Turnbull and Petty, 2013a), hypothermia occurs when an infant's temperature decreases below 36.5°C. The World Health Organisation (WHO; 2011) also defines mild hypothermia as a body temperature between 36.0° and 36.5°C; moderate hypothermia as a temperature between 32.0° and 36.0°C and severe hypothermia is as a temperature less than 32.0°C. Most current studies are using WHO definitions of hypothermia; infants' body temperature should be kept above a minimal standard of 36.5°C. Babies lose heat during birth, resuscitation and transportation. Air temperatures in the delivery room should be kept warm to avoid cold stress. Cold stress affects oxygenation by increasing pulmonary artery resistance and reducing surfactant production. Poor perfusion causes an increase in anaerobic metabolism leading to worsening acidosis. Acidosis itself increases pulmonary artery pressure, decreasing the amount of blood flow through the lungs leading to hypoxia. Surfactant, as well as being produced at lower rates, loses its ability to act as a surface tension lowering agent if body temperature drops below 35°C, which will give rise to atelectasis, thereby worsening hypoxia (Aylott, 2006a; 2006b; Turnbull and Petty, 2013a). The heightened utilisation of glucose caused by increased metabolism can lead to hypoglycaemia, which worsens acidosis and reduces energy available for growth. Acidosis can lead to the displacement of unconjugated bilirubin from albumin binding sites, causing an increase in the risk of **kernicterus** (see figure 11.3).

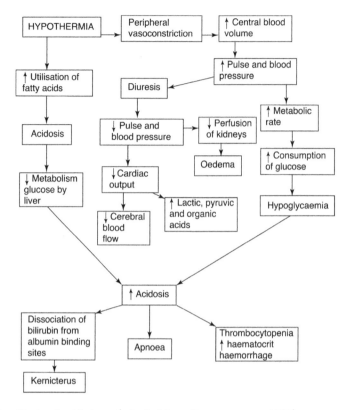

Figure 11.3 The effects of cold stress (adapted from Brueggemeyer, 1993)

Hyperthermia

Hyperthermia in the neonate is unusual and except when the infant is pyrexial due to sepsis, it is most likely due to inappropriate environmental situation. That is why it is important that all infants in the NNU should have their temperatures closely monitored. In sepsis there will be a large difference in the core and peripheral temperatures. The same factors that are responsible for hypothermia can also give rise to hyperthermia – large surface area, limited insulation and limited ability to sweat. Hypotension can occur secondary to the vasodilatation, and dehydration follows an increase in insensible water loss.

MANAGEMENT OF THERMAL STABILITY AT DELIVERY

In utero foetal temperature is at least one degree higher than that of the mother to allow a gradient to offload heat from the foetus to the mother via the placenta. The drop in ambient temperature at delivery is even more marked due to the wet infant being delivered into a cool environment.

McCall et al. (2014; 2018) published an extensive review of interventions studied to prevent heat loss following delivery in premature infants. They identified key interventions to reduce heat loss in the delivery room: increasing ambient temperature in the delivery room, using heated humidified gases, using exothermic or thermal mattresses, use of heat loss barriers such as head coverings or plastic body coverings, and skin-to-skin care. The recommended delivery room temperature should be at least 25°C (ideal range 25–28°C; WHO, 1993) which should be increased depending on the gestation of the infant being delivered. Delivery room environments rarely meet the basic temperature standard.

The healthy infant

A healthy newborn infant is faced with a substantial drop in environmental temperature at birth and will react by increasing heat production. Even term or near-term infants, if left naked and wet in a temperature of 25°C, will lose heat at a rate that exceeds heat production. However, if dried immediately and wrapped, or preferably, dried and placed on the mother's abdomen for skin-to-skin contact covered with a blanket in an optimum room temperature, they will be able to maintain their temperature adequately (Beiranvand et al., 2014). It is well documented that skin-to-skin contact immediately after birth and thereafter confers many benefits to both mother and infant (Baley, 2015; Gabriel et al., 2015; Kristoffersen et al., 2016; Petty, 2017) including the prevention of heat loss through the skin, and conductive heat gain from mother or father to the baby. In addition, a hat will reduce or even prevent heat loss through the head which has a large surface area. Early establishment of feeding will furthermore ensure that the infant has nutrition to support thermogenesis.

The high-risk infant

DELIVERY BY CAESAREAN SECTION

It is known that infants delivered by caesarean section are more likely to encounter problems with respiration and thermoregulation because they have not undergone the normal processes associated with vaginal delivery (Beiranvand et al., 2014).

PERINATAL HYPOXIA

The infant who is delivered following a hypoxic event or period of foetal distress requires particular attention, alongside effective airway management, towards effective thermal care. All wet towels should be removed, and warm, dry towels available for the baby to lie on under a radiant heat source (McCall et al., 2018).

INFANTS WITH CONGENITAL ANOMALIES

Certain conditions – such as gastroschisis, exomphalos and myelomeningocele – have increased surface areas for heat loss and increased evaporative loss (Sugarman et al., 2012), and management strategies should be geared to preventing hypothermia.

PRETERM OR LOW BIRTH WEIGHT INFANTS

This group of infants faces many problems (figure 11.4) and is most likely to become hypothermic because most delivery rooms are not an optimal thermal environment. Commonly, the room temperature is low; there may be draughts which increase convective heat loss;

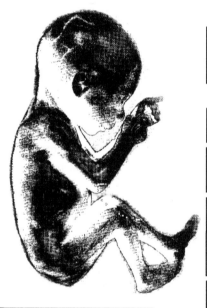

Pituitary unable to secrete adequate corticotrophins and the infant is unable to initiate gluconeogenesis

Cold stress leads to
↑ O$_2$ requirement
↑ pulmonary artery pressure
↓ surfactant production

Insufficient brown adipose tissue leading to poor heat production

Insufficient insulin, amino acids and poor glucose transporters leading to glucose intolerance

↓ Na$^+$K$^+$ATPase leading to hyperkalaemia

Adrenal glands small leading to low levels of catecholamines

Myelination of nervous system incomplete leading to poor conduction from skin sensors

Vasoconstriction is inefficient leading to heat loss through peripheries

Poor peripheral perfusion leading to acidosis which in turn can lead to > bilirubin and hypoglycaemia

Surface area is large in relation to its weight leading to heat loss

Poorly keratinised epidermis leading to water loss

Poor muscle development leading to an inability to change posture according to temperature

Figure 11.4 Thermal problems facing vulnerable infants

the air surrounding the infant has low humidity; and there is usually no source for warmed gas. The body temperature of an exposed 1kg infant can fall at the rate of 1°C every 5 minutes. Therefore, the first measure is to ensure a warm delivery room/theatre by setting the temperature to reflect the gestation of the infant about to be delivered, i.e. >25°C for infants <27 weeks' gestation (Kent and Williams, 2008). Ensuring that all windows and doors are shut at the time of delivery will reduce the air current passing over the infant. The radiant warmer should be set to its maximum output with warmed towels to limit heat loss.

All infants who are delivered at less than 30 weeks' gestation should be wrapped in polyethylene skin wrapping at delivery to prevent heat loss (Wyllie et al., 2016). They should be placed immediately in the bag without drying, covering the back of the head (which can be a major source of heat loss), adding a hat but leaving the face free and allowing clear sight of the chest (Björklund and Hellström-Westas, 2000; Vohra et al., 2004; Bredemeyer et al., 2005; McCall et al., 2014; 2018). This simple tool has been proven to be effective both at limiting/preventing heat loss (by 30–40%) and TEWL in the very LBW infant (Belghazi et al., 2006). It is also reported that the number of very LBW neonates admitted with temperatures less than 36°C was reduced, with increased overall admission temperatures for infants weighing less than 1500g with the addition of polyurethane-lined hats and chemical mattresses (Frazer et al., 2018). Yip et al. (2017) also described higher delivery room temperatures and use of full-body polyethylene wraps and woollen caps, implemented during initial stabilisation, to be beneficial in relation to thermal control. Skin-to-skin contact is also documented as beneficial in preterm infants in the NNU (Kristoffersen et al., 2016; Jones and Santamaria, 2018).

MANAGEMENT OF THERMAL STABILITY IN THE NEONATAL UNIT

Once the infant has been transferred to the NNU, it is vital that the correct thermal environment is provided, or, as stated earlier; thermal neutrality. Waldron and MacKinnon (2007) refer to the 'neutral thermal environment' (NTE) defined as an environmental temperature at which an infant with a normal body temperature has a minimal metabolic rate and minimal oxygen consumption. In setting standards for neutral temperature, the temperature at which infants can maintain an adequate core temperature at rest has been suggested to be between 36.7 and 37.3°C (Çınar and Filiz, 2006). The neonatal nurse has a responsibility to ensure that heat loss is minimised and that the thermal conditions are stable for the infant. In order to provide this, there are various well-developed warming devices, and it is important that such equipment is used appropriately. To reiterate a consistent theme throughout the book relating to any aspect of neonatal care, it must be remembered that the family is also an important part of thermal management (Turnbull and Petty, 2013b). Education and training are required to increase knowledge of and reinforce all these interventions in both delivery suite and the NNU along with an awareness of their importance for infant and family.

Radiant warmers

Radiant warmers limit heat loss during interventions because of ease of access and rapid radiant warmer responsiveness. During the stabilising period, the infant may be subjected to many interventions which may involve the infant being covered with sterile drapes, or the head of the operator may prevent the heat output reaching the infant, so it is a priority to ensure that these procedures are carried out as rapidly as possible to prevent heat loss.

Metabolic rates are higher under radiant heat due to the increased rate of evaporative and convective losses. Therefore, although an open radiant heat source can warm an infant more quickly, heat losses in the LBW infant are much higher and overall more fluctuant. A Cochrane review completed in 2003, with no recent updates, concluded that radiant warmers cause significant increases in insensible water loss and increases in oxygen consumption (Flenady and Woodgate, 2003), which is a disadvantage when caring for premature infants. This is more often seen in the LBW infant of low gestational age who has a poorly developed stratum corneum. It is essential to provide supplemental humidity and shielding to counteract water loss and prevent hypernatraemic dehydration.

Radiant warmers are still a good choice when it is necessary to reach the infant easily for a short period of time, such as stabilisation after birth and for surgical procedures (Knobel-Dail, 2014). Indeed, they can also facilitate closer proximity to the parents for a given time and enable parents to touch their baby without the barrier of incubator walls. However, time spent on a radiant warmer is usually temporary while procedures are carried out, given that incubator care provides a more conducive thermal environment; for example, it is difficult to create a humidified environment using a radiant warmer. (Ågren et al., 2006).

Incubators

Incubators have the advantage of providing an enclosed space in which the infant is protected from external noise and excessive handling. Most modern incubators are double-walled, which reduces the heat lost through radiation from the infant. Modern incubators can surround the baby with a curtain of heat, and endeavour to maintain warmth even with the doors open. Incubators are equipped with safe and efficient humidity systems which mean that prevention of TEWL can be more effectively managed. Temperature control with an incubator is either by skin servo-control, or setting of an air temperature. Servo-control self-adjusts according to the readings from a skin probe attached to the infant, whereas using the air temperature mode, settings are manually changed according to the infant's monitored temperature. A comparison of these methods indicated that either is effective at maintaining the skin temperature at 36.5–37.7°C (Sinclair, 2002).

Humidity

Humidity has been shown to reduce TEWL and improve the maintenance of body temperature. In contrast, infants nursed without humidity are known to become hypothermic in very high incubator temperatures. A method of coping with TEWL is to increase the fluid load to maintain normal serum sodium concentrations. However, this is known to precipitate sequelae such as patent ductus arteriosus, necrotising enterocolitis, intraventricular haemorrhage, and can increase the incidence of bronchopulmonary dysplasia (Bell and Acarregui, 2014). Preterm infants may lose up to 13% of their body weight as TEWL in the first day of life when nursed in 50% humidity.

Most incubators are equipped with an active source of humidity, which heats and evaporates water separately from the circulating air and then adds it to the incubator canopy, which prevents bacterial growth. Servo-control allows precise levels of humidity, and because it is an active system, when the portholes are opened, the recovery response is minimal as the vapour is continuously added to the circulating air. Providing humidity via an incubator is a relatively easy task (Ågren et al., 2006).

It is important to note that TEWL can increase during the delivery of phototherapy, whether by halogen spotlight or more conventional methods, with the most significant increases in the cubital fossa and groin. Therefore, close monitoring of electrolyte levels is essential, and fluid replacement must be considered. Table 11.1 outlines some guidance for humidity in the NNU.

Heated mattresses

Heated, water-filled mattresses have become a useful adjunct to caring for the healthy preterm infant in the nursery. They can help mothers overcome anxieties about their baby more easily and encourage bonding, compared to the experience of mothers of infants nursed

TABLE 11.1 GUIDELINES FOR HUMIDITY SETTINGS

26 weeks' gestation or less	27–30 weeks' gestation
80% humidity for at least 4 weeks may require higher percentage to cope with raised serum sodium levels	80% humidity for at least 2 weeks
The infant's skin should have keratinised fully at the end of this period; therefore, the humidity can be gradually reduced, as tolerated to maintain an axilla temperature within the normal range (Chiou and Blume-Peytavi 2004).	
Reduce the humidity gradually according to the infant's temperature until 20–30% is reached before discontinuing. Great Ormond Street recommend that humidity should be decreased after seven days, reducing the percentage relative humidity by approximately 5–10% each day and ceased on or before 14 days (Parsons, 2017).	

in incubators. McCall et al. (2014) found that heated mattresses were just as effective in warming premature infants as incubators. Where heated, water-filled mattresses have been compared to incubator care, mean body temperatures were similar, with no significant differences in the incidence of cold stress, weight gain or morbidity (Gray and Flenady, 2011).

Open cots

When a baby is ready to be transferred to an open cot from an incubator is another area of nursing assessment that needs to be undertaken. Clinically stable preterm infants may be transferred to unheated open cots at a weight of 1600g without adverse effects on temperature stability or weight gain, and earlier transfer does not necessarily result in being discharged earlier (New et al., 2011). Other specific guidance states a weight between 1500 and 1600g is appropriate once the incubator or mattress temperature has been weaned, and a baby no longer requires close monitoring, is gaining weight and can maintain a stable central temperature in 26–28°C room temperature (Barone et al., 2014; Parsons, 2017). Transition to an open cot is a significant milestone for the baby and family, meaning that parents can more easily touch, hold and have closer physical contact with their baby, as well as take part in his or her care without the barrier imposed by the incubator walls.

THERMAL STATUS DURING TRANSPORT

Prevention of heat loss is paramount during the transport of preterm/LBW and sick infants (Nordike et al., 2018). Engorn et al. (2017) demonstrated that infants undergoing procedures outside the neonatal intensive care unit requiring transport may be at risk of hypothermia. Moving the sick or small infant involves some inevitable heat loss due to moving between incubators at both ends of the journey, and strategies should be in place to reduce this negative impact, such as continual monitoring and a warming mattress for example, combined with a transport incubator (Libert et al., 2017). A probe should be securely placed in a skin-to-mattress site (intrascapular) and peripheral temperature should be monitored. Where possible, any existing hypothermia should be corrected before the journey.

Humidification systems designed for transport ventilators will reduce respiratory water loss and airway reactivity. The incubators themselves do not have humidification, and the small infant is at risk of high evaporative heat losses unless wrapped in polyethylene. If transferring a baby requiring surgical care, this technique can also be used to limit heat and water loss. TransWarmer© mattresses are a useful adjunct to transferring the hypothermic infant, and have been shown to be effective at stabilising temperatures. At the point of activation, they should be between 19 and 28°C to ensure optimal heat output, and the infant's temperature should be monitored constantly while cared for on the mattress (Carmichael et al., 2007).

TEMPERATURE MEASUREMENT

Finally, obtaining an accurate temperature is an integral part of the neonatal nurse's role and should be done using a device that has been designed to cause little disruption to the infant. The measurement of temperature plays an important part of clinical decision-making, and the nurse should be competent to carry out this action. Digital devices or chemical dot thermometers which are placed in the axilla remain a common option for use in NNUs (Smith et al., 2013; Smith, 2014). Frequency of intermittent central temperature recording depends on the clinical condition of the infant, as does whether they also receive continuous temperature monitoring, via servo or manual control as highlighted previously.

This will require individual nursing assessment and explanations to the parents (Turnbull and Petty, 2013b). In addition to training for the use of any device, infection control must also be considered.

CONCLUSION

In summary, hypothermia is an easily preventable condition, even in vulnerable newborns, and NNU staff need to know if an infant is too cold, so that they can take action to normalise the temperature (RCPCH, 2018). The neonatal nurse needs to have a working awareness of physiology in relation to thermoregulation, especially when caring for the very preterm infant. In the infant born early, the systems that are involved in thermal control are limited and poorly functioning. Knowledge of the mechanisms of heat production and losses will enable the nurse to choose the most appropriate way of providing a thermally stable environment for an infant in their care, whatever its gestation. Preventative action should be taken to reduce heat loss. Precautionary steps routinely include a warm delivery room; drying the newborn immediately, especially the head; wrapping in pre-warmed dry blankets that cover the head; pre-warming surfaces, and eliminating draughts (McCall et al., 2014; 2018). The temperature of newborn infants should be actively maintained between 36.5°C and 37.5°C after birth. unless a decision has been taken to commence therapeutic hypothermia (see chapter 14). The importance of achieving this has been highlighted and reinforced because of the strong association with mortality and morbidity. Even mild hypothermia that was once felt to be inevitable and therefore clinically acceptable carries a risk. The admission temperature should be recorded as a predictor of outcomes as well as a quality indicator (NHS Improvement, 2017).

Finally, thermal management must be given in the context of family-centred care and should be evidence-based. Current research should be incorporated into the care delivered; this has been demonstrated in the context of thermal care by the introduction of the polyethylene wraps for the very preterm infant at delivery. This relatively simple manouvre has dramatically improved temperature stability in this particularly vulnerable population and reminds the reader of an important message to end this chapter: that infants need 'simple things done well' (Wyllie et al., 2015).

CASE STUDIES

Case study 1: Thermal care in a premature infant

Simona arrived in the emergency department in early labour and within ten minutes delivered Jasmine at 26 weeks' gestation by precipitous vaginal delivery while she was in the toilet. The A&E staff attended to both Jasmine and Simona and fortunately, the neonatal team were called quickly and a resuscitaire brought to the scene.

With reference to the key points within the chapter, consider the following questions:

Q.1. What are the ways this infant will lose heat?
Q.2. What are the physiological factors that may lead to poor thermal control?
Q.3. What factors/strategies need to be considered in the thermal care of this infant?

Case study 2: Cold stress in the term infant

A term infant, Jake, has just arrived from the delivery suite with an admission core temperature of 35.7° Celsius. The infant had to be given inflation breaths in the delivery suite with a bag-valve mask for poor respiratory effort at birth. The resuscitaire had malfunctioned.

With reference to the key points within the chapter, consider the following questions:

Q.1. What are the potential effects of this infant being so cold?
Q.2. What is the physiological basis of your answer for Q.1?
Q.3. In line with cold stress, what interventions are needed for this infant?

Case study 3: Transition to going home

Premature twins born at 25 weeks are now 10 weeks old (35 weeks corrected) and have come off all respiratory support except for low flow oxygen. Time has arrived to prepare them towards discharge home, but they are still being nursed in incubators. What factors now require consideration for both the infants' thermal care and that of the family needs moving towards going home?

For suggested answer guides to the questions posed in these case studies, please refer to the web-based companion site specific to this chapter (see URL below).

WEB-BASED RESOURCES

For further information, online resources and greater detail on the case studies featured in this chapter go to www.routledge.com/cw/nicnursing

References

Ågren, J., Sjörs, G., & Sedin, G. (2006). Ambient humidity influences the rate of skin barrier maturation in extremely preterm infants. *The Journal of Pediatrics, 148*(5), 613–617.

Asakura, H. (2004). Fetal and neonatal thermoregulation. *Journal of Nippon Medical School, 71*(6), 360–370.

Aylott, M., (2006a). The neonatal energy triangle Part 1: Metabolic adaptation. *Nursing Children and Young People. 18*(6), 38–43.

Aylott, M. (2006b). The neonatal energy triangle Part 2: Thermoregulatory and respiratory adaptation. *Nursing Children and Young People, 18*(7).

Baley, J. (2015). Skin-to-skin care for term and preterm infants in the neonatal ICU. *Pediatrics, 136*(3), 596–599.

Barone, G., Corsello, M., Papacci, P., Priolo, F., Romagnoli, C., & Zecca, E. (2014). Feasibility of transferring intensive cared preterm infants from incubator to open crib at 1600 grams. *Italian Journal of Pediatrics, 40*(1), 41.

Beiranvand, S., Valizadeh, F., Hosseinabadi, R., & Pournia, Y. (2014). The effects of skin-to-skin contact on temperature and breastfeeding successfulness in full-term newborns after cesarean delivery. *International Journal of Pediatrics.*

Belghazi, K., Tourneux, P., Elabbassi, E. B., Ghyselen, L., Delanaud, S., & Libert, J. P. (2006). Effect of posture on the thermal efficiency of a plastic bag wrapping in neonate: assessment using a thermal "sweating" mannequin. *Medical physics, 33*(3), 637–644.

Bell, E. F., Acarregui, M. J. (2014). Restricted versus liberal water intake for preventing morbidity and mortality in preterm infants. *Cochrane Database of Systematic Reviews*, Issue 12. Art. No.: CD000503. DOI: 10.1002/14651858.CD000503.pub3

Björklund, L. J., & Hellström-Westas, L. (2000). Reducing heat loss at birth in very preterm infants. Journal of Pediatrics, 137: 739–740.

Bredemeyer, S., Reid, S., & Wallace, M. (2005). Thermal management for premature births. *Journal of Advanced Nursing, 52*(5), 482–489.

Brueggemeyer, A. (1993). Thermoregulation. In Kenner, C., Brueggemeyer, A., & Porter Gunderson, L. (Eds.) *Comprehensive Neonatal Nursing. A Physiologic Perspective*. Philadelphia, PA: Saunders.

Carmichael, A., McCullough, S., & Kempley, S. T. (2007). Critical dependence of acetate thermal mattress on gel activation temperature. *Archives of Disease in Childhood: Fetal and Neonatal Edition, 92*(1), F44–F45.

Carrascosa, A., Ruiz-Cuevas, P., Clemente, M., Salcedo, S., & Almar, J. (2008). Thyroid function in 76 sick preterm infants 30–36 weeks: Results from a longitudinal study. *Journal of Pediatric Endocrinology and Metabolism, 21*(3), 237–244.

Chiou, Y. B., & Blume-Peytavi, U. (2004). Stratum corneum maturation. *Skin Pharmacology and Physiology, 17*(2), 57–66.

Çınar, N. D., & Filiz, T. M. (2006). Neonatal thermoregulation. *Journal of Neonatal Nursing, 12*(2), 69–74.

Clemente, M., Ruiz-Cuevas, P., Carrascosa, A., Potau, N., Almar, J., Salcedo, S., & Yeste, D. (2007). Thyroid function in preterm infants 27–29 weeks of gestational age during the first four months of life: Results from a prospective study comprising 80 preterm infants. *Journal of Pediatric Endocrinology and Metabolism, 20*(12), 1269–1280.

Deguines, C., Dégrugilliers, L., Ghyselen, L., Chardon, K., Bach, V., & Tourneux, P. (2013). Impact of nursing care on temperature environment in preterm newborns nursed in closed convective incubators. *Acta Paediatrica*, *102*(3), e96–e101.

Doglioni, N., Cavallin, F., Mardegan, V., Palatron, S., Filippone, M., Vecchiato, L., ... & Trevisanuto, D. (2014). Total body polyethylene wraps for preventing hypothermia in preterm infants: a randomized trial. *The Journal of Pediatrics*, *165*(2), 261–266.

Elabbassi, E. B., Belghazi, K., Delanaud, S., & Libert, J. P. (2004). Dry heat loss in incubator: comparison of two premature newborn sized manikins. *European Journal of Applied Physiology*, *92*(6), 679–682.

Endo, T., & Kobayashi, T. (2008). Thyroid-stimulating hormone receptor in brown adipose tissue is involved in the regulation of thermogenesis. *American Journal of Physiology-Endocrinology and Metabolism*, *295*(2), E514–E518.

Enerbäck, S. (2010). Human brown adipose tissue. *Cell metabolism, 11*(4), 248–252.

Engorn, B. M., Kahntroff, S. L., Frank, K. M., Singh, S., Harvey, H. A., Barkulis, C. T., ... & Greenberg, R. S. (2017). Perioperative hypothermia in neonatal intensive care unit patients: Effectiveness of a thermoregulation intervention and associated risk factors. *Pediatric Anesthesia*, *27*(2), 196–204.

Fastman, B. R., Howell, E. A., Holzman, I., & Kleinman, L. C. (2014). Current perspectives on temperature management and hypothermia in low birth weight infants. *Newborn and Infant Nursing Reviews*, *14*(2), 50–55.

Flenady, V., & Woodgate, P. G. (2003). Radiant warmers versus incubators for regulating body temperature in newborn infants. *Cochrane Database of Systematic Reviews*, Issue 4. Art. No.: CD000435. DOI: 10.1002/14651858.CD000435

Frazer, M., Ciarlo, A., Herr, J., & Briere, C. E. (2018). Quality Improvement Initiative to Prevent Admission Hypothermia in Very-Low-Birth-Weight Newborns. *Journal of Obstetric, Gynecologic & Neonatal Nursing*, *47*(4), 520–528.

Gray, P. H., & Flenady, V. (2011). Cot-nursing versus incubator care for preterm infants. *Cochrane Database of Systematic Reviews*, Issue 8. Art. No.: CD003062. DOI: 10.1002/14651858. CD003062.pub2

Hall, J. E. (2011). *Guyton and Hall Textbook of Medical Physiology*. (12th Edition). Philadelphia: Saunders Elsevier.

Hammarlund, K., Sedin, G., & Strömberg, B. (1983). TRANSEPIDERMAL WATER LOSS IN NEWBORN INFANTS: VIII. Relation to Gestational Age and Post-natal Age in Appropriate and Small for Gestational Age Infants. *Acta Paediatrica*, *72*(5), 721–728.

Jones, H., & Santamaria, N. (2018). Physiological benefits to parents from undertaking skin-to-skin contact with their neonate, in a neonatal intensive special care unit. *Scandinavian Journal of Caring Sciences*, *32*(3), 1012–1017.

Kent, A. L., & Williams, J. (2008). Increasing ambient operating theatre temperature and wrapping in polyethylene improves admission temperature in premature infants. *Journal of Paediatrics and Child Health*, *44*(6), 325–331.

Knobel, R., Holditch-Davis, D., Schwartz, T., & Wimmer, J. E. (2009). Extremely low birth weight preterm infants lack vasomotor response in relationship to cold body temperatures at birth. *Journal of Perinatology*, *29*, 814–821.

Knobel, R. B. (2014). Fetal and neonatal thermal physiology. *Newborn and Infant Nursing Reviews*, *14*(2), 45–49.

Knobel-Dail, R. B. (2014). Role of effective thermoregulation in premature neonates. *Research and Reports in Neonatology*, *4*, 147–156.

Kristoffersen, L., Stoen, R., Hansen, L. F., Wilhelmsen, J., & Bergseng, H. (2016). Skin-to-skin care after birth for moderately preterm infants. *Journal of Obstetric, Gynecologic & Neonatal Nursing*, *45*(3), 339–345.

Laptook, A. R., Salhab, W., & Bhaskar, B. (2007). Admission temperature of low birth weight infants: Predictors and associated morbidities. *Pediatrics*, *119*(3), e643–e649.

Laptook, A. R., Bell, E. F., Shankaran, S., Boghossian, N. S., Wyckoff, M. H., Kandefer, S., ... & Higgins, R. (2018). Admission Temperature and Associated Mortality and Morbidity among Moderately and Extremely Preterm Infants. *The Journal of Pediatrics*, 192, 53–59.

Libert, J.-P., Delanaud, S., & Bach, V. (2017). Warming mattresses for newborns: Effectiveness and risks. *Biomedical Journal of Scientific & Technical Research* 1(7), 2011–2014.

McCall, E., Alderdice, F., Halliday, H., Johnston, L., & Vohra, S. (2014). Challenges of minimizing heat loss at birth: A narrative overview of evidence-based thermal care interventions. *Newborn and Infant Nursing Reviews*, 14(2), 56–63.

McCall, E. M., Alderdice, F., Halliday, H. L., Vohra, S., & Johnston, L. (2018). Interventions to prevent hypothermia at birth in preterm and/or low birth weight infants. *Cochrane Database of Systematic Reviews*, Issue 2. Art. No.: CD004210. DOI: 10.1002/14651858.CD004210.pub5

Marieb, E. N., & Hoehn, K. N. (2015). *Human Anatomy & Physiology* (10th Edition). Cambridge: Pearson.

Meyer, M. P., Hou, D., Ishrar, N. N., Dito, I., & te Pas, A. B. (2015). Initial respiratory support with cold, dry gas versus heated humidified gas and admission temperature of preterm infants. *The Journal of Pediatrics*, 166(2), 245–250.

Modi, N. (2004). Management of fluid balance in the very immature neonate. *Archives of Disease in Childhood: Fetal and Neonatal Edition*, 89(2), F108–F111.

NHS Improvement. (2017). *Reducing harm leading to avoidable admission of full-term babies into neonatal units. Findings and resources for improvement*. NHS Improvement.

New, K., Flenady, V., & Davies, M. W. (2011). Transfer of preterm infants from incubator to open cot at lower versus higher body weight. *Cochrane Database of Systematic Reviews*, Issue 9. Art. No.: CD004214. DOI: 10.1002/14651858.CD004214.pub4

Nordike, K., Nichols, E. A., Clark, T., & Murphy, C. (2018). Process Improvement of Thermoregulation for Elbw Neonates During Critical Care Transport.

Oranges, T., Dini, V., & Romanelli, M. (2015). Skin physiology of the neonate and infant: clinical implications. *Advances in Wound Care*, 4(10), 587–595.

Parsons, H. (2017). *Great Ormond Street Hospital for Children NHS Foundation Trust. Thermoregulation for neonates*. www.gosh.nhs.uk/health-professionals/clinical-guidelines/thermoregulation-neonates

Petty, J. (2010). Fact sheet: Normal postnatal adaptation to extrauterine life – b) Thermoregulation and glucose homeostasis. *Journal of Neonatal Nursing* 16, 198–199.

Petty, J. (2017). Kangaroo mother care' helps preterm babies survive ... but offers benefits for all. *The Conversation*. https://theconversation.com/kangaroo-mother-care-helps-preterm-babies-survive-but-offers-benefits-for-all-71644.

Royal College of Paediatrics and Child Health & Healthcare Quality Improvement Partnership. (2018). *National Neonatal Audit Programme 2018 Annual Report on 2017 data*. Royal College of Paediatrics and Child Health.

Sinclair, J. C. (2002). Servo-control for maintaining abdominal skin temperature at 36C in low birth weight infants. *Cochrane Database of Systematic Reviews*, Issue 1. Art. No.: CD001074. DOI: 10.1002/14651858.CD001074

Smith, J. (2014). Thermoregulation and temperature taking in the developing world: A brief encounter. *Journal of Neonatal Nursing*, 20(5), 218–229.

Smith, J., Alcock, G., & Usher, K. (2013). Temperature measurement in the preterm and term neonate: a review of the literature. *Neonatal Network*, 32(1), 16–25.

Sugarman, I., Stringer, M. D., & Smyth, A. G. (2012). Gastroenterology. Part 4: Congenital defects and surgical problems. In Rennie, J. M. (Ed.) *Rennie & Roberton's Textbook of Neonatology* (5th Edition). London: Elsevier Health Sciences.

Sweet, D. G., Carnielli, V., Greisen, G., Hallman, M., Ozek, E., Plavka, R., ... & Visser, G. H. (2017). European consensus guidelines on the management of respiratory distress syndrome-2016 update. *Neonatology*, 111(2), 107–125.

Turnbull, V., & Petty, J. (2013a). Evidence-based thermal care of low birth weight neonates. Part 2: Family-centred care principles. *Nursing Children and Young People*. doi: https://doi.org/10.7748/ncyp2013.04.25.3.26.e172

Turnbull, T., & Petty, J. (2013b). Understanding evidence-based thermal care in the low birth weight neonate: PART 1: An overview of principles and current practice. *Nursing Children and Young People*. doi: https://doi.org/10.7748/ncyp2013.03.25.2.18.e140

Vohra, S., Roberts, R. S., Zhang, B., Jens, M., & Schmidt, B. (2004). Heat loss prevention (HeLP) in the delivery room: A randomised control trial of polyethylene occlusive skin wrapping in very preterm infants, *Journal of Pediatrics 145*(6): 720–723.

Waldron, S., & MacKinnon, R. (2007). Neonatal thermoregulation. *Infant, 3*(3), 101–104.

World Health Organization. (1993). *Thermal control of the newborn: a practical guide* (No. WHO/FHE/MSM/93.2). Geneva: World Health Organization.

World Health Organization. (2011). *Preventing and treating hypothermia in severely malnourished children*. www.who.int/elena/titles/bbc/hypothermia_sam/en/

Wyllie, J., Bruinenberg, J., Roehr, C. C., Ruediger, M., Trevisanuto, D., & Urlesberger, B. (2015). Resuscitation and support of transition of babies at birth. *Notfall & Rettungsmedizin, 18*(8), 964–983.

Wyllie, J., Ainsworth, S., Tinnion, R., & Hampshire, S. (2016). *Newborn Life Support* (4th Edition). London: Resuscitation Council UK.

Yip, W. Y., Quek, B. H., Fong, M. C. W., Ong, S. S. G., Lim, B. L., Lo, B. C., & Agarwal, P. (2017). A quality improvement project to reduce hypothermia in preterm infants on admission to the neonatal intensive care unit. *International Journal for Quality in Health Care, 29*(7), 922–928.

12 MANAGEMENT OF RESPIRATORY DISORDERS

Breidge Boyle

CONTENTS

GUIDANCE ON HOW TO ENHANCE PERSONAL LEARNING FROM THIS CHAPTER

Key points covered in this chapter

❖ Common neonatal respiratory conditions.
❖ An overview of respiratory/ventilation strategies.
❖ Nursing care and assessment of infants requiring respiratory support.

Reflection

Reading through the chapter, you are encouraged to engage with the key points and related literature in an enquiring way. Ask these questions:

■ Which common respiratory conditions have you seen in practice and how should these be managed?

■ How will the content in this chapter inform or change your practice in caring for infants requiring respiratory support?

■ How can parents be involved in the respiratory care of their baby?

Implications for nursing care

■ Finally: how will this chapter enable you to consider best, evidence-based practice in the respiratory care of the high-risk infant in neonatal care? Consider the implications of what you learn for your nursing care relating to this area.

INTRODUCTION AND BACKGROUND

Despite advances in the treatment of respiratory disease in the newborn, respiratory compromise remains a very common cause for admission to the neonatal unit (NNU; Sweet, 2017). In this chapter, the most common respiratory disorders in the newborn will be presented, incorporating the pathophysiology of the conditions and the strategies that can be utilised in their management. Even less invasive methods of managing respiratory disease in the neonate are complex and not without risk and complications. As the respiratory support now available is more varied, an overview of non-invasive interventions, mechanical ventilation and related nursing care are also included.

THE PHYSIOLOGICAL BASIS OF NEONATAL RESPIRATORY CARE

Gas exchange is a prerequisite of life and, although most creatures are not born with completely mature lungs, sufficient development must have taken place by the time of birth to sustain independent functioning (Schittny, 2017).

Foetal lung development

The foetal lung has to develop sufficiently *in utero* in order to be able to support the gas exchange necessary for the baby following delivery. Lung development can be divided into five stages (Bhutani, 2006):

1 *The embryonic stage* (0–7 weeks' gestation). During this stage, the laryngotracheal groove develops from the foregut and a septum begins to form, which separates the trachea from the oesophagus. Primitive bronchi also begin to develop.

2   *The pseudoglandular stage* (8–16 weeks' gestation). During this stage, a network of narrow tubules develops, airway division commences, and terminal bronchioles are formed. Connective tissue, muscle and blood vessels also start to develop.

3   *The canalicular stage* (17–27 weeks' gestation). During this stage, respiratory bronchioles continue to branch and develop. A rich vascular supply is evident, with arteries and veins developing alongside the respiratory airways. By approximately 24 weeks, pulmonary gas exchange is theoretically possible (Hsia et al., 2016). Type I and Type II pneumocytes can be identified. Type I cells are flattened and form approximately 90% of the gas exchange surface of the mature lungs. Type II cells are cuboidal secretory cells containing surfactant.

4   *The saccular stage* (28–35 weeks' gestation). During this stage, the terminal air sacs multiply and their surface epithelium thins. This allows closer contact with the capillary bed, promoting greater gaseous exchange.

5   *The alveolar stage* (>36 weeks' gestation). This stage involves the further development of air sacs and the formation of true alveoli. This continues after birth and throughout early childhood.

Foetal lung fluid and foetal breathing movements

During foetal life, the lungs are full of fluid, which increases from 4–6mL/kg during the mid-trimester to 30mL/kg towards term. This fluid is important for cell maturation and development. It also helps to determine the size and shape of the developing lungs (Gahlot et al., 2009), and its volume is equivalent to the lung fluid's functional residual capacity (FRC) in the early postnatal period. Foetal breathing movements are evident from approximately 12 weeks' gestation, with strength and frequency increasing as the foetus matures. It is thought that foetal lung fluid and foetal breathing movements assist in the development of the diaphragm and chest wall muscles. Foetal development of the respiratory system is followed by a neonatal period of approximately two months, with full lung development completed by approximately 8 years.

Surfactant

Surfactant is produced by the alveolar type II cells. It is a complex mixture of phospholipids, neutral lipids and proteins, and its function is to reduce the surface tension in the lungs, aiding gaseous exchange (Chakraborty and Kotecha, 2013). Surfactant prevents the alveoli from collapsing completely (atelectasis) at the end of expiration, and helps to reduce the work of breathing for the infant. The synthesis and secretion of surfactant are regulated by a series of enzymes and hormones, e.g. glucocorticoids appear to accelerate the normal pattern of lung development. This illustrates the rationale for giving antenatal corticosteroids to women at risk of a premature delivery (Sweet, 2017). Catecholamines also increase surfactant production. In the infant who is small for gestational age, catecholamine response is increased, which explains why, despite their size, many of these infants do not develop respiratory problems. Insulin, on the other hand, inhibits the production of surfactant and consequently, infants of diabetic mothers are at an increased risk of developing respiratory distress syndrome (Mitanchez et al., 2015). Hypothermia and acidosis can also inhibit surfactant production, so the importance of keeping babies within an appropriate thermal neutral range, particularly around the time of delivery, cannot be overemphasised (Hillman, 2012). Acidaemic states should be recognised early and corrected immediately.

Respiratory changes at birth

The predominant stimuli for initiating the first breaths are:

- clamping or obstructing the umbilical cord which results in an 'asphyxial' event
- cooling – with the sudden drop from intrauterine temperature
- physical discomfort from touching and drying.

(Wyllie et al., 2015)

According to Hillman (2012), the average 3kg term baby will clear approximately 100mL of fluid from their airways following the initiation of respiration (approximately 30mL/kg). A healthy term infant generates high intrathoracic negative pressures to draw air into the lungs. This pressure is further increased when the baby cries, which helps to drive lung fluid out of the alveoli and into the pulmonary vascular circulation, and helps to establish the resting lung volume. A rapid labour or a caesarean section before the onset of labour does not allow the lungs to 'prepare' for their adaptation to extrauterine life. This partially explains why these babies have a higher incidence of respiratory problems at birth including transient tachypnoea of the newborn (TTN) and respiratory distress syndrome (RDS; Sun et al., 2013).

RESPIRATORY CONDITIONS IN THE NEONATE

Respiratory distress syndrome

RDS is predominantly a pulmonary disorder associated with the immaturity of the neonatal lungs, but the presentation has changed over time with the advent of new treatments and early, prophylactic interventions (Sweet, 2017). It is associated with a lack of surfactant, and the incidence and severity of RDS are inversely related to gestational age. This reflects the increase in surfactant production the nearer to term an infant is born.

RDS presents in the first four hours of life, and is characterised by an increase in the respiratory rate >60breaths/min (tachypnoea) and dyspnoea, which is evident by nasal flaring and subcostal and/or sternal recession (from a very compliant ribcage), with a predominantly diaphragmatic breathing pattern. Often there is an expiratory grunt which is caused by the infant forcing air past a partially closed glottis in an effort to retain some air or pressure in the alveoli at the end of each breath to prevent atelectatic collapse (Goldsmith et al., 2016). This classic presentation is not often witnessed these days, as the highest-risk infants are actively managed at delivery with intubation, exogenous surfactant, mechanical ventilation or continuous positive airway pressure (CPAP; Shetty and Greenough, 2014; Sweet 2017).

Traditionally, surfactant-deficient lungs require high pressure ventilation to maintain their capacity for gas exchange, which leads to inflammatory changes and protein leak on to the alveolar surface, which in turn form hyaline membranes. These membranes further inhibit gaseous exchange. The diagnosis of RDS can be suspected by the clinical picture and confirmed by radiological findings. The chest X-ray of an infant presenting with RDS traditionally illustrates a typical 'ground glass' or 'reticulogranular' pattern with air bronchograms evident. In severe RDS, the X-ray may show near total atelectasis with complete opacification or 'white-out'. In a non-intubated and ventilated infant, the chest X-ray can also show a reduction in the lung volume.

The blood gases of an infant with RDS show acidosis, demonstrated by a reduction in the blood pH. This may either be a respiratory acidosis, due to the retention of carbon dioxide (hypercapnia), metabolic acidosis from tissue hypoxia, or mixed acidosis, with both respiratory and metabolic components. It may be difficult to differentiate between RDS and congenital pneumonia. The loss of protein and impaired renal blood flow during the acute phase of the disease lead to the infant becoming oedematous. As surfactant synthesis commences (approximately 36–48 hours of age), the severity of the disease begins to decline. Characteristically, this period is associated with a spontaneous diuresis and a general improvement in the infant's condition.

The aim of treatment of RDS is to establish adequate gaseous exchange and prevent complications from arising by providing respiratory support until the type II pneumocytes regenerate and begin to produce surfactant. Much research has been carried out into methods of doing so while minimising the development of chronic lung disease (CLD), also known as bronchopulmonary dysplasia (BPD; Sweet et al., 2017). This condition will be discussed in the next section.

Infants with mild RDS, who have good, effective respiratory effort may only require supplemental oxygen to manage their condition. Oxygen administration is also discussed later in the chapter. Despite the increasing popularity of non-invasive methods, about half of infants with RDS still require intubation (Ambalavanan et al., 2010).

Traditionally, surfactant is delivered to the lungs via the endotracheal tube (ETT) over a period of a few seconds as a prophylactic treatment (Soll, 2009; McDonald and Ainsworth, 2004). Surfactant disseminates homogeneously and works by coating the alveolar surface of the lung, which primarily reduces surface tension, improving lung volume, pulmonary perfusion and oxygenation. However, the increasing use of non-invasive respiratory support has raised questions around the efficacy of surfactant versus the risks associated with intubation. To minimise the time spent on invasive ventilation, **In**tubation, administration of **Sur**factant and **E**xtubation following a very short period ventilated (INSURE) was proposed (Dani et al., 2015). A review by Stevens et al. (2007) included studies where intubation was carried out without sedation to allow early extubation, and so the efficacy of practice when an infant is sedated for intubation was questioned. Two methods of administering surfactant while an infant is on CPAP are now more universally in use. **L**ess **I**nvasive **S**urfactant **A**dministration (LISA), sometimes referred to as **M**inimally **I**nvasive **S**urfactant **T**reatment (MIST), involves passing a thin catheter into the trachea, with or without using Magill's forceps (Göpel et al., 2011; Dargaville and Copnell, 2006; Dargaville et al., 2013). Neither of these treatments has shown improved outcomes when compared to INSURE. Nebulised surfactant has been proposed as an alternative (Minocchieri et al., 2014), but trials are still in the very early stages with no positive results reported to date.

Those infants who 'fail' non-invasive respiratory support and are intubated to receive ventilation will usually be given surfactant on intubation, commonly called a rescue dose. Rojas-Reyes et al. (2012), in a systematic review, found less risk of chronic lung disease or death with early stabilisation using CPAP alongside selective surfactant administration to infants requiring intubation, rather than the practice of prophylactically administering it to all premature babies. The European consensus guidelines recommend that infants ≤26 weeks' gestation are given surfactant, using INSURE, LISA or MIST, when their FiO_2 requirement is >0.30, and those born at >26 weeks' gestation when their FiO_2 requirement is >0.40 (Sweet, 2017). The national recommendation is now to use minimally invasive methods of surfactant administration wherever possible (National Institute for Health and Care Excellence (NICE), 2019)

Initially, infants with RDS will require intravenous (IV) fluids and parental nutrition, as enteral feeding may compromise respiratory function. Small-volume milk feeds (ideally breast milk) can be introduced once the ventilatory status is more stable. These infants can have their clinical course affected by other problems associated with prematurity, e.g. intraventricular haemorrhage (IVH), infections, and necrotising enterocolitis (NEC).

Bronchopulmonary dysplasia

BPD, also known as CLD, is the most common long-term morbidity associated with prematurity, with an increased risk of mortality as well as of neurodevelopmental and pulmonary problems later in life (Kennedy et al., 2016; Javaid and Morris, 2018). The definition of BPD remains open to debate. Originally, prior to the late 1980s, this related to premature infants born with RDS, who required prolonged ventilation and high oxygen supplementation, leading to CLD. These infants required oxygen at 28 days of life and had consistent radiological changes including scarring and areas of both atelectasis and hyperinflation. An alternative definition emerged for infants who were receiving oxygen supplementation at 36 weeks postmenstrual age (PMA). However, with the advent of gentler modes of ventilation and other areas of current management, this classic presentation is much less common.

A newer definition from the National Institute of Child Health and Human Development (NICHD) was offered in 2000 (Jobe and Steinhorn, 2017) which is severity-based relating to infants who have received >21% oxygen for at least 28 days and are assessed at 36 weeks PMA or at discharge home: mild (breathing in air); moderate (<30% oxygen); severe (>30% oxygen). This definition places an emphasis on alveolar developmental arrest leading to fewer and larger alveoli, causing less effective gas exchange.

Aside from the lack of complete confirmation of a definition, it is well documented and now generally agreed that BPD is a complex, multifactorial condition (Donn, 2017) influenced by antenatal and postnatal factors, occurring in infants who are mechanically ventilated, and is inversely related to gestational age and birth weight. Inflammation is a key factor underlying the lung injury leading to the development of BPD (Nelin and Logan, 2017). Additional risk factors include male sex, significant hypothermia on admission, infection, and the use of formula milk (NICE, 2019).

Management of BPD should begin with prevention, commencing antenatally, including, where possible, preventing preterm birth, improving antenatal care and the advice to pregnant mothers and the administration of antenatal corticosteroids (Roberts et al., 2017), the single most effective intervention in promoting lung maturation and reducing rates of BPD. Delivery room management is also important in preventing BPD; for example, avoiding intubation and full ventilation, surfactant administration followed by gentle ventilation strategies, preferably non-invasive in nature (Shetty and Greenough, 2014; Boel et al., 2017). Regarding the use of postnatal corticosteroids, it may be prudent to reserve the use of late administration for infants who cannot be weaned from mechanical ventilation, and to minimise both dose and duration for any course of treatment (Doyle et al., 2017; NICE, 2019).

Nursing responsibilities should centre around minimising oxygen and careful control and titration of any ventilatory or oxygenation change. Parents should be reassured and supported when their baby receives any respiratory support (NICE, 2019). Nurses need to explain the rationale behind this area of care, so that parents are fully informed at all stages and they understand the need to give individualised care tailored to their baby to improve outcomes starting at the point of delivery if resuscitation is required (Baik et al., 2018) and beyond. They also need to be aware of the potential long-term implications of their baby's condition. This is particularly pertinent if their baby is likely to develop BPD and be discharged home in oxygen. Home oxygen therapy plays a key role in the management of BPD and local/national guidance should be followed when implementing this, along with good community nursing and outreach support (Nzirawa, 2018; NICE, 2019).

Given the complex antenatal and postnatal factors for the development of BPD, a combination of strategies should be the focus for future prevention of BPD (Aschner et al., 2017). This is of great importance given that, despite the advances in ventilation and management discussed here, the incidence of BPD has not changed, nor is it diminishing

(Hunt et al., 2018; Jarvaid and Morris, 2018), and remains a potential long-term problem for neonates born prematurely, impacting on the lives of their families at home.

Transient tachypnoea of the newborn

TTN is a lung disorder characterised by pulmonary oedema due to delayed reabsorption and clearance of foetal lung fluid. It is one of the most common causes of perinatal dyspnoea (Liu et al., 2014). TTN is a common cause of respiratory distress in the immediate newborn period, and infants usually present with tachypnoea and increased work of breathing lasting for 24 to 72 hours. Chest X-rays reveal excess fluid in the interstitial space, and occasionally **pleural effusions**. Management is supportive, likely including supplemental oxygen, and frequently CPAP is necessary to assist in maintaining alveolar patency and driving fluid into the infant's circulation. Blood gases may reveal a mild respiratory acidosis and hypoxaemia. The course of TTN is self-limiting and does not usually require mechanical ventilation (Reuter et al., 2014).

Pulmonary interstitial emphysema

A complication of RDS is pulmonary interstitial emphysema (PIE). Air is trapped outside the airways, e.g. in the interstitial spaces, rather than the alveoli due to terminal bronchiole rupture, usually following high pressure ventilation. PIE alters the pulmonary mechanics by decreasing lung compliance, making the lungs much stiffer. This in turn increases the residual volume within the lungs, and increases the dead space impeding pulmonary blood flow which reduces pulmonary perfusion and leads to hypoxaemia and hypercapnia. It can be localised, but is more commonly widespread throughout both lungs. Clinical signs of PIE include marked respiratory acidosis and hypoxaemia. Chest radiography reveals hyper-inflation with a characteristic cystic appearance. If PIE is advanced, the X-ray may show the formation of large bullae within the affected area of the lung. Transillumination of the chest wall with widespread PIE shows an increased transmission of light, similar to that seen with a **pneumothorax**.

Management is focused on preventing further barotrauma to the lungs. In conventional ventilation, this involves reducing the peak inspiratory pressure (PIP), reducing positive end-expiratory pressure (PEEP), and reducing the tidal volume, provided blood gases can be maintained. Higher than normal $PaCO_2$ levels may need to be tolerated (permissive hypercapnia; Thome et al., 2015). PIE is amenable to high frequency oscillatory ventilation (HFOV), as this form of ventilation is effective in treating lung injury (Bunnell, 2006). Localised PIE may resolve spontaneously; however, widespread PIE can take several weeks to improve. Infants with localised PIE should be nursed with the affected side down, to compress the lung on that side. Selective intubation of the non-affected side has been suggested to 'deflate' the hyperinflated areas. However, the real treatment for PIE is in its prevention, by avoidance of over-distension of the lungs when managing RDS.

Pneumothorax

Spontaneous pneumothorax can occur in a small number of infants. This incidence increases with both prematurity and the need for mechanical ventilation, especially where high inspiratory pressures are needed. Clinical signs include

- Pallor
- Deterioration in oxygenation
- Bradycardia and hypotension
- Unequal chest movement/air entry which can be rapid and dramatic in **tension** pneumothorax.

Transillumination of the chest may be helpful, especially in preterm infants and, while a chest X-ray will confirm the presence of free air in the chest, it may not be practicable to wait for this due to the infant's condition. A thoracic drain should be inserted and attached to an underwater seal drain. This drain should remain in situ until the air is drained, the lung re-expanded, so that the baby's clinical condition is sufficiently stable to allow for its removal.

Pulmonary haemorrhage

Infants receiving respiratory support may demonstrate some evidence of small amounts of blood in tracheal aspirates following trauma during intubation. The term pulmonary haemorrhage or haemorrhagic pulmonary oedema is usually reserved for significant bleeding into the lung structure and airways (Bendapudi et al., 2012). It is more common in extremely preterm and growth-restricted infants who have been ventilated and treated with exogenous surfactant. A patent ductus arteriosus is also a significant contributing factor, but pulmonary haemorrhage may present in any infant with underlying lung pathology. It is usually detected after an acute deterioration in the baby's condition associated with a degree of tube obstruction. On suctioning the ETT, a large volume of fresh blood-stained fluid may be present. Treatment is generally supportive. Ventilatory support needs to be increased with high PEEP (up to 8cm H_2O) to reduce further alveolar capillary leakage by tamponade, and a higher PIP to re-expand the fluid-filled airways to improve oxygenation and V/Q mismatch. HFOV may be beneficial. The rapid loss of blood can lead to shock, so that resuscitation with volume and blood may be necessary. The administration of fresh frozen plasma and/or platelets may be necessary to correct any clotting disorders, as disseminated intravascular coagulation may be an underlying factor (see chapter 15 for details). The prognosis is often poor and depends on the degree of respiratory and systemic deterioration following the blood loss (Raju, 2006).

Pneumonia

Neonatal pneumonia may be an isolated focal infection but is usually part of a more widespread illness. As pneumonia can be difficult to distinguish from RDS, all infants with respiratory symptoms at birth should be screened for infection and treated with appropriate antibiotics until proven negative (Sweet, 2017). Pneumonia in the neonatal period falls into three general categories: congenital or intrauterine pneumonia, early onset or intrapartum pneumonia, and late onset pneumonia.

CONGENITAL PNEUMONIA

This form of pneumonia usually occurs because of ascending infection and chorioamnionitis following premature or prolonged rupture of membranes. It can be difficult to distinguish from TTN on presentation, but the clinical course is different, with affected infants displaying higher morbidity and requiring treatment for longer (Costa et al., 2012). Congenital pneumonia has an incidence of 4.5 per 100,000 births in the UK (Tambe et al., 2015). Rarely, it may be viral in origin. Approximately 20–40% of infants with toxoplasmosis, cytomegalovirus, rubella and herpes simplex viruses present with respiratory symptoms and consequently, infants should be screened for these viruses as a matter of course (Parravicini and Polin, 2006).

EARLY ONSET PNEUMONIA

Early onset pneumonia presents within the first 48 hours of life. It is commonly due to pathogens acquired from the birth canal, with Group B streptococcus (GBS) being the most common pathogen accounting for many cases. Other pathogens include *Haemophilus influenzae*, *Streptococcus pneumoniae*, *Listeria monocytogenes* and *Escherichia coli*.

LATE ONSET PNEUMONIA

This type of pneumonia occurs after 48 hours of life, and is usually acquired nosocomially. It is most common in preterm infants who require some form of ventilatory support (Dear, 2005). The most common pathogens for late onset pneumonia include gram-negative bacilli, enterobacter and *E. coli*. The treatment for all forms of neonatal pneumonia includes the administration of IV antibiotics.

There is currently debate as to which antibiotic therapy should be administered. General consensus supports the use of ampicillin or penicillin with an aminoglycoside such as gentamicin. This regime tends to be for congenital and early onset pneumonia. For late onset pneumonia, the treatment is a third-generation cephalosporin plus vancomycin. Antibiotic therapy should be evaluated when sensitivities to the pathogens have been identified. According to Dear (2005), antibiotic treatment should continue for 10 days for a proven pneumonia unless the pathogen is *Staphylococcus aureus*, in which case a three-week course of antibiotics should be administered. However, antibiotic regimes and combinations for pneumonia in the NNU are varied in line with local policies and resistance profiles.

Ventilatory support required during the acute illness will be determined by the degree of respiratory compromise and may vary from supplemental oxygen to full mechanical ventilation.

Meconium aspiration syndrome

Meconium-stained amniotic fluid is observed in approximately 13% of all deliveries, yet only 4–5% of infants born through meconium-stained amniotic fluid go on to develop meconium aspiration syndrome (MAS; van Ierland et al., 2010). The overall incidence of MAS may be decreasing with changes in obstetric practice, but despite improvements in maternal and infant care, MAS continues to carry the risk of death or significant short- and long-term morbidity (Dargaville and Copnell, 2006; Vain and Batton, 2017).

MAS is generally a problem associated with term and post-term infants, with the risk increasing in post-term infants (Vain and Batton, 2017). *In utero* passage of meconium is often a sign of chronic and/or acute foetal compromise, mainly due to hypoxic stress. This hypoxic stress further leads to foetal gasping, which may cause the meconium-stained fluid to be inhaled into the foetal lungs (Vain and Batton, 2017). Postnatal aspiration is also possible, where the meconium-stained amniotic fluid is drawn into the lungs with the first breaths after birth, but generally meconium aspiration occurs secondary to perinatal foetal compromise (Wyllie et al., 2015). The presence of meconium-stained amniotic fluid in the preterm population was thought to be a marker of chorioamnionitis or infection with *Listeria monocytogenes*. This finding is now questioned; however, the presence of meconium at the delivery of preterm infants does appear to detrimentally affect their long-term outcome (Tybulewicz et al., 2004).

Meconium within the respiratory tract causes several problems:

■ The particulate matter creates a physical obstruction which can be complete, leading to atelectatic collapse of the alveoli; or partial, leading to air-trapping, over-distension, air leak and pneumothorax.
■ Surfactant inactivation by damage to type II cells, thus decreasing lung compliance.
■ Complex inflammatory response leading to chemical pneumonitis and parenchymal lung injury, further inactivating surfactant and increasing pulmonary vascular resistance (PVR).
■ Infection by inhibition of the action of alveolar **macrophages** (see chapter 18).

These pulmonary effects can lead to ventilation/perfusion (V/Q) mismatch, which can make oxygenation and ventilation of these infants difficult and hence MAS has a strong association with persistent pulmonary hypertension of the newborn (PPHN) (see p. 284). Most infants with MAS develop some signs of respiratory distress (e.g. tachypnoea, nasal flaring, sternal recession, cyanosis and grunting) soon after birth. In addition, the infant's chest can appear hyperinflated or barrel-shaped. These signs can be delayed due to the evolving disease process, so any infant delivering through meconium-stained amniotic fluid should have their respiratory status assessed regularly by the attending midwife.

Up to 50% of infants with MAS develop respiratory failure and can be complex infants to care for. Conventional care focuses on providing respiratory support to correct the hypoxia and hypercapnia. As oxygen is a potent pulmonary vasodilator, high concentrations of inspired oxygen can be used to create a normoxaemic state and, although unproven, some clinicians try to maintain a hyperoxaemic state in order to try to reduce the PVR (Wiswell, 2006; Vain and Batton, 2017). If CPAP or mechanical ventilation is required, then care must be taken, as the areas of over-distension combined with the parenchymal lung injury put these infants at high risk of air leak with rates of approximately 10% (Dargaville and Copnell, 2006). These infants may 'fight' the ventilator, even in synchronised modes, and there is often the need to sedate and administer muscle-relaxing agents for a period of time to achieve compliance and optimal ventilation and oxygenation. Acidosis also increases PVR, so ventilating to achieve a 'normal' pCO_2 (see table 12.1) will help to keep the pH normal. Both HFOV and pulmonary surfactant may have a role in the management of MAS by reducing its severity and reducing the need for extracorporeal membrane oxygenation (ECMO; El Shahed et al., 2007; Chen et al., 2015). There may be a role for chest physiotherapy if the X-ray shows areas of collapse or consolidation (Hough et al., 2008), although these infants are often sensitive to handling and may not tolerate the procedure.

If there has been a severe acute hypoxic-ischaemic insult, other body systems may require support. This may include the brain, kidneys, liver and heart. Measurement and monitoring of blood pressure, preferably by arterial access, are required to ensure that systemic pressure and organ perfusion are maintained. Infants who have suffered chronic intra-uterine stress may have undergone abnormal pulmonary vascular development, resulting in them being more at risk of PPHN.

Inotropic therapies may be required. Echocardiography can be helpful in determining which inotrope would be most beneficial by assessing myocardial contractility and cardiac output. It is also useful to confirm a structurally normal heart, determine the degree of PPHN present, and whether other drugs such as systemic pulmonary vasodilators or inhaled nitric oxide (iNO) would be beneficial. Hypotension and poor tissue perfusion may lead to metabolic acidosis, which may need correction by the administration of a base, e.g. sodium bicarbonate.

Renal compromise from peripartum insult or postnatal hypotension makes the accurate recording of fluid balance an important facet of care in these infants. Fluids are usually restricted to prevent volume overload, and consequently blood sugar levels should be regularly monitored, as hypoglycaemia can become a problem. As the bladder may not empty spontaneously, catheterisation may be required. An infection screen should be undertaken to exclude underlying infection, and antibiotics administered as appropriate until blood culture results are proven negative.

If the infant is receiving muscle relaxants, protection of the eyes is necessary to prevent drying and corneal abrasions; additionally, careful supported positioning should be used along with passive limb movements as tolerated. If this level of conventional support is not sufficient for the infant, further advice needs to be sought regarding the ongoing management which could include transfer to a specialist centre for iNO or extracorporeal membrane oxygenation ECMO.

Persistent pulmonary hypertension of the newborn

PPHN is the failure of the normal circulatory transition that occurs after birth (see chapter 13 for details). It is characterised by increased PVR, which results in a variable degree of right-to-left shunting of blood through the foramen ovale and ductus arteriosus, leading to severe hypoxaemia. PPHN is a pathophysiological feature often arising from other disease states affecting the infant and can be a result of any of the following (Gomella, 2004):

■   Primary or idiopathic PPHN +/− presence of mild neonatal lung disease. These babies are profoundly hypoxic with very little evidence of lung disease.
■   Secondary to severe intrapartum asphyxia. These babies present with hypoxia and severe acidosis. This combination results in pulmonary artery vasoconstriction preventing normal postnatal circulatory changes from occurring (Greenough et al., 2012). The right-to-left shunt may be exacerbated by systemic hypotension secondary to myocardial asphyxial damage.
■   Secondary to MAS leading to obstruction and inflammation of the airways.
■   Secondary to infection, GBS being the most prevalent organism.
■   Secondary to pulmonary hypoplasia in congenital diaphragmatic hernia or alveolar capillary dysplasia.
■   Secondary to congenital heart disease resulting in a right-to-left shunt.

The clinical appearance of a neonate presenting with PPHN is that of respiratory distress with cyanosis. Infants with primary PPHN present within the first 12 hours of life, and very rarely after 24 hours. Where PPHN is secondary to pre-existing lung disease such as infection or MAS, presentation is within the first few hours of life. Infants with PPHN are critically ill and despite mechanical ventilation and 100% oxygen may remain cyanosed with poor perfusion and acidosis. Simultaneous pre-ductal and post-ductal oxygen saturation monitoring is useful in diagnosing and managing PPHN. In the presence of right-to-left shunting through the ductus arteriosus, saturations in pre-ductal blood (right hand) will be higher than those in post-ductal (left hand/feet). A difference of >5% (Gomella, 2004; Kinsella et al., 2006) is considered indicative of a right-to-left ductal shunt. If invasive monitoring is used, a gradient of 20mmHg (2.7kpa) higher in the pre-ductal PaO_2 than post-ductal may indicate a right-to-left ductal shunt (Schumacher and Donn, 2006).

Oxygenation is often assessed by calculating the oxygenation index (OI):

$$OI = \frac{FiO_2 \times MAP \times 100}{PaO_2 \text{ (mmHg)}}$$

OI values of 30–40 are indicative of severe respiratory disease. Mortality often occurs with an OI greater than 80 (Gomella, 2004). The higher the OI, the more severe the degree of pulmonary hypertension. An OI level >40 is a useful indicator for considering ECMO as a management strategy for PPHN.

A full blood count should be undertaken as polycythaemia and hyperviscosity (demonstrated by a high haematocrit) aggravate PPHN. A white cell count is useful to determine whether an underlying infection or pneumonia is present. The platelet count is frequently depressed, particularly in newborns with MAS or asphyxia. Blood chemistry should be monitored to ensure hypoglycaemia and hypocalcaemia do not occur as they tend to worsen PPHN.

Chest radiography is useful in determining whether underlying parenchymal lung disease such as MAS or RDS is present. In newborns with idiopathic PPHN, the lung fields are clear with decreased vascular markings. The heart size is typically normal or slightly enlarged. Echocardiography is essential for neonates with PPHN, as it will rule out cyanotic congenital heart disease, and will give a definitive diagnosis of PPHN (Gomella, 2004). Echocardiography provides information about shunting at the arterial and ductal levels, and allows assessment of ventricular output and contractility, both of which may be depressed in neonates with PPHN.

The care of infants with PPHN requires meticulous attention to monitoring, oxygenation, blood pressure and perfusion. Mechanical ventilation is usually required to help maintain adequate oxygenation. Surfactant may need to be administered to reduce alveolar surface tension and decrease the work of breathing. Minimal handling and sedation, including analgesia and possibly muscle relaxants should be used for these infants to maintain compliance and synchrony with the ventilator. Maintenance of systemic arterial blood pressure is achieved using pharmacological vasopressor/inotropic support such as dopamine and dobutamine (see chapter 13). These agents act by increasing myocardial contractility and peripheral vasoconstriction, and reduce the right-to-left shunting of blood. This occurs when the systemic blood pressure is higher than the pulmonary blood pressure.

Pulmonary vasodilatation, aimed at lowering pulmonary blood pressure, can be attempted by the administration of drugs known to act on the pulmonary vascular bed, e.g. tolazoline, epoprostenol, and magnesium sulphate. These influence both pulmonary and systemic blood pressures, so can cause significant hypotension. Specific pulmonary vasodilators such as sildenafil are useful, however iNO is the most specific vasodilator modality for neonates with PPHN.

TRENDS IN NEONATAL RESPIRATORY CARE

It is now widely accepted that positive-pressure ventilation in the neonatal period can result in lung injury which increases the risk of respiratory morbidity including air leak and CLD. This has resulted in an increase in the use of non-invasive methods of respiratory support (see pp. 289–293). Several mechanisms for ventilator-induced lung injury have been proposed:

■ Volutrauma, where the alveoli are over-distended by the delivery of too much gas.

■ Barotrauma, where the alveoli are subjected to high pressures causing alveolar disruption.

■ Biotrauma, resulting from the injurious effects of inflammation, infection and oxidative stress.

■ Atelectotrauma, where there is alveolar collapse at the end of expiration, requiring re-recruitment with every breath.

■ Stretch trauma, where the rate of inflation of the alveoli is beyond their normal elastic capability (Donn and Sinha, 2006).

The modern trend in ventilating preterm newborns is to provide those who need it with the gentlest invasive ventilation possible for the shortest time possible. A strategy for protecting the lungs can be achieved through permissive hypercapnia, where the target $PaCO_2$ is higher than the previously accepted norm (usually defined together with a target pH), and permissive hypoxaemia, where the oxygen saturation target is lower than in a normal infant (Thorne et al., 2015). These strategies may decrease volutrauma and the duration of positive-pressure ventilation. The small group of term infants who require mechanical ventilation have different pathophysiology and require different targets. Example targets for both groups are shown in Table 12.1.

ACID-BASE BALANCE, GAS TRANSPORT AND MONITORING

In well infants, there are homeostatic control mechanisms within in the cardiorespiratory system, brain and kidneys that combine to maintain the acidity (pH) of the blood in the narrow range shown in Table 12.1. Sick infants are vulnerable to disturbances in their homeostasis caused by disease or treatment (Cifuentes and Carlo, 2007; Arias-Oliveras, 2016). Nurses caring for ventilated infants need to understand acid-base balance and blood gases in order to recognise abnormal results and act accordingly. Maintenance of the blood pH within acceptable parameters is necessary, since all bodily functions are controlled by enzymes and molecular proteins that are highly sensitive to its changes. Several factors contribute to the regulation of pH including:

■ CO_2 buildup (respiratory acidosis)
■ low CO_2 (respiratory alkalosis)
■ poor tissue perfusion leading to anaerobic metabolism (metabolic acidosis)
■ loss of organic acids from persistent removal of gastric secretions (metabolic alkalosis).

TABLE 12.1 ACCEPTABLE BLOOD GAS RESULTS FOR INFANTS REQUIRING RESPIRATORY SUPPORT

Parameter	Normal	Ventilated preterm infants[a]	Term targets
pH	7.35–7.45	>7.25	7.3–7.4
PaCO$_2$[b]	4.5–6 kPa	4.5–8.5 kPa (up to 10kPa from day 4)	4.5–6 kPa
PaO$_2$[b]	11–14 kPa	6.5–9.5 kPa	>8 kPa
SaO$_2$	100%	90–94%	>95%

(adapted from Greenough et al., 2012; NICE, 2019)
a Targets with permissive hypercapnia and permissive hypoxia
b arterial

TABLE 12.2 RELATIONSHIPS BETWEEN BLOOD GAS PARAMETERS AND ACID-BASE STATUS

	pH	PaCO$_2$	Bicarbonate	Base excess
Respiratory acidosis	Low	High	Normal	negative
Compensated respiratory acidosis	Normal	High	High	High positive
Metabolic acidosis	Low	Normal	Low	High negative
Respiratory alkalosis	High	Low	Normal	positive
Metabolic alkalosis	High	Normal or low	High	High positive
Mixed respiratory/ metabolic acidosis	Low	High	Low	High negative

The underlying cause for the alteration of the pH needs to be considered. If the pH reflects respiratory acidosis, an increase in ventilation is necessary; however, a low pH in the presence of normal CO$_2$ suggests a metabolic cause that should be treated by eliciting the underlying cause (e.g. hypotension) and treating accordingly, and/or infusion of base (usually sodium bicarbonate). Sodium bicarbonate therapy needs to be given with caution as it is a hyperosmolar, high sodium solution which can predispose to IVH if given too quickly and it can also lead to an increase in CO$_2$ levels. Over-correction can lead to a metabolic alkalosis. Low CO$_2$ states (hypocapnia) should be avoided as they lead to an increase in cerebral vascular resistance and poor cerebral perfusion, which can compound an ischaemic insult (Levene and Evans 2005; see table 12.2).

CO$_2$ is carried in the blood in three ways: (1) dissolved in plasma (10%); (2) bound to haemoglobin (30%); and (3) as bicarbonate (60%). CO$_2$ dissolved in water produces unstable carbonic acid, which in normal states dissociates rapidly to produce a hydrogen and bicarbonate balance. In pulmonary disease states, retention of CO$_2$ leads to a failure of this mechanism, and respiratory acidosis (low pH) results. Hypocapnia may lead to respiratory alkalosis (low levels of CO_2, high pH), which can lead to decreased cerebral blood flow and should be avoided or corrected expediently.

Four methods are available to assess an infant's CO_2 status:

- Arterial blood sampling to directly measure the infant's $PaCO_2$. This requires either insertion of an indwelling arterial line or regular arterial puncture.
- Heel prick capillary blood sample will directly measure the pCO_2. A warm, well-perfused foot will give an estimation of the arterial pCO_2 that is accepted by most clinicians.
- Transcutaneous pCO_2 ($TcpCO_2$) monitoring estimates the arterial pCO_2 by the attachment of a probe containing a heated electrode to the skin. The underlying skin is warmed (to 43°C) arterialising the underlying capillary bed; the CO_2 level is measured by its diffusion across the electrode's membrane. This method is useful for continuous trending, but the electrode needs regular calibration and site changes to avoid burning the skin. The more immature the infant, the greater the risk of skin damage from the heat and from the adhesive fixation rings. The trending is particularly helpful in infants who are changed from conventional ventilation to HFOV, as there can be significant drops in CO_2 during this time.
- End-tidal CO_2 monitoring is less commonly used in neonatal care but may be useful for confirming correct ET tube placement (by monitoring the presence of expired CO_2) and is useful for trending (Kugelman et al., 2008).

Oxygen crosses the alveolar capillary bed by diffusion and is then carried in the blood predominantly bound to haemoglobin (98%), with a small amount dissolved in the plasma (2%). Oxygen is required by all tissues for efficient cellular metabolism and the production of cellular energy adenosine triphosphate (ATP). Anaerobic metabolism, due to poor tissue perfusion, is less efficient and produces minimal ATP; it also generates the by-product of lactate, which accumulates in the tissues leading to metabolic acidosis. High levels of oxygen (hyperoxia) are injurious to tissues and carry risks of eye, lung and brain injury (Tin and Gupta, 2007).

Three methods are available to assess and monitor an infant's oxygenation:

- Arterial blood sampling to directly measure the PaO_2.
- Transcutaneous pO_2 (TcO_2) which is now rare.
- Oxygen saturation (SaO_2) monitoring provides a continuous measure of the haemoglobin that is saturated with oxygen. It is simple to apply, requires no calibration and gives instantaneous readings. Saturation monitoring is, however, prone to being affected by strong ambient light, movement and poor tissue perfusion affecting its accuracy and performance. The probe should have regular position changes (minimum four-hourly) to prevent pressure damage from too tight an application or in poor perfusion states. SaO_2 has become the commonest method of oxygen monitoring within the NNU. Oxygen saturation levels for preterm infants are discussed below.

RESPIRATORY SUPPORT STRATEGIES IN NEONATAL CARE

It is vital to follow the latest, national guidance for the respiratory care of premature infants (NICE, 2019) which will be referred to, where applicable in the following discussion of respiratory support strategies. However, it must be remembered that not all infants requiring ventilatory support are premature, and so all modes of ventilation will be discussed.

Oxygen therapy

Oxygen therapy is a common aspect of care in the NNU. Oxygen can be administered by several methods depending on the infant's clinical condition and specific requirements. For those requiring low concentrations, ambient oxygen can be administered via the incubator for short periods, or for longer-term administration via low flow nasal cannula (<1L/minute). In recent years, the use of high flow nasal cannula (HFNC) has developed with promising results (El-Farghali, 2017); for example, when weaning from ventilation (Sasi and Malhotra, 2015); this will be discussed shortly.

For sicker infants, oxygen of course is delivered via the chosen mode of ventilation. Oxygen administered to neonates for prolonged episodes needs to be warmed and humidified (Fallon, 2012), particularly at higher flow rates (NICE, 2019). Oxygen therapy contributes greatly to neonatal care but is not without its risks (Perrone et al., 2017). It is necessary to treat oxygen as the drug that it is, identify correctly the baby that needs oxygen, assess the baby's condition to administer the correct dose, use the most appropriate method of administration, and administer oxygen for the correct duration in order that the baby receives the greatest therapeutic benefit with the least risk. Oxygen administration requires careful consideration in preterm infants, as the correct therapeutic range has proven difficult to establish (BOOST II, 2013). A meta-analysis of data from five international trials comparing infants born at less than 28 weeks' gestation targeted to receive SpO_2 85–89% with similar infants targeted to receive SpO_2 90–95% included data from 4965 infants worldwide. The lower SpO_2 target range was associated with a higher risk of death and NEC, but a lower risk of retinopathy of prematurity treatment (Askie et al., 2018). The most recent national guidelines recommend that in preterm infants receiving oxygen the target SpO_2 level should be 91–95% (NICE, 2019).

Non-invasive respiratory support

Infants who are at high risk of developing RDS and those who display an increase in their work of breathing associated with hypercapnia and an increase in oxygen requirements will benefit from non-invasive respiratory support in the form of CPAP, nasal intermittent positive-pressure ventilation (NIPPV), or HFNC. Non-invasive support can be considered if the infant has a reasonable spontaneous respiratory effort with mild hypercapnia. Early trials showed that CPAP is comparable with intubation and mechanical ventilation as a treatment for RDS, even in very preterm infants (Morley et al., 2008).

Although research is ongoing, specifically in the extremely preterm population, little difference has been found between rates of death and CLD between the methods of delivering non-invasive respiratory support (Millar et al., 2016, Wilkinson et al., 2016). Those infants who 'fail' non-invasive support, either because they present with a decreased respiratory drive or apnoeas with a raised $PaCO_2$ and reduced PaO_2 will need to be intubated and ventilated. In line with the recent aim to provide protective lung strategies to prevent BPD, non-invasive ventilation strategies must be considered wherever possible (Petty, 2013a; Boel et al., 2017; NICE, 2019). An overview of the options available will now be discussed.

CONTINUOUS POSITIVE AIRWAY PRESSURE

CPAP is a method of delivering a predetermined continuous pressure and supplementary oxygen to the airways of a spontaneously breathing infant (see figure 12.1). CPAP helps reduce upper airway occlusion and decreases upper airway resistance by mechanically splinting the airways open. This improves ventilation by recruiting collapsed alveoli and increasing the surface area available for gas exchange. It also stabilises the chest wall and reduces the work of breathing. It was traditionally used post-extubation from invasive ventilation, decreasing extubation failure rates and decreased morbidity when compared to the now outdated oxygen administration through a headbox (Davis and Henderson-Smart, 2003). Following a study by Morley et al. (2008), CPAP was recognised as a first-line treatment for preterm infants with RDS, and a recent Cochrane review, including data from

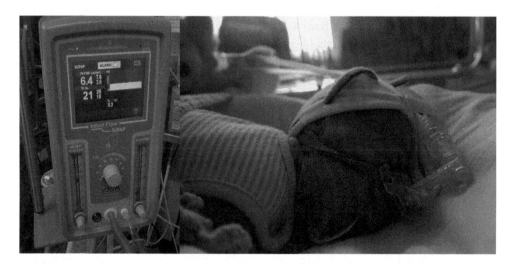

Figure 12.1 CPAP

seven studies and involving 3123 infants born at less than 32 weeks' gestation showed very inconsistent results when comparing CPAP to other forms of non-invasive respiratory support, but in the three studies (2354 infants) which compared CPAP to mechanical ventilation, with or without surfactant, CPAP resulted in a small reduction in the development of BPD and death associated with BPD (Subramaniam et al., 2016). The starting pressure for CPAP is usually in the range of 6–8cmH$_2$O. Bi-level CPAP is sometimes used, with small differences in pressure generated at the inspiratory and expiratory phases of respiration. This has not been shown to confer greater benefit than traditional CPAP (Lampland et al., 2015).

CPAP can be administered in a variety of ways. It has previously been administered through an ETT; however, this practice is deemed unsatisfactory, as the resistance from the ETT makes it difficult for the neonate to breathe effectively for more than a short period of time (Morley, 2006). Additionally, the ETT can get blocked with secretions.

Nasal CPAP (nCPAP) prongs were traditionally the most commonly applied means of delivering CPAP (Gomella, 2004). Similar prongs are used to deliver NIPPV. As newborn infants are inherent nasal breathers, nCPAP is easily facilitated and usually well tolerated. Prongs need to be carefully sized before insertion into the infant's nares and attaching to the CPAP delivery device, as they have been associated with erosion of the nasal septum resulting in facial disfigurement, which is generally due to poor, overzealous fixation. McCoskey (2008) acknowledges the presence of nares and nasal septum breakdown as a complication of CPAP. This can be primarily overcome using correctly fitting nasal CPAP hats and prongs (Fischer et al., 2010). Prongs and masks have developed over the intervening years, and are now made of more flexible plastic and in a wider variety of sizes, with no statistical difference observed in the efficacy of delivery by either method (Kieran et al., 2012)

Problems associated with the delivery of nCPAP include:

■ Obstruction of the nose and prongs from nasal secretions. Regular assessment and nasal suctioning, as necessary, will eliminate this problem.

■ Loss of pressure due to an open mouth. Chinstraps can be used with extreme caution, as they prevent the infant from clearing the mouth in the event of vomiting or regurgitation, and therefore increase the risk of aspiration. Pacifiers can be utilised, with parental permission.

■ Gastric distension increases when a baby is on CPAP and can be overcome by having a naso- or orogastric tube in situ and either leaving on free drainage or aspirating the tube on a regular basis to decompress the stomach. An orogastric tube is probably preferable in very small infants to prevent overcrowding of the nostril and potential notching disfigurement.

■ Air leak or pneumothorax can be a particular issue in the larger infant with RDS. Any infant suddenly deteriorating or having a significant increase in their oxygen requirements while on CPAP should be immediately investigated for pneumothorax.

Weaning practices from CPAP will vary, but in many NNUs pressures are gradually weaned until the baby is either switched to HFNC, or may attempt breathing without support or in nasal cannula oxygen only.

Historically, once the infant was stable on CPAP of approximately 4–5cmH$_2$O, time periods off CPAP were trialled and subsequently extended as tolerated. This is now uncommon practice but may still be observed in some NNUs.

NASAL INTERMITTENT POSITIVE-PRESSURE VENTILATION

NIPPV is a method of delivering ventilation through nasal prongs rather than through an ETT. The idea is not new (Llewellyn et al., 1970), and conventional ventilators are still used, meaning that, if synchronisation of breaths is to take place, external abdominal measurements of distension are required. NIPPV has be shown to be more effective than CPAP in preventing intubation in infants with apnoea, but other outcomes, including tissue damage to the nose, were similar (Bancalari and Claure 2013), with no difference in rates of BPD and death observed in infants treated with either synchronised or non-synchronised NIPPV compared to those treated with CPAP (Millar et al., 2016).

HIGH FLOW NASAL CANNULA

This non-invasive method of respiratory support allows for the administration of flows >1 L/min oxygen, or a blend of air and oxygen, as an alternative to other non-invasive ventilatory interfaces (see figure 12.2). It is unclear whether HFNC works because some CPAP

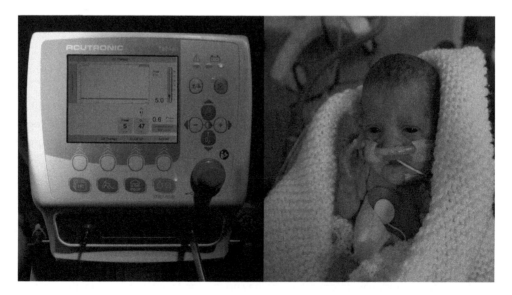

Figure 12.2 HFNC

is generated through the high flow of gas in relatively small infant nares, but emerging data shows that it confers similar benefits to traditional CPAP for infants weaning from invasive ventilation (Wilkinson et al., 2016). Its goal is to optimise spontaneous breathing through the reduction of dead space and the creation of positive distending airway pressure (El-Farghali, 2017). As the nasal cannula are not applied to the nose with the same pressure, there should be less incidence of tissue damage comparative to CPAP.

Modes of invasive ventilation

Decision-making in relation to the most appropriate respiratory mode and parameters should be undertaken on an individualised basis in conjunction with the parents. In this, the neonatal nurse plays an integral role (Petty, 2013b). The technology supporting invasive ventilation has improved remarkably in the past few decades with several strategies now available. The integration of real-time monitoring of inspiratory and expiratory flow (inspired tidal volume V_{Ti} and expired tidal volume V_{Te}), processed then to loops and waves (see figures 12.3–12.5 and box 12.1 for terminology), show the interaction between the infant and the ventilator, which can assist clinicians and nurses in optimising ventilatory support. These modes of ventilation potentially allow infant-regulated breath by breath changes in peak pressures, tidal volumes, inspiration times and rate. This is important as, while mean airway pressure is associated with controlling PaO_2, tidal volume is associated with controlling $PaCO_2$. While the need to control PaO_2 levels has been discussed above, hypercapnia

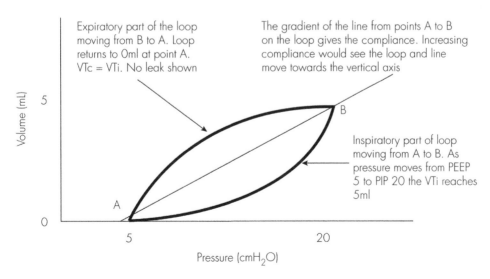

Pressure – Volume loop showing single ventilator cycle
Pressure $20/5cmH_2O$ achieving VT 4mL

Figure 12.3 Ventilation loop

Flow – Time wave through two ventilator cycles. The first cycle shows normal flow and the second shows expiratory flow changes from increasing resistance

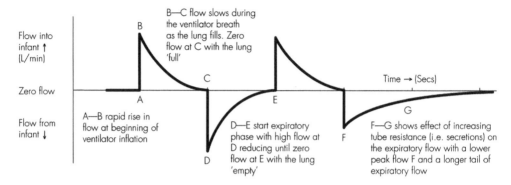

Figure 12.4 Ventilation waveform 1

Flow – Time wave through two ventilator cycles. Both cycles show a leak around ETT during the inspiratory phase. The second cycle also shows a leak in expiratory phase

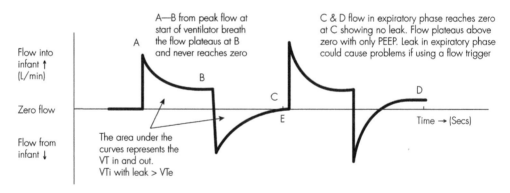

Figure 12.5 Ventilation waveform 2

and fluctuating levels of $PaCO_2$ in infants were both associated with severe intracranial hemorrhages, BPD and poor neurodevelopmental outcomes, independently of PaO_2 (Ambalavanan et al., 2015). Modern ventilation modes make it easier to control both PaO_2 and $PaCO_2$ while optimising the infant's comfort (figure 12.6). As various nomenclatures exist between manufacturers for the modes of ventilation being used, practitioners need to be aware of what is being utilised in their individual clinical settings. Synchronised time-cycled pressure-limited modes (although discussed in the following sections) are not recommended anymore without targeted tidal volumes (NICE, 2019).

BOX 12.1 TERMINOLOGY RELATING TO RESPIRATORY FUNCTION MONITORING THROUGH A VENTILATOR CYCLE

The pressure in the ventilator circuit rises to PIP. This causes a movement of gas towards the infant from the ventilator circuit through the ETT – inspiratory flow. During the period of the inspiration time this gas either collects in the infant's lungs or leaks out around the ETT up the trachea and is lost. The ventilator calculates the total volume that has gone through the ETT to give the inspiratory tidal volume (VTi).

The pressure in the ventilator circuit drops to PEEP, which is the pressure maintained in the lung at expiration. The movement of gas from the infant to the ventilator is the expiratory flow. During the period of the expiration time the gas in the infant's lungs returns to the ventilator circuit and little, if any, is lost around the ETT. The ventilator calculates the total volume that has gone through the ETT to give the expiratory tidal volume (VTe).

The ventilator will calculate the difference between VTi and VTe, giving the amount of leak. The VTe is generally accepted as the better measure of the infant's true tidal volume (VT) because of the lack of leak.

At the end of expiration, the alveoli and larger airways should still contain gas. The volume left is called the functional residual capacity (FRC).

The minute volume (MV) is theoretically the sum of all the individual VT measured over one minute (VT × rate per minute).

The behaviour of the lung and chest walls will also affect how much VT is achieved for the pressure delivered by the ventilator. Given the same pressure over the same time, a stiff lung will expand less than a normally functioning lung. This difference is expressed as the compliance.

The condition of the airway (ETT and bronchial tree) can affect the speed of the gas flow and therefore the VT. Increasing length and decreasing diameter of the airway will slow the speed by increasing the resistance to flow.

CONTINUOUS MANDATORY VENTILATION

Also known as intermittent mandatory ventilation (IMV), and intermittent positive-pressure ventilation (IPPV), continuous mandatory ventilation (CMV) is the longest-established form of neonatal ventilation. It is usually time-cycled, pressure-limited and with continuous flow. The clinician sets the inspiratory time (T_i), rate, PIP and PEEP. These parameters are unchanged by any action of the infant, and consequently this mode is best used in infants who are sedated and muscle-relaxed to prevent any asynchronous breathing from

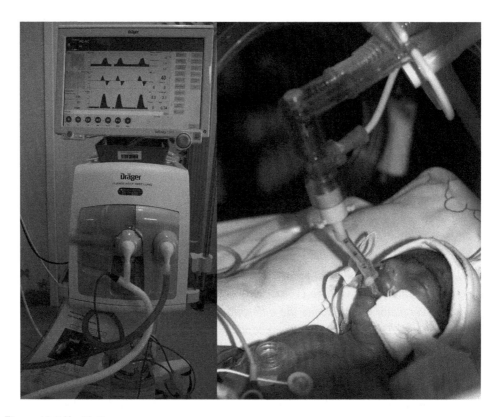

Figure 12.6 Ventilation

occurring. Infants can find this mode uncomfortable while weaning, and largely this mode of ventilation has been superseded by synchronised strategies.

VOLUME-TARGETED VENTILATION

Damage caused by lung over-distension (volutrauma) has been implicated in the development of BPD. Babies ventilated using volume-targeted modes of ventilation were more likely to survive free of lung damage (Klingenberg et al., 2017), and this is now the recommended mode of providing invasive ventilation to preterm infants (NICE, 2019). Modern neonatal ventilation modes can target a set tidal volume as an alternative to traditional pressure-limited ventilation using a fixed inflation pressure. Volume-targeted ventilation (VTV) aims to produce a more stable tidal volume in order to reduce lung damage and stabilise pCO_2.

In more detail, VTV is a mode that delivers time-cycled pressure-limited breaths, but allows the pressure to be adjusted to deliver a tidal volume in the range as set by the clinician. Potential advantages include reduced risk of volutrauma, as the set tidal volume is not exceeded when lung compliance improves, reduced peak pressures when baby makes significant contribution to tidal volume, more stable tidal volume delivery, and auto-weaning of PIPs, thus protecting against barotrauma (Gupta and Janakiraman, 2017)

VTV may also be known as volume guarantee, volume-assured and volume-limited ventilation, which is determined by the model of ventilator used. The clinician calculates the required tidal volume (4–6mL/kg in preterm infants; Greenough and Sharma, 2007) and sets the maximum PIP and T_i to achieve this. The ventilator will then deliver the predetermined tidal volume, but the pressure to deliver it will vary with each infant breath, as pulmonary compliance alters. This control can be added to all forms of ventilation. Due to the uncuffed nature of the neonatal ETT and its concomitant variable leak, an accurate volume cannot always be assured.

ASSIST-CONTROL VENTILATION

Also known as patient-triggered ventilation (PTV) and synchronised intermittent positive-pressure ventilation (SIPPV), assist-control (A/C) ventilation uses a signal from the infant to trigger the ventilator breath and hence determine the rate of ventilation. Originally, an abdominal capsule was used to detect inspiratory activity; however, there were problems with detection of breaths leading to delay in support and asynchrony. The commonest trigger today is the inspiratory flow. The PIP, PEEP, T_i, a back-up rate (in the event of apnoea) and the sensitivity of the trigger level are all set. This sensitivity needs to be at an appropriate level for each infant, and the nurse caring for the baby needs to be aware of the signs of trigger thresholds set too high or too low. Artefact from water or secretions in the sensors can cause auto-triggering and affect the infant–ventilator interaction. The T_i, PIP and PEEP are unchanged for each breath, but every breath the infant initiates which crosses the trigger threshold will be assisted by the ventilator, so the rate is determined by the infant. If the infant stops breathing, or if the effort is undetected, the back-up will be activated, and ventilation will continue.

SYNCHRONISED INTERMITTENT MANDATORY VENTILATION

Synchronised intermittent mandatory ventilation (SIMV) offers less support to the infant than A/C and may be used as a weaning tool. The setting of the trigger, T_i, PIP and PEEP is the same as A/C. The rate set is now effectively the maximum number of supported breaths the infant will receive per minute. Any breaths taken in addition to the assisted rate are supported only by PEEP.

PRESSURE SUPPORT VENTILATION

Pressure support ventilation (PSV) is a modified version of A/C offering less PIP support to the infant. Each infant breath triggers the ventilator in the usual way, but the duration of the assisted breath is variable. The trigger for the termination of the breath is usually when the inspiratory flow has dropped to a clinician-set percentage (e.g. 5%) of the peak flow. PSV can be used in conjunction with SIMV with a higher PIP, so that the infant receives a higher level of support for the SIMV breaths.

HIGH FREQUENCY OSCILLATORY VENTILATION

HFOV is the delivery of small tidal volumes to a neonate at supraphysiologic rates (10 Hz = 600breaths/minute). It is used to improve gas exchange in patients with severe respiratory failure (figure 12.7). As both inspiratory and expiratory phases are active, the likelihood of gas-trapping is reduced. The advantages of HFOV are said to be that it improves ventilation at lower pressure, reduces volutrauma to the lungs and produces a more uniform lung inflation which can reduce air leaks. It is the recommended mode of ventilation for preterm infants where VTV is not effective (NICE, 2019). Studies as yet have not shown any short- or long-term benefits in the use of HFOV over conventional ventilation in either term or preterm populations (Cools et al., 2015; Henderson-Smart et al., 2009; De Paoli et al., 2009). Disadvantages of HFOV are rapid reductions in CO_2 levels, which can lead to alterations in cerebral blood flow, and decreased venous return from increased pressure within the thorax, which in turn can lead to decreased cardiac output and a fall in blood pressure.

Two volume strategies can be used to deliver HFOV; those of low volume or high volume. A low-volume strategy in which the mean airway pressure (MAP) is limited with the aim of preventing damage due to barotrauma is used for infants with non-homogeneous lung disease, e.g. MAS, air leaks/pneumothorax, diaphragmatic hernia, PIE and PPHN. High-volume strategy in which MAP is elevated to promote optimum alveolar expansion

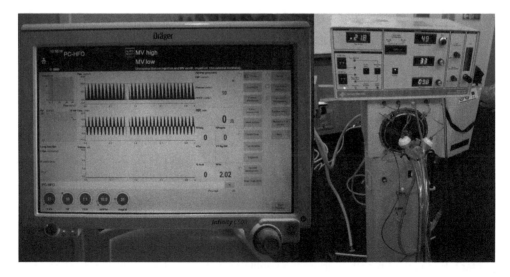

Figure 12.7 Two types of neonatal oscillator

consequently improving oxygenation is used for infants with more homogeneous disease states, e.g. severe RDS. If a high-volume strategy is used as rescue support, then the infant should commence HFOV with a MAP 2cmH$_2$O higher than that delivered on conventional ventilation. The MAP is then gradually increased to optimise oxygenation. Infants with severe RDS may need an increase in MAP by as much as 10cmH$_2$O. If oxygenation does not improve over the next few hours, additional therapies such as the use of iNO should be considered.

CO$_2$ elimination is primarily dependent on the oscillatory amplitude – delta P (ΔP). However, other factors such as frequency and I:E ratio will also affect CO$_2$ elimination. On commencing HFOV, the oscillatory amplitude is increased until chest wall 'wobbling' or vibration is apparent, and then adjusted to manage the CO$_2$ level. Infants receiving HFOV require frequent chest X-rays to check for over- or under-expansion of the lungs. Over-expansion is depicted by the presence of more than nine posterior rib ends and a flattened diaphragm, and can result in a rapid decrease in CO$_2$ levels and a drop in blood pressure. Under-expansion is demonstrated by fewer than eight posterior rib ends and poor aeration of the lung fields. Frequent blood gas analysis is also important for neonates on HFOV, as changes in parameters can be rapid.

Nursing care of neonates on HFOV is similar to that of any ventilated neonate (De Jesus and Petty, 2012; see below). However, there are salient points to consider: There may be increased secretions during HFOV due to the intrapulmonary percussion, so good humidification of the circuit is necessary to prevent blockage of the ETT. When undertaking suction, an in-line suction procedure should be utilised to avoid reduction in the MAP. If disconnection is necessary, it should be minimised to avoid de-recruitment of the alveoli. Post suction, it may be necessary to temporarily increase the MAP by 1–2cmH$_2$O if the infant's oxygenation has dropped in order to re-recruit the alveoli. As the infant's condition improves, the MAP and amplitude can be reduced according to blood gas results, and the infant switched to conventional ventilation or CPAP as tolerated.

Inhaled nitric oxide

Nitric oxide is a colourless gas with a half-life of approximately 2 seconds. It is delivered to the intubated and ventilated infant via the ETT, where it diffuses from the alveoli to pulmonary vascular smooth muscle causing it to relax, improving oxygenation and decreasing V/Q mismatch. Excess iNO diffuses into the bloodstream, where it is rapidly inactivated by binding to haemoglobin. This rapid inactivation limits its actions to the pulmonary vasculature and consequently it has no systemic effects.

iNO can improve short-term oxygenation and reduce the need for ECMO in term or near-term infants (Barrington et al., 2017). It has been used to treat both term and preterm infants with respiratory failure, and term infants with PPHN have been seen to respond to iNO with improvement in oxygenation indices and a decreased need for ECMO (Soll, 2009). Additional to the reduced need for ECMO, Clark et al. (2000) noted a reduction in the need for supplemental oxygen at 30 days of age in term infants who received iNO. The use of iNO in preterm infants remains controversial and inconclusive, and should only be considered in the presence of underlying pathology such as pulmonary hypoplasia or PPHN (NICE, 2019). It is thought to be of little benefit in the prevention of the evolution of CLD and may contribute to IVH due to its vasodilatory nature (Arul and Konduri 2009; Soll 2009).

Initial research studies reported starting doses of 80 parts per million (ppm). Following review of the studies, the recommended starting dose for iNO is now 20ppm in an infant ≥34 weeks. Increasing the dose to 40ppm does not appear to improve oxygenation in infants who do not respond to 20ppm. Infants who do respond to iNO can be weaned at a fairly rapid rate once oxygen requirements have fallen to approximately 40%. The basic criterion for weaning iNO is the maintenance of adequate oxygenation and stability of the infant without evidence of rebound pulmonary hypertension (Gomella, 2004). Complications associated with iNO include an increase in methaemoglobin (MetHb) which leads to the haemoglobin having a reduced oxygen-carrying capacity, resulting in cyanosis. Levels of MetHb need to be monitored on a regular basis. At levels of 20ppm and less, this is rarely a complication (figure 12.8).

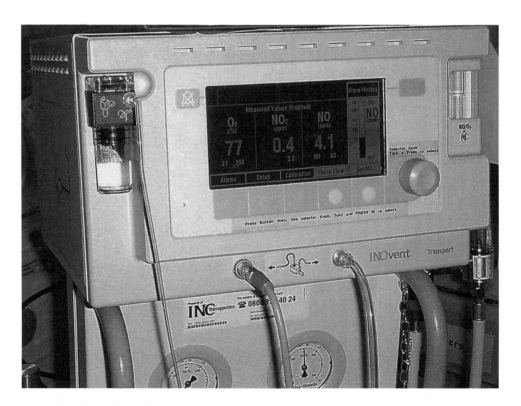

Figure 12.8 Nitric oxide delivery system

WEANING FROM INVASIVE VENTILATION

The large selection of ventilator modes available and the variation in their use between units mean that there is also a wide variation between individual NNUs in weaning methods. As blood gases and respiratory efforts improve, gradual reductions in the level of ventilation support are made (i.e. lowering PIP or tidal volume and rate, introducing SIMV and/or PSV). This is commonly followed by extubation to a non-invasive respiratory support mode. There have been several attempts to use some of the measured parameters of infant effort to determine readiness for extubation (Shalish et al., 2017), but most decisions are made following clinical assessment of the individual infant and experience of the clinician.

EXTRACORPOREAL MEMBRANE OXYGENATION

ECMO is a complex procedure of life support used in severe but potentially reversible respiratory failure in term or near-term infants (Mugford et al., 2008). It is generally reserved for when other conventional treatment modalities have failed.
Criteria for ECMO are:

■ Birth weight >2.0kg
■ Gestational age >34 weeks
■ No bleeding disorders
■ No congenital anomaly incompatible with quality of life
■ OI >40.

The latter index is the marker of the severity of the respiratory failure. ECMO is unsuitable for less mature infants, as the amount of anticoagulation required in the circuit makes preterm infants more prone to IVH. Benefits have been shown in terms of both the mortality and morbidity in infants receiving ECMO; however, there are still concerns surrounding the invasive nature of the technique, especially with its disruption to cerebral circulation. Half of the children who have received ECMO have died or are disabled at 4 years of age. This is thought, however, to reflect the severity of the underlying pathology rather than the technique *per se* (Mugford et al., 2008). As ECMO is generally instigated once conventional therapies have failed, earlier referral may result in improved outcomes.

NURSING CARE OF THE INFANT RECEIVING RESPIRATORY CARE

The nursing management of a ventilated baby can be challenging, as the majority of these infants will be initially sick and unstable. Nurses managing the ventilated neonate need to be vigilant to subtle variations in observations, as early recognition of changes may prevent a significant deterioration and collapse. Infants on respiratory support should have constant monitoring of their heart rate, blood pressure and oxygen saturation as a minimum. End-tidal CO_2 and transcutaneous monitoring can also help manage infants more effectively, but the latter may be difficult to achieve as the monitor must be fitted to the ETT, and monitors are comparatively heavy for infants, increasing the risk of accidental extubation. As the nurse is probably the infant's best monitor, no ventilated baby should ever be left unattended.

In line with this, respiratory assessment is a vital nursing skill. Nurses must ensure they understand how to assess the respiratory system and identify the deteriorating condition in the case of respiratory or ventilatory compromise, including clinical observation, vital sign monitoring and blood gas analysis (see chapter 2 on assessment).

Maintenance of patency and security of the ETT is a prime consideration. The ETT may be introduced nasally, but more commonly orally with the size appropriate to the weight of the infant (see chapter 20). The largest appropriate tube should be used, as the smaller its diameter, the greater the resistance to flow and increased risk of leak around the ETT resulting in suboptimal ventilation. However, when using a larger-diameter tube, there is a greater risk of complications from pressure damage to the nose, larynx and tracheal walls. The correct tip position for an ETT is below the larynx and above the **carina** (approximately T2–3). This distance is small in very low birth weight infants and increases their risk of tube displacement. The tube size and position should be clearly documented in the infant's notes. The ETT can be secured in many ways (Lai et al., 2014), each having their advantages and disadvantages, but failure of secure tube fixation is the commonest reason for accidental extubation (Veldman et al., 2006) and means the infant is subjected to emergency reintubation, which may cause trauma and destabilisation.

When an ETT is in situ, the normal mucociliary action is suppressed, and removal of secretions will be necessary if tube patency and optimal ventilation are to be maintained. Good humidification is necessary in order to liquefy secretions and prevent drying and damage to the mucosa (Petty, 2013b). Inspired gases should be delivered at 37°C and as close to 100% relative humidity as possible. Endotracheal suctioning should not be performed as routine but rather according to the needs of the baby (LaMar, 2006).

Indications for suction include:

■ Secretions visible in ETT
■ Reduced or coarse breath sounds
■ A decrease in oxygen saturation
■ Deterioration in blood gases
■ Change in pulmonary graphics.

Complications of ET suctioning include:

- Hypoxia
- Bradycardia
- Raised intra-cranial pressure
- Atelectasis
- Trauma
- Sepsis
- Dislodgement of the ETT.

Deep suctioning, where the catheter goes beyond the end of the ETT can cause mucosal damage and perforation of the carina. To avoid this, the length of insertion of the suction catheter should be carefully measured (e.g. the length of the ETT plus the connector prior to the procedure) and the depth adhered to. If resistance is met following insertion, the catheter should be withdrawn slightly before suction is applied. The suction pressure should not exceed 10kPa, and suction only applied during withdrawal of the catheter. The duration of the procedure should be less than 20 seconds. The use of saline as a lavage during the procedure is contentious. The instillation of saline was thought to loosen secretions and aid their removal. According to Puchalski (2007), this practice does not thin secretions or improve pulmonary function and can further reduce oxygen saturation and increase the risk of bacterial colonisation of the lower airways.

Suctioning can be performed using the open method (infant disconnected from the ventilator circuit) or closed (suction catheter is integrated into the ventilator circuit). In a review of available literature, Woodgate and Flenady (2001) reported that there was insufficient evidence at that time to ascertain the best approach; they concluded, however, that the procedure should only be undertaken by practitioners proficient in the technique. Recording of the nature, colour and volume of the secretions should be undertaken, as this is useful clinical information that may lead to a review or change in current management.

Infants requiring respiratory support should be nursed in a thermal neutral environment, as hypothermia can result in a decrease in surfactant production, and an increase in oxygen consumption (Turnbull and Petty, 2013). The environment should also be conducive to rest, enabling the baby's condition to improve. Minimal handling should be observed with the baby in a quiet environment protected from bright lights and noise. Additional to this, a pain assessment scoring chart may be useful in gauging the level of sedation the baby may need in order to maintain safety and comfort.

Finally, as stated earlier, the family must be a prime consideration in any care, and respiratory care is no exception. Parents with a baby who requires respiratory support must be made aware of the rationale for interventions performed and be fully informed and included in the care of their baby (NICE, 2019; see chapters 4 and 5).

CONCLUSION

Respiratory failure from prematurity or underlying disease processes are the most common reasons for admission to NNU. With decreasing gestational age, clinicians need to correlate therapies to the stage of development of the infant in order to optimise efficacy and prevent further ventilation-associated lung injury. While there have been significant technological advancements in the provision of respiratory support, it is clear from a review of the literature that more research is necessary to define the best way to ventilate this vulnerable population.

CASE STUDY

CASE STUDIES

For the three case studies below, consider the following questions:

Q.1. Considering the current literature and guidelines on neonatal respiratory management, what are the strategies required for these three case studies below?

Q.2. What are your reasons for your answer to Q.1, for each case study?

Q.3. What factors will benefit these infants' outcomes and why?

Q.4. What are the risks associated with respiratory management in these cases and how can these be minimised?

Case study 1: Ventilatory management of the premature infant

Thomas is 27^{+3} weeks' gestation and weighs 810g. He was delivered by lower segment caesarean section for maternal pregnancy-induced hypertension. His mother is a primigravid and received a full course of antenatal steroids prior to delivery. At birth, Thomas had a heart rate over 100 but had a very weak respiratory effort. His cord blood gas at 10 minutes old was pH = 7.16, $PaCO2$ = 8.6kpa $PaO2$ = 2.4kpa. Bicarbonate 14 mmol/L Base excess = −7

Case study 2: Weaning from ventilation

Gabriella was born at 30 weeks' gestation, birth weight 900g and required resuscitation at birth due to respiratory distress. She was diagnosed with an early onset infection and has required full ventilation as she did not tolerate CPAP. She has failed one previous attempt at intubation extubation at 4 days old. She is now 7 days old and her blood gas is pH 7.49, $PaCO2$ = 3.4 kpa $PaO2$ = 10.5kpa. Bicarbonate 20 mmol/L Base excess = +3

Case study 3: Weaning from CPAP

Sanjeet, born at 26 weeks' gestation, has chronic lung disease and has been on bi-level CPAP now for 5 weeks after an unstable period of ventilation. He has an oxygen requirement of 55%. He is now 9 weeks old and the decision is made to wean and discontinue the CPAP as soon as his condition allows. His blood gas is pH 7.33, PaCO2 = 9kpa PaO2 = 8.6kpa (in oxygen) Bicarbonate 30 mmol/L Base excess = +4.

For suggested answer guides to the questions posed in these case studies, please refer to the web-based companion site specific to this chapter (see URL below).

WEB-BASED RESOURCES

For further information, online resources and greater detail on the case studies featured in this chapter go to www.routledge.com/cw/nicnursing

References

Ambalavanan, N., Carlo, W. A., Wrage, L. A., Das, A., Laughon, M., Cotten, C. M., ... & Higgins, R. D. (2015). PaCO2 in surfactant, positive pressure, and oxygenation randomised trial (SUPPORT). *Archives of Disease in Childhood: Fetal and Neonatal Edition, 100*(2), F145–F149.

Arias-Oliveras, A. (2016). Neonatal blood gas interpretation. *Newborn and Infant Nursing Reviews, 16*(3), 119–121.

Arul, N., & Konduri, G. G. (2009). Inhaled nitric oxide for preterm neonates. *Clinics in Perinatology, 36*(1), 43–61.

Aschner, J. L., Bancalari, E. H., & McEvoy, C. T. (2017). Can we prevent bronchopulmonary dysplasia? *The Journal of Pediatrics, 189*, 26–30.

Askie, L. M., Darlow, B. A., Finer, N., Schmidt, B., Stenson, B., Tarnow-Mordi, W., ... & Das, A. (2018). Association between oxygen saturation targeting and death or disability in extremely preterm infants in the neonatal oxygenation prospective meta-analysis collaboration. *Jama, 319*(21), 2190–2201.

Baik, N., O'Reilly, M., Fray, C., van Os, S., Cheung, P., & Schmölzer, G. M. (2018). Ventilation strategies during neonatal cardiopulmonary resuscitation. *Frontiers in Pediatrics, 6*(18), 1–7

Bancalari, E., & Claure, N. (2013). The evidence for non-invasive ventilation in the preterm infant. *Archives of Disease in Childhood: Fetal and Neonatal Edition, 98*(2), F98–F102.

Barrington, K. J., Finer, N., Pennaforte, T., & Altit, G. (2017). Nitric oxide for respiratory failure in infants born at or near term. *Cochrane Database of Systematic Reviews*, Issue 1. Art. No.: CD000399. DOI: 10.1002/14651858.CD000399.pub3

Bendapudi, P., Narasimhan, R., & Papworth, S. (2012). Causes and management of pulmonary haemorrhage in the neonate. *Paediatrics and Child Health, 22*(12), 528–531.

Bhutani, V. K. (2006). Development of the respiratory system. In Donn, S. M., & Sinha, S. K. (Eds.) *Manual of Neonatal Respiratory Care* 2nd Edition. Philadelphia: Mosby Elsevier.

Boel, L., Broad, K., & Chakraborty, M. (2017). Non-invasive respiratory support in newborn infants. *Paediatrics and Child Health. 28*(1), 6–12.

BOOST II UK, Australia, and New Zealand Collaborative Groups. (2013). Oxygen saturation and outcomes in preterm infants. *New England Journal of Medicine, 368*(22), 2094–2104.

Bunnell, J. B. (2006). High-Frequency Ventilation: General Concepts. In Donn, S. M., & Sinha, S. K. (Eds) *Manual of Neonatal Respiratory Care*, 2nd Edition (pp. 315–328). Philadelphia: Mosby Elsevier.

Chakraborty, M., & Kotecha, S. (2013). Pulmonary surfactant in newborn infants and children. *Breathe, 9*(6), 476–488.

Chen, D. M., Wu, L. Q., & Wang, R. Q. (2015). Efficiency of high-frequency oscillatory ventilation combined with pulmonary surfactant in the treatment of neonatal meconium aspiration syndrome. *International Journal of Clinical and Experimental Medicine, 8*(8), 14490.

Cifuentes, J., & Carlo, W. (2007). Respiratory system. In Kenner, C., & Lott, J. (Eds.) *Comprehensive Neonatal Care* 4th Edition (pp. 1–4). Missouri: Saunders Elsevier.

Clark, R. H., Kueser, T. J., Walker, M. W., Southgate, W. M., Huckaby, J. L., Perez, J. A., … & Kinsella, J. P. (2000). Low-dose nitric oxide therapy for persistent pulmonary hypertension of the newborn. *New England Journal of Medicine, 342*(7), 469–474.

Cools, F., Offringa, M., & Askie, L. M. (2015). Elective high frequency oscillatory ventilation versus conventional ventilation for acute pulmonary dysfunction in preterm infants. *Cochrane Database of Systematic Reviews*, Issue 3. Art. No.: CD000104. DOI: 10.1002/14651858.CD000104.pub4

Costa, S., Rocha, G., Leitão, A., & Guimarães, H. (2012). Transient tachypnea of the newborn and congenital pneumonia: a comparative study. *The Journal of Maternal-Fetal & Neonatal Medicine, 25*(7), 992–994.

Dani, C., Corsini, I., Bertini, G., Fontanelli, G., Pratesi, S., & Rubaltelli, F. F. (2010). The INSURE method in preterm infants of less than 30 weeks' gestation. *The Journal of Maternal-Fetal & Neonatal Medicine, 23*(9), 1024–1029.

Dargaville, P. A., & Copnell, B. (2006). The epidemiology of meconium aspiration syndrome: Incidence, risk factors, therapies, and outcome. *Pediatrics, 117*(5), 1712–1721.

Dargaville, P. A., Aiyappan, A., De Paoli, A. G., Kuschel, C. A., Kamlin, C. O. F., Carlin, J. B., & Davis, P. G. (2013). Minimally-invasive surfactant therapy in preterm infants on continuous positive airway pressure. *Archives of Disease in Childhood: Fetal and Neonatal Edition, 98*(2), F122–F126.

Davis, P. G., & Henderson-Smart, D. J. (2003). Nasal continuous positive airway pressure immediately after extubation for preventing morbidity in preterm infants. *Cochrane Database of Systematic Reviews*, Issue 2. Art. No.: CD000143. DOI: 10.1002/14651858.CD000143

Dear, P. (2005). Infection in the newborn. In Rennie, J. M. (Ed.) *Roberton's Textbook of Neonatology* 4th Edition. Philadelphia: Elsevier Churchill Livingstone.

De Jesus, H., & Petty, J. (2012). High frequency ventilation: A reflective case study. *Journal of Neonatal Nursing, 18*, 112–120.

De Paoli, A. G., Clark, R. H., Bhuta, T., & Henderson-Smart, D. J. (2009). High frequency oscillatory ventilation versus conventional ventilation for infants with severe pulmonary dysfunction born at or near term. *Cochrane Database of Systematic Reviews*, Issue 3. Art. No.: CD002974. DOI: 10.1002/14651858.CD002974.pub2

Donn, S. M., & Sinha, S. K. (2006). Minimising ventilator induced lung injury in preterm infants. *Archives of Disease in Childhood: Fetal and Neonatal Edition, 91*(3), F226–F230.

Donn, S. M. (2017, October). Bronchopulmonary dysplasia: Myths of pharmacologic management. In *Seminars in Fetal and Neonatal Medicine* (Vol. 22, No. 5, pp. 354–358). WB Saunders.

Doyle, L. W., Cheong, J. L., Ehrenkranz, R. A., & Halliday, H. L. (2017). Late (> 7 days) systemic postnatal corticosteroids for prevention of bronchopulmonary dysplasia in preterm infants. *Cochrane Database of Systematic Reviews*, Issue 10. Art. No.: CD001145. DOI: 10.1002/14651858.CD001145.pub4

El-Farghali, O. G. (2017). High-Flow Nasal Cannula in Neonates. *Respiratory Care. 62*(5), 641–642.

El Shahed, A. I., Dargaville, P. A., Ohlsson, A., & Soll, R. (2007). Surfactant for meconium aspiration syndrome in full term/near term infants. , Issue 3. Art. No.: CD002054. DOI: 10.1002/14651858. CD002054.pub2

Fallon, A. (2012). Oxygen therapy in neonatal care. Journal of Neonatal Nursing, *18*(6), 198–200.

Fischer, C., Bertelle, V., Hohlfeld, J., Forcada-Guex, M., Stadelmann-Diaw, C., & Tolsa, J. F. (2010). Nasal trauma due to continuous positive airway pressure in neonates. *Archives of Disease in Childhood: Fetal and Neonatal Edition*, *95*(6), F447–F451.

Gahlot, L., Green, F. H., Rigaux, A., Schneider, J. M., & Hasan, S. U. (2009). Role of vagal innervation on pulmonary surfactant system during fetal development. *Journal of Applied Physiology*, *106*(5), 1641–1649.

Goldsmith, J. P., Karotkin, E., Suresh, G., & Keszler, M. (2016). *Assisted Ventilation of the Neonate E-Book*. Elsevier Health Sciences.

Gomella, T. L. (2004). *Neonatology. Management, Procedures, On-Call Problems, Diseases, and Drugs* 5th Edition. New York: McGraw-Hill.

Göpel, W., Kribs, A., Ziegler, A., Laux, R., Hoehn, T., Wieg, C., … & Groneck, P. (2011). Avoidance of mechanical ventilation by surfactant treatment of spontaneously breathing preterm infants (AMV): An open-label, randomised, controlled trial. *The Lancet*, *378*(9803), 1627–1634.

Greenough, A., Milner, A. D., Hannam, S., Fox, G. F., Turowski, C., Davenport, M., & Morrison, G. (2012). Pulmonary disease of the newborn. In Rennie, J. M. (Ed.) *Rennie & Roberton's Textbook of Neonatology* (5th Edition). London and New York: Elsevier Health Sciences.

Greenough, A., & Sharma, A. (2007). What is new in ventilation strategies for the neonate? *European Journal of Pediatrics*, *166*(10), 991–996.

Gupta, S., & Janakiraman, S. (2017). Volume ventilation in neonates. *Paediatrics and Child Health*. *28*(1), 1–5.

Hillman, N. H., Kallapur, S. G., & Jobe, A. H. (2012). Physiology of transition from intrauterine to extrauterine life. *Clinics in Perinatology*, *39*(4), 769–783.

Hough, J. L., Flenady, V., Johnston, L., & Woodgate, P. G. (2008). Chest physiotherapy for reducing respiratory morbidity in infants requiring ventilatory support. *Cochrane Database of Systematic Reviews*, Issue 3. Art. No.: CD006445. DOI: 10.1002/14651858.CD006445.pub2

Hsia, C. C., Hyde, D. M., & Weibel, E. R. (2016). Lung Structure and the Intrinsic Challenges of Gas Exchange. *Comprehensive Physiology*, *6*(2), 827–895.

Hunt, K. A., Dassios, T., Ali, K., & Greenough, A. (2018). Prediction of bronchopulmonary dysplasia development. *Archives of Disease in Childhood – Fetal and Neonatal Edition,* *103*(6), F598–F599.

Javaid, A., & Morris, I. (2018). Bronchopulmonary dysplasia. *Paediatrics and Child Health, 28*(1), 22–27.

Jobe, A. H., & Steinhorn, R. (2017). Can we define bronchopulmonary dysplasia? *The Journal of Pediatrics*, *188*, 19–23.

Kennedy, K. A., Cotten, C. M., Watterberg, K. L., & Carlo, W. A. (2016). Prevention and management of bronchopulmonary dysplasia: Lessons learned from the neonatal research network. *Seminars in Perinatology*, *40*(6), 348–355.

Kieran, E. A., Twomey, A. R., Molloy, E. J., Murphy, J. F., & O'Donnell, C. P. (2012). Randomized trial of prongs or mask for nasal continuous positive airway pressure in preterm infants. *Pediatrics – English Edition*, *130*(5), e1170.

Kinsella, J. P., Cutter, G. R., Walsh, W. F., Gerstmann, D. R., Bose, C. L., Hart, C., … & George, T. N. (2006). Early inhaled nitric oxide therapy in premature newborns with respiratory failure. *New England Journal of Medicine*, *355*(4), 354–364.

Klingenberg, C., Wheeler, K. I., McCallion, N., Morley, C.J., & Davis, P. G. (2017). Volume-targeted versus pressure-limited ventilation in neonates. *Cochrane Database of Systematic Reviews*, Issue 10. Art. No.: CD003666. DOI: 10.1002/14651858.CD003666.pub4

Kugelman, A., Zeiger-Aginsky, D., Bader, D., Shoris, I., & Riskin, A. (2008). A novel method of distal end-tidal CO_2 capnography in intubated infants: Comparison with arterial CO_2 and with proximal mainstream end-tidal CO_2. *Pediatrics*, *122*(6), e1219–e1224.

Lai, M., Inglis, G. D. T., Hose, K., Jardine, L. A., & Davies, M. (2014). Methods for securing endotracheal tubes in newborn infants. *Cochrane Database of Systematic Reviews*, Issue 7. Art. No.: CD007805. DOI: 10.1002/14651858.CD007805.pub2

LaMar, K. (2006). Nursing care of the ventilated neonate. In Donn, S. M., & Sinha, S. K. (Eds.) *Manual of Neonatal Respiratory Care* 2nd Edition. Philadelphia: Mosby Elsevier.

Lampland, A. L., Plumm, B., Worwa, C., Meyers, P., & Mammel, M. C. (2015). Bi-level CPAP does not improve gas exchange when compared with conventional CPAP for the treatment of neonates recovering from respiratory distress syndrome. *Archives of Disease in Childhood: Fetal and Neonatal Edition*, *100*(1), F31–F34.

Levene, M., & Evans, D. J. (2005). Hypoxic-ischaemic brain injury. In Rennie, J. M. (Ed.) *Roberton's Textbook of Neonatology* 4th Edition. Philadelphia: Elsevier Churchill Livingstone.

Llewellyn, M. A., Tilak, K. S., & Swyer, P. R. (1970). A controlled trial of assisted ventilation using an oro-nasal mask. *Archives of Disease in Childhood*, *45*(242), 453–459.

Liu, J., Wang, Y., Fu, W., Yang, C. S., & Huang, J. J. (2014). Diagnosis of neonatal transient tachypnea and its differentiation from respiratory distress syndrome using lung ultrasound. *Medicine, 93*(27), e197.

McCoskey, L. (2008). Nursing care guidelines for prevention of nasal breakdown in neonates receiving nasal CPAP. *Advances in Neonatal Care*, *8*(2), 116–124.

McDonald, C. L., & Ainsworth, S. B. (2004). An update on the use of surfactant in neonates. *Current Paediatrics*, *14*(4), 284–289.

Millar, D., Lemyre, B., Kirpalani, H., Chiu, A., Yoder, B. A., & Roberts, R. S. (2016). A comparison of bilevel and ventilator-delivered non-invasive respiratory support. *Archives of Disease in Childhood: Fetal and Neonatal Edition*, *101*(1), 21–25.

Minocchieri, S., Knoch, S., Schoel, W. M., Ochs, M., & Nelle, M. (2014). Nebulizing poractant alfa versus conventional instillation: Ultrastructural appearance and preservation of surface activity. *Pediatric Pulmonology*, *49*(4), 348–356.

Mitanchez, D., Yzydorczyk, C., Siddeek, B., Boubred, F., Benahmed, M., & Simeoni, U. (2015). The offspring of the diabetic mother – short- and long-term implications. *Best Practice & Research Clinical Obstetrics & Gynaecology*, *29*(2), 256–269.

Morley, C. (2006). Continuous positive airway pressure. In Donn, S. M., & Sinha, S. K. *Manual of Neonatal Respiratory Care* 2nd Edition. Philadelphia: Mosby Elsevier.

Morley, C. J., Davis, P. G., Doyle, L. W., Brion, L. P., Hascoet, J. M., & Carlin, J. B. (2008). Nasal CPAP or intubation at birth for very preterm infants. *New England Journal of Medicine*, *358*(7), 700–708.

Mugford, M., Elbourne, D., & Field, D. (2008). Extracorporeal membrane oxygenation for severe respiratory failure in newborn infants. *Cochrane Database of Systematic Reviews*, (3).

National Institute for Health and Care Excellence. (2019). *Specialist neonatal respiratory care for babies born preterm. NG124.* NICE.

Nelin, L. D., & Logan, J. W. (2017, October). The use of inhaled corticosteroids in chronically ventilated preterm infants. In *Seminars in Fetal and Neonatal Medicine* (Vol. 22, No. 5, pp. 296–301). WB Saunders.

Nzirawa, T., Haque, A., & Mas, A. (2017). Primary care givers of infants on home oxygen therapy. *Journal of neonatal nursing*, *23*(4), 185–187.

Parravicini, E., & Polin, R. A. (2006). Pneumonia in the newborn infant. In Donn, S. M., & Sinha, S. K. (Eds.) *Manual of Neonatal Respiratory Care* 2nd Edition. Philadelphia: Mosby Elsevier.

Perrone, S., Bracciali, C., Di Virgilio, N., & Buonocore, G. (2017). Oxygen Use in Neonatal Care: A Two-edged Sword. *Frontiers in Pediatrics*, *4*, 143.

Petty, J. (2013a). Fact sheet: Understanding neonatal non invasive ventilation. *Journal of Neonatal Nursing*, *19*(1), 10–14.

Petty, J. (2013b). Understanding neonatal ventilation: strategies for decision making in the NICU. *Neonatal Network*, *32*(4), 246–261.

Pulchalski, M. (2007). Should normal saline be used when suctioning the endotracheal tube of the neonate? Retrieved from www.medscape. com/viewarticle/552862.

Raju, T. N. K. (2006). Neonatal pulmonary hemorrhage. In Donn, S. M., & Sinha, S. K. (Eds.) *Manual of Neonatal Respiratory Care* 2nd Edition. Philadelphia: Mosby Elsevier.

Reuter, S., Moser, C., & Baack, M. (2014). Respiratory distress in the newborn. *Pediatrics in Review*, *35*(10), 417–428.

Roberts, D., Brown, J., Medley, N., & Dalziel, S.R . (2017). Antenatal corticosteroids for accelerating fetal lung maturation for women at risk of preterm birth. *Cochrane Database of Systematic Reviews*, Issue 3. Art. No.: CD004454. DOI: 10.1002/14651858.CD004454.pub3

Rojas-Reyes, M. X., Morley, C. J., & Soll, R. (2012). Prophylactic versus selective use of surfactant in preventing morbidity and mortality in preterm infants. *Cochrane Database of Systematic Reviews*, Issue 3. Art. No.: CD000510. DOI: 10.1002/14651858.CD000510.pub2

Sasi, A., & Malhotra, A. (2015). High flow nasal cannula for continuous positive airway pressure weaning in preterm neonates: A single-centre experience. *Journal of Paediatrics and Child Health*, *51*(2), 199–203.

Schumacher, R. E., & Donn, S. M. (2006). Persistent hypertension of the newborn, in Donn, S. M., & Sinha, S. K. (Eds.) *Manual of Neonatal Respiratory Care* 2nd Edition (pp. 183–190). Philadelphia: Mosby Elsevier.

Shalish, W., Kanbar, L. J., Rao, S., Robles-Rubio, C. A., Kovacs, L., Chawla, S., ... & Sant'Anna, G. M. (2017). Prediction of Extubation readiness in extremely preterm infants by the automated analysis of cardiorespiratory behavior: study protocol. *BMC Pediatrics*, *17*(1), 167.

Shetty, S., & Greenough, A. (2014). Neonatal ventilation strategies and long-term respiratory outcomes. *Early Human Development*, *90*(11), 735–739.

Schittny, J. C. (2017). Development of the lung. *Cell and Tissue Research*, *367*(3), 427–444.

Soll, R. F. (2009). Inhaled nitric oxide in the neonate. *Journal of Perinatology*, *29*(S2), S63.

Stevens, T. P., Blennow, M., Myers, E. H., & Soll, R. (2007). Early surfactant administration with brief ventilation vs. selective surfactant and continued mechanical ventilation for preterm infants with or at risk for respiratory distress syndrome. *Cochrane Database of Systematic Reviews*, (4).

Subramaniam, P., Ho, J. J., & Davis, P. G. (2016). Prophylactic nasal continuous positive airway pressure for preventing morbidity and mortality in very preterm infants. *Cochrane Database of Systematic Reviews*, Issue 6. Art. No.: CD001243. DOI: 10.1002/14651858.CD001243.pub3

Sun, H., Xu, F., Xiong, H., Kang, W., Bai, Q., Zhang, Y., ... & Zhu, C. (2013). Characteristics of respiratory distress syndrome in infants of different gestational ages. *Lung*, *191*(4), 425–433.

Sweet, D. G., Carnielli, V., Greisen, G., Hallman, M., Ozek, E., Plavka, R., ... & Visser, G. H. (2017). European consensus guidelines on the management of respiratory distress syndrome-2016 update. *Neonatology*, *111*(2), 107–125.

Thome, U. H., Genzel-Boroviczeny, O., Bohnhorst, B., Schmid, M., Fuchs, H., Rohde, O., ... & Timme, K. (2015). Permissive hypercapnia in extremely low birthweight infants (PHELBI): A randomised controlled multicentre trial. *The Lancet Respiratory Medicine*, *3*(7), 534–543.

Tambe, P., Sammons, H. M., & Choonara, I. (2015). Why do young children die in the UK? A comparison with Sweden. *Archives of disease in childhood*, *100*(10), 928–931.

Tin, W., & Gupta, S. (2007). Optimum oxygen therapy in preterm babies. *Archives of Disease in Childhood: Fetal and Neonatal Edition*, *92*(2), F143–F147.

Turnbull, T., & Petty, J. (2013). Understanding evidence-based thermal care in the low birth weight neonate: Part 1: An overview of principles and current practice. *Nursing Children and Young People*.

Tybulewicz, A. T., Clegg, S. K., Fonfé, G. J., & Stenson, B. J. (2004). Preterm meconium staining of the amniotic fluid: Associated findings and risk of adverse clinical outcome. *Archives of Disease in Childhood – Fetal and Neonatal Edition*, *89*(4), F328–F330.

Vain, N. E., & Batton, D. G. (2017, August). Meconium 'aspiration' (or respiratory distress associated with meconium-stained amniotic fluid?). In *Seminars in Fetal and Neonatal Medicine* (Vol. 22, No. 4, pp. 214–219). WB Saunders.

van Ierland, Y., de Boer, M., & de Beaufort, A. J. (2010). Meconium-stained amniotic fluid: discharge vigorous newborns. *Archives of Disease in Childhood – Fetal and Neonatal Edition, 95*(1), F69–F71.

Veldman, A., Trautschold, T., Weiß, K., Fischer, D., & Bauer, K. (2006). Characteristics and outcome of unplanned extubation in ventilated preterm and term newborns on a neonatal intensive care unit. *Pediatric Anesthesia, 16*(9), 968–973.

Wilkinson, D., Andersen, C., O'Donnell, C. P. F., De Paoli, A. G., & Manley, B. J. (2016). High flow nasal cannula for respiratory support in preterm infants. *Cochrane Database of Systematic Reviews*, Issue 2. Art. No.: CD006405. DOI: 10.1002/14651858.CD006405.pub3

Wiswell, T. E. (2006). Meconium aspiration syndrome. In Donn, S. M., & Sinha, S. K. (Eds.) *Manual of Neonatal Respiratory Care* 2nd Edition. Philadelphia: Mosby Elsevier.

Woodgate, P. G., Flenady, & V. (2001). Tracheal suctioning without disconnection in intubated ventilated neonates. *Cochrane Database of Systematic Reviews*, Issue 2. Art. No.: CD003065. DOI: 10.1002/14651858.CD003065

Wyllie, J., Bruinenberg, J., Roehr, C. C., Rüdiger, M., Trevisanuto, D., & Urlesberger, B. (2015). European Resuscitation Council Guidelines for Resuscitation (2015). Section 7. Resuscitation and support of transition of babies at birth.

13 MANAGEMENT OF CARDIOVASCULAR DISORDERS

Nicky McCarthy and Karen Hoover

CONTENTS

GUIDANCE ON HOW TO ENHANCE PERSONAL LEARNING FROM THIS CHAPTER

Key points covered in this chapter

■ An overview of embryological development of the cardiovascular system, foetal circulation and physiology of the heart.

■ Types of congenital heart disease, their diagnosis and management.

■ Cardiovascular disorders such as blood pressure disturbances and dysrhythmias, and their management.

Reflection

Reading through the chapter, you are encouraged to engage with the key points and related literature in an enquiring way. Ask these questions:

■ How does what you have learned about embryology and cardiac function help you understand the problems of the cardiovascular system newborns can present with?

■ How can you carry out a comprehensive assessment of the cardiovascular system, which may help with the diagnosis of any problems?

■ What do you need to know about the management strategies of the various conditions, to provide good nursing care to affected babies?

Implications for nursing care

■ Finally: how will this chapter enable you to approach the assessment, management and nursing care of neonates with cardiac problems? Consider the implications of what you learn for your daily practice relating to this area.

INTRODUCTION AND BACKGROUND

Cardiovascular disorders are one of the most common challenges that present in the neonatal period. All knowledge of cardiac anatomy and physiology must be considered in the context of a cardiovascular system that is undergoing rapid changes which do not occur at any other time in life. It is imperative to understand the implications of this transition. This chapter will revise embryology, anatomy and physiology, as well as examine common disorders, congenital heart disease and their current management.

INCIDENCE OF CARDIOVASCULAR DISORDERS

Structural heart disease occurs in 8 per 1000 live births (Anderson, 2002), however, the number of newborns affected by acquired heart disease such as endocarditis, metabolic disorders which may involve the heart muscle, as well as neonatal arrhythmias have no reliable data and therefore the true incidence of all neonatal heart disease is as yet unquantifiable (Yates, 2012).

EMBRYOLOGY

The heart is the first functioning organ, beating rhythmically as early as day 22 (Schoenwolf et al., 2014). The heart functions as an efficient organ providing oxygen and nutrients and disposing of carbon dioxide and waste to and from the mother's blood (Moore et al., 2016). Most of the development, remodelling and separation occurs while the heart is pumping blood (Schoenwolf et al., 2014). The development of the heart begins with the formation of two endocardial tubes which fuse, forming a thin endothelial tube which is separated from a thick myocardium by a gelatinous matrix of connective tissue, the cardiac jelly (Moore et al., 2016). Between weeks 4 and 8, the primitive heart tube undergoes a process of looping, remodelling, realignment and separation that transforms the single lumen into four regions which will further develop into the more recognised chambers of the adult heart. As the heart tube lengthens, it develops a series of expansions and shallow sulci that will subdivide into heart chambers at the earliest stages of their development (Schoenwolf et al., 2014). Starting at the caudal end, which is towards the tail of the embryo, these sections of the primitive heart are the sinus venosus, the primitive atrium, the primitive ventricle, the bulbus cordis and the truncus arteriosus (see figure 13.1).

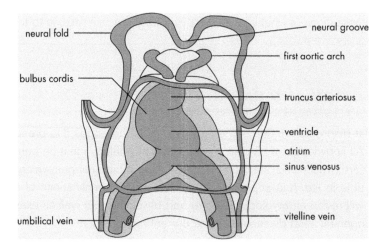

Figure 13.1 Differentiation of the regions in the primitive heart tube

The bulbus cordis and the ventricle grow more rapidly than the other regions, which are restricted by the pericardium. This causes the tube to loop and fold, resulting in an S-shaping (Tortora and Derrickson, 2011). Essentially, the heart folding involves the bulbus cordis and truncus arteriosus travelling forwards and downwards, and the primitive atrium and primitive ventricles being pushed upwards and backwards. The end result of this cardiac modulation is to bring the four chambers of the future heart into the correct position (figure 13.2). The remainder of the heart development consists of remodelling these chambers, developing the septa and valves between them, and forming the epicardium, coronary vasculature and cardiac innervation and conducting system (Schoenwolf et al., 2014).

Partitioning of the heart into four chambers is accomplished through the formation of walls (septa) in the primitive atrium, ventricles and outflow tract (Schoenwolf et al., 2014). By the 5th week, endothelial cushions appear and function as primitive valves that assist the forward propulsion of blood (Carlson, 2014). The primitive atrium is divided into the right and left atria by the formation of two septa; the septum primum and septum secundum. The septum primum develops downwards from the roof of the common atrium towards the endocardial cushions. Before a complete closure of the connection between the right and left atrium, an opening develops in the mid-section in this newly formed wall; this is called the foramen secundum (Moore et al., 2016). As the septum secundum, a more muscular structure, then begins a similar descent from the roof alongside the septum primum, a communication between both atria remains open; this is called the foramen primum. Once both septa have formed, they leave an oval-shaped orifice, the foramen ovale (FO), through which for the rest of foetal development, blood shunts from the right atrium across to the left atrium. Blood cannot travel back in the opposite direction, as the foramen secundum acts as a block when pushed against the muscular septum secundum (Schoenwolf et al., 2014; Moore et al., 2016).

While the interatrial septa are forming, a muscular interventricular septum begins to grow between the ballooning right and left ventricle towards the atrioventricular cushions.

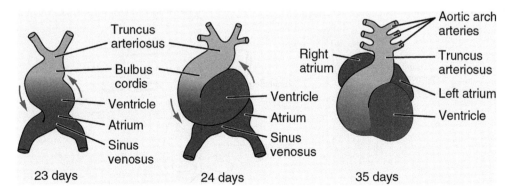

Figure 13.2 Bending of the primitive heart and orientation of the atria and ventricles in their final adult position (Source: Creative Commons)

The intraventricular foramen is present initially, but this is obliterated by the growth of the muscular interventricular septum (Carlson, 2014). The protrusion of the muscular interventricular septum is formed as the expanding walls of the right and left ventricles become more closely opposed to each other (Schoenwolf et al., 2014). The formation of the outflow tracts begin with the single lumen, the bulbus cordis. By the time the interventricular septum begins to form, this single tube has elongated and divided. Although initially there is a single channel within this tube, due to the direction of flow through it, the tract divides into separate aortic and pulmonary channels. As they are shaped by the spiral flow of blood during the partitioning, they develop into a helical arrangement, the ridges finally meeting and separating the lumen into two channels (figure 13.3) (Schoenwolf et al., 2014). The sinus venosus becomes integrated with the right atrium and forms the **inferior** vena cava (IVC) and **superior** vena cava (SVC) by the end of the fifth week (Schoenwolf et al., 2014). Aortic and pulmonary artery valves and the atrioventricular valves, namely the mitral and triscuspid valves, form from subendothelial tissue, and their function is to prevent blood from washing back (Carlson, 2014).

The heart has to function as soon as it forms. Rhythmic waves of electric depolarisation that trigger the myocardium to contract spontaneously arise from the cardiac muscle itself and spread from cell to cell (Schoenwolf et al., 2014). This results in the primitive heart tube cardiomyocytes contracting asynchronously. A cluster of cells that migrate from the sinus venosus into the right atrium take over the pacemaker activity and develop into the sinoatrial node. Soon after the development of the sinoatrial node, cells within the atrioventricular junction begin to form a secondary pacemaker: the atrioventricular node. This node regulates the conduction of impulses from the atrium to the ventricles. Simultaneously, from the atrioventricular node, the bundle of His is then formed and this is followed by the development of the Purkinje fibres. This produces a conductive system for the heart (Schoenwolf et al., 2014).

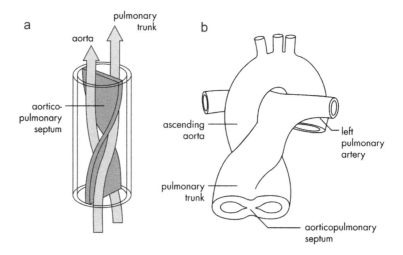

Figure 13.3 Heart development

PHYSIOLOGY

The understanding of cardiovascular physiology will assist the neonatal nurse's ability to assess, interpret and plan management for the neonate displaying signs and symptoms of a congenital or an acquired cardiovascular disorder.

Foetal circulation

The foetal circulation is quite different from the neonatal circulation; it comprises two umbilical arteries bringing deoxygenated blood to the placenta, and a single umbilical vein carrying oxygenated blood back to the heart (Levene et al., 2008). Oxygenated blood travels from the placenta through the umbilical vein, where it meets the first of three foetal shunts: the ductus venosus which diverts the blood away from the liver. The blood then moves to the right atrium, where most of it flows through the second foetal shunt, the FO, straight into the left atrium. This foetal shunt effectively bypasses the pulmonary circulation. The blood then flows into the left ventricle, where it is pumped into the aorta and around the body. Not all of the blood that enters the right atrium is shunted through the FO; instead, it enters the right ventricle and leaves the heart via the pulmonary artery, where it meets the third and final foetal shunt, the ductus arteriosus (DA). This shunt directs most of the blood away from the lungs and into the aorta (figure 13.4). Only 7% of the combined ventricular output of blood actually passes into the lungs (Levene et al., 2008). The mechanism allowing blood to be shunted away from the lungs is facilitated by the high pulmonary pressure as a result of the fluid-filled foetal lung. Therefore, the blood is taking the path of least resistance in every case. Consequently, unlike in the adult heart, the right ventricle is the dominant chamber *in utero*, and is ejecting 66% of the combined ventricular output (Levene et al., 2008).

Cardiovascular adaptations are required to survive extrauterine life. When an infant breathes for the first time at birth, the fluid in the lungs is expelled by the generation of significant negative pressures (60–90cmH$_2$O). This fluid is absorbed through the pulmonary lymphatics and capillaries over the first 6–12 hours of life (Levene et al., 2008). Lung aeration triggers the cardiovascular transition at birth by decreasing pulmonary vascular resistance, which allows for increased pulmonary blood flow. There is a decrease in the pressure on the right side of the heart due to the reduction in pulmonary pressure. As a consequence of this pressure change, blood no longer crosses from the right to the left atrium through the FO, which results in its closure. Hereafter it is referred to as the fossa ovalis. There is decreased blood flow in the IVC resulting in the closure of the ductus venosus, which becomes the ligamentum teres. The umbilical vessels take longer to become obliterated and may still be cannulated up to 10 days after birth (Levene et al., 2008). The increase in the concentration of oxygen in the blood leads to a decrease in circulating prostaglandins and causes the closure of the DA. Blood is now prevented from bypassing the pulmonary circulation, and the newly operational lungs must oxygenate the infant's blood.

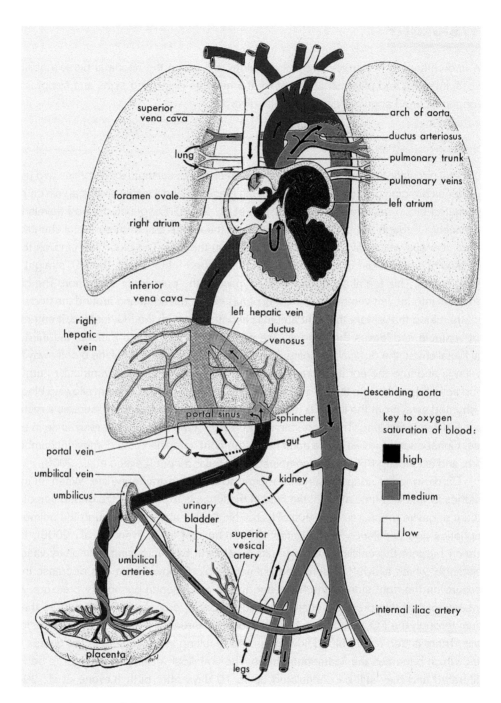

Figure 13.4 Foetal circulation

Cardiac cycle

A single cardiac cycle includes all of the events associated with one heartbeat. One full cardiac cycle consists of systole and diastole of the atria, plus systole and diastole of the ventricles (Tortora and Derrickson, 2011). During atrial systole, the atria are contracting, and at the same time the ventricles are relaxed. During atrial diastole the atria are relaxed while at the same time ventricular systole is occurring, which means the ventricles are contracting (Tortora and Derrickson, 2011). Blood fills both atria simultaneously: the IVC and SVC fill the right atrium, and the pulmonary veins fill the left atrium. The sinoatrial node is stimulated and sends an impulse to contract across the atria; this causes the blood to be ejected into the ventricles through the atrioventricular valves. The atrioventricular node is then stimulated by this contraction, and it in turn emits an impulse of contraction down the Purkinje fibres, stimulating the contraction of the ventricles and the expulsion of the blood into the pulmonary artery and aorta. The heart relaxes, and this is the completion of one cardiac cycle (Tortora and Derrickson, 2011).

Cardiac output

Cardiac output (CO) is the total amount of blood ejected from both ventricles, and is dependent upon **stroke volume** (SV) and heart rate (HR)

$$CO = SV \times HR$$

SV is the total amount of blood leaving the ventricles in one heart beat and is dependent upon the stretch undergone by individual heart myofibres.

$$SV = preload + afterload + contractility$$

Preload represents the passive stretching of the resting heart prior to ventricular filling. The myocardium contracts efficiently at certain preload volumes. If filling increases, the cardiac muscle fibres are stretched, leading to an increase in the force of the ventricular muscle contraction. This is known as the Frank-Starling Law (Noble, 2009). Overfilling or underfilling can cause the contractions to be less effective (Levene et al., 2008).

Afterload is pressure against which the heart has to work to eject the blood from both ventricles. The afterload effect on the left ventricle is determined by the aortic pressure, and the afterload effect on the right ventricle must exceed the pressure in the pulmonary trunk. Essentially, afterload is the resistance the heart must pump against and is dependent on peripheral vascular resistance and the viscosity of the blood (Sinha et al., 2018).

Contractility is the metabolic state of the heart muscle itself and is independent of pre- and afterload. CO can be increased by increasing myocardial contractility (inotropy) or increasing the HR (chronotropy). These changes are mediated through adrenergic receptors, either α, β, or dopaminergic receptors. β_1 stimulation increases myocardial contractility and heart rate; β_2 stimulation increases pulmonary and systemic vasodilation; and α_1 stimulation causes arteriolar constriction. Dopaminergic stimulation causes vasodilation

TABLE 13.1 ADRENERGIC RECEPTORS, THEIR AGONISTS AND ANTAGONISTS

	α_1	α_2	β_1	β_2	β_3
Adrenaline	+	+	+	+	+
Noradrenaline	+	+	+		
Isoprenaline			+	+	+
Dopamine	+	+	+		
Dobutamine			+		
Salbutamol				+	
Propranolol			-	(-)	
Labetalol	-		-	-	

in vascular beds such as the kidney, brain and gut (Sinha et al., 2018). The increase in contractility produced by β-adrenoceptor stimulation can be mimicked by drugs such as dopamine and dobutamine, which are described as positive inotropes (ibid). A complete list of drugs used in the management of cardiovascular disorders appears in table 13.1.

Heart rate

Cardiac excitation originates in the sinoatrial node, spreads through the atrial muscle to the atrioventricular node and after a short delay progresses down the bundle of His to bring about depolarisation of the ventricular muscle (Noble, 2009). The individual parts of the heart each have an intrinsic rhythm of their own, but the rate of the heart is dominated by the part with the faster rhythm, the sinoatrial node. The sympathetic and parasympathetic nerves modify HR (Noble, 2009). The accelerans nerve provides sympathetic input to the heart by releasing noradrenaline onto the cells of the sinoatrial node, which in turn increases HR, while the vagus nerve provides parasympathetic input on the sinoatrial node by releasing acetylcholine, reducing HR (Tortora and Derrickson, 2011). This effect can be mimicked by agonists such as adrenaline and isoprenaline and can be blocked by propranolol (see table 13.1; Noble, 2009). Other sensory receptors that provide input into the cardiovascular centre include **chemoreceptors** which monitor chemical changes in the blood, and **baroreceptors** which monitor the stretching of major arteries and veins (Tortora and Derrickson, 2011). Receptors in the arch of the aorta and carotid arteries detect changes in blood pressure and provide this information to the cardiovascular centre. There are also chemicals that regulate HR: hypoxia, acidosis and alkalosis all depress cardiac activity.

Cations (positively charged ions) modulate HR. Sodium and potassium are crucial for the production of action potentials in all nerve and muscle fibres; it is important to know that ionic imbalances can quickly compromise the pumping effectiveness of the heart (Tortora and Derrickson, 2011).

Blood pressure

Blood pressure (BP) is the product of flow and resistance according to the formula

Blood pressure = blood flow x peripheral resistance (Levene et al., 2008)

The resistance in peripheral circulation is controlled by the pressure in the arterioles. They constitute the greatest resistance to flow of any segment of the circulation. This means that the peripheral circulatory control is dependent on arteriolar smooth muscle contraction (Noble, 2009). They are stimulated to contract or dilate by various endothelial factors, local metabolites, blood-borne hormones and neuronal stimulus.

■ *Endothelial factor* Nitric oxide (NO) has a vasodilator action and is produced continuously in the blood vessel walls. The main stimulus is the friction of the blood flowing within the vessels, as well as some blood-borne agonists such as acetylcholine, bradykinin and thrombin. Chemical mediators such as cytokines also stimulate NO (Noble, 2009). Cytokines are released during an inflammatory response, as for example in septic shock; if substantial amounts are released, cytokines cause excessive vasodilation, which can in turn cause the blood pressure to drop. This is seen commonly in babies with sepsis.

■ *Local metabolites* During periods of increased metabolic activity, accumulation of hydrogen, carbon dioxide and lactic acid will have a local effect and relax the smooth muscle around it, leading to increased blood flow in that area, which will flush out these accumulated metabolites (Noble, 2009).

■ *Blood-borne hormone* The rennin-angiotensin system is a potent systemic pressor. The renin system is functional in the foetus, and activity increases at birth helping to maintain BP. Figure 13.5 details the function of the renin-angiotensin system.

■ *Neural control* The baroreceptor reflex is guided by the major receptors of high pressure located in the carotid sinus and the aortic arch. Baroreceptors are modified nerve endings sensitive to stretch – when arterial pressure rises, the vessel becomes inflated and the nerve endings are stretched. In the glossopharyngeal nerve for example, the increase in stretch passes along via the cranial nerve into the medulla of the brain. The medulla and hypothalamus process this information and organise an autonomic response (Noble, 2009).

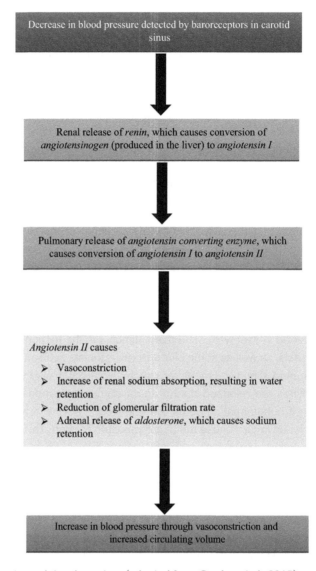

Figure 13.5 The renin-angiotensin system (adapted from Gordan et al., 2015)

CONGENITAL HEART DEFECTS

Congenital heart disease (CHD) is the most common congenital anomaly. 25% of all CHD cases are classified as critical (CCHD, see table 13.2), meaning defects that require surgery or will result in death in the first 28 days of life (Carvalho, 2016). Such defects rely on the patency of the DA to maintain pulmonary or systemic blood flow. Affected infants show little evidence of cardiovascular compromise on examination in the first 24–48 hours while the DA is open and may not become unwell until discharged home. CCHD is increasingly diagnosed antenatally, facilitating planning of the baby's delivery in a tertiary centre with access to paediatric cardiology, to optimise neonatal management (Mellander, 2013). Babies with CCHD delivered outside tertiary units, where appropriate intervention is not immediately available, have much higher mortality rates (Eckersley et al., 2016), unless there is close liaison with paediatric cardiology (Anagnostou et al., 2013). Improved outcomes for babies who not so long ago died in infancy mean that there is now a population of adult CHD survivors who outnumber the children born with CHD. Many of these adults have lifelong health problems (Mussa and Baron, 2017).

TABLE 13.2 CRITICAL CONGENITAL HEART DISEASE

	Defect	Presentation
Duct-dependent pulmonary circulation	Pulmonary Atresia or Critical Pulmonary **Stenosis** Tetralogy of Fallot (ToF) Tricuspid Atresia	Cyanosis unresponsive to oxygen and worsening hypoxia as DA closes
Duct-dependent systemic circulation	Coarctation of Aorta (CoA) Interrupted Aortic Arch (IAA) Critical Aortic Stenosis Hypoplastic Left Heart Syndrome (HLHS)	Shock as DA closes, but usually normal oxygen saturation Absent or reduced femoral pulses
Duct-dependent pulmonary and systemic circulation	Transposition of the Great Arteries (TGA)	Severe cyanosis and deterioration from birth
Non-duct-dependent	Obstructed Total Anomalous Pulmonary Venous Return (TAPVR)	Similar to severe persistent pulmonary hypertension of the newborn (PPHN)

(adapted from Morris, 2015)

Risk factors for congenital heart defects

- *Prematurity* Excluding isolated patent DA, the risk of CHD is higher in babies born prior to 37 weeks' gestation (Tanner et al., 2005).
- *Family history* The risk of CHD increases threefold when a first-degree relative (parent or sibling) is affected (Øyen et al., 2009).
- *Genetic syndromes* Around 20% of babies with CHD have chromosomal abnormalities or a syndrome, see table 13.3 (Hartman et al., 2011).
- *Maternal conditions* A number of maternal conditions are associated with CHD, and these include diabetes mellitus, connective tissue disorders and systemic lupus erythematosus. Maternal medications known to cause foetal cardiac defects (such as lithium, sodium valproate) are no longer prescribed for pregnant women (Liu et al., 2013).

Presentation

DYSMORPHIC FEATURES

Any dysmorphic features can cause anxiety for the parents and healthcare professionals. Such babies must be examined carefully, and a full cardiac examination is indicated if any features associated with congenital heart disease (CHD) are noted.

TABLE 13.3 COMMON GENETIC SYNDROMES AND THEIR ASSOCIATION WITH CHD

Disorder	Most common CHD	Percentage affected
Trisomy 21	Atrioventricular septal defect (AVSD)	45% of babies with Trisomy 21 have an AVSD, but 80% of babies with AVSD will have Trisomy 21
Turner's syndrome (XO)	Coarctation of the aorta	50% have CHD, of which 15% will have coarctation of the aorta
22q11 deletion syndrome	Tetralogy of Fallot Interrupted aortic arch	74% have CHD, of which 20% have tetralogy of Fallot Up to 90% of interrupted aortic arch patients will have 22q11 deletion
Williams syndrome (7q11.23 deletion)	Supravalvular aortic stenosis	80% have CHD, of which 75% have aortic stenosis
Noonan's syndrome	Pulmonary stenosis	60% have pulmonary stenosis

(adapted from Metcalfe, 2018)

If CHD is diagnosed, the baby must be carefully examined for additional birth defects in other systems, as identifying a pattern of defects can indicate a specific syndrome (Aboliras et al., 2018).

ABNORMAL PULSE OXIMETRY

At present there is no mandatory national policy for newborns to have pulse oximetry screening (POS) routinely. It has increased diagnosis of babies with CCHD, where the baby may be liable to collapse in the first week after birth when the DA closes. It measures the oxygen saturation in the right hand (pre-ductal) and either foot (post-ductal). Both saturation levels should be greater than 95% *and* the difference between them less than 3%.

POS is performed on babies in the UK as early as 4–6 hours after birth, and this has resulted in a higher false positive rate (i.e. an abnormal POS that is not due to CHD) compared to countries where the screening is done after 24 hours. The reason for this is that in the first 12–24 hours, the baby is in a transitional circulatory state, and the foetal high pulmonary pressures may not have fallen enough to enable full oxygenation in the early postnatal period. POS is best at diagnosing cyanotic CHD, where low saturations will be apparent from birth but the baby does not show any signs of distress because the DA is allowing pulmonary blood flow (Ewer et al., 2011; Ismail et al., 2017). It is not so accurate at detecting defects that result in obstruction of blood flow to the systemic circulation, because these babies often have normal saturations in the first few days while the DA is open (Lannering et al., 2015). However, in conjunction with antenatal scans and the post-natal examination, POS markedly increases detection of CCHD in babies before discharge, reducing the risk of potential collapse at home (Ismail et al., 2017).

CYANOSIS

The appearance of blue or purple colouration of the skin or mucous membranes best defines cyanosis, and in a newborn is usually perceived when arterial oxygen saturation is less than 85% (Steinhorn, 2008). Peripheral cyanosis is common in the newborn, but central cyanosis may be caused by a structural cardiac disease. Facial **petechiae** may give the appearance of cyanosis as well as severely polycythaemic infants. The grey pallor of anaemia and/or desaturation or the slate black or grey colour of methaemoglobinaemia may mistakenly be taken for cyanosis (Yates, 2012).

RESPIRATORY EFFORT

The presence of respiratory signs often makes the differentiation of cardiac problems from respiratory problems challenging. As in infants with pulmonary disease, the infant with CHD may present with signs such as tachypnoea, recession and nasal flaring. A slow breathing pattern with increased respiratory depth, however, has been described in infants with poor pulmonary blood flow as found in cyanotic lesions. Grunting is not usually a sign of CHD, unless the baby's condition is rapidly deteriorating, so that this should trigger the investigation of pulmonary causes for respiratory distress (Theorell, 2002).

MURMUR

A heart murmur is a noise additional to the normal heart sounds, often described to have a 'whooshing' quality, caused by turbulent blood flow. In the case of an 'innocent' (non-pathological) murmur, this is the normal flow of blood through the heart (Frank and Jacobe, 2011). Murmurs are detected during routine examination in approximately 3–4% of newborns. Of these cases, 50% are due to CHD (Ainsworth et al., 1999; Mirzarahimi et al., 2011). Four areas on the chest are auscultated during examination; as these relate to the locations of the cardiac valves, they can provide some information about the potential cause of the murmur. The murmur is furthermore evaluated according to its loudness, duration, pitch and the presence of any added sounds, and some such 'grades' of murmurs may be more strongly associated with underlying CHD than others (Frank and Jacobe, 2011). However, as very serious cardiac conditions may have an unimpressive or even no murmur, careful examination of the infant is necessary in every case, and further investigations may be indicated (Yates, 2012).

PULSES

A neonate's pulses should be equal in upper and lower limbs, and right and left. While weak pulses may be a sign of shock, they can also be indicative of an impairment of systemic blood flow. This is particularly the case if upper limb pulses are stronger than lower limb pulses, so that they should be palpated simultaneously. Very easily palpable, or 'bounding' pulses are found in conditions with wide pulse pressures, such as a PDA. This may be better appreciated in the palmar and pedal pulses than the commonly palpated femoral pulses (Theorell, 2002).

FAILURE TO THRIVE

As infants with CHD have increased metabolic demands, one of the presenting signs may be failure to thrive (Teitel, 2016). This would not be apparent in the immediate neonatal period but may be seen in the infant who does not regain birth weight, or some longer-term neonatal unit (NNU) patients. A detailed feeding history obtained from the parents may contain further clues – CHD often results in breathlessness during feeding (Theorell, 2002).

DIAPHORESIS

Neural and hormonal mechanisms are activated to maintain the increased CO, and this results in tachycardia and **diaphoresis** (sweating). Diaphoresis occurs mainly on the forehead and scalp when the baby is feeding (Teitel, 2016).

HEPATOMEGALY

Babies with increased pulmonary blood flow present in heart failure in the first 2–6 weeks after birth when the pulmonary vascular resistance falls and pulmonary blood flow increases. This increased blood volume results in hepatomegaly – the liver enlarges to accommodate excess fluid (Teitel, 2016).

Diagnosis of CHD

ANTENATAL SCREENING SCANS

Foetal ultrasound scans are a routine element of antenatal care. In the UK, pregnant women are offered two ultrasound scans; first, the dating scan at 8–14 weeks, and second, the anomaly scan at 18–21 weeks. The dating scan includes a nuchal translucency measurement, which is part of the combined screening for Down's syndrome. The anomaly scan includes a screen of the cardiac anatomy, with a four-chamber view. The four-chamber view will detect less than 50% of cases of structural heart lesions even in experienced hands (Bull, 1999; Singh and McGeoch, 2016). Particularly defects such as coarctation of the aorta are notoriously difficult to diagnose (Singh and McGeoch, 2016). If views of the outflow tract are obtained in addition to the four-chamber view, the range of abnormalities detected is increased (Carvalho et al., 2002). Foetuses with a suspicion of cardiac defects or other abnormalities are referred for a foetal echocardiogram (Singh and McGeoch, 2016).

NEWBORN EXAMINATION

This is done for all babies within the first 72 hours of birth, and usually earlier, before discharge from hospital. Part of the examination is evaluation of the cardiovascular system for murmurs and palpation of the femoral pulses. However, this examination only detects up 50% of babies with CHD, because a murmur may not be present even in the most serious defects, and many infants with murmurs do not have CHD (Ainsworth et al., 1999; Mirzarahimi et al., 2011). Also, the femoral pulses are present in babies with CCHD due to obstruction to the systemic blood flow until the DA closes, which may not be until after discharge from hospital (Wren et al., 1999).

The incorporation of POS into the newborn examination has improved detection rates of CCHD (see above).

HYPEROXIA TEST

This, now less commonly utilised diagnostic tool, is used to support a diagnosis of cyanotic CHD. The baby is placed in 100% oxygen for 10 minutes. A PaO_2 (arterial) less than 15kPa is seen in cyanotic CHD, but this cannot exclude lesions where there is a lot of mixing of deoxygenated and oxygenated blood, such as total anomalous pulmonary venous return (TAPVR) and tetralogy of Fallot. Nor can it exclude pulmonary disease (Morris, 2015).

CHEST X-RAY AND ELECTROCARDIOGRAM

Chest X-rays are easily available, and – at little cost – allow the additional information of visceral situs (the arrangement of the organs relative to the midline), cardiac position, cardiac size and shape, and bony abnormalities. A 12-lead electrocardiogram (ECG) provides information on the rhythm, atrial position and any enlargement, as well as the ventricular position, hypertrophy and ischaemia (Yates, 2012). Neither, however, are usually helpful in the immediate diagnosis of CCHD and can appear normal in life-threatening duct-dependent lesions (Mellander, 2013).

ECHOCARDIOGRAM

This is the gold standard diagnostic tool to rule out or definitively confirm CCHD. It is a non-invasive investigation which provides information about cardiac structure and overall function (Yates, 2012). Most NNUs have access to this and staff trained to perform it in an emergency (Mellander, 2013).

Duct-dependent pulmonary circulation

When there is an obstructive lesion affecting the right side of the heart, this means that the baby is dependent on a patent DA to perfuse the lungs (pulmonary circulation). Unlike the other foetal shunts, the DA does not close as soon as the cord is cut, but constricts over 12–48 hours (Rudolph, 2010). In duct-dependent pulmonary circulation, blood can only reach the lungs by travelling from the aorta through the DA and into the pulmonary arteries (refer back to figure 13.4 for foetal circulation). Obstruction to blood flow in the right side of the heart means that deoxygenated blood coming back from the head (via the SVC) and body (via the IVC) cannot get to the lungs to be oxygenated. It is shunted through the FO to the left side of the heart to enter the aorta and subsequently returns to the lungs via the DA.

Babies with duct-dependent pulmonary circulation usually have cyanosis, which is unresponsive to oxygen supplementation, from birth or within the first few days, and deteriorate as the DA closes. Detection is usually by POS in the first day of life, or as babies are noted to be cyanotic soon after birth. They may be tachypnoeic but are often described as 'comfortably tachypnoeic' without other signs of respiratory distress, and a normal carbon dioxide level even though oxygen saturations may be around 80–85% (Teitel,

2016). However, once the DA closes, the blood flow to the lungs is severely compromised and the baby will rapidly deteriorate with increasing hypoxia and metabolic acidosis (Mellander, 2013).

A number of heart defects associated with obstruction to blood flow to the lungs from the right side of the heart are discussed below.

PULMONARY ATRESIA OR CRITICAL PULMONARY STENOSIS

The pulmonary artery is blocked or severely narrow, and blood can only reach the lungs by access to the left ventricle (see figure 13.6). This can be via a large ventricular septal defect (VSD), patent FO or, in many cases, is totally dependent on blood flow in the aorta entering the DA and subsequently the lungs. Surgical management is usually total repair with valve replacement, although catheter intervention to dilate the valve may be used in pulmonary stenosis (Mellander, 2013).

TETRALOGY OF FALLOT

Tetralogy of Fallot is a severe form of pulmonary atresia where there are four defects: pulmonary stenosis (or atresia), a large VSD, an overriding aorta which sits over the VSD, and right ventricular hypertrophy (see figure 13.7). The degree of cyanosis will depend on how obstructed the pulmonary artery is; the greater the obstruction, the earlier the presentation. Complete repair is usually done in the neonatal period, but some patients may need a pulmonary artery shunt to increase pulmonary blood flow (Mellander, 2013). Tetralogy of Fallot is associated with a number of genetic syndromes (Burger et al., 2015; see table 13.3).

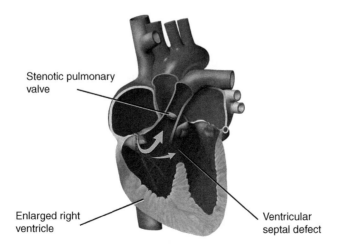

Stenotic pulmonary valve

Enlarged right ventricle

Ventricular septal defect

Figure 13.6 Pulmonary atresia (Source: Centers of Disease Control and Prevention, National Center on Birth Defects and Developmental Disabilities)

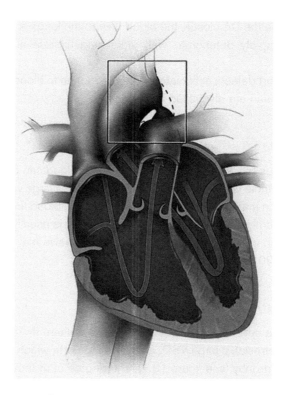

Figure 13.7 Tetralogy of Fallot (Source: Centers of Disease Control and Prevention, National Center on Birth Defects and Developmental Disabilities)

TRICUSPID ATRESIA

In tricuspid atresia the tricuspid valve has not formed so there is obstruction to blood entering the right ventricle. In the most common form, these babies have a large VSD and pulmonary stenosis, so although blood can get to the pulmonary artery via the FO and through the VSD, flow up the pulmonary artery is restricted by the narrowing and instead it enters the aorta and through the DA flows to the lungs. These patients often require staged operations in the first few years to achieve suitable systemic and pulmonary circulation (Mellander, 2013).

Duct-dependent systemic circulation

Babies with left heart obstructions are usually well until the DA closes, as this is the only means of blood reaching the aorta and thus systemic circulation from the pulmonary artery. Thereafter, blood flow through the aorta to the body is reduced or absent, and metabolic acidosis rapidly ensues. Femoral pulses will be absent or severely reduced in volume. These babies usually pass POS, as there is no problem with blood flow to the lungs and, while the DA is open, adequate systemic blood flow is present. All newborns who present with a sepsis-like picture with metabolic acidosis, tachycardia, tachypnoea and poor perfusion (i.e.

grey, mottled skin with slow capillary refill time) should have a left heart obstruction ruled out and prostaglandin commenced if they continue to deteriorate despite adequate management strategies (Mellander, 2013).

The heart defects associated with obstruction to blood flow to the body from the left side of the heart are described below.

COARCTATION OF THE AORTA

In coarctation of the aorta, there is a narrowing of the aorta usually opposite the DA (see figure 13.8). When the DA is open, flow to the lower body from the aorta is normal, but once it closes the narrowing is 'unmasked' and flow to the lower limbs severely compromised. This results in tissue hypoxia leading to a metabolic acidosis, which presents initially with tachypnoea with rapid progression to hypotension, and worsening acidosis (Joshi et al., 2017). Half of all infants with coarctation of the aorta have a normal newborn examination and pass POS, but present in cardiovascular failure after discharge home (Wren et al., 1999). Babies with aortic coarctation present with weak or absent femoral pulses and oxygen saturations higher in the upper compared to the lower limbs. Non-invasive measurement

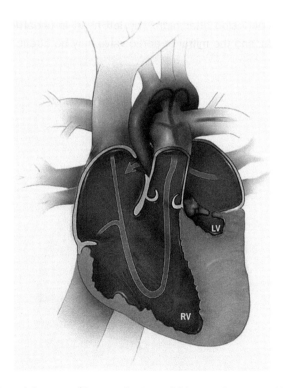

Figure 13.8 Coarctation of the aorta (Source: Centers of Disease Control and Prevention, National Center on Birth Defects and Developmental Disabilities)

of 4-limb blood pressures may show decreased values in the legs compared to the arms, however, these results may not be reliable due to factors such as movement, and incorrect sizing and placement of the cuff. Therefore, it has been proposed that comparing pulse volume in upper and lower limbs provides the same information with less scope for error (Joshi et al., 2017). Surgical repair of coarctation of the aorta is done in the newborn period (Mellander, 2013).

INTERRUPTED AORTIC ARCH

Interrupted aortic arch (IAA) is an extreme form of coarctation of the aorta, where a segment of the aortic arch is missing. It nearly always occurs with other cardiac defects and is strongly associated with 22q11 deletion syndrome (Hartmann et al., 2011). The DA forms the 'arch' to supply blood to the lower body, but when it closes, flow ceases and the baby rapidly deteriorates, presenting with signs of low CO as in coarctation of the aorta. Surgical repair is usually done in the newborn period (Mellander, 2013).

HYPOPLASTIC LEFT HEART SYNDROME

Hypoplastic left heart syndrome (HLHS) is the most common defect that presents with inadequate systemic perfusion after birth. The left heart is underdeveloped, with a small left ventricle and aorta, and the mitral or aortic valve may be atretic (see figure 13.9). This

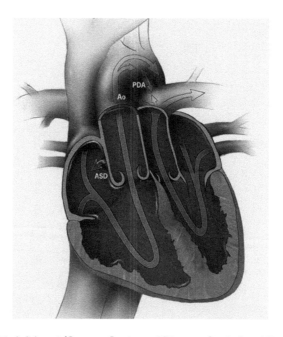

Figure 13.9 Hypoplastic left heart (Source: Centers of Disease Control and Prevention, National Center on Birth Defects and Developmental Disabilities)

means the left side of the heart cannot support the systemic circulation and survival is only possible when some of the blood entering the pulmonary artery goes through the DA to reach the brain and lower body. In addition, blood returning to the left atrium from the lungs can only reach the systemic circulation by crossing into the right atrium through the FO and up the pulmonary artery to the DA, and again to the brain and rest of the body. Without a patent DA, the baby will die soon after birth (Mussa and Barron, 2017).

These babies are often well initially because the DA allows flow to the systemic circulation. However, pulmonary blood flow is increased because blood destined for the aorta is entering the pulmonary artery, and the baby will develop respiratory symptoms as pulmonary vascular resistance decreases and blood flow to the lungs increases (Mellander, 2013). Compounding this developing situation, as the DA closes and flow to the systemic circulation is reduced, the baby presents with signs of shock. Babies with HLHS deteriorate much more quickly if they are administered oxygen because its vasodilatory effect allows increased blood flow to the lungs at the expense of the systemic circulation. This results in a paradoxical situation where the baby has oxygen saturations near 95% because of the high pulmonary blood flow yet looks pale and mottled with an increasing metabolic acidosis and elevated lactate as the systemic circulation is compromised.

Oxygen saturations are therefore maintained at 75–85% in HLHS preoperatively, as any higher can indicate pulmonary over-circulation and clinical deterioration (Daily et al., 2018).

Improving antenatal diagnosis has led to a reduction in the number of babies born with HLHS (Mellander, 2013). However, surgical repair involves three major operations in the first few years of life, and although prognosis has improved over the past 5–10 years, many of these children have ongoing health problems, placing considerable strain on families (Mussa and Baron, 2017).

CRITICAL AORTIC STENOSIS

In this condition, the aortic valve is narrowed and flow to the systemic circulation is markedly reduced when the DA closes. This presents in neonates when the narrowing is severe, and it is likely to be associated with HLHS. The valve can be dilated through catheter-based intervention (Mellander, 2013).

Duct-dependent pulmonary and systemic circulation

TRANSPOSITION OF THE GREAT ARTERIES

Transposition of the great arteries (TGA) is the most common cyanotic CHD in the neonatal period. The aorta and pulmonary artery are 'transposed' to the wrong ventricle and therefore result in a parallel circulation, where blood returning from the lungs into the left heart goes up the pulmonary artery (when it should be the aorta) and back to the lungs; and blood returning back from the body to the right heart goes up the aorta (when it should be the

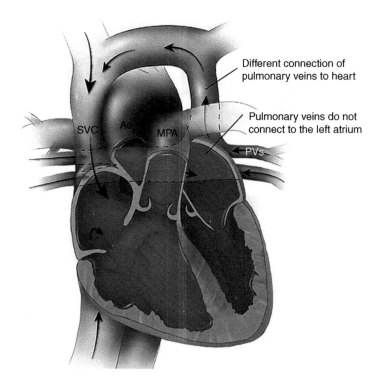

Figure 13.10 Transposition of the great arteries (Source: Centers of Disease Control and Prevention, National Center on Birth Defects and Developmental Disabilities)

pulmonary artery; see figure 13.10). This is demonstrated in saturations which are higher in the feet (post-ductal) than the right hand (pre-ductal) because of the reversed relationship of the great arteries (Teitel, 2016). These babies present with profound cyanosis and hypoxaemia after birth, and survival depends on the degree of mixing of the circulation; the less this occurs, the sooner the baby will present. In fact, the earlier the cyanosis in babies with CHD, the more likely it is due to TGA (Teitel, 2016).

In most cases, the only way blood can mix is through a patent FO, and this can be very small (restrictive) in some cases, allowing little mixing. The DA shunt indirectly increases aortic blood flow via higher pulmonary blood flow (Vaujois et al., 2017) and keeping it patent with a prostaglandin infusion will help the baby with a non-restricted FO, but it will not sustain life if this is restrictive. In these babies, the FO must be widened as a matter of urgency. This is done by with a Raskind's septostomy and can be done at the bedside under ultrasound guidance. A catheter with a balloon is inserted in the femoral vein and threaded into the IVC and right atrium and across the FO to the left atrium. The balloon is then inflated, and the catheter pulled back sharply, causing a tear in the atrial wall. This allows mixing of oxygenated blood in the left atrium with blood in the right atrium and stabilises the baby prior to surgery to 'switch' the arteries around to their correct place (Mellander, 2013).

Non-duct-dependent CCHD

OBSTRUCTED TOTAL ANOMALOUS PULMONARY VENOUS RETURN

In this uncommon defect, the four pulmonary veins, which normally bring oxygenated blood back from the lungs to the left atrium, enter the right atrium (see figure 13.11). The veins can take a number of routes to do this, but in obstructed total anomalous pulmonary venous return (TAPVR) this is via a connecting vein which runs down to below the diaphragm through the ductus venosus, and into the IVC. Once blood is in the right atrium, it will cross the FO to enter the left heart and be pumped to the systemic circulation. The ductus venosus becomes obstructed at birth, because as a foetal shunt it allows blood from the placenta to bypass the liver and enter the right atrium. However, once the cord is cut, it begins to constrict, and this results in blood from the connecting vein backing up into the lungs, resulting in severe pulmonary oedema and hypoxaemia (Mellander, 2013.)

These babies present in a critical condition soon after birth, with marked respiratory distress and cyanosis, and are often thought to have PPHN. Although it can be difficult to differentiate between these two causes, the history of poor condition at birth or meconium aspiration may point to PPHN. However, an echocardiogram should be performed on all babies with suspected PPHN, especially if they do not improve with conventional therapy such as nitric oxide. Prostaglandin will help dilate the ductus venosus to relieve the obstruction to blood flow back to the heart, but it may not improve the situation, so that these babies need urgent surgery to connect the pulmonary veins to the left atrium. Although

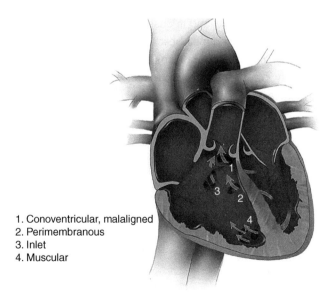

1. Conoventricular, malaligned
2. Perimembranous
3. Inlet
4. Muscular

Figure 13.11 Total anomalous pulmonary venous return (Source: Centers of Disease Control and Prevention, National Center on Birth Defects and Developmental Disabilities)

unobstructed TAPVR, where the veins enter the right atrium from above the diaphragm, is increasingly being picked up by failed POS, these babies are not usually symptomatic at birth, but present later with signs of heart failure, with poor feeding and failure to thrive (Artman et al., 2011).

Prostaglandin in duct-dependent CCHD

Prostaglandin causes the DA to dilate and is lifesaving for newborns with CCHD. It also allows time for diagnosis and evaluation.

The indications for prostaglandin are:

- To increase pulmonary blood flow in right heart obstruction (pulmonary atresia/stenosis, tetralogy of Fallot, tricuspid atresia)
- To increase systemic blood flow in left heart obstruction (coarctation, interrupted aortic arch, hypoplastic left heart, critical aortic stenosis)
- To increase pulmonary blood flow in TGA
- To dilate the ductus venosus in TAPVR and relieve obstruction to blood flow.

Therefore, babies with a suspicion of CCHD due to the above should be commenced on prostaglandin without delay. The risks of administering prostaglandin when it is not needed are small. There are two different preparations of prostaglandin in the UK: alprostadil or Prostaglandin E1 (PGE1) and dinoprostone or Prostaglandin E2 (PGE2). Both are potent vasodilators and as the infusion starts, the DA widens, and the infant rapidly becomes pink when there is an obstruction to pulmonary blood flow, and in cases with systemic blood flow obstruction, the femoral pulses become palpable and metabolic acidosis starts to resolve (Singh and Mikrou, 2018). Dosing is the same for both preparations of prostaglandin (see table 13.4).

Prostaglandin may be administered centrally or peripherally, but two intravenous routes should be available at all times.

TABLE 13.4 PROSTAGLANDIN DOSING

Presentation	Dose
Antenatal diagnosis Cyanotic, but not acidotic	5–10nanograms/kg/min
Absent femoral pulses, but not acidotic	10–15nanograms/kg/min
Unwell or acidotic with suspected duct-dependent CCHD	50nanograms/kg/min Dose can be doubled to a maximum of 100nanograms/kg/min

(adapted from Singh and Mikrou, 2018)

The baby needs to be carefully monitored for side effects:

- Apnoea usually in doses > 15 nanograms/kg/min or if the dose is increased
- Hypotension
- Pyrexia
- Tachycardia
- Flushing.

Less commonly, the following may be observed:

- Hypothermia
- Bradycardia
- Seizures (ibid.).

CHD resulting in heart failure

Signs of heart failure, such as respiratory distress, failure to thrive and hepatomegaly were discussed above in the presentation of CHD. The most common conditions associated with heart failure are babies with a large VSD or a complete atrioventricular septal defect (AVSD), with the latter seen in babies with Trisomy 21 (Teitel, 2016).

VENTRICULAR SEPTAL DEFECT

This is the most common CHD, where part of the septum between the ventricles has not formed (see figure 13.12). Babies with an isolated VSD rarely present in the first weeks, as the pulmonary vascular resistance is high and the excess blood entering the right ventricle is prevented from entering the pulmonary artery. But as the pulmonary vascular resistance falls, pulmonary blood flow increases, resulting in signs of heart failure (Teitel, 2016).

ATRIOVENTRICULAR SEPTAL DEFECT

AVSD (see figure 13.13) is highly associated with Trisomy 21 and is usually diagnosed antenatally. However, all newborns with Trisomy 21 should have a postnatal echocardio- gram. These babies have very high pulmonary blood flow and develop heart failure sooner than babies with simple VSDs.

MANAGEMENT

- Diuretics to decrease fluid overload are the first-line treatment while planning for sur- gical intervention
- Furosemide 1 mg/kg and spironolactone 2 mg/kg daily with electrolyte monitoring

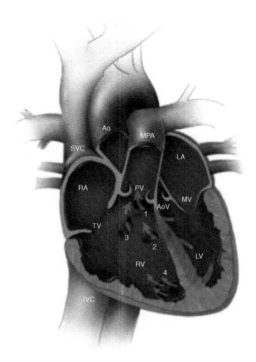

Figure 13.12 Ventricular septal defect (Source: Centers of Disease Control and Prevention, National Center on Birth Defects and Developmental Disabilities)

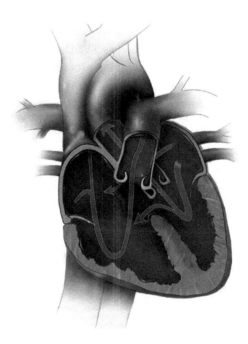

Figure 13.13 Atrioventricular septal defect (Source: Centers of Disease Control and Prevention, National Center on Birth Defects and Developmental Disabilities)

- Captopril, an ACE inhibitor can be used if signs of heart failure persist, but it causes hypotension which must be monitored
- Fluid restriction but need to maintain calorie intake for growth
- Daily weight to monitor fluid overload
- Reduce energy expenditure by nasogastric tube feeding
- Provide oxygen and nurse upright to help decrease work of breathing (Teitel, 2016).

OTHER CARDIOVASCULAR DISORDERS AND THEIR MANAGEMENT

Hypotension

Periods of low BP are an extremely common occurrence in the neonatal period, especially for babies born at a lower gestation. This could be attributed to the lack of agreement as to what level defines hypotension in the preterm population. The consensus is to target the gestational age, plus days of life (up to 4 days old); an example would be a 2-day-old baby born at 27 weeks requiring a mean arterial BP of at least 29mmHg (Levene et al., 2008). Importantly, it is not only the numerical figure which must be reviewed, but in fact it is the assessment of organ perfusion that will inform the urgency of treatment. Box 13.1 contains the clinical indicators of poor organ perfusion.

BOX 13.1 CLINICAL SIGNS OF POOR ORGAN PERFUSION

- Skin and superficial tissue perfusion: in low CO states, blood supply to the skin is diverted to vital organs. Skin perfusion can be assessed by timing capillary refill and measuring central-peripheral temperature gap. Both of these can be affected by the thermal environment (Farrugia et al., 2013).
- Metabolic acidosis: tissue hypoxia leads to anaerobic metabolism and lactate production (Levene et al., 2008).
- Reduced urine output: a urine output < 1ml/kg/hour is indicative of inadequate kidney perfusion.
- Reduced conscious level: with severe hypotension comes a loss of autoregulation of blood flow in the brain so that babies may become encephalopathic (Sinha et al., 2018).
- Reduced gut perfusion: the splanchnic blood vessels may constrict to maintain central BP, a mechanism which can predispose to necrotising enterocolitis (NEC; Levene et al., 2008).

Management of hypotension must be targeted to the underlying cause. If the cause is a diminished preload as seen in hypovolemia and septic shock, then the first action would be to fill the vascular compartment with volume.

If afterload has been compromised, for example by depleted vascular resistance in septic shock/NEC, then dopamine may cause a sufficient increase in peripheral vascular resistance.

If the myocardium is in a poor metabolic state and contractility is diminished, as seen in hypoxic injury, then dobutamine is an inotrope which improves cardiac function.

Finally, if the heart rate is not adequate to sustain a good CO, noradrenaline may be indicated to induce tachycardia as well as increase contractility and vascular resistance.

VOLUME REPLACEMENT

Cautious volume administration of 10–20mL/kg of a normal saline bolus is reasonable (Seri 2006; Ibrahim, 2008). Sick premature infants may become hypovolaemic due to insensible water loss, however overall hypovolemia is a less common cause in the preterm infant. Therefore, the response to this may be minimal (Seri, 2006). Importantly, overzealous administration of fluids to premature infants may be harmful (Gupta and Donn, 2014).

INOTROPES

- *Dopamine* produces a mixture of cardiovascular effects, the main being vasodilation in the renal circulation as well as increased CO (Rang et al., 2012). In low doses (1–5mcg/kg/minute), it has a primary dopaminergic effect and vasodilates renal, coronary and possibly cerebral circulation. In higher doses (5–10mcg/kg/minute), it stimulates β_1 receptors, which enhances myocardial contractility and increases HR. At the highest dose (10–20mcg/kg/minute), the effects are almost exclusively α-adrenergic, and thus increase peripheral vascular resistance and reduce renal blood flow (Levene et al., 2008).
- *Dobutamine* (5–20mcg/kg/minute) has mainly β_2 effects, increasing BP by increasing myocardial contractility, but with some reduction in systemic vascular resistance, therefore it may be of some value in a failing heart (Levene et al., 2008).
- *Noradrenaline* (norepinephrine, 0.1–1mg/kg/minute) is sometimes used once dopamine and dobutamine have been given at their maximum dose. It has both α- and β-receptor effects, equating to increased contractility and tachycardia. The main effect is vasoconstriction, thus increasing SVR. The use of noradrenaline has been associated with compromised peripheral perfusion, so that the baby needs to be carefully monitored for signs of this.
- *Adrenaline* (epinephrine) acts on both α- and β-receptors increasing the contractility of the myocardium as well as HR.

> ## BOX 13.2 POTENTIAL CAUSES OF HYPOTENSION
>
> ■   Technical problem with BP measurement (cuff size, zero transducer)
> ■   Prescription or administration error (check all infusions and doses)
> ■   Pneumothorax
> ■   Pericardial tamponade
> ■   Extreme hypovolemia
> ■   High mean airway pressure (especially on high frequency oscillatory ventilation)
> ■   Hidden blood loss (IVH or scalp, bowel, twin-to-twin transfusion or foeto-maternal haemorrhage)
> ■   PPHN (check pre- and post-ductal oxygen saturation)
> ■   Congenital heart defect
> ■   Drug side effects
>
> (adapted from Levene et al., 2008)

■   *Hydrocortisone* 2.5mg/kg can be used to treat apparently incurable hypotension in extremely preterm babies, as they may have adrenal dysfunction. It is, however, slow to work and has been associated with small bowel perforation (Levene et al., 2008).

NURSING CONSIDERATIONS

A significant proportion of hypotensive newborns will be receiving invasive ventilation, which increases their risk of pneumothorax or pneumopericardium, both of which could impair venous return (Farrugia et al., 2013). It is imperative that if nursing a baby who is not responding to inotropes, other possible causes of hypotension be considered (see box 13.2).

Hypertension

The incidence of neonatal hypertension is low, and its causes are varied. It can be associated with coarctation of the aorta, endocrine disorders, chronic lung disease and steroid therapy (Levene et al., 2008). The most common cause is renovascular disease caused by umbilical artery catheter placement (Batisky, 2014) which may require renal or aortic surgery. Sustained BP over the 99th percentile (see table 13.5 for normal values) is likely to be harmful over time, and a blood pressure above the 95th percentile should have treatment with antihypertensives considered (Beaulieu et al., 2014).

TABLE 13.5 BP VALUES IN INFANTS

Postconceptional age		95th percentile	99th percentile
40 weeks	Systolic BP	95 mmHg	100 mmHg
	Diastolic BP	65 mmHg	70 mmHg
	MAP	75 mmHg	80 mmHg
30 weeks	Systolic BP	80 mmHg	85 mmHg
	Diastolic BP	55 mmHg	54 mmHg
	MAP	65 mmHg	63 mmHg
26 weeks	Systolic BP	72 mmHg	77 mmHg
	Diastolic BP	50 mmHg	56 mmHg
	MAP	57 mmHg	63 mmHg

(adapted from Dionne et al., 2012)

Circulatory maladaptation at birth

PERSISTENT DUCTUS ARTERIOSUS

Patency of the DA is maintained *in utero* through prostaglandins and low levels of oxygen; thus following birth increased blood oxygenation and lower concentrations of prostaglandins lead to constriction of the DA, usually within 72 hours in well term infants (Kenney et al., 2010). In preterm infants, however, ductal closure is often delayed due to immaturity-related physiological differences (Yates, 2012). Postnatal changes to the pressure gradients within the neonatal cardiovascular system subsequently lead to shunting of blood from the systemic to the pulmonary circulation across the DA. This results in reduced renal, gastrointestinal and cerebral perfusion, associated with increased risks of NEC, intestinal perforation and intraventricular haemorrhage. Simultaneously, there is circulatory overload of the lungs, leading potentially to a prolonged need for mechanical ventilation, pulmonary haemorrhage, exacerbation of respiratory distress syndrome and possibly chronic lung disease (Benitz, 2010; Ohlsson et al., 2018).

Apart from a heart murmur, clinical signs of a patent DA (PDA) observable by the neonatal nurse may include apnoeas, bounding pulses, an active praecordium, significant systolic/diastolic blood pressure difference and fluctuating oxygen saturations. A PDA may also give rise to a clinical course of respiratory distress syndrome which does not respond to supportive treatment, or respiratory deterioration in the first two weeks of life (Yates, 2012). Asymptomatic infants should be monitored for any evidence of heart failure, failure to thrive, increasing oxygen requirements, or other complications (Kenney et al., 2011).

Controversy remains as to whether active treatment of a PDA is preferable to no intervention (Benitz, 2010). PDA management consists of pharmacological or surgical treatment, with the latter generally implemented when drug therapy has been unsuccessful (Yates, 2012).

There are currently three options for pharmacological management: indometacin, ibuprofen or paracetamol. Indometacin and ibuprofen function via inhibition of prostaglandin synthesis. Paracetamol has a similar but weaker effect on the same enzymes as the above, so that its effect on the DA may be secondary to yet unidentified mechanisms (Ohlsson and Shah, 2018).

As reduced prostaglandin synthesis results in vasoconstriction not only of the DA, the risks associated with pharmacological treatment are similar to those posed by the PDA itself, i.e. NEC/bowel perforation, poor renal function and increased risk of IVH. A side effect observed with indometacin and ibuprofen is furthermore thrombocytopaenia, so that therapy should not be commenced in infants with low platelet levels (Yates, 2012).

In view of these potentially hazardous side effects, prophylactic pharmacological management of the PDA has not become standard practice, as an improvement of long-term outcomes has not been demonstrated (Fowlie et al., 2010). Multiple trials have shown ibuprofen to be as effective as indometacin in achieving ductal closure, but with less severe adverse effects (Ohlsson et al., 2018). The efficacy of paracetamol needs yet to be addressed in further research trials, but there is evidence that it causes ductal constriction with fewer renal and gastrointestinal side effects than ibuprofen or indometacin, even in infants where these drugs have not been effective. Further research, particularly taking into consideration long-term neurodevelopmental outcomes, is required in light of suggestions of an association of prolonged paracetamol use and autism spectrum disorders (Ohlsson and Shah, 2018).

From a nursing perspective, careful observation of the infant throughout the duration of treatment, including for abdominal concerns, signs of bleeding and measurements of urine output, is vital.

Surgical intervention – ligation – is reserved for infants with haemodynamically significant PDAs, for example ventilator-dependent babies; those who are not eligible for medical treatment; where this is not effective; or where the DA reopens following initial pharmacological closure (Yates, 2012). The surgery is not without risk: potential side effects include chylothorax, left vocal cord paresis and prolonged period of intensive care (Engeseth et al., 2018).

PERSISTENT PULMONARY HYPERTENSION OF THE NEWBORN

This subject is covered in detail in chapter 12, management of respiratory disorders.

Dysrhythmias

Disorders of the HR and rhythm may occur in the antenatal or postnatal period. It is important for neonatal nurses to be able to detect an abnormal HR or rhythm, to enable

---

BOX 13.3 MANAGEMENT OF SVT

1. Vagal stimulation by applying an ice pack to the face
2. Adenosine (150–300microgram/kg) by rapid intravenous/intraosseous injection
3. Direct current cardioversion (0.5–1J/kg).

(adapted from Kleinman et al., 2010; Chu et al., 2015)

---

swift remedial or supportive action. The three commonest dysrhythmias encountered in the neonatal period are described below.

SUPRAVENTRICULAR TACHYCARDIA

Supraventricular tachycardia (SVT) is considered in HR greater than 220 beats per minute and can be a result of either a congenital cause such as an aberrant electrical pathway re-entering the atrioventricular node causing it to depolarise in asynchrony with the cardiac cycle; or an iatrogenic cause, for example a misplaced umbilical catheter in the right atrium stimulating the sinoatrial node. Recurrent SVTs can also affect the foetus during pregnancy, often lead to the development of hydrops and can result in death (Kothari and Skinner, 2006). To avoid heart failure in the neonate, remedial action (see box 13.3) is required.

CONGENITAL ATRIOVENTRICULAR BLOCK

Congenital heart block can be due to a cardiac abnormality, such as transposition of the great arteries (see above), or damage to the conducting system from maternal antibodies secondary to connective tissue disorders such as systemic lupus erythematosus. Third-degree heart block, known as complete heart block, presents as profound bradycardia and is predominantly treated with isoprenaline to increase HR. Mostly these infants recover without further intervention; some, however, will require a pacemaker (Wren, 2006).

VENTRICULAR TACHYCARDIA

Ventricular tachycardia (VT) is rare in the neonate, and often presents with cardiac arrest rather than notable tachycardia. It is not always easy to differentiate from SVT, even with the aid of an ECG (Kothari and Skinner, 2006). Pulseless VT, where the infant presents arrested, requires full resuscitation and direct current cardioversion. In infants who appear otherwise well, pharmacological management with lidocaine or amiodarone can be attempted (Yates, 2012).

CONCLUSION

Cardiovascular management in the neonatal period is a vast and complex subject, which requires a good understanding of the underlying embryology, anatomy and physiology. While many congenital heart defects do not present in the immediate neonatal period, the neonatal nurse with an awareness of their pathophysiology will be able to proactively participate in their diagnosis and management, as well as facilitate parent support during a very difficult time. Understanding the clinical signs indicative of poor cardiac function will furthermore enable the neonatal nurse to recognise and escalate subtle changes in his or her patient's condition, thus contributing to optimisation of cardiovascular management.

Case studies Case study 1: The term baby with failed pulse oximetry screening

Neil is a 6-hour-old term baby who has failed pulse oximetry screening with both upper and lower saturation reading 78%. He is tachypnoeic but has no other signs of respiratory distress.

Q.1. What are the cyanotic defects presenting with failed pulse oximetry?

Q.2. What defect can present with higher post-ductal saturations compared to pre-ductal?

Neil is commenced on a prostaglandin infusion

Q.3. What is the aim of the prostaglandin infusion in this case?

Q.4. What are the side effects of prostaglandin?

Q.5. What particular nursing care does this baby need?

Case study 2: The term baby with absent femoral pulses

Ryan is a 5-day-old term baby who is completing a course of antibiotics for pneumonia on the postnatal ward. On his discharge examination, the femoral pulses cannot be felt. The baby is otherwise well and feeding normally.

Q.1. What congenital heart defect is most commonly associated with absent femoral pulses?

Q.2. Is the pulmonary or systemic circulation affected?

Q.3. What could you do to provide more information regarding the possible diagnosis before the echocardiogram is performed?

A prostaglandin infusion is commenced.

Q.4. What is the aim of the prostaglandin infusion in this case?
Q.5. What would you expect to happen once prostaglandin is commenced?

Case study 3: Hypotension in a preterm infant

Bryony is a 25-week gestation infant who is now 8 hours old. She has been stable since admission, minimally ventilated, has commenced parenteral nutrition and has umbilical lines in situ. You notice that for the past 10 minutes her MABP has been reading 22–24mmHg.

Q.1. What are your first steps to verify if this is a true reflection of Bryony's BP? What else would your clinical assessment include?
Q.2. What would the initial pharmacological management of her hypotension be?

Bryony has been commenced on a dopamine infusion. There is suboptimal response to this at 10mcg/kg/minute, so a dobutamine infusion is also started at initially 5mcg/kg/minute

Q.3. Other than the desired increase in BP, what other changes in Bryony's parameters might you observe?
Q.4. In the case of a poor response, what other causes of hypotension would you need to consider? Which investigations could aid in the diagnosis of these?

Case study 4: The baby with a VSD

Shelley is a 2-week-old term baby admitted for poor feeding and has been found to have a heart murmur due to a ventricular septal defect (VSD). Over the past few days she has become increasingly tachypnoeic and in need of nasal cannula oxygen.

Q.1. What is happening and why?
Q.2. What other signs would you expect to see?
Q.3. What medical treatment would you expect this baby to have?
Q.4. What are the principles of nursing care for this baby?

For suggested answer guides to the questions posed in these case studies, please refer to the web-based companion site specific to this chapter (see URL below).

WEB-BASED RESOURCES

For further information, online resources and greater detail on the case studies featured in this chapter go to www.routledge.com/cw/nicnursing

References

Aboliras, E. T., Hijazi, Z. M., Lopex, C. L., & Hagler, D. J. (2018). *Visual guide to Neonatal Cardiology.* Oxford: Wiley Blackwell.

Ainsworth, S. B., Wyllie, J. P., & Wren, C. (1999). Prevalence and clinical significance of cardiac murmurs in neonates. *Archives of Disease in Childhood: Fetal and Neonatal Edition, 80*(1), F43–F45.

Anagnostou, K., Messenger, L., Yates, R., & Kelsall, W. (2013). Outcome of infants with prenatally diagnosed congenital heart disease delivered outside specialist paediatric cardiac centres. *Archives of Disease in Childhood: Fetal and Neonatal Edition, 98*(3), F218–F221.

Anderson, R. H., Baker, E. J. Macartney, F. J., Rigby, M. L., Shinebourne, E. A., & Tynan, M. (Eds.) (2002). *Paediatric Cardiology.* 2nd Edition. London: Churchill Livingstone.

Artman, M, Mahoney, L., & Teital, D. F. (2011). *Neonatal Cardiology* (2nd Edition). New York: McGraw-Hill Medical.

Batisky, D. L. (2014). Neonatal hypertension. *Clinics in Perinatology, 41*(3), 529–542.

Beaulieu, M. J., & Carsello, C. (2014). A review of drug therapy for neonatal hypertension. *Neonatal Network, 33*(2), 95–100.

Benitz, W. E. (2010). Treatment of persistent patent ductus arteriosus in preterm infants: Time to accept the null hypothesis? *Journal of Perinatology, 30*(4), 241.

Bull, C. (1999). Current and potential impact of fetal diagnosis on prevalence and spectrum of serious congenital heart disease at term in the UK. *The Lancet, 354*(9186), 1242–1247.

Burger, N. B., Bekker, M. N., de Groot, C. J., Christoffels, V. M., & Haak, M. C. (2015). Why increased nuchal translucency is associated with congenital heart disease: A systematic review on genetic mechanisms. *Prenatal Diagnosis, 35*(6), 517–528.

Carlson, B. M. (2014). *Human Embryology and Developmental Biology* (5th Edition). Philadelphia, PA: Mosby.

Carvalho, J. S., Mavrides, E., Shinebourne, E. A., Campbell, S., & Thilaganathan, B. (2002). Improving the effectiveness of routine prenatal screening for major congenital heart defects. *Heart, 88*(4), 387–391.

Carvalho, J. S. (2016). Antenatal diagnosis of critical congenital heart disease. Optimal place of delivery is where appropriate care can be delivered. *Archives of Disease in Childhood, 101*(6), 505–507.

Chu, P. Y., Hill, K. D., Clark, R. H., Smith, P. B., & Hornik, C. P. (2015). Treatment of supraventricular tachycardia in infants: Analysis of a large multicenter database. *Early Human Development, 91*(6), 345–350.

Daily, J. A., Bolin, E., & Eble, B. K. (2018). Teaching pediatric cardiology with meaning and sense. *Congenital Heart Disease, 13*(1), 154–156.

Dionne, J. M., Abitbol, C. L., & Flynn, J. T. (2012). Hypertension in infancy: Diagnosis, management and outcome. *Pediatric Nephrology, 27*(1), 17–32.

Eckersley, L., Sadler, L., Parry, E., Finucane, K., & Gentles, T. L. (2016). Timing of diagnosis affects mortality in critical congenital heart disease. *Archives of Disease in Childhood, 101*(6), 516–520.

Engeseth, M. S., Olsen, N. R., Maeland, S., Halvorsen, T., Goode, A., & Røksund, O. D. (2018). Left vocal cord paralysis after patent ductus arteriosus ligation: A systematic review. *Paediatric Respiratory Reviews, 27*, 74–85.

Ewer, A. K., Middleton, L. J., Furmston, A. T., Bhoyar, A., Daniels, J. P., Thangaratinam, S., ... & PulseOx Study Group. (2011). Pulse oximetry screening for congenital heart defects in newborn infants (PulseOx): A test accuracy study. *The Lancet, 378*(9793), 785–794.

Farrugia, R., Rojas, H., & Rabe, H. (2013). Diagnosis and management of hypotension in neonates. *Future Cardiology, 9*(5), 669–679.

Fowlie, P. W., Davis, P. G., & McGuire, W. (2010). Prophylactic intravenous indomethacin for preventing mortality and morbidity in preterm infants. *Cochrane Database of Systematic Reviews*, Issue 7. Art. No.: CD000174. DOI: 10.1002/14651858.CD000174.pub2

Frank, J. E., & Jacobe, K. M. (2011). Evaluation and management of heart murmurs in children. *American Family Physician, 84*(7), 793.

Gordan, R., Gwathmey, J. K., & Xie, L. H. (2015). Autonomic and endocrine control of cardiovascular function. *World Journal of Cardiology, 7*(4), 204.

Gupta, S., & Donn, S. M. (2014). Neonatal hypotension: Dopamine or dobutamine? *Seminars in Fetal and Neonatal Medicine, 19*(1), 54–59.

Hartman, R. J., Rasmussen, S. A., Botto, L. D., Riehle-Colarusso, T., Martin, C. L., Cragan, J. D., … & Correa, A. (2011). The contribution of chromosomal abnormalities to congenital heart defects: A population-based study. *Pediatric Cardiology, 32*(8), 1147–1157.

Ibrahim, C. H. (2008). Hypotension in preterm infants. *Indian Pediatrics, 45*(4), 285.

Ismail, A. Q. T., Cawsey, M., & Ewer, A. K. (2017). Newborn pulse oximetry screening in practice. *Archives of Disease in Childhood-Education and Practice, 102*(3), 155–161.

Joshi, G., Skinner, G., & Shebani, S. O. (2017). Presentation of coarctation of the aorta in the neonates and the infant with short and long term implications. *Paediatrics and Child Health, 27*(2), 83–89.

Kenney, P., Hoover, D., Williams, L.C., & Iskersky, V. (2010). Cardiovascular diseases and surgical interventions. In Merenstein, G. B., & Gardner, S. L. (Eds.) *Handbook of Neonatal Intensive Care*. (7th Edition). St Louis, MO: Mosby.

Kleinman, M. E., Chameides, L., Schexnayder, S. M., Samson, R. A., Hazinski, M. F., Atkins, D. L., … & Hickey, R. W. (2010). Part 14: Pediatric advanced life support: 2010 American Heart Association guidelines for cardiopulmonary resuscitation and emergency cardiovascular care. *Circulation, 122* (18 suppl 3), S876–S908.

Kothari, D. S., & Skinner, J. R. (2006). Neonatal tachycardias: an update. *Archives of Disease in Childhood: Fetal and Neonatal Edition, 91*(2), F136–F144.

Lannering, K., Bartos, M., & Mellander, M. (2015). Late diagnosis of coarctation despite prenatal ultrasound and postnatal pulse oximetry. *Pediatrics, 136*(2), e406–e412.

Levene, M. I., Tudehope, D. I., & Sinha, S. (2008). *Essential Neonatal Medicine* (4th Edition). Oxford: Blackwell.

Liu, S., Joseph, K. S., Lisonkova, S., Rouleau, J., Van den Hof, M., Sauve, R., & Kramer, M. S. (2013). Association between maternal chronic conditions and congenital heart defects: A population-based cohort study. *Circulation, 128*(6), 583–589.

Mellander, M. (2013). Diagnosis and management of life-threatening cardiac malformations in the newborn. *Seminars in Fetal and Neonatal Medicine, 18*(9), 302–310.

Metcalfe, K. (2018). Cardiac problems in genetic syndromes. *Paediatrics and Child Health, 28*(12), 574–578.

Mirzarahimi, M., Saadati, H., Doustkami, H., Alipoor, R., Isazadehfar, K., & Enteshari, A. (2011). Heart murmur in neonates: How often is it caused by congenital heart disease? *Iranian Journal of Pediatrics, 21*(1), 103.

Moore, K. L., Persaud, T. V. N., & Torchia, M. G. (2016). *The Developing Human. Clinically Orientated Embryology* (10th Edition). Philadelphia, PA: Elsevier.

Morris, I. (2015). *Duct Dependent Congenital Heart Disease. Neonatal Transfer Service London (NTS)* (Clinical Guideline). https://london-nts.nhs.uk/wp-content/uploads/2015/01/Duct-Dependent-Cardiac-Lesions-NTS-Guideline.pdf

Mussa, S., & Barron, D. J. (2017). Hypoplastic left heart syndrome. *Paediatrics and Child Health, 27*(2), 75–82.

Noble, A. (2009). The Cardiovascular System. In Hall, M., Noble, A., & Smith, S. (Eds.) *A Foundation for Neonatal Care.* Oxford: Radcliffe.

Ohlsson, A., & Shah, P. S. (2018). Paracetamol (acetaminophen) for patent ductus arteriosus in preterm or low birth weight infants. *Cochrane Database of Systematic Reviews*, Issue 4. Art. No.: CD010061. DOI: 10.1002/14651858.CD010061.pub3

Ohlsson, A., Walia, R., & Shah, S. S. (2018). Ibuprofen for the treatment of patent ductus arteriosus in preterm or low birth weight (or both) infants. *Cochrane Database of Systematic Reviews*, Issue 9. Art. No.: CD003481. DOI: 10.1002/14651858.CD003481.pub7

Øyen, N., Poulsen, G., Boyd, H. A., Wohlfahrt, J., Jensen, P. K., & Melbye, M. (2009). Recurrence of congenital heart defects in families. *Circulation, 120*(4), 295–301.

Rang, H. P., Dale, M. M., Ritter, J. M., Flowers, R. J., & Henderson, G. (2012). *Rang and Dale's Pharmacology.* (7th Edition). Philadelphia: Elsevier Churchill Livingstone.

Rudolph, A. M. (2010). Congenital cardiovascular malformations and the fetal circulation. *Archives of Disease in Childhood: Fetal and Neonatal Edition, 95*(2), F132–F136.

Schoenwolf, G. C., Bleyl, S. B., Brauer, P. R., & Francis-West, P. H. (2014). *Larsen's Human Embryology.* Philadelphia, PA: Elsevier Health Sciences.

Seri, I. (2006). Management of hypotension and low systemic blood flow in the very low birth weight neonate during the first postnatal week. *Journal of Perinatology, 26*(S1), S8.

Singh, Y., & McGeoch, L. (2016). Fetal anomaly screening for detection of congenital heart defects. *Journal of Neonatal Biology, 5*(2), 100–115.

Singh, Y., & Mikrou, P. (2018). Use of prostaglandins in duct-dependent congenital heart conditions. *Archives of Disease in Childhood-Education and Practice, 103*(3), 137–140.

Sinha, S., Miall, L., & Jardine, L. (2018). *Essential Neonatal Medicine* (6th Edition). Oxford: Wiley.

Steinhorn, R. H. (2008). Evaluation and management of the cyanotic neonate. *Clinical Pediatric Emergency Medicine, 9*(3), 169–175.

Tanner, K., Sabrine, N., & Wren, C. (2005). Cardiovascular malformations among preterm infants. *Pediatrics, 116*(6), e833–e838.

Teitel, D. (2016). Recognition of undiagnosed neonatal heart disease. *Clinics in Perinatology, 43*(1), 81–98.

Theorell, C. (2002). Cardiovascular assessment of the newborn. *Newborn and Infant Nursing Reviews, 2*(2), 111–127.

Tortora, G. J., & Derrickson, B. (2011). *Principles of anatomy and physiology* (13th Edition). Chichester: John Wiley & Sons.

Vaujois, L., Boucoiran, I., Preuss, C., Brassard, M., Houde, C., Fouron, J. C., & Raboisson, M. J. (2017). Relationship between interatrial communication, ductus arteriosus, and pulmonary flow patterns in fetuses with transposition of the great arteries: prediction of neonatal desaturation. *Cardiology in the Young, 27*(7), 1280–1288.

Wren, C., Richmond, S., & Donaldson, L. (1999). Presentation of congenital heart disease in infancy: implications for routine examination. *Archives of Disease in Childhood: Fetal and Neonatal Edition, 80*(1), F49–F53.

Wren, C. (2006, June). Cardiac arrhythmias in the fetus and newborn. *Seminars in Fetal and Neonatal Medicine, 11*(3), 182–190.

Yates, R. W. M. (2012). Cardiovascular disease. In Rennie, J. M. (Ed.) *Rennie & Roberton's Textbook of Neonatology* (5th Edition). London: Elsevier Health Sciences.

14 NEONATAL BRAIN INJURY

Debbie Webster

CONTENTS

GUIDANCE ON HOW TO ENHANCE PERSONAL LEARNING FROM THIS CHAPTER

Key points covered in this chapter

■ An overview of neonatal conditions affecting the brain and neurological system.

■ Physiological basis and vulnerability of the infant brain.

■ Nursing care and assessment of infants with neurological compromise.

Reflection

Reading through the chapter, you are encouraged to engage with the key points and related literature in an enquiring way. Ask these questions:

■ How have neurological problems affected the condition of babies you have encountered in your clinical practice?

■ How can you minimise potential insults to the neurological system and brain?

■ How might neurological compromise influence infants' outcomes?

Implications for nursing care

■ Finally: how will this chapter enable you to consider and understand the nature of vulnerability of the neonatal brain and nervous system? Consider the implications of what you learn for your nursing care relating to this area, both in the short term and in relation to long-term outcomes.

INTRODUCTION AND BACKGROUND

Normal function of the central nervous system (CNS) is critical to the working of all other organs and systems in the body and therefore any injury to the brain will have implications for both physical and cognitive outcomes. Despite great advances in the understanding of the mechanisms of injury to the developing brain and the many attempts at prevention, perinatal cerebral brain injury remains a major cause of neonatal morbidity and mortality. Of preterm survivors, 5–10% have major motor defects and around half have significant cognitive, behavioural or sensory impairment (Volpe, 2009; Back, 2015). Preterm infants are particularly at risk of intraventricular haemorrhage (IVH), periventricular haemorrhagic infarction (PVHI) and periventricular leucomalacia (PVL). More recently, with the increased availability of magnetic resonance imaging (MRI), the importance of white matter injury (WMI) and its significance in preterm brain injury is being realised (Volpe, 2009). There is currently ongoing debate around the contribution of impaired maturation of the brain versus specific injury causing poor neurodevelopmental outcome (Penn, 2016). In addition, in the term infant, encephalopathy occurs in 1–3 per 1000 births (Hagberg, 2016). Neonatal Encephalopathy (NE) is defined as a condition of disturbed neurological function in the newborn period that may be identified through altered tone or consciousness, abnormal reflexes, cardiorespiratory compromise or seizures (Martinello, 2017; Battin and Sadler, 2018). A variety of causes can result in encephalopathy; hypoxic-ischaemic perinatal events is the most common, but other causes such as cerebral haemorrhage, infection and metabolic disturbances should be considered, particularly if a history for hypoxic-ischaemic encephalopathy (HIE) is not clear or does not fit the clinical picture. This chapter provides an overview of both the preterm and term infant in relation to a range of neurological conditions with reference to how they can be prevented to minimise any impact on future outcomes.

VULNERABILITY OF THE NEONATAL BRAIN

To better understand neonatal brain injury, it is important to recognise that there are specific vulnerabilities that distinguish the response of the immature or neonatal brain, from that of the mature adult brain. Brain development begins in the embryonic period of development from 4–8 weeks of gestation and continues well into childhood. Development is in an organised, linear fashion of proliferation, migration, differentiation and maturation of neurons culminating in myelination, the success of which depends on the function of oligodendrocytes. At this critical time the brain is sensitive to harmful exposures such as drugs, poor nutrition, infection and environmental stressors (Tau, 2010). In particular, when hypoxia and ischaemia occur, oxygen free radicals are released which affect the normal development of oligodendrocytes. This can lead to **apoptosis** (programmed cell death) and impaired myelination (Back, 2015).

A further issue for premature infants is the presence of the fragile germinal matrix that lines the brain ventricles (see figure 14.1) which is prone to rupture due to the limited capacity of the immature brain to induce autoregulation in the event of systemic hyper- or hypotension. However, neurons in the preterm brain appear to have some resistant properties as they are less susceptible to degeneration following hypoxic-ischaemic damage than those in the term brain (Back, 2015; Blackburn, 2016).

For infants of any gestation who spend their first few weeks or even months on a neonatal unit (NNU) there is the added issue of being in a non-nurturing environment during a critical period of brain development, which may have implications for later life. Synaptic connections in the cortical plate increase at a rate of 4% a week until around 26–28 weeks' gestation, when there is acceleration in synaptogenesis, so that by 34 weeks' gestation there are 40,000 new synapses being formed every second (Tau, 2010). Exposure to an increased number of stressful events secondary to neonatal care is associated with decreased brain size in the frontal and parietal regions and corresponding poorer neurodevelopmental scores (Smith, 2011).

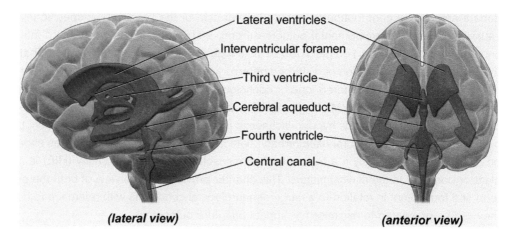

Figure 14.1 Ventricular system of the brain (Source: Creative Commons)

The importance of this crucial period of brain development, which lasts from conception to the age of 2 years, and how this impacts the future of the child, is well recognised. Nursing and medical management must aim to support vulnerable infants and their families during this time; for example, developmental care strategies as seen in chapter 5. All infants spending time on a NNU are at risk of developing neurological sequelae due to the harsh environment and possible delayed attachment to a specific primary caregiver.

INTRAVENTRICULAR HAEMORRHAGE AND PERIVENTRICULAR HAEMORRHAGIC INFARCTION

IVH is the most common type of intracranial haemorrhage seen in the neonatal period and is almost exclusively confined to infants <32 weeks or <1500g. It is the leading cause of neurological and cognitive impairment in preterm infants with an incidence that increases with increasing prematurity (Mahmoudzadeh et al., 2018). In the preterm infant the haemorrhage arises from the subependymal germinal matrix, while in the rarer cases of near-term IVH/PVHI it stems from the **choroid plexus**. IVH/PVHI is traditionally classified into grades according to severity (see box 14.1; Volpe, 2001).

The outcome for grades I and II is good; the outcome for grade III is dependent on the flow of cerebrospinal fluid (CSF) – if this is blocked by blood clots at the Aqueduct of Sylvius or Foramen of Monro causing further ventricular dilatation, outcome is much worse, as these infants usually go on to develop post-haemorrhagic **hydrocephalus**. Any involvement of the parenchyma (grade IV) carries a higher incidence of poor neurodevelopmental outcome.

BOX 14.1 CATEGORIES OF INTRAVENTRICULAR HAEMORRHAGE

Grade I: The bleed is confined to the periventricular germinal matrix, a highly vascularised area which supports the development of the brain. It contains neurons and glial cells which migrate out during embryological development.

Grade II: The bleed has extended from the germinal matrix into the ventricles, with no evidence of ventricular dilatation.

Grade III: The haemorrhage occupies more than 50% of one or both ventricles with evidence of dilatation.

Grade IV: Extension from the ventricles into the brain parenchyma.

The term hydrocephalus refers to a progressive dilatation of the cerebral ventricular system due to a production of CSF that exceeds the absorption rate. In the infant suffering an IVH, a particulate blood clot may occlude or obliterate the microscopic arachnoid villi rendering them non-functional, resulting in insufficient absorption of CSF. In many infants, ventricular dilatation occurs slowly. Increased intracranial pressure does not usually occur due to the neonate's soft malleable skull, open sutures and fontanelles that, for a period of time, allow head size to increase without an appreciable rise in pressure. In approximately half of all infants, ventricular dilatation spontaneously arrests within about 30 days. However, for the remaining infants, dilatation continues with accompanying signs of rising intracranial pressure such as bulging fontanelles, setting sun eye sign, dilated scalp veins and widely spaced sutures. Progressive ventricular dilatation may be managed with a ventriculo-peritoneal shunt or temporary ventricular drainage via needle aspiration if the infant is too small or unwell for surgery.

It is important to note that grade IV is not simply blood in the ventricles bursting out into the parenchyma but a consequence of a secondary ischaemic injury (PVHI). Although PVHI has a relatively low (5%) incidence in very low birth weight infants, this rises to 20–30% in babies <750g, and the poor outcome makes it a significant diagnosis (Volpe, 2009).

Aetiology of IVH/PVHI

The pathophysiology of IVH/PVHI involves a combination of intravascular, vascular and extravascular factors. The germinal matrix is a transient structure which involutes by 36 weeks' gestation. Here neuroectodermal cells (precursors for neurons) and glial cells develop before migrating to the cerebral cortex. Due to the high activity in this region during foetal life the area is highly vascularised, with a significant proportion of cerebral blood flowing through. In the preterm brain normal cerebral autoregulation may not be developed enough to maintain a steady blood flow with changes in systemic blood pressure resulting in possible under- or over-perfusion of this delicate area. Increased venous pressure can also directly affect the capillaries of the germinal matrix, impeding venous return and leading to reduced cerebral blood flow. The combination of these events, compounded by episodes of hypoxia and fragility of the immature and extremely thin-walled, irregularly shaped vessels of the germinal matrix lead to rupture of the area with various degrees of haemorrhage. Antenatal events that increase the risk of IVH include antepartum haemorrhage, foetal compromise/hypoxia, prolonged labour, and malpresentation. Following birth, hypoxic events such as respiratory problems, apnoea and hypotension are associated with an increased risk.

Episodes of high systemic blood pressure, linked to increased cerebral blood flow, can be caused by noxious stimulation, spontaneous over-activity or handling, crying, tracheal suctioning, excessive light and noise, over-infusion of inotropes, hypercapnia, pneumothorax and rapid volume expansion. Systemic hypotension significantly decreases cerebral blood flow and can be caused by cardiac dysfunction, sepsis and hypovolaemia. The most severe form of preterm brain injury, PVHI, occurs when an IVH is further complicated with an associated venous infarction that destroys the white matter leaving porencephalic cysts and possible secondary damage due to subsequent reduction in neuronal proliferation and migration (Volpe, 2009).

As gestation increases, the capillary walls thicken and from 32 weeks onwards, cell proliferation and migration reduce as does the risk of IVH.

Diagnosis of IVH/ PVHI

IVH is usually detected within the first week of life, with diagnosis at the bedside. In the newborn infant, the anterior fontanelle provides an ideal window through which cranial ultrasound scanning (CUSS) may be performed. CUSS is especially helpful in identifying brain injury in newborn infants and allows grading of the injury according to the location and severity of the haemorrhage. For more than 90% of newborn infants with IVH, bleeding occurs within the first 72 hours after birth, with 50% of haemorrhages occurring in the first 24 hours. For approximately 10–20% of infants, there is a progressive increase in the size of the haemorrhage over a 24–48-hour period. Late haemorrhages may be seen after a few days or weeks in a small number of infants; however, these are seen primarily in those preterm infants with a more complicated history, such as severe, prolonged respiratory problems.

The clinical manifestations of a IVH are non-specific. Volpe (2001) describes three classic syndromes: catastrophic, salutatory, or silent. The catastrophic syndrome occurs most infrequently, but is one of sudden dramatic deterioration with a decrease in blood pressure and haematocrit, a full fontanelle and seizure activity. Catastrophic deterioration usually involves major haemorrhages that evolve rapidly over several minutes or hours. Some infants exhibit a more protracted or salutatory course where symptoms 'wax and wane' over a period of time. Findings include changes in alertness and tone, abnormal eye position and movement, an abnormally tight popliteal angle, with respiratory distress progressing to apnoea. These signs evolve over many hours and may cease, only to begin again. They may also be so subtle they are missed. Infants with a clinically silent syndrome, the most common of the three, fail to show any neurological signs but may have an unexplained fall in haematocrit or failure of haematocrit to rise following red blood cell transfusion. Diagnosis of silent haemorrhages is usually by CUSS.

PERIVENTRICULAR LEUKOMALACIA AND WHITE MATTER INJURY

PVL occurs following necrosis of the white matter behind and to the sides of the **lateral** ventricles (Huang et al., 2017; Lee, 2017). The area is susceptible to ischaemic damage from reduced blood flow, as this border zone is furthest away from arterial supply (Tsuji, 2014). PVL can be classified as cystic or non-cystic. In cystic PVL, early CUSS shows a bright area (periventricular brightness, also called 'flare') that later develops into macroscopic cysts which can be detected on ultrasound. In non-cystic PVL the damage is diffuse, and the microscopic cysts cannot be seen and evolve into glial scars. In later MRI scans this non-cystic PVL manifests itself with reduced growth of the cerebellum and is thought to be a possible cause of poor neurodevelopment in preterm infants, especially when earlier CUSS showed little or no abnormality (Volpe, 2009).

Previously, cystic PVL was a common occurrence on NNUs, but with improving perinatal care, most preterm WMI is non-cystic and diffuse (Penn, 2016). Poor function of the glial cells and the vulnerability of the oligodendrocyte precursors to inflammation and ischaemia are thought to lead to hypomyelination, a common characteristic of WMI on MRI scans. This supports the argument that neonatal brain injury nowadays is as likely due to dysmaturation as specific injury (Volpe, 2009; Back, 2015; Penn, 2016).

PREVENTION OF PRETERM BRAIN INJURY

Prevention or risk reduction begins in the perinatal period with the forestalling of preterm birth, the single most important method of preventing brain injury of any type. National standards dictate that high-risk pregnancies should be managed in a tertiary centre able to provide optimal delivery, resuscitation and neonatal intensive care; consequently *in utero* transfer may be required. Antenatal administration of corticosteroids is associated with a decreased risk and incidence of IVH, as these aid maturation of the foetal lungs, decreasing the incidence of respiratory distress syndrome (RDS) with its concomitant acid-base balance disturbances (Ballabh, 2014). Additionally, antenatal corticosteroids may also decrease IVH by promoting cardiovascular stability postnatally, and may contribute to maturation of the germinal matrix itself.

Magnesium sulphate has been shown in many studies to protect the brain of the foetus and is now recommended practice (Royal College of Obstetricians and Gynaecologists (RCOG), 2011). Delayed clamping of the umbilical cord for up to 2 minutes has been shown to be associated with a lower incidence of IVH and suggest improved outcomes (Mercer et al., 2006; Duley et al., 2018).

Numerous prophylactic regimes including the administration of phenobarbital and vitamin K have been evaluated as prenatal and postnatal interventions; however, none have proved to be effective enough interventions to warrant their use. Likewise, although the administration of indometacin has been shown to reduce the incidence of severe IVH and the need for surgical ligation of a patent ductus arteriosus, its administration has not resulted in improvements in long-term neurocognitive outcomes as hoped. Many practitioners feel the potential unwanted side effects of indometacin, such as reduced organ perfusion, particularly to the renal and gastrointestinal tract, outweigh the clinical benefit (Ballabh, 2014).

Caffeine is one of the most widely used drugs in NNUs, its primary objective being the prevention of apnoea of prematurity. However, in the trial designed to investigate its use, it was found that infants in the caffeine arm had a lower incidence of cerebral palsy and cognitive delay (Schmidt, 2006).

Sodium bicarbonate should be used cautiously as a buffer due to its effect of causing an abrupt rise in arterial carbon dioxide following administration that leads to vasodilation of the cerebral arteries and a subsequent increase in cerebral perfusion. The neonatal team should work together to carefully control weaning of ventilation, maintain blood gases within a normal range, manage optimal blood pressure and ensure good fluid balance in order to achieve stability of the infant and reduce the risk of IVH. Traditionally seen as nursing responsibilities, good positioning, careful handling, pain management and teaching parents behavioural cues and comforting techniques cannot be underestimated as a vital part of neuro-protective care that must be adopted by the entire multidisciplinary team to improve long-term outcome.

MANAGEMENT OF PRETERM BRAIN INJURY

Acute management of the infant once IVH has occurred is supportive in nature, with control of ventilation, fluids, metabolic and nutritional states, temperature, and, if a catastrophic bleed, management of seizures. The outcome for an infant suffering an IVH is largely determined by the severity and extent of the haemorrhage and the presence of associated problems, such as RDS, perinatal hypoxic-ischaemic injury and sepsis, which all increase morbidity and mortality. Parents should be kept fully updated and be aware that their child may have some developmental delay; assurance should be given that close follow-up will identify any specific needs promptly and early intervention will be given if required. Community support and follow-up should be coordinated, and the importance of attending follow-up appointments must be stressed.

BRAIN INJURY IN THE TERM INFANT

As previously mentioned, the most common cause of NE in the term infant is hypoxic-ischaemic encephalopathy (HIE), a devastating consequence of a spectrum of antenatal and birthing complications (Ralphe, 2016). A diagnosis of HIE can be made where there is cardiovascular compromise manifesting itself as either an Apgar score of 5 or less, or continued need for resuscitation at 10 minutes of age, or acidosis at 60 minutes age accompanied by signs of encephalopathy including abnormal electroencephalography (EEG; Azzopardi, 2009). The potential causes of hypoxia can be seen in table 14.1.

However, for a confident diagnosis of HIE, there should be a clear history of a hypoxic-ischaemic event and, although therapeutic hypothermia may be started in the absence of a clear diagnosis, other causes of encephalopathy should be investigated. These include neo-natal stroke, sepsis, metabolic, neuromuscular or cardiac disorders. When a sentinel event to cause HIE is not apparent, further tests should commence using a structured approach.

Pathophysiology of hypoxic-ischaemic encephalopathy

The hypoxic-ischaemic event results in primary injury that significantly depletes adenosine triphosphate (ATP) stores and increases lactate production. The low ATP causes disruption of cell functions, particularly to the sodium-potassium pump and the mechanism to maintain low intracellular calcium. The failure of the sodium-potassium pump results in depolarisation of neurons and the release of glutamate (a neuro-transmitter) that further increases intracellular calcium and sodium. The detrimental effects of this process include cerebral oedema and microvascular damage leading to necrosis and apoptosis (Allen, 2011). Around 6 hours following this initial period of damage there is a latent period where many of the damaged

TABLE 14.1 CAUSES OF HYPOXIC BRAIN INJURY

Failure of gas exchange across the placenta	Prolonged or excessive uterine contractions Placental abruption Ruptured uterus
Interruption of umbilical blood flow	Cord compression (including tight nuchal cord, shoulder dystocia, cord prolapse, true knots)
Inadequate placental perfusion	Maternal hypo-/hypertension
Impaired maternal oxygenation	Asthma Pulmonary embolism Pneumonia
Compromised foetus	Intrauterine growth restriction Anaemia
Failure of cardiorespiratory adaptation at birth	

neurons partially recover and there is a transient improvement in cerebral metabolism. This is followed by a secondary phase of injury, and the severity of this is linked with long-term outcome (Davidson, 2015). Understanding of the mechanisms of the secondary phase is continually evolving, however it is recognised that excitotoxicity, mitochondrial impairment, intracellular calcium regulation, oxidative stress and inflammation all contribute to the process of further and possible catastrophic cell death (Hagburg, 2016).

TREATMENT

Following results of three large trials (TOBY, CoolCap, NICHD) there is now robust evidence that moderate hypothermia following a perinatal hypoxic-ischaemic event results in improved neurodevelopmental outcome for survivors (Gluckman et al., 2005; Shankaran, 2005; Azzopardi et al., 2009). Furthermore, the TOBY study group has shown that this improvement continues into middle childhood (Azzopardi et al., 2014).

Therapeutic hypothermia is now a standardised treatment for HIE and should be followed in all NNUs (National Institute for Health and Care Excellence (NICE), 2010). Active cooling to a core temperature of 33–34°C for a period of 72 hours (Azzopardi et al., 2009) with a servo-control mattress should be commenced as soon as diagnosis is confirmed, so transport to a tertiary centre is time-critical. The aim of treatment is to prevent the secondary phase of damage, and therefore starting cooling within six hours of birth is essential to ensure this crucial window is not missed. This has been based on animal data, which suggest the effectiveness of cooling diminishes as the time increases from the hypoxic-ischaemic insult to initiation of cooling. There are a number of postulated mechanisms by which hypothermia is thought to be neuroprotective. It may safeguard neurons by reducing cerebral metabolic rate, attenuating the release of excitatory amino acids, ameliorating the ischaemia-impaired uptake of glutamate, and lowering production of toxic nitric oxide and free radicals. Hypothermia may also modify cells programmed for apoptosis, leading to their survival.

Hypothermia appears to be well tolerated. Adverse effects such as sinus bradycardia, increased blood pressure and increased oxygen requirement are generally transient and reversible with re-warming. Severe hypotension may be problematic, but generally only occurs with too rapid re-warming (Thoresen, 2008). Due to the potential effect of hypoxia on other body organs, the infant being treated for HIE should be closely monitored; poor renal, hepatic and intestinal function, deranged clotting and cardiac and respiratory deficiencies are all commonly seen. Pain management and sedation must be considered. Once at a tertiary centre, EEG monitoring should commence.

Maintaining physiological stability in a critically ill, hypothermic infant is challenging, requiring labour-intensive and skilful care. Enteral feeds are generally withheld to relieve the burden on a gastrointestinal tract made vulnerable by hypoxia-ischaemia and the additional risk factor of hypothermia. Perceptions of patient discomfort during cooling, with anecdotal experiences of restlessness and shivering, have arisen in those caring for these infants. Clinicians have acknowledged this as a major barrier for nursing staff and provision for providing comfort with sedation is standard in protocols. Support of the family, especially following the often-traumatic events of a hypoxic-ischaemic insult, is paramount.

The most effective intervention against hypoxic-ischaemic brain injury remains prevention with vigilant intrapartum monitoring to help detect those foetuses at risk. The hallmarks of intrapartum hypoxia-ischaemia are the occurrence of foetal heart rate abnormalities and the passage of meconium *in utero*. Robust intrapartum assessment allows appropriate obstetric management and effective resuscitation following delivery. A better understanding of the biological processes contributing to the secondary phase of neuronal cell death have led to investigation of several pharmacological treatments such as xenon gas, calcium channel blockers, free-radical scavengers, glutamate receptor blockers, anti-inflammatory agents and growth factors to advance repair (Dixon et al., 2015). Currently none of these has been shown to be beneficial.

CEREBRAL FUNCTION MONITORING

Amplitude-integrated EEG (aEEG) is almost universally used in the neonatal intensive care unit today. aEEG uses a limited number of channels to record raw EEG signals which are filtered and displayed on an amplitude and time-compressed scale (see figure 14.2; Glass,

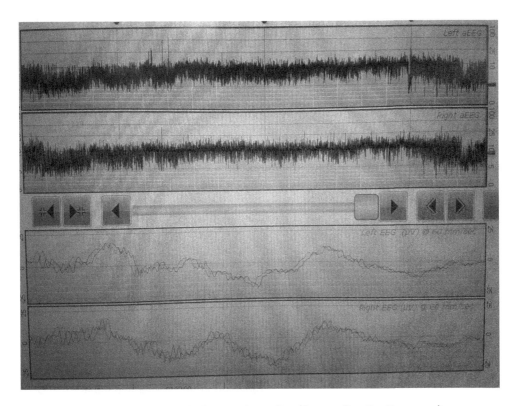

Figure 14.2 Normal aEEG trace with sleep–wake cycling (Source: Creative Commons)

2013). This can be monitored continuously at the bedside without interruption of daily care, and extensive formal training is not required. Primarily, the aEEG is used to detect seizure activity, gauge response to anticonvulsant therapy, and as part of routine clinical monitoring, especially for those infants pharmacologically paralysed.

Studies have shown that the aEEG is very accurate in outcome prediction of term infants with HIE between 3 and 48 hours' postnatal age, especially when the early aEEG is combined with clinical evaluation. Continuous activity with a lower amplitude of around 5 microvolts (µV) and maximum up to 50µV is considered normal; sleep–wake cycling should be seen. An abnormal background pattern persisting beyond the first 12–24 hours after birth is known to carry a poor prognosis (Spitzmiller et al., 2007; Toet and de Vries, 2008).

OUTCOME

HIE can be classified according to the following criteria in box 14.2.

Utilising the definitions above, for those term infants with mild neonatal encephalopathy in the first few days of life, there is a high likelihood of being completely normal at follow-up. For those with moderate encephalopathy there is a 20–35% risk of neurological sequelae, although those with normal neurological examination and effective feeding within two weeks of birth are likely to have normal outcomes. Infants with severe encephalopathy have a 75% risk of dying with coma persisting or progressing to brain death by 72 hours of life. If the infant survives for longer than 72 hours without losing all cerebral function, a variable amount of improvement may be seen; however, there is an almost universal risk of poor neurological outcome in survivors (Wu et al., 2008). Permanent sequelae may be mild, such as learning difficulties or attention deficit disorder, or may be severe and disabling, including cerebral palsy, epilepsy, visual impairment and severe cognitive and developmental disorders.

Clinical evaluation including aEEG and neurological examination, and MRI are useful means of long-term prognostication. However, they should not be relied on in isolation – all the details of a baby's individual case, including antenatal and perinatal history, clinical course and neurological status at discharge must be taken into consideration to allow for as accurate a prognosis as possible (Uria-Avellanal et al., 2013).

BOX 14.2 HYPOXIC-ISCHAEMIC ENCEPHALOPATHY CLASSIFICATION

Mild: hyperalert, hyperexcitable, normal or increased muscle tone, no seizures.
Moderate: hypotonia, decreased movements, often seizures.
Severe: stuporous, flaccid, absent primitive reflexes, usually with seizures.

(adapted from Lissauer and Fanaroff, 2006)

OTHER MECHANISMS OF BRAIN INJURY

Subdural haemorrhage

Subdural and subarachnoid haemorrhages are difficult to diagnose with routine CUSS and are consequently most likely underdiagnosed. The causes are usually related to delivery injury, and with improved obstetric care the incidence has reduced. Signs include lethargy, apnoea and seizures accompanied by a full fontanelle. Management is symptom control and close developmental follow-up (Buonacore, 2012).

Neonatal stroke

Neonatal stroke is a rare occurrence presenting in the majority of infants in the first 48 hours of life. It can be defined as a focal disruption of cerebral blood flow secondary to arterial ischaemia or sinovenous thrombosis (Van der Aa, 2014), which can occur secondary to the fact that the neonate is relatively thrombophilic. Conditions such as polycythaemia, dehydration, congenital vascular or cardiac anomalies, meningitis, and transplacental passage of an **embolus** have been described as causative of neonatal stroke. Symptoms can be subtle and non-specific, or sudden and dramatic, ranging from lethargy and poor feeding to seizures. If suspected, an EEG and CUSS should be carried out as soon as possible followed by MRI when practical. Management is primarily symptom control and ensuring stability of all body systems as required (Shah and Rennie, 2012).

Chorioamnionitis

Strong epidemiologic data link maternal infection with neonatal brain injury. Chorioamnionitis is associated with premature delivery and low gestational age. Cytokines play a part in this process. These are produced by, or act on, the immune system mediating responses associated with infection, inflammation and tissue injury. Recent work links increased amniotic fluid or blood concentrations of cytokines with perinatal brain injury. It is thought that maternally or foetally derived circulating inflammatory mediators may cross the immature blood–brain barrier, either directly injuring neurons or increasing their vulnerability to subsequent hypoxic-ischaemic insults. Alternatively, intrauterine infection could initiate injury by producing septic shock *in utero* with its resultant decreased cerebral perfusion. The neurological outcome linked most commonly with chorioamnionitis is cerebral palsy (Rocha, 2007).

Metabolic disorders

When a newborn infant presents with a sudden illness which may include signs from almost every system, inborn errors of metabolism should be considered. Although rare, outcome is very much linked to speed of diagnosis and initiation of treatment. When neurological symptoms are present with no explanation from antenatal or perinatal history, then metabolic screening should be carried out and advice sought from a specialist paediatrician. Relevant symptoms include hypotonia, encephalopathy, seizures and sudden respiratory collapse (Buonacore, 2012).

NEONATAL SEIZURES

Seizures are the most common neurological sign during the neonatal period resulting from abnormal electrical impulses generated by the brain. Excessive synchronous electrical discharge or depolarisation in the brain produces stereotypic, repetitive behaviours which may be the first, and at times only, sign of CNS dysfunction. Although the precise mechanism that causes neonatal seizures is unknown, they are thought to result from one or more of these mechanisms: disturbances in the sodium-potassium pump, altered neuronal permeability to sodium, or imbalance in excitatory (glutamate) and inhibitory (GABA) neurotransmitters (Mruk, 2015). Seizures are important, as they indicate a potentially serious underlying disease process and may have a detrimental effect on the developing brain. They also interfere with supportive care and result in an increase in glucose metabolism and altered cerebral blood flow. Repetitive seizures may eventually alter brain lipid, protein and energy metabolism or result in damage from hypoxia or oedema, however although neonates have a lower seizure threshold than children or adults, it is thought that the developing neurons are more resistant to the toxic effects of seizure activity (Mruk, 2015).

Seizures occur more often in the newborn infant than at any other period of life, with the incidence in term infants being 0.7 to 2.8 per 1000 live births, and more common than this in the preterm population. The clinical manifestations of neonatal seizures differ from those of older children with five major varieties described: subtle, generalised tonic, multifocal clonic, focal clonic and myoclonic (see table 14.2). Seizures generally indicate an underlying, potentially treatable, aetiology. Therefore, determining and treating the cause of the seizures are the priority in preventing further seizures and neurological injury. Timing of the onset of seizures (box 14.3) may provide insight into possible aetiology.

The time of onset of seizures following a hypoxic-ischaemic event may add some clarity to the timing of the insult. With a pre-labour insult, the first seizures generally occur before 12 hours of age, whereas in infants with a peripartum insult, the onset of seizures is generally after 18–20 hours of age (Filan, 2005).

The issue of when to treat with anticonvulsant drugs and for how long, however, remains controversial. Generally, if a seizure is longer than 3 minutes' duration, or occurs at a frequency of more than three per hour, treatment is required. The first-line anticonvulsant remains phenobarbital, despite the known long-term effects on brain growth. Other drugs often used include phenytoin, and benzodiazepines such as midazolam (Glass et al., 2012). Newer agents, such as levetiracetam look promising with no evidence of neurotoxicity in the developing brain at anticonvulsant concentrations in experimental studies (Rennie and Boylan, 2007). As anticonvulsants can be respiratory, myocardial and CNS depressants, the infant's respiratory effort and heart rate must be assessed to maintain adequate ventilation and perfusion. Anticonvulsants also compete with bilirubin for albumin binding sites, so the infant must be monitored for signs of jaundice.

Neonatal seizures must be differentiated from non-seizure behaviours of the newborn, which can at times be problematic. Normal behaviour such as stretching, yawning,

TABLE 14.2 NEONATAL SEIZURES[a]

Type of seizure	Manifestation	Comments
Subtle seizures	Horizontal deviation of the eyes or repetitive blinking/fluttering of eyelids.	Most common seizure in newborns especially preterm infants.
	Drooling, sucking and/or tongue thrusting, lip smacking, yawning. Swimming or rowing movements of limbs or cycling movements of legs.	Difficult to distinguish from normal movements; therefore may be missed.
Tonic seizures	Tonic extension or flexion (less common) of all extremities or may be limited to one.	Generalised tonic seizures may be mistaken for decerebrate (extension of arms and legs) or decorticate posturing (extension of legs, flexion of arms) where there are no EEG changes.
	May be accompanied by eye deviations, apnoea, occasional clonic movements.	Seizure most frequently seen in preterm infant especially following IVH and asphyxia.
Clonic seizures	Rhythmic jerky movements. Multifocal – migration in non-ordered fashion.	More frequent in term infants. More frequent in term infants. Often associated with: ■ CNS injury ■ Severe acidosis ■ Asphyxia.
	Focal – usually focal injury.	
Myoclonic seizures	Sudden single or multiple jerks with flexion of upper (more common) or lower extremities.	Uncommon in term infants. Rarely seen in preterm infants. Often associated with: ■ inborn errors of metabolism ■ other metabolic problems.
Benign myoclonic seizures	Brief, intermittent jerk (no EEG changes).	Seen during sleep only.

a listed in order of decreasing incidence

jitteriness, startling and clonus may raise suspicions of seizure activity. Traditionally, diagnosis in the NNU has been based upon clinical observation; however, in recent years, continuous cerebral function monitoring has become increasingly acknowledged as a method for evaluation of brain activity in neonates and is now a daily part of clinical surveillance of sick newborn infants (Hellström-Westas and Rosén, 2006). Overall, accurate and prompt diagnosis is pivotal in providing optimal outcomes for infants with neonatal seizures. As clinical signs may be subtle or lacking altogether, effective management should involve continuous aEEG or EEG monitoring (see table 14.3)

> **BOX 14.3 CAUSES OF NEONATAL SEIZURES BY TIMING OF ONSET**
>
> *Day 1* HIE, hypoglycaemia, congenital infection, subarachnoid haemorrhage.
> *Day 2* Intracerebral bleed, HIE, hypoglycaemia.
> *Day 3* Hypoglycaemia, inborn errors of metabolism.
> *Day 4–7* Hypocalaemia, meningitis, drug withdrawal, 'fifth day fits'.

TABLE 14.3 CLASSIFICATION OF aEEG TRACES IN FULL-TERM INFANTS

Continuous normal voltage pattern	Continuous activity with lower margin of amplitude around 5 to 10µV and maximum amplitude around 10 to 25µV (up to 50). Sleep–wake cycling should be present.
Discontinuous normal voltage pattern	Discontinuous background, with variable minimal amplitude, but < 5µV and maximum amplitude greater than 10µV.
Burst suppression	Discontinuous background with minimum amplitude without variability at 0 to 2µV.
Continuous low voltage	Continuous background pattern of extremely low voltage (less than or around 5µV).
Inactive flat trace	Mainly inactive (isoelectric tracing) background less than 5µV.

depending on local availability and identification of the underlying potential cause (Chalia and Austin, 2018).

NURSING CARE OF INFANTS WITH NEUROLOGICAL COMPROMISE

Nursing and medical care in relation to the neonatal brain and nervous system should focus on preventative, protective and supportive strategies. In more detail, minimising brain injury in premature infants should start in the perinatal period with the prevention of preterm birth, birth trauma and hypoxic events. After birth, nurses have a key role in the prevention of brain injury in premature infants during the neonatal period and the worsening of injuries that have occurred already. Nursing management includes interventions to reduce activities that can lead to hypoxic events, rapid changes to cerebral blood pressure, flow and pressures. Recognition and management of pain and stress are furthermore of vital importance, as well as developmentally supportive care, including handling and positioning techniques

TABLE 14.4 NEUROPROTECTIVE NURSING CARE

Type of care	Strategies	Rationale
Preventative care	■ Assessment of oxygenation and perfusion. ■ Optimise ventilation and oxygenation levels, avoiding fluctuations in pressure and oxygen. ■ Avoid routine endotracheal tube suctioning. ■ Careful fluid bolus administration. ■ Close monitoring – EEG. ■ Assist with preparation of the infant for regular scanning and/or timely brain imaging.	To avoid sudden changes to oxygenation, blood pressure and volume. To prevent potentially catastrophic sequelae of this, and improve the clinical outcome (Lee, 2017). To identify any problem as early as possible and any worsening of injuries that have occurred already. Brain imaging is an important step in the diagnosis and management of sick infants: e.g. post-haemorrhagic ventricular dilatation, encephalopathy, seizures and suspected structural brain abnormalities (Sorokan et al., 2018).
Protective care	■ Neurological assessment including tone, consciousness, activity level, behaviour changes as well as vital signs: blood pressure, oxygenation, blood gases. Correction of imbalances ■ Avoid unnecessary handling, stress/pain and stimulation ■ Careful handling ■ Avoid transportation if possible.	As above, to identify any changes early and ensure appropriate care is given. To protect the immature, vulnerable brain. The seven neuroprotective core measures are ■ healing environment ■ partnering with families ■ positioning and handling ■ safeguarding sleep ■ minimising stress and pain ■ protecting skin ■ optimising nutrition (Altimier and Phillips, 2016).
Supportive care	■ Optimise the environment ■ Give developmentally supportive care in partnership with parents ■ Ensure comfortable and supportive positioning ■ Reduce and manage stress and pain (e.g. containment and pain relief) during procedures.	To provide a nurturing supportive environment without undue stress that optimises the developmental capabilities of the developing infant. Noise, light, invasive treatment and caring activities are among disturbing factors in the NNU (Mahmoodi et al., 2016). See also chapters 5 and 6.

(Blackburn, 2016). These interventions can promote physiological stability during and after caregiving and reduce environmental stress and so protect the infant. Table 14.4 outlines examples in relation to these areas. Parents must also be consistently involved in any individualised, developmental care programmes that aim to reduce any external stressors on their vulnerable baby and promote the best future outcomes.

CONCLUSION

Newborn infants at risk of or suffering from a brain injury present a significant challenge to neonatal nurses. Across the range of gestational ages, the nature of brain injuries and their aetiologies are variable and require different approaches to nursing care. The neonatal nurse must therefore be equipped with a sound knowledge base of the types of brain injury covered in this chapter, to be able to plan optimal care of affected or at-risk infants. A knowledge of the nature and implications of types of brain injury covered in this chapter aids the planning of optimal care of these infants. For parents, ongoing support is needed in understanding and dealing with their baby's serious illness, the changes in responsiveness or irritability, the possibility of death, or potential implications for future poor neurological outcome.

CASE STUDIES

Case study 1: The infant with IVH

Kwame is a 25-week gestation infant born by precipitous vaginal delivery, weighing 720g. During pregnancy, there had been some intermittent vaginal bleeding at 12–16 weeks' gestation and then again at 24 weeks. However, before Margaret, his mother, could be transferred to a tertiary perinatal centre, she began to feel unwell with uterine tenderness and fever, and on admission to her local hospital, Kwame was delivered. Margaret also experienced a significant antepartum haemorrhage. Kwame required resuscitation at birth including intubation and positive-pressure ventilation and after being given a dose of surfactant, he was transferred to the neonatal intensive care unit (NICU). On admission to NICU, he was commenced on volume-targeted ventilation and in the first 24 hours of life, his blood pressure was problematic, requiring two doses of volume expansion followed by inotropic support. As his condition was very unstable, Kwame was transferred to a level 3 neonatal intensive care unit, 26 miles from the local hospital. His parents are Margaret and Oko, a Ghanian married couple with three other children.

Q.1. What antenatal factors placed Kwame at risk of brain injury?
Q.2. What postnatal factors in the first few hours of life placed Kwame at further risk of brain injury?

On day three of life, Kwame became more hypotensive and a murmur presented on auscultation. A patent ductus arteriosus was confirmed on cardiac echo. On day 7, a head ultrasound scan identified evidence of intraventricular haemorrhage (IVH) with blood present in both right and left ventricles (grades 3 and 2 respectively). The right ventricle was also enlarged.

Q.3. Describe the mechanisms for injury that were present in this situation.
Q.4. What potential caregiving practices need addressing in the prevention and management of IVH?

Follow-up head ultrasound scan at 14 days of age revealed further bleeding on the left side and ventricles were slightly dilated. However, he was extubated to continuous positive airways pressure (CPAP) on day 15 and further regular ultrasounds were planned as the parents had been told there was a risk of post-haemorrhagic hydrocephalus. Successive scans did show progressive dilation of the ventricles. He also remained on low flow oxygen for chronic lung disease.

Q.5. How should the team prepare the parents, Margaret and Oko, for Kwame's discharge and how can they all work together to optimise his outcome?
Q.6. What is Kwame's likely long-term outcome?

Case study 2: The infant with HIE

Chloe is a 41[+3]-week gestation female infant born by emergency caesarian section subsequent to her mother being admitted due to antepartum bleeding and foetal bradycardia presenting during prolonged second stage of labour. Chloe was born pale, floppy, with no respiratory effort, and a heart rate of less than 60. She required inflation breaths followed by bag and mask ventilation, chest compressions, intubation and adrenaline. A fluid bolus of 10ml/kg/dose of normal saline was given for poor perfusion. Her first spontaneous respiration was noted at 10 minutes of age. Apgar scores were 1, 1, 5 and 7 at 1, 5, 10 and 15 minutes respectively. On admission to NICU her breathing pattern was stabilising but she was irritable with abnormal posturing. On the first arterial gas obtained, her pH was 6.9 with a base deficit of 16mEq/L.

Q.1. Why is therapeutic cooling likely to be beneficial to Chloe and what are the initial actions that must be taken at this point?
Q.2. Describe the reasons for this in line with the criteria for this treatment.
Q.3. What should be explained to the parents?

The aEEG initially showed a discontinuous pattern without sleep–wake cycling; however, at 18 hours of age she was noted to have repetitive jerky movements of her upper extremities with eye flickering lasting 45 seconds. She was given a loading dose of phenobarbital for recurrent episodes of jerking movements correlating to seizure activity on aEEG.

Q.4. Describe the significance of seizures including their nature and timing.
Q.5. Identify and explain caregiving practices required while Chloe is being cooled.

Over the next 12 hours her seizures stopped. She was re-warmed after 72 hours of cooling and was extubated to room air. Over the course of the next 10 days Chloe established breastfeeding well.

Q.6. What is Chloe's long-term outcome likely to be and what do the parents need to be told?

Case study 3: The infant with uncertain neurological outcome

Andreas is one of triplets born at 25 weeks' gestation and is now 12 weeks old. Following a long period of respiratory support and stabilisation, he is now progressing in the special care are of the neonatal unit along with the other triplets, Marcos and Paul who are due to go home in the next few days. Andreas however has been much slower to get to this point and suffered periods of being much more unstable both from a ventilation and blood pressure perspective. He also has two periods of infection requiring antibiotics which set his progress back. Andreas' mother Beth also showed signs of infection during her pregnancy. The last few head ultrasound scans show that there are bilateral white, cystic appearances around the ventricular areas of the brain. He is presenting with some abnormal neurological signs.

Q.1. What is the significance of the information presented here in relation to a possible diagnosis relating to the brain?
Q.2. What factors leading up to this point have predisposed Andreas to neurological compromise?
Q.3. In relation to the 'abnormal' neurology mentioned above, what might this be in relation to your nursing assessment of this infant?
Q.4. What is the potential long-term outcome for Andreas?
Q.5. What should the parents be told about this situation and how will they be facilitated/supported to improve future outcome?

For suggested answer guides to the questions posed in these case studies, please refer to the web-based companion site specific to this chapter (see URL below).

WEB-BASED RESOURCES

For further information, online resources and greater detail on the case studies featured in this chapter go to www.routledge.com/cw/nicnursing

References

Allen, K. A., & Brandon, D. H. (2011). Hypoxic ischemic encephalopathy: pathophysiology and experimental treatments. *Newborn and Infant Nursing Reviews, 11*(3), 125–133.

Altimier, L., & Phillips, R. (2016). The neonatal integrative developmental care model: Advanced clinical applications of the seven core measures for neuroprotective family-centered developmental care. *Newborn and Infant Nursing Reviews, 16*(4), 230–244.

Azzopardi, D. V., Strohm, B., Edwards, A. D., Dyet, L., Halliday, H. L., Juszczak, E., ... & Thoresen, M. (2009). Moderate hypothermia to treat perinatal asphyxial encephalopathy. *New England Journal of Medicine, 361*(14), 1349–1358.

Azzopardi, D., Strohm, B., Marlow, N., Brocklehurst, P., Deierl, A., Eddama, O., ... & Levene, M. (2014). Effects of hypothermia for perinatal asphyxia on childhood outcomes. *New England Journal of Medicine, 371*(2), 140–149.

Back, S. A. (2015). Brain injury in the preterm infant: New horizons for pathogenesis and prevention. *Pediatric Neurology, 53*(3), 185–192.

Ballabh, P. (2014). Pathogenesis and prevention of intraventricular hemorrhage. *Clinics in Perinatology, 41*(1), 47–67.

Battin, M., & Sadler, L. (2018). Neonatal encephalopathy: How can we improve clinical outcomes? *Journal of Paediatrics and Child Health, 54*(11), 1180–1183.

Blackburn, S. (2016). Brain injury in preterm infants: Pathogenesis and nursing implications. *Newborn and Infant Nursing Reviews, 16*(1), 8–12.

Buonacore. G., Bracci, R., & Weindling, M. (2012). *Neonatology: A practical approach to neonatal management*. New York: Springer Publishing Company.

Chalia, M., & Austin, T. (2018). Practice guide to neonatal seizures. *Paediatrics and Child Health, 28*(10), 488–491.

Davidson, J. O., Wassink, G., van den Heuij, L. G., Bennet, L., & Gunn, A. J. (2015). Therapeutic hypothermia for neonatal hypoxic-ischemic encephalopathy–where to from here? *Frontiers in Neurology, 6*, 198.

Dixon, B., Reis, C., Ho, W., Tang, J., & Zhang, J. (2015). Neuroprotective strategies after neonatal hypoxic ischemic encephalopathy. *International Journal of Molecular Sciences, 16*(9), 22368–22401.

Duley, L., Dorling, J., Pushpa-Rajah, A., Oddie, S. J., Yoxall, C. W., Schoonakker, B., ... & Fawke, J. A. (2018). Randomised trial of cord clamping and initial stabilisation at very preterm birth. *Archives of Disease in Childhood: Fetal and Neonatal Edition, 103*(1), F6–F14.

Filan, P., Boylan, G. B., Chorley, G., Davies, A., Fox, G. F., Pressler, R., & Rennie, J. M. (2005). The relationship between the onset of electrographic seizure activity after birth and the time of cerebral injury in utero. *BJOG: An International Journal of Obstetrics & Gynaecology, 112*(4), 504–507.

Glass, H. C., Kan, J., Bonifacio, S. L., & Ferriero, D. M. (2012). Neonatal seizures: treatment practices among term and preterm infants. *Pediatric Neurology, 46*(2), 111–115.

Glass, H. C., Wusthoff, C. J., & Shellhaas, R. A. (2013). Amplitude-integrated electro-encephalography: The child neurologist's perspective. *Journal of Child Neurology, 28*(10), 1342–1350.

Gluckman, P. D., Wyatt, J. S., Azzopardi, D., Ballard, R., Edwards, A. D., Ferriero, D. M., ... & Gunn, A. J. (2005). Selective head cooling with mild systemic hypothermia after neonatal encephalopathy: Multicentre randomised trial. *The Lancet, 365*(9460), 663–670.

Hagberg, H., Edwards, A. D., & Groenendaal, F. (2016). Perinatal brain damage: The term infant. *Neurobiology of Disease, 92*, 102–112.

Hellström-Westas, L., & Rosén, I. (2006). Continuous brain-function monitoring: state of the art in clinical practice. *Seminars in Fetal and Neonatal Medicine, 11*(6), 503–511.

Huang, J., Zhang, L., Kang, B., Zhu, T., Li, Y., Zhao, F., … & Mu, D. (2017). Association between perinatal hypoxic-ischemia and periventricular leukomalacia in preterm infants: A systematic review and meta-analysis. *PloS One, 12*(9), e0184993.

Lee, Y. A. (2017). White matter injury of prematurity: its mechanisms and clinical features. *Journal of Pathology and Translational Medicine, 51*(5), 449.

Lissauer, T., & Fanaroff, A. (2006). *Neonatology at a Glance.* Oxford: Blackwell Publishing.

Mahmoodi, N., Arbabisarjou, A., Rezaeipoor, M., & Mofrad, Z. P. (2016). Nurses' awareness of preterm neonates' sleep in the NICU. *Global Journal of Health Science, 8*(6), 226.

Mahmoudzadeh, M., Dehaene-Lambertz, G., Kongolo, G., Fournier, M., Goudjil, S., & Wallois, F. (2018). Consequence of intraventricular hemorrhage on neurovascular coupling evoked by speech syllables in preterm neonates. *Developmental Cognitive Neuroscience, 30*, 60–69.

Martinello, K., Hart, A. R., Yap, S., Mitra, S., & Robertson, N. J. (2017). Management and investigation of neonatal encephalopathy: 2017 update. *Archives of Disease in Childhood: Fetal and Neonatal Edition, 102*(4), F346–F358.

Mercer, J. S., Vohr, B. R., McGrath, M. M., Padbury, J. F., Wallach, M., & Oh, W. (2006). Delayed cord clamping in very preterm infants reduces the incidence of intraventricular hemorrhage and late-onset sepsis: A randomized, controlled trial. *Pediatrics, 117*(4), 1235.

Mruk, A. L., Garlitz, K. L., & Leung, N. R. (2015). Levetiracetam in neonatal seizures: A review. *The Journal of Pediatric Pharmacology and Therapeutics, 20*(2), 76–89.

National Institute for Health and Care Excellence. (2010). *Therapeutic hypothermia with intracorporeal temperature monitoring for hypoxic perinatal brain injury.* NICE

Penn, A. A., Gressens, P., Fleiss, B., Back, S. A., & Gallo, V. (2016). Controversies in preterm brain injury. *Neurobiology of Disease, 92*, 90–101.

Ralphe, J. L. (2016). Neonatal Hypoxic Ischemic Encephalopathy: A Case Study. *Newborn and Infant Nursing Reviews, 16*(1), 25–27.

Rennie, J., & Boylan, G. (2007). Treatment of neonatal seizures. *Archives of Disease in Childhood – Fetal and Neonatal Edition, 92*, F148–F150.

Rocha, G., Proença, E., Quintas, C., Rodrigues, T., & Guimarães, H. (2007). Chorioamnionitis and brain damage in the preterm newborn. *The Journal of Maternal-Fetal & Neonatal Medicine, 20*(10), 745–749.

Royal College of Obstetricians and Gynaecologists. (2011). *Magnesium sulphate to prevent cerebral palsy at birth. Scientific impact paper number 29.* London: RCOG.

Schmidt, B., Roberts, R. S., Davis, P., Doyle, L. W., Barrington, K. J., Ohlsson, A., … & Tin, W. (2006). Caffeine therapy for apnea of prematurity. *New England Journal of Medicine, 354*(20), 2112–2121.

Shah, D.K. & Rennie, J.M. (2012). Neurological problems in the newborn. Part 3: Intracranial haemorrhage and perinatal stroke (arterial and venous) at term. In Rennie, J. M. (Ed.) *Rennie & Roberton's Textbook of Neonatology* (5th Edition). London: Elsevier Health Sciences.

Shankaran, S., Laptook, A. R., Ehrenkranz, R. A., Tyson, J. E., McDonald, S. A., Donovan, E. F., … & Finer, N. N. (2005). Whole-body hypothermia for neonates with hypoxic-ischemic encephalopathy. *New England Journal of Medicine, 353*(15), 1574–1584.

Smith, G. C., Gutovich, J., Smyser, C., Pineda, R., Newnham, C., Tjoeng, T. H., … & Inder, T. (2011). Neonatal intensive care unit stress is associated with brain development in preterm infants. *Annals of Neurology, 70*(4), 541–549.

Sorokan, S. T., Jefferies, A. L., & Miller, S. P. (2018). Imaging the term neonatal brain. *Paediatrics & child health, 23*(5), 322–328.

Spitzmiller, R. E., Phillips, T., Meinzen-Derr, J., & Hoath, S. B. (2007). Amplitude-integrated EEG is useful in predicting neurodevelopmental outcome in full-term infants with hypoxic-ischemic encephalopathy: a meta-analysis. *Journal of Child Neurology*, *22*(9), 1069–1078.

Tau, G. Z., & Peterson, B. S. (2010). Normal development of brain circuits. *Neuropsychopharmacology*, *35*(1), 147.

Thoresen, M. (2008). Supportive care during neuroprotective hypothermia in the term newborn: adverse effects and their prevention. *Clinics in Perinatology,* 35, 749–63.

Toet, M. C., van Rooij, L. G., & de Vries, L. S. (2008). The use of amplitude integrated electroencephalography for assessing neonatal neurologic injury. *Clinics in Perinatology*, *35*(4), 665–678.

Tsuji, T., Okumura, A., Kidokoro, H., Hayakawa, F., Kubota, T., Maruyama, K., ... & Watanabe, K. (2014). Differences between periventricular hemorrhagic infarction and periventricular leukomalacia. *Brain and Development*, *36*(7), 555–562.

Uria-Avellanal, C., Marlow, N., & Rennie, J. M. (2013). Outcome following neonatal seizures. *Seminars in Fetal and Neonatal Medicine,18*(4), 224–232.

Van der Aa, N. E., Benders, M. J. N. L., Groenendaal, F., & de Vries, L. S. (2014). Neonatal stroke: A review of the current evidence on epidemiology, pathogenesis, diagnostics and therapeutic options. *Acta Paediatrica*, *103*(4), 356–364.

Volpe, J .J. (2001). Intracranial hemorrhage: germinal matrix-intraventricular hemorrhage of the premature infant. In Volpe, J. J. (Ed.) *Neurology of the Newborn* (4th Edition). Philadelphia: WB Saunders.

Volpe, J. J. (2009). Brain injury in premature infants: A complex amalgam of destructive and developmental disturbances. *The Lancet Neurology*, *8*(1), 110–124.

Wu, Y., Nordli, D. R., Weisman, L. E., & Dashe, J. F. (2019). Clinical features, diagnosis, and treatment of neonatal encephalopathy. Up *To Date*. www.uptodate.com/contents/clinical-features-diagnosis-and-treatment-of-neonatal-encephalopathy

15 MANAGEMENT OF HAEMATOLOGICAL DISORDERS

Lynne Wainwright and Annette Rathwell

CONTENTS

GUIDANCE ON HOW TO ENHANCE PERSONAL LEARNING FROM THIS CHAPTER

Key points covered in this chapter

■ An overview of the main haematological disorders that present in neonatal care.

■ The causes and clinical presentation of these disorders.

■ The assessment, management and nursing care associated with caring for infants with a range of haematological disorders.

Reflection

Reading through the chapter, you are encouraged to engage with the key points and related literature in an enquiring way. Ask these questions:

■ Have you observed infants who have had abnormal blood results? What were these and the underlying causes?

■ How did these infants present?

■ How were these infants managed?

Implications for nursing care

■ Finally: how will this chapter enable you to consider how to best care for high-risk infants with haematological conditions? Consider the implications of what you learn for your nursing care relating to this area.

INTRODUCTION AND BACKGROUND

Caring for babies with haematological disorders presents the neonatal nurse with many challenges. To correctly interpret clinical signs, monitor changes and provide information to support parents, a background knowledge of the haematological system is necessary. This chapter will review a range of common haematological disorders in the newborn: jaundice, polycythaemia, coagulation disorder including vitamin K deficiency bleeding (VKDB, also known as haemorrhagic disease of the newborn), thrombocytopaenia, disseminated intra-vascular coagulation (DIC), and finally, anaemia. The pathophysiology and treatment of each condition will be discussed, to enable the nurse to anticipate problems, assess the effect-iveness of treatment and limit complications that may impact on the infant.

JAUNDICE

Jaundice in a newborn is extremely common, estimated to occur in roughly two-thirds of all newborns in the first week of life (Magyar et al., 2017). Approximately 60% of term and 80% of preterm infants will develop jaundice during the first week of life (Rennie et al., 2010). It is usually harmless, but high levels of unconjugated bilirubin can be damaging. Jaundice can also be a sign of serious liver disease. It is vital, therefore, that jaundice is recognised early, to ensure treatment of any underlying condition to be instigated.

Jaundice is the yellow discolouration of the skin and sclerae seen when there is a buildup of bilirubin, produced from the breakdown of red blood cells (RBC). If levels of bili-rubin in the circulation are high, this is known as hyperbilirubinaemia (National Institute for Health and Care Excellence (NICE), 2015a; 2016). Neonates have higher levels of bilirubin than adults due to their higher concentration of RBC, which also have a shorter lifespan. When RBC break down, unconjugated bilirubin is formed. Unconjugated bilirubin is bound to albumin in the circulation and is then metabolised by the liver to produce conjugated (water-soluble) bilirubin which can then be excreted in the stool (NICE, 2016). Elevated levels of serum bilirubin (SBR) are common in the newborn and usually harmless. However, jaundice occurring in the first 24 hours of life, lasting for more than two weeks, or reaching excessive levels is more concerning. This will be discussed in the relevant sections.

Physiology of bilirubin metabolism

In utero, the placenta manages the excretion of unconjugated bilirubin. Following delivery, the neonatal liver assumes responsibility for bilirubin metabolism. The main source of bili-rubin is the breakdown of haem-containing proteins; 75% of bilirubin is formed by the breakdown of haemoglobin (Hb), a major constituent of RBC (Bhandari, 2018). One gram of Hb produces approximately 600μmol of unconjugated, fat-soluble bilirubin, which cannot be excreted via the gut or kidney but can easily pass through the lipid membranes of cells such as fatty tissue and the brain. Infants produce higher rates of bilirubin than adults, as their RBC have a short lifespan of 40–70 days compared with 120 days in adults, and they have an increased circulating red cell mass. Newborns produce 6mg/kg/day of bilirubin, double the amount produced by an adult (Maisels and McDonagh, 2008). Bilirubin production is a two-stage process within the reticuloendothelial system. During the first stage, haem is degraded by the enzyme haem oxygenase, which causes the release of iron and the formation of biliverdin and carbon monoxide. Biliverdin is then broken down by biliverdin reductase to form unconjugated bilirubin.

Unconjugated bilirubin is transported in the circulation bound with albumin. Once bound, the bilirubin enters the smooth endoplasmic reticulum in the liver with the help of carrier proteins Y (a ligandin) and Z. A series of reactions then occur, catalysed by the enzyme uridine diphosphate glucuronyl transferase (UGT), resulting in the joining of bilirubin with two molecules of glucuronic acid to produce conjugated bilirubin (figure 15.1). Conjugated bilirubin is a component of bile and enters the gut via the biliary system. During its passage through the intestinal tract, bacterial enzymes convert bilirubin into urobilinogen and stercobilinogen. As these compounds are now water-soluble, they can be excreted in the stools (Mitra and Rennie, 2017).

Physiological jaundice

Neonatal jaundice is classified as either physiological or pathological.

Physiological jaundice can be a result of:

■ An increased bilirubin production due to increased RBC volume, decreased RBC life span, or increased enterohepatic circulation
■ Decreased uptake by the liver because of decreased ligandins or binding of ligandins to other **anions**
■ Decreased conjugation in the liver because of decreased uridine diphosphoglucuronyl transferase (UDPGT) activity
■ Decreased excretion into bile (Mitra and Rennie, 2017).

Physiological jaundice may be exacerbated by prematurity, administration of albumin-bound medications, bruising, polycythaemia, short life span of foetal red blood cells, inadequate oral intake, delayed passage of stool and breastfeeding (Truman, 2006; NICE, 2015a).

Sick and premature infants are more susceptible to the neurotoxic effects of high bilirubin levels (Mitra and Rennie, 2017). Hyperbilirubinaemia can cause neurological damage including deafness, neurodevelopmental and cognitive problems (Shortland et al., 2008). Kernicterus occurs when unconjugated bilirubin passes through the blood–brain barrier

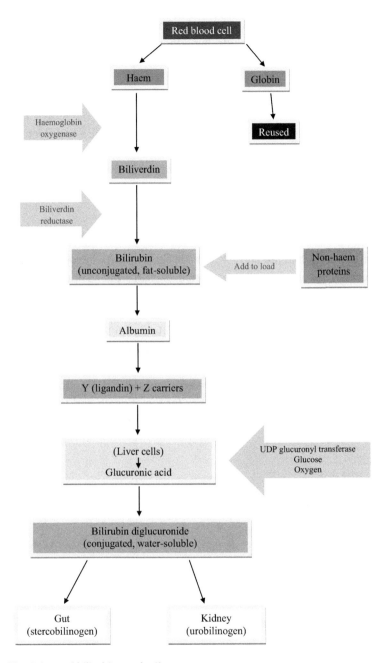

Figure 15.1 Physiology of bilirubin production

causing a yellow staining of the basal ganglia. The damage is irreversible. The symptoms of this clinical encephalopathy include hypertonia, an abnormally high-pitched cry, poor feeding, seizures and abnormal posture. Risk factors for developing kernicterus are:

■ Serum bilirubin >340 µmol/L in a term infant (>37 weeks)
■ A rapid rise in the SBR level (>8.5µmol/litre/hour)
■ Clinical signs suggestive of bilirubin encephalopathy (Mitra and Rennie, 2017).

In addition, the threat of neurologic damage always remains, especially with very high bilirubin level, in presence of certain risk factors (Singh et al., 2016).

Pathological jaundice

Jaundice that occurs within the first 24 hours is likely to be pathological (Mitra and Rennie, 2017) and usually results from the presence of exacerbating factors in addition to the mechanisms leading to physiological jaundice (Shortland et al., 2008). Underlying disease processes may cause haemolysis, which increases the bilirubin levels due to the increased breakdown of RBC; or other conditions may interfere with the normal bilirubin metabolism pathway. This can occur for several reasons (see table 15.1), the most common being haemolytic disease highlighted below. Haemolytic Disease of the Foetus and Newborn (HDFN) is caused by maternal alloimmunisation against RBC **antigens**. In severe cases, HDFN may lead to foetal anaemia with a risk for foetal death and to severe forms of neonatal hyperbilirubinaemia with a risk for kernicterus (De Haas et al., 2015).

TABLE 15.1 CAUSES OF PATHOLOGICAL JAUNDICE

Pathology	Mechanism
ABO/Rhesus incompatibility (haemolytic disease) Haemoglobinopathies G6PD deficiency	Increased red cell breakdown leading to hyperbilirubinaemia
Trauma	Sequestered blood
Hypothyroidism Galactosaemia	Interfere with metabolism and excretion
Drugs	Need albumin binding sites
Infection	May affect hepatic function +/− increase haemolysis
Biliary atresia Cystic fibrosis Tumours	Impair ability to excrete conjugated bilirubin

Rhesus incompatibility

Rhesus (Rh) haemolytic disease of the newborn (HDN), also known as erythroblastosis foetalis, occurs when there is maternal red cell alloimmunisation, and is one of the common pathological causes of hyperbilirubinaemia (Singh et al., 2016). Maternal **antibodies** are directed against foetal red cells when foetal RBC positive for an antigen (often Rhesus D) pass into the circulation of a mother who is negative for that antigen (Smits-Wintjens et al., 2008). The foetal and maternal circulations, although closely positioned in the placenta, are essentially separate from one another. Small tears in the placental capillaries or placental separation during delivery may facilitate the passage of foetal cells into the normally separate maternal circulation. Where a mother is Rh negative and is carrying a Rh positive foetus, passage of Rh positive foetal cells into the Rh negative maternal circulation generates an immune response and the production of anti-Rh antibodies. These maternal antibodies cause destruction of the Rh positive foetal red blood cells (see figure 15.2).

This maternal sensitisation to foetal Rh antigens occurs when there is foetal-maternal blood transfusion during pregnancy, delivery, miscarriage, termination or **amniocentesis**. During the first pregnancy this does not cause any issues, however, during subsequent pregnancies the risk of foetal red cell haemolysis is present due to the elevated level of maternal anti-Rh antibodies. Breakdown of foetal RBC then results in raised bilirubin levels. During pregnancy, this excess bilirubin is excreted via the placenta, but after birth haemolysis

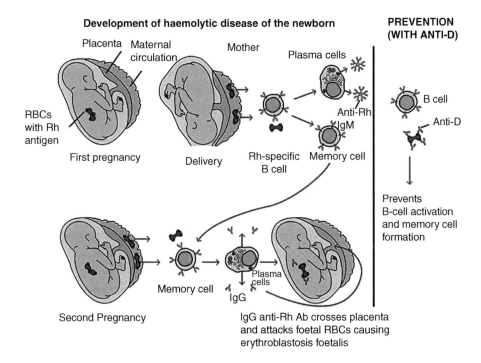

Figure 15.2 Haemolytic disease of the newborn

continues, and the immature neonatal liver is unable to cope with the conjugation of large amounts of bilirubin, resulting in severe hyperbilirubinaemia appearing in the first 24 hours (De Haas et al., 2015).

Severe HDN in the foetus due to Rh incompatibility can cause anaemia of the foetus and promotes RBC production from unusual sites such as the liver. The most severe form of HDN causes foetal hypoxia and cardiac failure, which in turn results in hydrops foetalis with generalised oedema and pleural, pericardial and/or peritoneal effusions (Bagwell, 2007). Due to the production of therapeutic anti-D **immunoglobulin** that binds to foetal cells and promotes their destruction prior to the initiation of a maternal immune response, this is now a rare occurrence. Routine administration of anti-D was introduced in the 1960s and dramatically reduces maternal alloimmunisation in subsequent pregnancies (De Haas et al., 2015). The routine administration of anti-D immunoglobulin to Rh negative mothers during the second trimester (28–34 weeks) and following any high-risk event during pregnancy is now accepted obstetric practice.

ABO incompatibility

ABO incompatibility occurs in the following situations:

■   Maternal blood type is O and infant's blood type A (most common type) or B (results in most severe haemolysis).
■   Maternal blood type is B and infant's blood type is A or AB.
■   Maternal blood type is A and infant's blood type is B or AB (Mundy, 2005).

Naturally occurring maternal antibodies attach to the antigens on the incompatible foetal RBC, causing haemolysis and the production of bilirubin. The infant presents with anaemia and jaundice. The direct antiglobulin (Coombs) test (DAT), which detects the presence of antibodies on the surface of RBC, is positive.

G6PD deficiency

Glucose-6-phosphate dehydrogenase is an enzyme responsible for maintaining the integrity of the red cell membrane. A deficiency of this enzyme renders the cell liable to haemolyse. This is most common in infants of Mediterranean, Asian or African origin (Luzzatto et al., 2016). G6PD deficiency presents after 48 hours. In affected individuals, this can occur during ingestion of or exposure to oxidants such as naphthalene (moth balls), sulphonamide medications, fava beans (broad beans), or during periods of infection. Newborns are usually symptom-free until exposed to an oxidant, which triggers haemolysis. This condition has a sex-linked recessive inheritance pattern, which means that heterozygous females are carriers and males are affected. Once diagnosis is established, the family need to be advised on how to avoid the oxidants. G6PD deficiency is usually only clinically significant in infancy where there is a risk of developing kernicterus, and is not a clinical problem in adults.

The most frequent clinical manifestations of G6PD deficiency are neonatal jaundice and acute haemolytic anaemia, which is usually triggered by an exogenous agent. Some G6PD variants cause chronic haemolysis, leading to congenital non-spherocytic haemolytic anaemia. The most effective management of G6PD deficiency is to prevent haemolysis by avoiding oxidative stress (Cappellini and Fiorelli, 2008).

Measurement of bilirubin levels

Jaundice becomes clinically evident when serum levels of bilirubin reach 90µmol/L (Mitra and Rennie, 2017). Assessment of jaundice and bilirubin measurement is an important nursing role. The visual progression of jaundice may indicate the level of bilirubin; however, it should not replace actual SBR measurement. NICE guidance advises checking for signs of jaundice, especially in the first 72 hours. The naked infant should be viewed in bright, ideally natural light. The sclerae, gums and skin should be examined (Ford, 2010), but visual inspection alone is not enough to estimate the bilirubin level (Allen, 2016). Transcutaneous bilirubinometers (TcB) are an accurate and non-invasive screening method for clinically significant jaundice in the well term infant (Mitra and Rennie, 2017). The device measures the presence of yellow pigment in the skin of the forehead or over the sternum (Ives, 2011). Although these measurements correlate well with SBR in the lower range, and their use as a screening device to detect clinically significant jaundice decreases the need for frequent blood sampling in the well term infant, accuracy is reduced above 250µmol/L. NICE (2016) recommends checking an SBR if transcutaneous reading is above 250µmol/L. Serum measurement of total bilirubin remains the gold standard for diagnosing and treating hyperbilirubinaemia. SBR should be used for infants in the first 24 hours of life or in infants below 35 weeks' gestation (NICE, 2016). In infants who are over 35 weeks' gestation and over 24 hours old, TcB can be used, or in the absence of a bilirubinometer, SBR can be measured. SBR should be measured where bilirubin levels are at or above treatment thresholds and for subsequent measurements (Amos et al., 2017).

Thresholds are depicted as a line on graphs on which SBR levels are plotted over time. They differ according to gestation. A link to the phototherapy threshold graphs provided by NICE, now almost universally used in neonatal units (NNUs) in the UK, can be found in the web-based companion.

Phototherapy

Developed following recognition that sunshine appeared to reduce the jaundice pigment in the skin of an infant reported by Cremer in 1958 (Shortland et al., 2008), phototherapy is universally used as a safe and convenient way of lowering SBR levels. It causes reactions that convert bilirubin into water-soluble isomers which can then be excreted more easily from the body as the products of breakdown do not need conjugation in the liver (Rennie et al., 2010; Bhandari, 2018). It is effective only once bilirubin enters the skin and the SBR is above 80µmol/L (Ives, 2011; Mitra and Rennie, 2017). Phototherapy works in three ways; the first is structural isomerisation, when irreversible photo-alteration of bilirubin produces a water-soluble structure (lumirubin) that can be excreted in urine and bile. Configurational isomerisation turns the bilirubin isomer into water-soluble non-toxic products. Finally, photo-oxidation results in the destruction of bilirubin molecules, but only a small amount of bilirubin is excreted in this way (Shortland et al., 2008).

Phototherapy lamps/units emitting visible blue light in the wavelength of 425–475 nanometres are the most effective in reducing serum bilirubin (see figure 15.3). The efficacy of phototherapy is dependent on dose and wavelength of the light used and the surface area of the infant's skin which is exposed to the light. The dose can be increased by placing the lights at the minimum safe distance from the infant, by using more than one unit, or by combining overhead lamps with a fibreoptic system under the infant.

Conventional phototherapy units use fluorescent tubes to administer light at the blue end of the spectrum. These lights are placed above the infant. Newer phototherapy units utilise multiple light-emitting diodes (LEDs) which can be used closer to the infant's skin as they do not generate infrared or ultraviolet radiation (Ives, 2011). Fibreoptic systems are used via a body pad or wrap, and have made phototherapy more versatile. In this case, phototherapy is delivered using a single light source that comprises a light generator, a fibreoptic cable through which the light is carried, and a flexible light pad on which the infant is placed, or that is wrapped around the infant. Although a Cochrane review found that fibreoptic phototherapy was as effective as conventional phototherapy in preterm infants, it suggested that this was less so in term infants (Mills and Tudehope, 2001). NICE guidance (2016) advises that phototherapy can be delivered with light-emitting diodes, fibreoptic or fluorescent lamps, tubes or bulbs, no specific device is recommended.

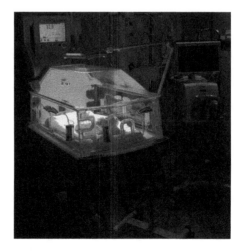

Figure 15.3 Phototherapy

Gestational age-specific treatment threshold graphs should be used to determine the need for treatment (NICE, 2016). These graphs show two clear lines indicating the phototherapy and exchange transfusion thresholds for infants in the first two weeks of life. Term infants over 24 hours of age who have a bilirubin reading below the treatment line, but within 50μmol/L, should have a SBR measurement repeated within 18 hours if they have risk factors for jaundice (a sibling who required phototherapy, or where the mother intends to exclusively breastfeed), or within 24 hours if they have no risk factors (NICE, 2016).

Nursing management of the jaundiced infant not only includes assessment, but the administration of phototherapy with its own set of specific care interventions, outlined in table 15.4.

In infants who require phototherapy, SBR should be checked 4–6 hours after commencement of treatment and then every 6–12hours if stable or falling. Phototherapy should be continued until the SBR is at least 50μmol/L below the treatment threshold, and rechecked 12–18 hours later to check for rebound. In cases where SBR levels are rising rapidly, are within 50μmol/L below the exchange transfusion threshold after 72 hours, or fail to respond to initial phototherapy within 6 hours, intensified phototherapy should be considered (NICE, 2016).

Phototherapy is a generally safe treatment although it is not without side effects. These include:

- Diarrhoea
- Increased transepidermal water loss: hydration and fluid balance should be monitored by daily weighing of the infant and assessment of weight of nappies
- Unstable temperature: the temperature should be monitored, and the infant should be nursed in a thermoneutral environment (see chapter 11)
- Skin rashes and discolouration (Bronze infant syndrome and tanning): Bronze infant syndrome occurs due to an interaction between cholestatic jaundice and photo-therapy. The brown pigment stains the skin and may linger after discontinuation of treatment for some weeks
- Potential retinal damage: Early animal studies suggested that retinal damage may occur following exposure to phototherapy lights. Although these studies were conducted over 40 years ago, it has never been conclusively established that this may or may not occur in humans and thus infants' eyes should be shielded during phototherapy (Bhandari, 2018; Shortland et al., 2008). Eye shields should be removed at regular intervals to check for abrasions or infection. The shields need to be tight enough to prevent slipping and potential airway obstruction, but not so tight as to restrict blood flow or cause tissue damage. Orange-tinted head boxes or shields can be used as an alternative to eye shields in term infants (NICE, 2016).

Lotions, creams or oils should not be applied to an infant's skin if they are having phototherapy.

Parental support during phototherapy is essential. Explanations and reassurance for the need for phototherapy are vital for parents of infants undergoing treatment (Turnbull and Petty, 2012). Encouraging parents to continue feeding, caring for and visiting their baby may be necessary. NICE (2016) identify the need to give parents written and verbal information. Lactation support should be continued. During phototherapy, short breaks should be encouraged for feeding and cuddles. If intensified phototherapy is required, it should not be stopped for feeding, but intravenous fluids or enteral feeds of breast milk should be given dependent on clinical need.

Intravenous immunoglobulin

Administration of intravenous immunoglobulin (IVIG) combined with phototherapy has been shown to significantly reduce the need for exchange transfusion, length of phototherapy and overall length of stay in infants with severe Rhesus or ABO isoimmunisation (Ives, 2011). Infants are, however, more likely to need top-up transfusions for late anaemia. It has been suggested that the main role of IVIG is to 'buy time' before commencing exchange transfusion (Mitra and Rennie, 2017). NICE (2016) guidelines state that 500mg/kg over 4 hours should be given alongside intensified phototherapy when infants have severe Rhesus or ABO haemolytic disease and the SBR continues to increase by more than 8.5µmol/L per hour. IVIG works by blocking receptors on macrophages, reducing the breakdown of antibody-coated red cells, and by increasing the clearance of maternal antibodies (Louis et al., 2014). IVIG is a human-derived blood product and has potential side effects, including transfusion reactions, infection transmission, association with necrotising enterocolitis (NEC) and acute renal failure. Louis and colleagues' (2014) systematic review showed that the efficacy of IVIG was inconclusive in Rh disease.

Exchange transfusion

Exchange transfusion is a specialist procedure with associated risks of morbidity and mortality from vascular injuries, cardiovascular complications, biochemical and haematological disturbances, in addition to a small risk of blood-borne infection. However, exchange transfusions are now infrequently performed in NNUs, mainly due to the use of prophylactic anti-D for Rh negative mothers (New et al., 2016).

Aims of exchange transfusion:

■ To lower the SBR level and reduce the risk of brain damage and kernicterus
■ To correct anaemia and increase the oxygen-carrying capacity of the baby's blood
■ To remove damaged and antibody-coated red cells
■ To control the blood volume and relieve potential heart failure
■ To correct life-threatening electrolyte imbalance.

Double volume exchange transfusion should be used to treat infants whose SBR indicates its necessity, or where there are clinical signs of acute bilirubin encephalopathy (NICE, 2016). This will remove up to 50% of intravascular bilirubin.

Parents should be fully informed of the rationale for the procedure and its associated risks, and consent obtained. An exchange transfusion should normally be undertaken in neonatal intensive care, with the baby under a radiant heater. Intensified phototherapy should be continued. Nursing responsibilities include continuous monitoring and frequent recording of heart rate, respiratory rate, oxygen saturation, blood pressure and temperature during the procedure. A baseline set of observations encompassing colour, tone and blood sugar should be documented before the procedure starts. Enteral feeds should be stopped to reduce the risk of NEC. A specific red cell component for neonatal exchange transfusion is provided by UK Blood Services, usually group O, and should also be compatible with any maternal antibody (New et al., 2016). Twice the infant's blood volume should be exchanged (2 × 80mL/kg). Intravenous and arterial access is required via umbilical and/or peripheral lines. Aliquots of less than 5mL/kg are removed over 3–5 minutes with simultaneous continuous infusion of blood to the infant. After the exchange transfusion, intensified phototherapy should be continued and the SBR measured within 2 hours. Management is then maintained in accordance with the threshold graph.

Prolonged jaundice

Prolonged jaundice is defined as jaundice that is still evident in a term infant at 2 weeks of age, or in a premature infant at 3 weeks of age (Weng et al., 2018). This is most commonly unconjugated hyperbilirubinaemia, such as that seen in breastfed infants with around 9% of breastfed infants still jaundiced at 28 days of life. (Shortland et al., 2008; Ives, 2011; Mitra and Rennie, 2017). However, prolonged jaundice may occur due to an underlying disease or a condition that requires diagnosis and treatment, such as dehydration, infection, congenital hypothyroidism, inherited metabolic conditions and pyloric stenosis (Andre and Day, 2016). Suggested initial investigations for prolonged jaundice (NICE, 2016) are as follows:

- Evaluation of urine colour – is it dark and does it stain the nappy?
- Check stool colour – whether yellow or pale and chalky
- Measure total and split bilirubin
- Full blood count, blood group and DAT (Coombs test)
- Liver function test
- Urine culture
- Routine metabolic screening (ensure newborn bloodspot test has been sent)
- Thyroid function test
- G6PD level

Jaundice associated with breast milk/breastfeeding

The likelihood of a newborn developing hyperbilirubinaemia has been suggested to increase with the maternal intention to breastfeed exclusively (NICE, 2016). This type of jaundice usually reaches its peak between 14 and 21 days and is resolved by 3 months. The infant is generally well and gaining weight. This type of jaundice can occur for two reasons:

■ Newborns who are breastfed tend to have a lower fluid intake compared with formula-fed infants in the first few days, and as such have relatively higher levels of SBR. When a newborn has an insufficient intake of breast milk, their meconium output is decreased, increasing the reabsorption of bilirubin. Newborns have slower intestinal transit times increasing exposure to beta-glucuronidase as well as the unconjugation process via the enterohepatic circulation. A baby who is not feeding well is inclined to be lethargic and less likely to feed, therefore perpetuating the issue (Clark, 2013). Promotion of good milk supply in the early days will help the infant to take in sufficient amounts of colostrum, which is important, as it is a natural laxative and is an effective method of ensuring passage of meconium and prevention of a buildup of meconium. Breastfeeding mothers require support and education if they are to be successful.

■ The other proposed reason is thought to be due to constituents of breast milk. Breast milk is rich in beta-glucuronidase which increases the reuptake of unconjugated bilirubin. Additionally, epidermal growth factors have been found to be higher in breastfed infants, and these increase intestinal absorption in the newborn (Clark, 2013).

The potential harms of stopping breastfeeding outweigh any risks of mild or moderate hyperbilirubinaemia. If the infant is well, and no other pathologies are identified, breast milk jaundice is not known to result in bilirubin encephalopathy (Alex and Gallant, 2008). In an otherwise well infant, it is a benign and self-limiting condition (Preer and Philipp, 2011).

Conjugated hyperbilirubinaemia

If the serum conjugated bilirubin is greater than 25μmol/L, the infant should be referred for expert review as this may indicate serious liver disease, for example biliary atresia (NICE, 2016). This is often associated with pale, chalky stools and dark urine. Preterm infants on parenteral nutrition often have a marked conjugated hyperbilrubinaemia which improves gradually after parenteral nutrition is stopped. However, it may also be as a result of more permanent changes to the gut anatomy following surgery; for example, cholestasis, defined as a defect in either formation or excretion of bile, results in an increase in the serum of retained biliary components (bilirubin, bile acids, or cholesterol; Weiss and Vora, 2018), presenting as jaundice. Treatment is to address the primary cause of this conjugated type of jaundice, as listed below:

- Intrauterine infections
- Perinatal asphyxia
- Sepsis
- Severe haemolysis
- Prolonged use of parenteral nutrition
- α-1antitrypsin deficiency
- Cystic fibrosis
- Biliary atresia
- Choledochal cyst
- Spontaneous bile duct perforation
- Cholestasis
- Intrahepatic biliary hypoplasia
- Progressive familial idiopathic cholestasis
- Galactosaemia
- Tyrosinaemia.

Investigations for jaundice are outlined in Table 15.2.

TABLE 15.2 INVESTIGATIONS FOR JAUNDICE RELATED TO TIMING OF ONSET

Jaundice in the first 24 hours	Serum bilirubin levels including conjugated fraction (level >20μmol/L may indicate biliary atresia)
	Full blood count with haematocrit/packed cell volume
	Blood group and direct antiglobulin test
	Maternal blood group
	G6PD screening (be aware that this can be false during acute haemolysis)
	Galactose-l-phosphate uridyl transferase (to detect galactosaemia)
	TORCH screen for evidence of congenital infection (to detect toxoplasmosis, hepatitis, HIV, parvovirus, rubella, cytomegalovirus and herpes)
Jaundice appearing at 2–5 days	Same as for jaundice in first 24 hours as well as Blood cultures Urine metabolic screening looking for metabolic disorders
'Prolonged' jaundice (persisting for more than 14 days)	Same as for jaundice in first 24 hours, as well as Liver function tests Thyroid function tests

POLYCYTHAEMIA

Neonatal polycythaemia is defined as an excess of RBC. This results in raised haematocrit (>65%), otherwise known as packed cell volume (PCV). This, in turn increases blood viscosity, which can impair the circulatory flow to and in organs, and can cause neurological, cardiopulmonary and gastrointestinal symptoms. Many infants may be asymptomatic or may present with signs related to the organ affected by decreased perfusion (Gordon, 2003). Polycythaemia can be the result of a physiological condition, such as antenatal or intrapartum hypoxia, or a passive process (from RBC transfusion). Infants born post-term or small for gestational age, infants of diabetic mothers, recipient twins in twin-to-twin transfusion syndrome, are all at a higher risk of the condition (Remon et al., 2011).

A key nursing responsibility is to observe the affected infant for potential signs and symptoms and ensure that treatment is started, if applicable, as soon as possible to avoid complications such as diminished blood supply to organs and/or thrombosis. Symptoms include cyanosis, lethargy, poor feeding, and tremors, and apnoea may also be present.

Thrombocytopaenia and/or hyperbilirubinaemia may pose an issue. Respiratory distress, tachypnoea, and pleural or cardiac effusions may be complicating factors (Purves, 2005).

Treatment of polycythaemia is by partial exchange transfusion, which reduces the PCV. Partial exchange transfusion is carried out by withdrawing blood from a vein and replacing it with a diluent such as sodium chloride leading to diluted plasma volume. Further details about nursing care can again be found in table 15.4.

COAGULATION DISORDERS

Neonates are susceptible to bleeding for several reasons, including immaturity of the haemostatic system because of quantitative and qualitative deficiency of coagulation factors; maternal disease and medication use; birth trauma; and conditions such as sepsis and asphyxia. Coagulation disorders include those that involve haemorrhage, such as VKDB, thrombocytopaenia and DIC or, conversely, thrombosis. To understand the processes involved in coagulation disorders, it is important to appreciate the underlying physiology.

Coagulation physiology

Coagulation (clotting) and haemostasis (stopping the flow of blood) in the neonatal period are in a unique state of balance, due to the altered levels of procoagulants and anticoagulants common of this age group (Purves, 2005). Term infants have immature livers and associated levels of clotting factors in early life. Infants who are born prematurely or who are sick often present with even lower levels of clotting factors and further deranged clotting processes. The normal process is outlined below.

TABLE 15.3 BLOOD CLOTTING FACTORS

Factor I	Fibrinogen
Factor II*	Prothrombin
Factor III	Thromboplastin
Factor IV	Calcium ions
Factor V	Pro-accelerin
Factor VI	Is no longer recognised in the clotting pathway
Factor VII*	Pro-convertin (Serum prothrombin conversion accelerator)
Factor VIII	Antihaemophilic factor
Factor IX	Plasma thromboplastin component* (Christmas factor)
Factor X*	Thrombokinase (Stuart–Power factor)
Factor XI	Plasma thromboplastin antecedent
Factor XII	Hageman factor
Factor XIII	Fibrin stabilising factor
Other- Platelets	

* Vitamin K-dependent

When blood vessel injury occurs, platelets adhere to the damaged area and release adenosine diphosphate which activates the process of clotting. Platelets are pulled together due to an affinity for the blood protein fibrinogen, and in combination they form a mesh over the injury. In order to prevent the mesh from being pulled away, platelets contribute to the release of thromboxane, which encourages vasoconstriction and decreased blood flow in the damaged area. A process known as the clotting cascade is then initiated, in which a series of proteins and enzymes are activated sequentially through a variety of complex bio-chemical reactions to produce a blood clot. In addition, vitamin K is essential for the function of several proteins involved in blood coagulation (prothrombin, factors VII, IX and X, protein C, protein S and protein Z; see table 15.3). The importance of vitamin K in haemostasis arises from the fact that all vitamin K-dependent coagulation factors require carboxylation of glutamic acids to enable binding of calcium and attachment to phospholipid membranes.

Vitamin K deficiency bleeding

VKDB, formerly haemorrhagic disease of the newborn, can cause bleeding in an infant in the first few weeks of life. Vitamin K is necessary for the synthesis of coagulation factors. Term infants, especially those who are exclusively breastfed, are deficient in vitamin K and consequently may have VKDB. Preterm infants are potentially at greater risk for VKDB because of delayed feeding and subsequent delay in the colonisation of their gastrointes-tinal system with vitamin K-producing microflora, as well as immature hepatic and haemo-static function (Ardell et al., 2018). Vitamin K was first discovered in the early 1930s by the Danish biochemist Henrik Dam who observed – while studying cholesterol metabolism in chickens – that chicks fed with a diet free of sterols and low in fat tended to develop subcutaneous and intramuscular haemorrhages (Lippi and Franchini, 2011). Dietary deficiency in adults is extremely rare. Vitamin K deficiency in neonates is much more frequent due to both endogenous and exogenous deficiency. Endogenous vitamin K deficiency has been attributed to insufficient intestinal colonisation by bacteria. Many bacteria that colonise the human intestine synthesise vitamin K_2 (menaquinone). There is, however, debate on whether bacterial synthesis of vitamin K in the intestine provides a significant supply of this vitamin in humans (Shearer, 2009). Exogenous deficiency arises from poor placental transport of the vitamin and its low concentration in breast milk. The main source in neonates, which is almost exclusively breast milk, cannot adequately compensate for deficient endogenous production, since breast milk contains 1–4µg/L of vitamin K_1, and even lower amounts of vitamin K_2 (Lippi and Franchini, 2011).

Neonates are prone to vitamin K deficiency due to the limited stores at birth and insufficient intake (Van Winckel et al., 2009). VKDB is defined as a bleeding disorder in which the coagulation is rapidly corrected by vitamin K supplementation. In the UK, VKDB is very rare with most cases occurring in breastfed infants whose parents have refused prophylaxis (Knott, 2019). VKDB is usually classified by aetiology and by the age of onset.

- *Early onset* The least common form of VKDB presents within the first 24 hours and is associated with maternal intake of medications which interfere with vitamin K metabolism. These include anticonvulsants (phenytoin, carbemazepam and barbiturates), antituberculosis drugs (isonizid, rifampicin), some antibiotics (cephalosporins) and vitamin K antagonists (warfarin). The clinical presentation is often severe with cephalic haematoma and intracranial and intra-abdominal haemorrhages (Pichler and Pichler, 2008). Postnatal administration of vitamin K cannot prevent early neonatal bleeding. In pregnant women receiving anticonvulsant therapy, oral vitamin K (10mg) for 10 days prior to delivery may be of benefit to the infant (Bagwell, 2007).
- *Classical onset* This usually presents between 2 and 7 days of life and is associated with delayed or insufficient feeding. The clinical presentation is often mild, with bruises, gastrointestinal blood loss or bleeding from the umbilicus and puncture sites. Blood loss can be significant and intracranial haemorrhage has been described (Shearer, 2009).
- Late onset is associated with exclusive breastfeeding. It occurs between the ages of 2 and 12 weeks. The clinical presentation is severe with a mortality rate of 20% and intracranial haemorrhage occurring in 50%. In fully breastfed infants who did not receive vitamin K at birth, the incidence is between 1/15,000 and 1/20,000. Infants with cholestasis or malabsorption syndromes are at particular risk (Autret-Leca et al., 2001).

Babies who are entirely breastfed have a twentyfold risk of developing VKDB than those who receive formula milk, due to the low level of vitamin K in breast milk, and also the low levels of bacteria which help to synthesise vitamin K in the guts of breastfed infants.

If VKDB is suspected, it is important to review certain aspects of history:

■ Drugs taken in pregnancy
■ Gestation at delivery
■ Type and length of delivery
■ Feeding history (breastfed or formula-fed)
■ Maternal diseases e.g. idiopathic thrombocytopenic purpura, pre-eclampsia and diabetes
■ Family history of bleeding disorders
■ Previous affected siblings
■ Confirmation of vitamin K administration.

Investigations

■ Full blood count
■ Clotting screen, including prothrombin time (prolonged), coagulation time and partial thromboplastin time, D-dimer
■ Chest X-ray or ultrasound may confirm intrathoracic bleed
■ CT or MRI scan if intracranial haemorrhage or other major haemorrhage is suspected.

MANAGEMENT OF VITAMIN K DEFICIENCY BLEEDING

Vitamin K is commonly given prophylactically after birth for the prevention of VKDB. Since the 1950s, the use of artificial vitamin K, Konakion® 1mg to prevent VKDB has been common practice. Intramuscular (IM) administration continued until the 1980s, when it became more prevalent to give the IM preparation via the oral route. During the 1990s, administration of IM vitamin K to all newborn infants became routine. In 1992, Golding et al. (1992) reported an association between IM (not oral) vitamin K and childhood cancer, which caused controversy at the time, resulting in many parents not wishing their infants to receive the drug. Golding's studies were criticised for their methodology, and subsequent large-scale international studies have not supported the association of vitamin K to malignancy.

In accordance with current recommendation, healthy newborn infants who are not at particular risk of bleeding disorders should receive an IM injection of 1mg vitamin K at birth; or 1mg by mouth for 1 dose at birth and then 1mg every week for 12 weeks for infants who are exclusively breastfed (NICE, 2015b). For the preterm neonate, a single dose of 400 micrograms/kg (maximum dose 1mg) is to be given at birth. The intravenous route may be used with very low birth weight infants if IM injection is not possible. However, it may not provide the prolonged protection of IM administration, and the infant may require subsequent oral doses. Ardell et al. (2018) recommend further research on appropriate dosing and route for preterm infants. Many units require informed parental consent prior to any administration of vitamin K.

Thrombocytopaenia

The normal platelet count of a healthy newborn infant is 150 × 10^9/L and above; therefore, a count below this represents thrombocytopaenia (Roberts and Murray, 2003). The two underlying pathological mechanisms for this condition are decreased production or increased destruction of platelets. Thrombocytopaenia that presents early, for example, in the first 72 hours of life, is usually secondary to placental insufficiency leading to reduced platelet production. This can be mild to moderate in severity and should resolve spontaneously. Presentation after 72 hours of age is more likely secondary to sepsis or more serious conditions such as NEC. This is usually more severe and prolonged. Platelet transfusion is the treatment and administered either to prevent or to treat haemorrhage (Cremer et al., 2016).

Disseminated intravascular coagulation

DIC can be defined as a systemic thrombohaemorrhagic disorder (Veldman et al., 2010). Endothelial tissue damage from a variety of underlying disorders (sepsis, trauma) activates the coagulation cascade, which promotes fibrin production and consumption of clotting factors (figure 15.4). Neonates, especially preterm infants, are one of the highest-risk groups to develop DIC secondary to labile blood pressure and cardiac output, intravascular volume contraction after birth, immature mucosal and skin barriers and multiple invasive procedures. The most common conditions that lead to DIC in the neonatal population are probably infection/sepsis, NEC and hypoxic-ischaemia (Shetty and Givner, 2014). The

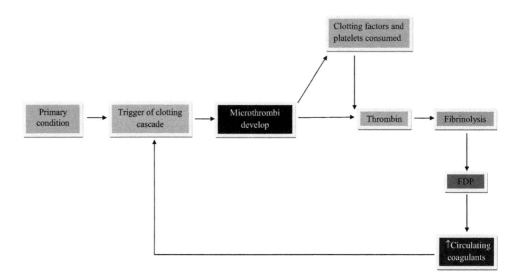

Figure 15.4 Disseminated intravascular coagulation

incidence of DIC is difficult to establish since it is a secondary disease process, but mortality rates are reported as 60–80% in infants with severe DIC who experience significant bleeding (Bagwell, 2007).

Clinical manifestations include petechiae, unexplained anaemia, bleeding from the gastrointestinal tract and puncture sites. In severe cases, intrapulmonary and intraventricular haemorrhages occur. Laboratory investigations should be interpreted in context of normal findings for gestation and postnatal age. Findings include consumption of coagulation factors and platelets and combined prolonged APTT and PT +/- low fibrinogen.

The importance of meticulous nursing observation for the presence of bleeding in the unwell NNU resident must not be underestimated. Haemorrhage may be evident, or more subtly noted in gastric/endotracheal aspirates or urine.

MANAGEMENT OF DISSEMINATED INTRAVASCULAR COAGULATION

Correction of the underlying disease process triggering the condition is the key to successfully treating the infant with DIC. Strategies such as early antibiotic therapy and identification and control of the source of disease in cases of NEC and sepsis should always precede interventions directed at normalising the coagulation system (Veldman et al., 2010). To improve oxygen delivery in the microcirculation, any form of circulatory compromise needs to be treated (Dellinger et al., 2013). Coagulation-based therapeutic approaches are mainly focused on preventing the formation of micro-thrombi in the capillary bed or preventing/stopping haemorrhage. Guidelines and protocols recommend the use of fresh frozen plasma (FFP) in the treatment of DIC (Mueller et al., 2002). However, prophylactic use of FFP in preterm neonates who are at high risk of haemorrhagic complications has not produced benefit, and a meta-analysis shows no advantage in survival or long-term outcome (Osborn et al., 2004). In recent years, the use of highly purified, virus-inactivated, plasma-derived proteins (factor XIII, factor XI, protein C and fibrinogen) has replaced FFP in Europe (Goldenberg and Manco-Johnson, 2006).

Nursing care related to DIC is outlined in table 15.4.

Thrombosis

There is an increased risk of thrombosis in high-risk infants (Meyer, 2016). Thromboses in neonates are often related to central venous catheters or arterial lines. All intravascular access acts to disrupt blood flow and damage endothelial cells and vessel walls, leading to **thrombus** formation. Venous or arterial catheters are especially risky and have led to concerns about using them too frequently due to this common complication. Renal vein thrombosis and portal vein thrombosis have also been reported as common in high-risk infants and nurses should be vigilant of potential complications (Greenway et al., 2004).

TABLE 15.4 NURSING CARE IN NEONATAL HAEMATOLOGICAL CONDITIONS

Condition	Nursing management
Jaundice (Hyperbilirubinaemia)	Clinical observation for presence of hyperbilirubinaemia, e.g. yellow skin and sclerae. Bilirubin monitoring via transcutaneous or blood sampling methods. Plotting bilirubin on threshold graph over time. Care during phototherapy or exchange transfusion as applicable.
Polycythaemia	Clinical observation for presence of polycythaemia- appearance, plethoric appearance/cyanosis, tachypnoea. PCV monitoring – be aware that the blood sampling site and perfusion of the sampling site may impact values; free-flowing venous sample is preferred.
Coagulation abnormalities 1 – Bleeding disorders (VKDB, Thrombocytopaenia, DIC)	Observe for signs of bleeding – via urine, bowel, stomach, bruises, at line insertion sites, procedures. Abnormal bruising, petechiae, purpura, bleeding and intracranial haemorrhage. Observe for signs such as poor feeding, pallor, poor weight gain, tachypnoea, and lethargy. Be familiar with normal clotting values and haemoglobin/platelet levels. Coagulation monitoring.
Coagulation abnormalities 2 – Thrombosis	Careful assessment and meticulous line care is essential in the prevention of thromboses, and other serious complications. Venous access should be initiated only when necessary. The nurse caring for the neonate with a venous or arterial thrombosis should carefully assess the affected limb and be aware of subtle changes in perfusion or patient status that could occur because of clot extension or embolism.
Anaemia	Clinical observation for presence of anaemia – pallor, changes to oxygenation, lethargy, apnoea. Be familiar with normal haemoglobin values. Haemoglobin monitoring.

ANAEMIA

Anaemia is a deficiency in the concentration of RBC and Hb in the blood and can result in tissue hypoxia and acidosis. An infant may be considered anaemic if the Hb or haematocrit value is more than two standard deviations below normal for their gestational age group

(Colombatti et al., 2016). All term and preterm infants experience a degree of physiological anaemia due to the conversion of foetal Hb to adult Hb during the first few weeks of post-natal life. Certain conditions may exacerbate this and lead to acute and chronic anaemia. These include acute or chronic blood loss/sampling and acute or chronic RBC haemolysis (Widness, 2008; Kolb and Levy, 2009; Kett, 2012). Delayed clamping of the umbilical cord (not earlier than 1 minute after birth) has been recommended to improve iron status in the infant for up to six months after birth (World Health Organization, 2014).

Physiological anaemia

During the first weeks of life, all infants will experience a decrease in the number of cir-culating RBC from that of the *in utero* level. It is universally acknowledged that healthy term infants will experience a drop in Hb to 110–120g/L at 10–12 weeks of age, which is well tolerated. The Hb will then remain low for most of the first year of life. This postnatal decrease in Hb is commonly referred to as physiological anaemia (Strauss, 2010).

Iatrogenic anaemia due to repeated blood sampling is an important consideration in the NNU. Measures which may reduce blood volume depletion and the incidence of iatro-genic anaemia include diagnostic testing based on individual infant condition rather than routine testing; micro sample laboratory techniques; non-invasive monitoring methods; and documentation of blood sample volumes collected. All the above may reduce the need for blood transfusion therapy.

Anaemia of prematurity

Erythropoiesis decreases after birth as a result of increased tissue oxygenation with the onset of breathing and closure of the ductus arteriosus, and a reduced production of erythropoietin. The primary cause of anaemia of prematurity (AOP) is the impaired ability to increase serum erythropoietin appropriately in the setting of anaemia and decreased tissue availability of oxygen. The majority of extremely low birth weight infants develop a normocytic, normochromic, hypoproliferative anaemia characterised by inadequate produc-tion of erythropoietin. This is in addition to blood sampling losses causing low haematocrit (Bishara and Ohls, 2009). Nutritional deficiencies of iron, vitamin E, vitamin B12 and folic acid may furthermore exaggerate the degree of anaemia.

Anaemia of prematurity typically occurs at 4–6 weeks after birth in infants of less than 32 weeks' gestation (Strauss, 2010). Many infants are asymptomatic despite having Hb values less than 70g/L (Zagl et al., 2012). Signs associated with AOP include tachycardia, poor weight gain, increased requirement of supplemental oxygen, or increased episodes of apnoea and bradycardia. Identification of the cause of anaemia through maternal and perinatal history review, laboratory data analysis and signs and symptoms will guide man-agement and treatment options.

MANAGEMENT OF ANAEMIA OF PREMATURITY

Clinicians who care for preterm infants should anticipate the development of AOP. Optimal nutrition (e.g. iron supplementation) should be provided, and patients monitored for signs of anaemia. Nurses also have a vital role in observing the infant for progressive anaemia, both clinically and by analysis of blood haemoglobin and PCV levels. This is summarised in table 15.4. Blood sampling should be limited to essential testing and micro techniques should be used to minimise blood loss due to phlebotomy (Madsen et al., 2000).

The following management strategies of AOP are available in NNUs in the UK:

■   *Iron supplementation* Iron content at birth is lower in preterm infants than in term infants, and the iron stores are often depleted by 2–3 months of age. As a result, all preterm infants who are breastfed should receive iron supplementation of 2–4mg/kg per day through the first year of life (Kleinman and Greer, 2014). Infants who receive iron-fortified formula need less additional supplementation than those who are exclusively breastfed, and this should be taken into account in a NNU's supplementation guidelines. Concurrent administration of calcium and phosphorus supplements should be avoided, as together with iron they form insoluble compounds which reduce the bioavailability of each mineral (Jones and King, 2005).

■   *Transfusion therapy* RBC transfusion is the most rapidly effective treatment for AOP. This is usually performed when anaemia is associated with clinical signs or is thought to compromise adequate oxygen delivery. Although no clearly defined biological markers have been identified to indicate when a RBC transfusion should be given, an absolute reticulocyte count <100,000/microL or Hb <70g/L are often used as criteria. However, transfusion is a temporary measure and has the disadvantages of further inhibiting erythropoiesis as well as being associated with risks of transmitted infection, graft versus host disease and toxic effects of anticoagulants and preservatives. To minimise these risks, blood is screened for many of the known organisms including hepatitis B and C, human immunodeficiency virus (HIV) and cytomegalovirus (CMV). Irradiation of blood products prevents transfusion-associated graft versus host disease, which results from a potentially fatal incompatibility between recipient and donor cells. This rare condition is said to be more likely when the recipient receives blood from multiple donors (Choi et al., 2010), and the use of smaller packs of irradiated blood produced from one donor, stored for as long as possible, may help to prevent this (Strauss, 2010).

■   *Erythropoiesis-stimulating agents* Erythropoietin is a glycoprotein which regulates the production rate of RBC. Studies in the USA and the UK have demonstrated that erythropoiesis-stimulating agents (ESAs) including recombinant erythropoietin, are effective in raising Hb levels and maintaining haematocrit levels during the normal phase of anaemia in the preterm infant (Bagwell, 2007; Ohlsson and Aher, 2017). ESAs have also been proposed as neuroprotective agents that reduce poor long-term neurodevelopment outcome (Ohls et al., 2013). Treatment with ESAs is usually commenced when infants are stable, receiving enteral feeds and can tolerate iron supplementation. It is administered for approximately 6 weeks or until 36 weeks postconceptional age is reached.

Pathological anaemia

Foeto-maternal transfusion, twin-to-twin transfusion, obstetric difficulties and internal haemorrhage are causes of acute neonatal blood loss or haemorrhage (Bagwell, 2007; Widness, 2008; Kett, 2012). Chronic anaemia may be associated with red cell destruction and haemolysis secondary to maternal–foetal blood group incompatibilities as well as acquired or congenital defects of red blood cells. Neonatal haemolysis is now most commonly caused by G6PD deficiency and less commonly with isoimmunisation, as seen in ABO and Rh incompatibilities. Haemolysis may occur as a result of bacterial sepsis and viral infections, and drug ingestion (maternal or direct administration of the drug to the newborn). Other rare causes of RBC haemolysis are thalassaemia and hereditary spherocytosis (Kolb and Levy, 2009; Kim et al., 2017).

NURSING CARE OF INFANTS WITH HAEMATOLOGICAL DISORDERS

The management of each condition within this chapter has been covered where applicable regarding specific elements of treatment and care. Speaking more generally about nursing care responsibilities within this area, monitoring neonates with signs and symptoms of a haematological condition is a key nursing intervention. Neonatal nurses should be familiar with normal blood values and be able to identify any concerns or abnormalities that may indicate a haematological condition. Blood sampling that is safe and timely is also a key component in good haematological care which can be advocated by the neonatal nurse. This should be done as part of an infant's holistic assessment in line with observation of clinical signs and associated changes in monitoring parameters. A summary of key areas of nursing assessment and care for each of the conditions in this chapter is outlined in table 15.4.

Understanding the pathophysiology, signs and symptoms, and basics of treatment is important in providing appropriate care in the NNU (Purves, 2005). This also ensures that healthcare professionals are in possession of the necessary information to support parents appropriately (Turnbull and Petty, 2012). The nurse has an important role in supporting families and, in the context of this chapter, answering questions about any haematological condition as they may struggle with not only the care of a new baby, but one with haematological problems.

CONCLUSION

Newborn haematology is a complex area of neonatal care that combines the unique aspects of maternal and foetal factors and the distinctive physiological conditions of the early post-natal period. This chapter has outlined specific haematological disorders that commonly present in the neonatal period including pathophysiology, signs and symptoms, treatment strategies and implications for nursing care.

CASE STUDIES

Case study 1: The infant with jaundice on day 1 of life

Amy is an infant girl born at 37 weeks' gestation, birth weight 2.4kg, second child to parents Bob and Karen. She has developed hyperbilirubinaemia on day 1 of life and is transferred to the special care unit for observation and investigation. She looks visibly jaundiced.

With reference to the key points within the chapter, consider the following questions:

Q.1. What type of jaundice is Amy presenting with and what are the potential causes?
Q.2. Can you explain the pathophysiology of this type of jaundice?
Q.3. What other types of jaundice are there and what is the associated physiology?
Q.4. What management and nursing care does this infant require?
Q.5. What information do you require from the parents and what do you need to explain to them?

Case study 2: The infant with abnormal blood results

Hassan is a 6-day-old premature infant born at 29 weeks' gestation who has been very unstable in his first few days of life and continues to show a fluctuating oxygen requirement, metabolic acidosis, possible signs of infection. He has umbilical catheters in situ and is fully monitored. His blood results show a low haemoglobin, prolonged clotting time and a low level of platelets.

With reference to the key points within the chapter, consider the following questions:

Q.1. What possible conditions is Hassan presenting with here and what are the underlying reasons for these blood results?

Q.2. What is the associated management and nursing care of this infant in relation to theses specific findings?

Q.3. How would you explain this to his parents to reassure them?

Case study 3: The infant who has a high red cell load

Thomas is a 35 weeks' gestation infant with intrauterine growth restriction who is 1 day old. His blood results show he has a high packed cell volume (PCV) of > 65% and is experiencing respiratory distress at present, grunting and tachypnoea.

With reference to the key points within the chapter, consider the following questions:

Q.1. What condition is Thomas presenting with here and what could be the potential underlying reasons for this blood result?

Q.2. What is the appropriate management and nursing care of this infant?

Q.3. What is the associated risk with this condition and how would you explain this to parents to reassure them?

For suggested answer guides to the questions posed in these case studies, please refer to the web-based companion site specific to this chapter (see URL below).

WEB-BASED RESOURCES

For further information, online resources and greater detail on the case studies featured in this chapter go to www.routledge.com/cw/nicnursing

References

Alex, M., & Gallant, D. P. (2008). Toward understanding the connections between infant jaundice and infant feeding. *Journal of Pediatric Nursing*, 23(6), 429–438.

Allen, D. (2016). Neonatal jaundice. *Nursing Children and Young People*, 28(6), 11.

Amos, R. C., Jacob, H., & Leith, W. (2017). Jaundice in newborn babies under 28 days: NICE guideline 2016 (CG98). *Archives of Disease in Childhood-Education and Practice*, 102(4), 207–209.

Andre, M., & Day, A. S. (2016). Causes of prolonged jaundice in infancy: 3-year experience in a tertiary paediatric centre. *Breast*, 140, 83–88.

Ardell, S., Offringa, M., Ovelman, C., & Soll, R. (2018). Prophylactic vitamin K for the prevention of vitamin K deficiency bleeding in preterm neonates. *Cochrane Database of Systematic Reviews*, Issue 2. Art. No.: CD008342. DOI: 10.1002/14651858.CD008342.pub2

Autret-Leca, E., & Jonville-Béra, A. P. (2001). Vitamin K in neonates. *Paediatric Drugs*, 3(1), 1–8.

Bagwell, G. (2007). A Hematologic System. In Kenner, C., & Lott, J. W. (Eds.) *Comprehensive Neonatal Care: An Interdisciplinary Approach* (4th Edition). Philadelphia: WB Saunders.

Bhandari, V. (2018). *BMJ Best Practice. Neonatal Jaundice.* www.bestpractice.bmj.com

Bishara, N., & Ohls, R. K. (2009). Current controversies in the management of the anemia of prematurity. *Seminars in Fetal and Neonatal Medicine, 33*(1), 29–34.

Cappellini, M. D., & Fiorelli, G. (2008). Glucose-6-phosphate dehydrogenase deficiency. *The Lancet, 371*(9606), 64–74.

Choi, S. W., Levine, J. E., & Ferrara, J. L. (2010). Pathogenesis and management of graft-versus-host disease. Immunology and allergy clinics of North America, 30(1), 75–101. DOI:10.1016/j.iac.2009.10.001

Clark, M. (2013). Clinical update: Understanding jaundice in the breastfed infant. *Community Practitioner*, 86(6), 42–45.

Colombatti, R., Sainati, L., & Trevisanuto, D. (2016). Anemia and transfusion in the neonate. *Seminars in Fetal and Neonatal Medicine, 21*(1), 2–9.

Cremer, M., Sallmon, H., Kling, P. J., Bührer, C., & Dame, C. (2016). Thrombocytopenia and platelet transfusion in the neonate. *Seminars in Fetal and Neonatal Medicine, 21*(1), 10–18.

De Haas, M., Thurik, F. F., Koelewijn, J. M., & van der Schoot, C. E. (2015). Haemolytic disease of the fetus and newborn. *Vox Sanguinis, 109*(2), 99–113.

Dellinger, R. P., Levy, M. M., Rhodes, A., Annane, D., Gerlach, H., Opal, S. M., … & Osborn, T. M. (2013). Surviving Sepsis Campaign: International guidelines for management of severe sepsis and septic shock, 2012. *Intensive Care Medicine, 39*(2), 165–228.

Ford, K. L. (2010). Detecting neonatal jaundice: New NICE guidance to recognise and treat neonatal jaundice and community settings. *Community Practitioner*, 83(8), 40–43.

Goldenberg, N. A., & Manco-Johnson, M. J. (2006). Pediatric hemostasis and use of plasma components. *Best Practice & Research Clinical Haematology*, 19(1), 143–155.

Golding, J., Greenwood, R., Birmingham, K., & Mott, M. (1992). Childhood cancer, intramuscular vitamin K, and pethidine given during labour. *British Medical Journal, 305*(6849), 341–346.

Gordon, E. A. (2003). Polycythemia and hyperviscosity of the newborn. *The Journal of Perinatal & Neonatal Nursing, 17*(3), 209–221.

Greenway, A., Massicotte, M. P., & Monagle, P. (2004). Neonatal thrombosis and its treatment. *Blood Reviews, 18*(2), 75–84.

Ives, N. K. (2011). Management of neonatal jaundice. *Paediatrics and Child Health, 21*(6), 270–276.

Jones, E., & King, C. (Eds.) (2005). *Feeding and Nutrition in the Preterm Infant.* Oxford: Elsevier.

Kett, J. C. (2012). Anemia in infancy. *Blood, 1599*(1678), 2.

Kim, Y., Park, J., & Kim, M. (2017). Diagnostic approaches for inherited hemolytic anemia in the genetic era. *Blood Research, 52*(2), 84–94.

Kleinman, R. E., & Greer, F. R. (2014). Nutritional needs of the preterm infant. In *Paediatric Nutrition Handbook.* (7th Edition). Itasca, IL: American Academy of Paediatrics.

Knott, L. (2009). Vitamin K deficiency bleeding. https://patient.info/doctor/vitamin-k-deficiency-bleeding

Kolb, E. A., & Levy, A. S. (2009). Anemia and Pallor. In McInerny, T. K., Adam, H. M., Campbell, D. E., Kamat, D. M., & Kelleher, K. J. (Eds.) *American Academy of Pediatrics Textbook of Pediatric Care.* Elk Grove Village: American Academy of Pediatrics.

Lippi, G., & Franchini, M. (2011). Vitamin K in neonates: Facts and myths. *Blood Transfusion, 9*(1), 4.

Louis, D., More, K., Oberoi, S., & Shah, P. S. (2014). Intravenous immunoglobulin in isoimmune haemolytic disease of newborn: An updated systematic review and meta-analysis. *Archives of Disease in Childhood: Fetal and Neonatal Edition, 99*(4), F325–F331.

Luzzatto, L., Nannelli, C., & Notaro, R. (2016). Glucose-6-phosphate dehydrogenase deficiency. *Hematology/Oncology Clinics, 30*(2), 373–393.

Madsen, L. P., Rasmussen, M. K., Bjerregaard, L. L., Nøhr, S. B., & Ebbesen, F. (2000). Impact of blood sampling in very preterm infants. *Scandinavian Journal of Clinical and Laboratory Investigation, 60*(2), 125–132.

Magyar, M. A., Metropulos, D., & Antoon, J. W. (2017). Direct Hyperbilirubinemia in an Infant. *Clinical Pediatrics, 56*(7), 696–699.

Maisels, M. J., & McDonagh, A. F. (2008). Phototherapy for neonatal jaundice. *New England Journal of Medicine, 358*(9), 920–928.

Meyer, S., Röhr, S., Duppré, P., Bay, J., Gortner, L., & Poryo, M. (2016). Neonatal thrombosis: Etiology and associated risk factors. *The Journal of Pediatrics, 175*, 242–243.

Mills, J. F., & Tudehope, D. (2001). Fibreoptic phototherapy for neonatal jaundice. *Cochrane Database of Systematic Reviews*, Issue 1. Art. No.: CD002060. DOI: 10.1002/14651858.CD002060

Mitra, S., & Rennie, J. (2017). Neonatal jaundice: Aetiology, diagnosis and treatment. *British Journal of Hospital Medicine, 78*(12), 699–704.

Mueller, M. M., Bomke, B., & Seifried, E. (2002). Fresh frozen plasma in patients with disseminated intravascular coagulation or in patients with liver diseases. *Thrombosis Research, 107*, S9–S17.

Mundy, C. (2005). Intravenous immunoglobulin in the management of hemolytic disease of the newborn. *Neonatal Network, 24*(6), 17–24.

National Institute for Health and Care Excellence. (2015a). *Jaundice in the Newborn. Clinical Knowledge Summary (CKS)*. NICE.

National Institute for Health and Care Excellence. (2015b). *Postnatal care up to 8 weeks after birth (CG37)*. NICE.

National Institute for Health and Care Excellence. (2016). *Jaundice in newborn babies under 28 days (QS57)*. NICE.

New, H. V., Berryman, J., Bolton-Maggs, P. H., Cantwell, C., Chalmers, E. A., Davies, T., ... & Stanworth, S. J. (2016). Guidelines on transfusion for fetuses, neonates and older children. *British Journal of Haematology, 175*(5), 784–828.

Ohls, R. K., Christensen, R. D., Kamath-Rayne, B. D., Rosenberg, A., Wiedmeier, S. E., Roohi, M., ... & Schrader, R. (2013). A randomized, masked, placebo-controlled study of darbepoetin alfa in preterm infants. *Pediatrics, 132*(1), e119.

Ohlsson, A., & Aher, S. M. (2017). Early erythropoiesis-stimulating agents in preterm or low birth weight infants. *Cochrane Database of Systematic Reviews*, Issue 11. Art. No.: CD004863. DOI: 10.1002/14651858.CD004863.pub5

Osborn, D. A., Evans, N., & Kluckow, M. (2004). Clinical detection of low upper body blood flow in very premature infants using blood pressure, capillary refill time, and central-peripheral temperature difference. *Archives of Disease in Childhood: Fetal and Neonatal Edition, 89*(2), F168–F173.

Pichler, E., & Pichler, L. (2008). The neonatal coagulation system and the vitamin K deficiency bleeding – a mini review. *Wiener Medizinische Wochenschrift, 158*(13–14), 385–395.

Preer, G. L., & Philipp, B. L. (2011). Understanding and managing breast milk jaundice. *Archives of Disease in Childhood: Fetal and Neonatal Edition, 96*(6), F461–F466.

Purves, E. (2005). Neonatal hematologic disorders. *Journal of Pediatric Oncology Nursing, 22*(3), 168–175.

Remon, J. I., Raghavan, A., & Maheshwari, A. (2011). Polycythemia in the Newborn. *NeoReviews, 12*(1), e20–e28.

Rennie, J., Burman-Roy, S., & Murphy, M. S. (2010). Neonatal jaundice: Summary of NICE guidance. *British Medical Journal, 340*, c2409.

Roberts, I., & Murray, N. A. (2003). Neonatal thrombocytopenia: causes and management. *Archives of Disease in Childhood: Fetal and Neonatal Edition, 88*(5), F359–F364.

Shearer, M. J. (2009). Vitamin K in parenteral nutrition. *Gastroenterology, 137*(5), S105–S118.

Shetty, A. K., & Givner, L. B. (2014). Disseminated neonatal herpes simplex virus infection presenting with pneumonia and progressive respiratory failure. *Journal of Clinical Neonatology, 3*(4), 211.

Shortland, D. B., Hussey, M., & Dey Chowdhury, A. (2008). Understanding neonatal jaundice: UK practice and international profile. *The journal of the Royal Society for the Promotion of Health, 128*(4), 202–206.

Singh, S. K., Singh, S. N., Kumar, M., Kumar, A., Tripathi, S., Bhriguvanshi, A., & Chandra, T. (2016). Etiology and clinical profile of neonates with pathological unconjugated hyperbilirubinemia with special reference to rhesus (rh) D, C, and E incompatibilities: A tertiary care center experience. *Clinical Epidemiology and Global Health, 4*(2), 95–100.

Smits-Wintjens, V. E. H. J., Walther, F. J., & Lopiore, E. (2008). Rhesus haemolytic disease of the newborn: Postnatal management, associated morbidity and long-term outcome. *Seminars in Fetal & Neonatal Medicine, 13*, 265–271.

Strauss, R. G. (2010). Anaemia of prematurity: Pathophysiology and treatment. *Blood Reviews. 24*(6), 221–225.

Truman, P. (2006). Jaundice in the preterm infant. *Paediatric Nursing, 18*(5), 20–22.

Turnbull, V., & Petty, J. (2012). Early onset jaundice in the newborn: Understanding the ongoing care of mother and baby. *British Journal of Midwifery, 20*(9), 615–622.

Van Winckel, M., De Bruyne, R., Van De Velde, S., & Van Biervliet, S. (2009). Vitamin K, an update for the paediatrician. *European Journal of Pediatrics, 168*(2), 127.

Veldman, A., Fischer, D., Nold, M. F., & Wong, F. Y. (2010). Disseminated intravascular coagulation in term and preterm neonates. *Seminars in Thrombosis and Hemostasis, 36*(4), 419–428.

Weiss, A. K., & Vora, P. V. (2018). Conjugated Hyperbilirubinemia in the Neonate and Young Infant. *Pediatric Emergency Care, 34*(4), 280–283.

Weng, Y., Cheng, S., Yang, C., & Chiu, Y. (2018). Risk assessment of prolonged jaundice in infants at one month of age: A prospective cohort study. *Scientific Reports, 8*(1), 1–6.

Widness, J. A. (2008). Pathophysiology of anemia during the neonatal period, including anemia of prematurity. *Neoreviews, 9*(11), e520–e525.

World Health Organization. (2014). *Optimal timing of cord clamping for the prevention of iron deficiency anaemia in infants.* The WHO Reproductive Health Library.

Zagol, K., Lake, D. E., Vergales, B., Moorman, M. E., Paget-Brown, A., Lee, H., … & Kattwinkel, J. (2012). Anemia, apnea of prematurity, and blood transfusions. *The Journal of Pediatrics, 161*(3), 417–421.

16 MANAGEMENT OF NEONATAL FLUID AND ELECTROLYTE BALANCE

Alli Mitchell and Ella Porter

CONTENTS

GUIDANCE ON HOW TO ENHANCE PERSONAL LEARNING FROM THIS CHAPTER

Key points covered in this chapter

■ The physiological basis of fluid and electrolyte balance in neonatal care.

■ An overview of the causes and implications of neonatal fluid and electrolyte imbalances.

■ The nursing management, including the assessment of an infant's fluid and electrolyte status.

Reflection

Reading through the chapter, you are encouraged to engage with the key points and related literature in an enquiring way. Ask these questions:

■ How would you recognise fluid depletion or fluid overload in the babies you care for?

■ Why is fluid balance and management in the neonatal unit challenging and why is it so important?

■ How does fluid balance relate to the other important topic of nutrition?

Implications for nursing care

■ Finally: how will this chapter enable you to consider and understand neonatal fluid and electrolyte balance when delivering holistic care to the infant and family? Consider the implications of what you learn for your nursing care relating to fluid management.

INTRODUCTION AND BACKGROUND

The aims of this chapter are to highlight the relevant aspects of fluid and electrolyte balance to enable the nurse to anticipate problems, to assess the adequacy of renal function, and subsequently to plan the management of infants in neonatal care. Many physiological, environmental, gestational and iatrogenic factors influence fluid and electrolyte balance. Fluid and electrolyte therapies play an important role in the management of preterm and term infants who are admitted to the neonatal unit (NNU). An understanding of this helps to form a rationale for management, as it is the role of the neonatal nurse to administer fluid therapy and monitor fluid balance. Providing maintenance fluid to these infants, including careful assessment to avoid excessive fluid administration that may increase the risk of neonatal morbidities (Oh, 2012) is an essential nursing responsibility. Therefore, meticulous attention to detail should highlight imbalances early to avoid potential serious complications; for example, intraventricular haemorrhage (IVH), chronic lung disease (Rocha et al., 2010; Bell and Acarregui, 2014; Barrington et al., 2017) and symptomatic patent ductus arteriosus (Harish Madhava and Settle, 2009). This chapter provides an overview of fluid and electrolyte balance and management in the NNU.

PHYSIOLOGICAL BASIS OF FLUID AND ELECTROLYTE BALANCE

Water and electrolytes are vital components of physiological stability at any point in life. In the newborn infant, this stability is often impaired due to immaturity or altered function, in the term infant, by an underlying disease process such as hypoxia or sepsis. These problems can be further compounded by the administration of **nephrotoxic** drugs. Fluid and electrolyte imbalances in the newborn period can lead to significant morbidity if not detected early.

Moreover, before considering the potential problems for the infant in the NNU, it is important to understand the vital role and function of the kidneys, which have been described as the major determinant of blood composition (Stafford-Smith, 2007). At term, each kidney contains the adult complement of approximately 1,000,000 nephrons. In the preterm infant, nephrogenesis may continue at the same rate as *in utero*. Development can continue up to forty days postpartum, with anatomical abnormalities occurring at any stage. Low birth weight (LBW), small size for gestational age and prematurity are all factors which can reduce the number of nephrons (Low Birth Weight and Nephron Number Working Group, 2017). An infant born at 24 weeks' gestation will not complete this process for 10–12 weeks. At 24 weeks, the kidney measures 2.5cm and grows to 4.5cm at term. The adult size of 6cm is achieved post-natally by the elongation of the **proximal** renal tubules and the loops of Henle. Maturation of renal function is completed by two years of age. However, particularly in the extremely preterm population, this may remain comparatively impaired even in later life (Sutherland et al., 2011).

Urine production begins with the process of glomerular filtration. As the blood flows through the afferent arteriole into the glomerulus, non-selective filtration occurs, in which fluid and **solutes** pass through the capillary membrane into Bowman's capsule. The rate of filtration is affected by several factors, but the most important is hydrostatic pressure. **Glomerular filtration rate** (GFR) is low in newborns compared with adults. The GFR rises after birth due to a progressive rise in systemic blood pressure, fall in renal vascular resistance, and an increase in renal blood flow from 4% of the cardiac output to 10%. This will further rise to the adult level of 25% in the first few days of life. GFR appears to increase in a programmed way at least from 26 weeks' gestation, and from the second postnatal day, unaffected by the gestation at birth. Estimating GFR using a single serum endogenous biomarker such as creatinine is considered more clinically useful than the alternative exogenous marker (Pasala and Carmody, 2017). The preterm infant should produce a minimum of 25–60mL of urine per kilogram every 24 hours, which can rise to a maximum of 300mL/ kg per 24 hours with acute increases in fluid intake. The minimum value on day 1 (0.51mL/ kg/hr) represents the lowest acceptable volume, as below this level solute accumulation will occur. Between days two and three, 2–3mL/kg/hour is acceptable; infants producing a lower volume warrant further investigation as a matter of urgency (Bezerra et al., 2013).

Most infants (95%) pass urine in the first 24 hours of life. Approximately 21% will pass urine at delivery, and as this may be missed or not recorded, it is advisable for the neonatal nurse to communicate to the professional who was present at the delivery of the infant to ascertain this information.

Physiological changes in neonates are not static. Following birth, several adaptive processes from intrauterine to extrauterine life occur. The structural and functional development of the kidney is responsible for a significant impact on postnatal adaptation to extrauterine life (Saint-Faust et al., 2014). All neonates continue to adapt postnatally. Body fluids are split into specific body compartments, the extracellular and the intracellular compartments. Extracellular fluid is found in plasma and the circulatory system. Intracellular fluids are inside the body's cells. Both control the movement of fluid and electrolytes within the body. Changes to the intracellular and extracellular compartments occur 12–48 hours following birth. After birth, the percentage of total body water gradually decreases, primarily as a result of decreasing extracellular fluid. Intracellular fluid proportionately increases postnatally (Lindower, 2017).

Initial adaptations to total body water, which encompasses both the intracellular and extracellular compartments, occur to compensate for the newborn's high metabolic demand, body temperature and growth (Bhatia, 2006). It is expected that a term infant will lose 5–10% body weight, while a preterm infant may lose 10–15% of their body weight in the first seven days of life. For sick, extremely premature neonates, 'third spacing' may occur. This is fluid which moves from the extracellular compartment into the interstitial spaces (between the skin and fascia). The result is a lower circulating volume, which causes hypotension and oedema, and requires senior medical advice and management.

FLUID AND ELECTROLYTE MANAGEMENT

It is not unusual to identify fluid and electrolyte disturbances, and many neonates who are admitted to a NNU are likely to require intravenous (IV) fluids during their stay.

TABLE 16.1 INSENSIBLE WATER LOSSES ACCORDING TO BIRTH WEIGHT

Birth weight	IWL (ml/kg/day)
<1000 grams	60–80
1000–1500 grams	40–60
>1500 grams	20

Insensible water loss (IWL) is the evaporation of water though mucous membranes and the skin. Greater water permeability occurs for infants who are low birth weight and premature due to higher skin permeability and a higher surface to body weight ratio (table 16.1). Insensible water losses are not readily measured, approximately 70% are lost through the skin and 30% via the respiratory tract. In the extreme premature infants, the IWL increases. There are many factors which contribute to an increase/reduction in IWL and fluid losses.

Increased IWL may occur in the following circumstances:

At delivery

- Increased environmental temperature
- Radiant heat sources (resuscitaire)
- Extremely LBW infants (large surface area to body weight ratio, less subcutaneous fat)
- Low gestational age.

Neonatal unit

- Heated mattresses
- Forced convection, radiation, evaporation, conduction – draughts, open windows and doors
- Hyperthermia
- Tachypnoea
- Surgical malformations (neural tube defects, gastroschisis, exomphalos – this is part of the rationale to cover such lesions with cling film)
- Phototherapy
- Frequent opening of incubator doors
- Crying
- Increased motor activity.

Strategies to reduce IWL include:

At delivery

- Thin transparent plastic bags/wraps
- Reduced staff traffic
- Closed doors and windows
- Ambient temperature 24–25°C
- Covering the baby during transportation.

Following admission to NNU

- High ambient humidity incubator
- Humidified gases
- Double-walled incubator
- Minimal handling
- Reduce staff traffic
- Tracheal intubation with humidification
- Good skin care.

It is important to maintain normothermia to reduce radiation, conduction, convection, and evaporative losses as they contribute to adverse effects in a neonate (Sinha et al., 2017). The management of thermal stability is explored in chapter 11.

Fluid requirements

Fluid intake is usually calculated on the infant's birth weight, until that weight is exceeded, unless weight gain is thought to be due to fluid retention and/or oedema. Sodium and water requirements in the first few days of life are low and should be increased after the postnatal diuresis (O'Brien and Walker, 2014). The fluid requirement for growth in a preterm infant is thought to be 120–150mL/kg in 24 hours, but until postnatal diuresis begins, much less is required, and usual starting figures are 60mL/kg in a well-humidified environment (Bell and Acarregui, 2014). Careful restriction of fluid intake is advised, so that physiological requirements are met, to prevent dehydration. Some infants may require a more rapid increase in fluid volumes, for example, very preterm infants with high insensible losses that are not minimised, while term infants, following asphyxial injury, require a more cautious approach and may undergo fluid restriction. When calculating an infant's fluid requirement, the weight, disease state, general condition, urine output, fluid losses and blood biochemistry need to be taken into consideration.

There are significant fluid shifts in a neonate from birth to 48 hours postnatal age. For neonates who are sick, preterm or compromised, calculating the daily fluid and electrolytes requires an individualised approach (Modi, 2004; 2012a; Oh, 2012). An alternative fluid and electrolyte regime may be necessary for neonates with the following conditions:

- Neonatal encephalopathy
- Hypoxic-ischaemic encephalopathy
  - likely renal compromise and oedema
  - decrease fluid volume to reduce the risks of cerebral oedema
- Acute renal injury
- High insensible losses (especially neonates <28 weeks)
- Ascites
- Hypoglycaemia
  - may require a higher fluid volume and or glucose concentration to normalise blood glucose
- Hyperglycaemia
  - may require a decrease in glucose concentration or fluid volume to normalise blood glucose
- Following surgery.

Prior to prescribing and administering any IV fluids and electrolytes, it is important to assess the following:

- Clinical history of the neonate's previous 24 hours to provide a basis for the following 24-hour fluid and electrolyte regime
- Physical examination
  - clinical condition
  - general wellbeing
- Cardiovascular system
  - heart rate, blood pressure
  - capillary refill time
  - oedema
- Weight trend
  - signs of dehydration and skin turgor
  - moist mucous membranes
  - fontanelles soft and flat, not sunken
- Fluid input/output
  - weigh all nappies
  - urine evaluation – output and specific gravity
  - gastric, chest drain losses etc.
  - stool
- Activity
  - good tone
- Assessment of current fluids, maintenance and additional infusions
  - assess patency of all intravenous lines
  - fluid prescriptions

- Review laboratory results
  - full blood count, serum urea, electrolytes, creatinine, glucose, urinary electrolyte concentrations
- Blood gas
  - acidosis, alkalosis
  - base excess and lactate.

The principles of fluid and electrolyte balance are to provide enough fluid to prevent dehydration, enough calories to prevent ketosis, allow growth and to provide correct electrolytes to maintain homeostasis.

Calculation of required daily fluid intake follows the formula below:

$$\frac{BW\,(kg) \times volume\,per\,day}{24} = hourly\,input$$

Example: Fiona was born today at 24 weeks' gestation at a birth weight of 600g. She requires 90mL/kg/day of 10% glucose. What is her hourly rate of IV glucose?

Answer:

$$\frac{0.6 \times 90}{24} = 2.25mL\,/\,hour$$

Fluids are calculated using the birth weight, until this is exceeded, to optimise fluid balance and electrolyte stability. Birth weight is usually regained by 7–10 days.

Routine maintenance IV fluid intake per day according to the neonate's gestation and birth weight can be calculated as seen in table 16.2 (guide only).

Depending on the neonatal age, gestation, birth weight and clinical condition, 10% glucose is the IV fluid of choice if the criteria for parenteral nutrition are not met, until full enteral feeds are established. Potassium and sodium are not required in the first 48 hours, as neonates

TABLE 16.2 MAINTENANCE INTRAVENOUS FLUID REGIMES

Postnatal age	<26 weeks GA or <750g birth weight	≥26 weeks GA or ≥750g birth weight
Day 1	90 ml/kg/day	60–90 ml/kg/day
Day 2	120 ml/kg/day	90 ml/kg/day
Day 3	150 ml/kg/day	120 ml/kg/day
Day 4	150–180 ml/kg/day	120–150 ml/kg/day
Day 5 onwards	150–210 ml/kg/day	150 ml/kg/day

(adapted from NICU guidelines, St Mary's Hospital, Manchester)

TABLE 16.3 PROBLEMS ASSOCIATED WITH FLUID IMBALANCE

Too much fluid will contribute to	Too little fluid will contribute to
Over-hydration	Under-hydration
■ Hyponatraemia	■ Hypernatraemia
■ Peripheral and pulmonary oedema	■ Hypovolaemia and hypotension
■ Pulmonary haemorrhage	■ Worsening jaundice
■ Increased respiratory illness	■ Metabolic acidosis
■ Symptomatic persistent ductus arteriosus	■ Low cardiac preload and impaired function
■ Heart failure	■ Impaired renal function and urine output
■ Hyperglycaemia	
■ Impaired renal function and urine output	

have a low GFR (thus producing small quantities of urine), and are therefore unable to tolerate additional sodium, as this can cause fluid retention). After 48 hours, GFR increases with a corresponding diuresis (Hartnoll et al., 2001; Hartnoll, 2003), so that thereafter electrolytes can be added to the maintenance fluids. Rigorous surveillance of urea and electrolytes should be closely monitored 8–12 hourly. The extremely premature neonate's electrolytes and weight may fluctuate within a given 24-hour period. Adjustments must be tailored accordingly to maintain normal thresholds. The problems associated with fluid imbalance are outlined in table 16.3.

In accordance with laboratory guidelines for fluid and electrolyte therapies, IV fluids may be increased in addition to normal requirements based on postnatal age in the presence of

- Increased weight loss (>3% per day, or a cumulative loss of more than 15%)
- Increased serum sodium (Na^+ >150 mmol/L)
- Increased specific gravity (>1.020) or urine osmolality (400mOsm/L)
- Decreased urine output (<1mL/kg/hr over 24 hours).

Conversely, IV fluids may need to be restricted in the presence of

- Decreased weight loss (<1% or a cumulative loss <5%)
- Decreased sodium content in the presence of weight gain (Na^+ <130mmol/L)
- Decreased urine specific gravity (1.005) or urine osmolality (<100mOsm/L).

ELECTROLYTE REQUIREMENTS

Sodium

Sodium (Na^+)
The normal value is 135–145mmol/L

Daily requirement varies 1–8mmol/kg/day
Average 2–4mmol/kg/day
Usually not required in the first 48 hours life

Sodium is an essential nutritional electrolyte. Prolonged deficiency is associated with poor growth, sensorineural hearing impairments and neurological sequalae (Bolisetty et al., 2015). The extremely preterm baby is known to have high rates of growth failure (Ofek et al., 2014). Sodium is the major cation in extracellular fluid and is vital for the regulation of circulating blood volume as well as weight gain and tissue growth. There is a lack of consensus for the assessment of total body sodium content in newborns. Evidence to support alternative sodium supplementation regimes in comparison with adults is unfounded (Bischoff et al., 2016). The newborn term kidney can filter and reabsorb sodium reasonably efficiently. Utilising approximately 9% of the infant's oxygen consumption for energy, sodium and water are reabsorbed from the nephron back into the circulation. Due to the high concentration gradient of sodium, it is the first ion to move from the filtrate in the tubular lumen to the tubular epithelial cell. A normal physiological negative balance of sodium and water has been found to occur in healthy newborn infants during the first few days of life.

The preterm infant has a poor capacity to excrete and reabsorb sodium, thus being at risk of early hypernatraemia (Gawlowski et al., 2006) and late hyponatraemia (Mannan et al., 2012; Kim et al., 2015). The very preterm infant is also at risk of high transepidermal water losses increasing the propensity for hypernatraemia. Reported risk factors for hyponatraemia include prematurity coupled with a birth weight of less than 1kg (Mannan et al., 2012), administration of fortified breast milk, as well as receiving loop diuretics and indometacin (Kim et al., 2015). The introduction and benefits of enteral feeds will be explored in chapter 17. In sick preterm infants, early intake of sodium is unnecessary and possibly harmful, and should be avoided until the physiological postnatal diuresis, or a weight loss of 6% of the birth weight has occurred. Thereafter, normal maintenance requirements are 2–4mmol/kg/day. Sick infants' requirements, however, will vary according to several factors, and this requires careful clinical assessment prior to supplementation. The serum sodium level should be measured 8-hourly in the acutely sick infant. Reasons for sodium imbalances are shown in table 16.4, while box 16.1 outlines the calculation for the correction of a sodium deficit.

HYPONATRAEMIA

Low sodium levels are often evident at birth, reflecting the maternal value (Modi, 2004). Hyponatraemia occurring during the first week of life may be due to water retention or sodium wastage, although opinion is mixed as to which is the most likely (Mannan et al., 2012). Inappropriate antidiuretic hormone (IADH) syndrome is frequently implicated as the factor responsible for hyponatraemia (Mattson Porth, 2011). Elevated antidiuretic hormone (ADH) levels are often seen along with hyponatraemia; this may be due to infant

TABLE 16.4 CAUSES OF SODIUM IMBALANCE

Hyponatraemia	Hypernatraemia
Excess maternal fluid intake during labour/ delivery	Excess insensible water loss (particularly very preterm)
Excess renal loss (particularly very preterm)	Insufficient fluid replacement
Insufficient replacement	■ While under phototherapy or radiant heaters
■ Sodium-poor intravenous therapy	■ Diarrhoea
■ Expressed breast milk with low sodium fortifiers	■ Glycosuria causing osmotic diuresis
Medication	Drugs or parenteral nutrition/ fluids containing excessive sodium
■ Diuretics (especially loop diuretics)	
■ Xanthines (i.e. caffeine)	
Inappropriate ADH secretion	
Excess sodium losses	
■ Diarrhoea, gastric, pleural, CSF	
■ Salt-losing congenital adrenal hyperplasia (17 hydroxyprogesterone deficiency)	
■ Adrenocortical failure	
■ Acute tubular necrosis	
■ Barter's syndrome (associated with hypokalaemia)	
Haemolysis	
Hyperlipidaemia	

(adapted from Modi, 2012a)

BOX 16.1 CALCULATION FOR CORRECTING A SODIUM DEFICIT

To calculate an infant's sodium deficit, the following formula is used:

0.7 x body weight (kg) x (140 − serum sodium) = sodium deficit

To correct the deficit, aim to replace two-thirds of this within 24 hours, while concurrently monitoring plasma and urine electrolytes at least daily, to determine subsequent replacement. Where the sodium deficit is due to inappropriate ADH secretion, fluids are restricted along with sodium replacement.

conservation of water to maintain circulating volume at the expense of the plasma osmolality. It is likely that in these situations secretion of ADH is physiologically appropriate. This differentiation is important, as a true case of IADH requires restriction of fluids, whereas in physiological adaptation due to low circulating volume an increase of fluid volume and sodium may be what is necessary. Irrespective of the cause of the hyponatraemia, an appropriate positive sodium balance is vital, since a chronic deficiency is associated with poor skeletal and tissue growth with adverse neurodevelopmental outcome (Bolisetty et al., 2015).

HYPERNATRAEMIA

A rising serum sodium (>145mmol/L) should prompt senior review and an increase in maintenance fluids by 10–30mL/kg/day in the extremely LBW neonate. Hypernatraemia usually presents in the very preterm infant secondary to TEWL, or due to 'hidden' sodium supplementation from saline infusions for arterial lines, IV flushes following drugs, or sodium bicarbonate infusions. In moderate hypernatraemia (serum level of up to 155mmol/L), sodium supplements are best avoided, and appropriate fluid replacement should correct the imbalance. At higher levels (Na$^+$ >155mmol/L), care must be taken not to lower the plasma concentration faster than 10mmol/day. Rapid falls in sodium concentration can precipitate cerebral oedema and convulsions. Judicious additional sodium may be required, while the fall in plasma sodium is carefully monitored.

Potassium

> Potassium (K$^+$)
> The normal value at 0–7days is 3.5–5.5/mmol/L
> at 8–24 days 3.4–6.0mmol/L
> Usually not required in the first 48 hours of life
> Daily requirement 1–2 mmol/kg/day

Potassium is the principal intracellular cation and is required for maintenance of the intracellular fluid volume. Potassium reabsorption, which occurs mainly in the **distal** tubule, is mediated by aldosterone, which regulates the sodium-potassium-pump to maintain cellular electroneutrality. Renal regulation of potassium is linked to the arterial pH. In a metabolic alkalotic state, the kidney will excrete potassium in exchange for sequestering bicarbonate within the cells, resulting in hypokalaemia. In a metabolic acidotic state, potassium is exchanged for hydrogen ions in the proximal tubule, increasing the plasma concentration. In infants requiring parenteral fluids, potassium supplementation should commence when urine output is adequate, providing that the plasma level is not elevated (Cairns, 2012). Serum potassium levels should be measured 8-hourly in the acutely sick infant. Reasons for potassium imbalances are shown in table 16.5.

TABLE 16.5 CAUSES OF POTASSIUM IMBALANCE

Hypokalaemia	Hyperkalaemia
Insufficient replacement	Tissue damage
Excess losses	Excessive bruising
■ Renal	Nephrotoxic drugs
■ polyuric states	Renal impairment/failure:
■ chronic diuretics	■ Acute tubular necrosis
■ renal tubular acidosis	■ Renal vein thrombosis
■ Bartter's syndrome (with hyponatraemia)	■ Congenital chronic renal failure
■ Medication	Rhabdomyolysis
■ salbutamol	
■ insulin	
Hyperaldosteronism	
Alkalosis	
Gastrointestinal causes	
■ Gastric aspiration	
■ Vomiting	
■ Stoma losses	
■ Diarrhoea	

HYPOKALAEMIA

It has been found that extreme variations in the plasma concentration of potassium can occur in neonates, both above and below the normal range of 3.8–5.0mmol/L, indicating rapid changes between the intracellular and extracellular compartments. A deficiency invariably involves an excessive loss via either the intestinal or renal routes, or both, or a lack of appropriate supplementation.

Potassium supplements should be commenced on the third postnatal day at a rate of 1–2mmol/kg/day, provided an adequate urine output (over 1mL/kg/hr) has been observed and the plasma level is not elevated. Administration of appropriate replacements as indicated is recommended, with estimation of ongoing losses and careful monitoring of serum levels (Vemgal and Ohlsson, 2012).

HYPERKALAEMIA

Hyperkalemia (K^+ >6.5mmol/L) is usually associated with a failure of the renal excretory mechanisms or secondary to an overwhelming situation arising from acidosis or severe infection. Elevated levels can also occur if there has been extensive bruising or ischaemic insult (Mahoney et al., 2005). Any potassium supplements must be omitted until the normal range of potassium is achieved. Spurious hyperkalaemia can also be reported following haemolysis of blood cells during sampling. Capillary potassium values are generally higher than arterial potassium values, so low potassium on a capillary sample indicates significantly lower arterial potassium values. Hyperkalaemia may be one of the earliest manifestations of congenital adrenal hyperplasia. True hyperkalaemia is extremely serious and potentially a lethal condition; the management must be prompt. All potassium supplementation or drugs containing potassium must be stopped and increased echocardiographic (ECG) surveillance commenced, closely observing for arrhythmias. Arrhythmias are unlikely unless the potassium level is >7.5mmol/L. A continued rise may lead to ventricular tachycardia, ventricular fibrillation or asystole (Paediatric Formulary Committee, 2018). A senior medical opinion should be sought. There are a number of drug therapies to reduce the levels of potassium in the short term.

Calcium gluconate may be infused slowly to counteract the excitatory effects of potassium on the myocardium. As calcium gluconate extravasation injury causes severe and permanent tissue damage, it is best infused via a central line. If it is infused peripherally, the infusion site should be clearly visible and carefully observed (Royal College of Nursing (RCN), 2016). Rectal calcium resonium reduces the serum potassium level by altering the cell membrane threshold to move potassium back into the cell. This can be achieved by the IV infusion of sodium bicarbonate (4.2% solution over 5–10 minutes), glucose and insulin solutions (with concurrent careful blood glucose monitoring), or salbutamol (O'Hare and Molloy, 2008). Ideally, neonates who are at risk of NEC should not receive rectal calcium resonium. IV sodium bicarbonate (1mmol/kg) is said to be effective in reducing serum potassium levels even if the patient is not acidotic (Haycock, 2003). Before effects of the drug therapies take place, it may be prudent to consider exchange transfusion or renal dialysis (Masilamani and van der Voort, 2012). Further details on drug therapies to normalise elevated potassium levels can be found in the web-based resources.

Chloride

Chloride (Cl⁻)
The normal value is 96–110mmol/L
Average requirement 2–4mmol/kg/day

Chloride is an anion abundant in extracellular fluid. Hypochloraemia may result from increased losses from gastric aspiration due to obstruction, or surgery leading to metabolic alkalosis. Hyperchloraemia can occur in infants who are hypernatraemic or receiving parenteral nutrition, and results in metabolic acidosis. High chloride levels are not linked to impaired neurological outcomes. There is a relationship between chloride and sodium balance; for instance, prematurity can influence chloride levels (Iacobelli et al., 2012).

Calcium and phosphate

Calcium (Ca^{2+})
The normal value is 1.8–2.9mmol/L

Calcium is bound to serum albumin, and thus monitored in conjunction

Phosphate (PO_4^{3-})

The normal values at day 2–3 are 1.8–3.0mmol/L

from day 21 1.7–2.6mmol/L

Requirements vary depending on gestational age, co-morbidities and type of enteral feeds

Raised alkaline phosphatase levels +/- hypercalcaemia in the presence of hypophosphataemia may be indicative of developing metabolic bone disease

Calcium and phosphate are essential minerals required for normal growth, development and bone mineralisation. Prolonged imbalances are associated with metabolic bone disease, which particularly the preterm population is at risk of. Serum ionised calcium is considered a true reflection of the body's calcium status (Sava et al., 2005). Hypocalcaemia in the newborn is defined as Ca^{2+} <2mmol/L in term infants and <1.75mmol/L in preterm infants. Clinical manifestations normally become apparent with an ionised calcium <0.75mmol/L. There is active transport of calcium and phosphate via the placenta to the foetus, with a gradient of 1:1.4, consequently the foetus is relatively hypocalcaemic in relation to the mother (Cheetham and Schenk, 2012). Perinatal asphyxia can also lead to a fall in calcium levels due to altered cell metabolism and phosphorus release, with alkalosis either from alkali therapy or over-ventilation, reducing the ionised serum calcium levels further. Manifestations of hypocalcemia are primarily neurological in nature, with tremors, twitching, irritability, laryngospasm, high-pitched cry, apnoea or seizures dominating the clinical picture. To offset this imbalance, an IV dose of 2mL/kg of 10% calcium gluconate over 10 minutes can be administered (Cheetham and Schenk, 2012). However, administration should be extremely closely monitored under strict ECG surveillance, as bradycardia and asystole can occur if given too rapidly. Ideally, infusion should be via a central line, as calcium is notorious for severe extravasation injury and scarring. Thus, if it is given via peripheral line, close observation of the cannula site is mandatory.

Magnesium

Magnesium (Mg^{2+})

The normal value is 0.7–1.0mmol/L

Daily requirement varies

Magnesium, along with phosphorous and calcium is the major cation in a newborn. Magnesium is primarily stored in the bones and has many functions, which include bone matrix development, nerve conduction, muscle, heart function and production of DNA/RNA. Magnesium is also an important cation which stabilises cell membranes. Complex homeostatic mechanisms regulate magnesium, calcium and phosphate via the kidney, bone and intestine to ensure parathyroid function and synthesis of vitamin D. Serum magnesium levels vary in preterm infants in the first week of life. Levels are influenced by maternal and neonatal health, such as renal perfusion and GFR. Infants with surgical conditions may have large losses of magnesium via stomas and thus require careful monitoring. Magnesium administration via injection, infusion, parenteral nutrition, formula and human breast milk contribute to normal levels (Rigo et al., 2017). Magnesium is primarily excreted via the kidneys.

GLUCOSE HOMEOSTASIS

Monitoring blood glucose levels of infants, both on admission and subsequently, is a primary responsibility of the nurse and should be undertaken if the adverse event of glucose instability is to be avoided. It is important therefore that neonatal nurses have an understanding of the factors surrounding maintenance of blood glucose levels. The more premature a baby is, the smaller the reserves are, increasing susceptibility to hypoglycaemia. At birth, the newborn infant undergoes a shift from an intrauterine **anabolic**-dominant state to a postnatal catabolic state (Blackburn, 2003), as separation from the maternal supply occurs. All newborns, therefore, have a potential for glucose instability but the susceptibility increases in certain situations, and is probably greatest in infants requiring admission to NNU.

Glucose is the main substance required by the body to create adenosine triphosphate, referred to as the 'energy currency' (Mobasheri, 2012). After birth, the infant has to regulate his or her own glucose metabolism. To survive, the newborn infant utilises the processes of glycogenolysis, the breakdown of stored glycogen to glucose, and gluconeogenesis, which is glucose produced from non-carbohydrate sources, such as alanine from skeletal muscle. Additionally, it is also recognised that ketone bodies and lactate are also metabolised by the foetal and neonatal brain as an energy source. This pathway is impaired in most of the infants admitted to NNU, e.g. preterm or growth-restricted infants, and those following hypoxic insults.

The ability of the renal tubules to reabsorb glucose is decreased in the preterm infant and increases towards term. The preterm infant has a low renal threshold for glucose conservation, and varying degrees of glycosuria are not uncommon. Glycosuria in conjunction with hyperglycaemia may cause an osmotic diuresis, whereby water is lost due to the high urinary solute concentration. This is unlikely to occur unless blood glucose levels exceed 12mmol/L.

> Glucose
> The normal value is 2.6–6.0mmol/L
> Daily requirement varies (6–8mg/kg/minute)
> Requirements may be increased in the presence of persistent hypoglycaemia

The usual requirement for glucose in a newborn is 6–8mg/kg/minute. This may be adjusted on an individual basis, as some infants require a higher percentage of glucose concentration to maintain normal plasma glucose levels. A neonate who persistently requires 10mg/

kg/minute of glucose and above requires senior medical review. The formula below is used to calculate an infant's glucose requirement.

$$\frac{\%glucose \times hourly\ rate}{(6 \times weight\ (kg))} = glucose\ load\ mg/kg/minute$$

Hypoglycaemia

The definition of hypoglycaemia remains a contentious area for debate. Definitive evidence for an agreed operational threshold remains inconclusive (Harding et al., 2017). Hypoglycaemia is considered if serum glucose concentrations are <2.6mmol/L, though there remains significant controversy around this definition. Hypoglycaemia is a common biochemical disturbance seen in the newborn. During the neonatal period, the pancreas remains in a relatively immature state with regard to glucagon and insulin secretion, leading to transient hypoglycaemia (Ghandi, 2017). Clinical manifestations have both autonomic and neuroglycopaenic origins: tachycardia, sweating, tremors and hypothermia suggest sympathetic activation, whereas lethargy, motor and sensory disturbances relate to a decreased availability of glucose (Halaby and Steinkrauss, 2012). Infants experiencing perinatal complications as in those admitted to NNU should have their glucose levels maintained at >2.5mmol/L (Cornblath et al., 2000; Stanley et al., 2015). It is recommended that in infants with profound, recurrent or persistent hyperinsulinaemic hypoglycaemia, a higher level of 3.3mmol/L should be maintained.

Close surveillance, early identification, and the instigation of prophylactic measures for the prevention of hypoglycaemia in the high-risk population constitute by far the best management strategy. Reasons for hypoglycaemia can be seen in table 16.6. Commencement of early feeding, either enterally or IV with 10% glucose at 3mL/kg/hour (5mg/kg/min) should be sufficient for most infants (Hawdon, 2012). If hypoglycaemia occurs despite this, a bolus of 10% glucose at 3–5mL/kg should be given slowly, followed by continuous glucose infusion (Hawdon, 2007; 2012). Higher concentrations should be avoided due to the risk of tissue injury and rebound hypoglycaemia. If higher concentrations are required to maintain blood glucose levels, the infusion must be administered via a central venous line in order to prevent vessel damage, extravasation injury and scarring (RCN, 2016). Vigilant observation of the infusion site and infusion pump pressures must be undertaken. Hypoglycaemia resistant to high glucose infusions are usually secondary to hyperinsulinaemia. For infants with proven hyperinsulinaemia, drug therapies need to be instigated under regular liaison with the local endocrine team. Close frequent monitoring of fluid and electrolyte therapies is paramount to highlight changes to the infant's condition. (National Institute for Health and Care Excellence (NICE), 2015; 2017).

While the consequences of asymptomatic hypoglycaemia are not well established (Cornblath et al., 2000), lower motor and mental development scores following five episodes

TABLE 16.6 INFANTS AT RISK OF HYPOGLYCAEMIA

Infant group	Mechanism	Expected duration
Decreased stores Preterm	Decreased stores of glycogen and fat Enteral feed intolerance Fluid (caloric) restriction Impaired hormonal responses	Transient
Intrauterine growth restriction	Decreased stores of glycogen and fat Impaired hormonal responses	Transient
Inborn errors of metabolism	Glycogen storage disease Enzyme deficiencies impairing glycogenolysis and gluconeogenesis	Prolonged
Increased utilisation Perinatal hypoxia	Anaerobic cellular metabolism exhausting stores	Transient
Sepsis	Increased metabolic rate	Transient
Hypothermia	Increased metabolic rate and brown fat metabolism	
Infant of diabetic mother	Hyperinsulinaemia	Transient
Beckwith–Wiedemann syndrome	Hyperinsulinaemia from islet hyperplasia	Prolonged
Erythroblastosis fetalis	Hyperinsulinaemia from islet hyperplasia	Transient
Exchange transfusion	Excess insulin secretion due to glucose level in stored blood	Transient
Islet cell dysplasias	Hyperinsulinaemia	Prolonged
Other causes Iatrogenic	'Tissued' IVs abruptly reducing supply Glucose infusion via UVC if tip is close to the coeliac access	Transient
Maternal drugs	β-receptor antagonists (e.g. labetalol)	Transient

of blood glucose levels below 2.6mmol/L in the very LBW population have been reported (Hay, 2006). Any neonate with a low blood sugar who is demonstrating seizure activity warrants urgent IV glucose treatment.

Hyperglycaemia

Neonatal hyperglycaemia is a metabolic disorder, defined as a blood glucose level >7mmol/L in term infants and >8mmol/L in the preterm population (Hawdon, 2012), and is a much less common neonatal condition than hypoglycaemia. Reasons for hyperglycaemia in the infant can be seen in table 16.7. Neonatal diabetes mellitus manifests postnatally in either a transient or permanent nature, but is rare (Fredrick et al., 2016). The incidence of 'transient

TABLE 16.7 INFANTS AT RISK OF HYPERGLYCAEMIA

Infant group	Mechanism	Expected duration
Extremely low birth weight infants	High intravenous glucose concentration Immature insulin and regulatory mechanisms	Transient
Medication	E.g. methylxanthines, caffeine citrate, corticosteroids	Transient
Infants undergoing surgery	Release of stress-related hormones Infusion of high glucose-containing solutions Transfusion of blood with high glucose levels	Transient
Neonatal diabetes mellitus	Decreased insulin production	Prolonged

diabetes' is more common, however, and appears to be increasing as more extremely LBW infants are actively managed within NNU. Hyperglycemia is associated with a higher incidence of IVH, and ultimately increased mortality if serum osmolality is increased due to the high serum glucose levels (Hay, 2006). It must be remembered that hyperglycaemia without a significant change in infused glucose concentration may be an indicator of infection and should be investigated.

Glycosuria in conjunction with hyperglycaemia may cause an osmotic diuresis, whereby water is lost due to the high urinary solute concentration. This situation can result in other electrolyte instabilities, such as hypernatraemia. Osmotic diuresis, however, is unlikely to occur in blood glucose levels below 12mmol/L. Reducing the concentration of infused glucose to a level that will reduce the blood glucose level is often all that is required. Infants not responding to this measure may be prescribed IV insulin therapy. While this practice appears to occur relatively frequently, there have been no controlled studies to validate it, and it must therefore be undertaken with caution (Hawdon, 2007).

ASSESSMENT AND MONITORING OF FLUID AND ELECTROLYTE BALANCE

Neonatal nurses must ensure vigilance and record, measure and monitor all IV therapies following in accordance with national guidelines (NICE, 2015). Any unexpected changes to a neonate's condition should be reported to senior medical staff for review.

Fluid balance

Recording and monitoring the fluid balance of infants in intensive care is an important area of practice in deciding how to manage these infants (Bhatia, 2006; Petty, 2015), and is principally the role of the nurse caring for the baby (Diacon and Bell, 2014). This aspect of care is as important as any other type of physiological monitoring, as imbalances and inaccuracies in fluid balance can cause serious deterioration or impair the infant's recovery. Fluid balance charts are commonplace, even though their usefulness has been questioned (Bekhof et al., 2013). Nonetheless, monitoring input and output is necessary to assess the infant's needs and fluid requirements.

ACCURATE MEASUREMENT OF BODY WEIGHT

Monitoring fluid balance includes accurate measurement of body weight. Monitoring of the infant's weight is important and particularly helpful in managing rehydration (Lander, 2016). Weight correlates very well with total body water content during the first few days of life. While infants in NNU are physiologically unstable and warrant minimal handling, weighing is an important marker for fluid balance and should be undertaken daily in most instances. The risks of the procedure, for example, accidental extubation, temperature instability and brief disconnection from invasive ventilation, have to be balanced against the infant's condition and benefits from the information gained. Several incubators on the market have inbuilt scales. While this weight may not be as accurate as taking the infant out of an incubator, it does allow for trending of weight if it is undertaken around the same time each day with the same equipment in situ.

MEASUREMENT OF URINE VOLUME

Urine output must be accurately measured, as it is a marker for not only water balance but also renal perfusion (Maddock and Gottstein, 2007; NICE, 2015). The volume voided can be estimated in several ways. Weighed nappies provide the simplest method and provide a degree of accuracy assuming the relative humidity is greater than 40% (Oddie et al., 2004). However, evaporation of urine into the environment, or further damping of the nappy by incubator humidity may create spurious results. Commercially available adhesive bags may be used, but fixation and retention without leakage can be a problem. Additionally, when the bag is removed, significant epidermal stripping can occur. The use of the finger of a polythene glove fixed to the skin with a smear of soft paraffin is sometimes successful in small inactive males, and some success can be achieved in female infants by using the thumb of a glove applied in the same way (Modi, 2012b). Urine output should be in the region of 1 mL/kg/hour on day 1, rising to >2–3 mL/kg/hour subsequently.

URINALYSIS

Urinalysis is a valuable procedure nurses undertake from very early in their clinical practice experience, and yet it is often overlooked in its importance in renal compromise and the recognition of renal disease (Falakaflaki et al., 2011). A small amount only is needed for urinalysis; simply placing a cotton wool ball in the infant's nappy, and then aspirating the absorbed urine with a syringe, is sufficient for the task and avoids skin damage from the application of adhesive urine bags.

■ *Specific gravity* This reflects the ability to concentrate and dilute urine. Urinary specific gravity is also a good but underused guide to hydration status (Petty, 2015; Lander, 2016). As the ability to concentrate urine is limited, the maximum specific gravity is usually 1015 to 1020, but the minimum may be as low as 1001 to 1005. As other factors such as glucose and protein can alter specific gravity, osmolality measurement of both blood and urine should be undertaken and compared if concentrating ability is in question. Urine osmolality determines movement of water into and out of the plasma. It varies from 50–600mOsm/kg in preterm neonates and 800mOsm/kg in term neonates; 200–400mOsm/kg implies the fluid intake is adequate. Healthy infants should be able to adjust urine excretion with daily fluid intake 90–200mL/kg when sodium is constant. A preterm infant has a limited capacity to concentrate their urine beyond 500mOsm/kg. (NB: specific gravity of 1020–1030 is equivalent to 400mOsm/L; Modi, 2012b).

■ *Urine pH* The pH reflects the kidneys' ability to acidify urine, but in neonates it is usually relatively alkalotic at 6.0. Many infants can acidify the urine to 5.0 by 1–2 weeks of age. In extreme prematurity, urinary bicarbonate losses may be high, increasing the pH to 7.0 or above.

■ *Glycosuria* This estimation reflects the kidneys' ability to handle glucose and is usually associated with a high blood glucose level. Hyperglycaemia associated with renal losses can contribute to osmotic diuresis and dehydration. A dipstick test will alert the nurse to the presence of glucose.

■ *Proteinuria* This is frequently seen in small amounts and is related to gestational age. Neonatal proteinuria is considered within physiological range at $68–309mg/m^2/24hrs$; values in excess of this may indicate a pathology and warrant medical review (Joseph and Gattineni, 2016).

■ *Haematuria* The presence of blood in the urine is not a normal finding and may be associated with renal damage following asphyxia, embolisation in the renal artery from umbilical arterial catheterisation, renal vein thrombosis, coagulopathies, or congenital abnormality such as cystic disease or obstruction. Again, senior medical review is justified where haematuria is present.

ACID-BASE BALANCE

Maintaining a stable acid-base balance involves complex synergy of the lungs, kidneys and brain. The kidneys are part of a buffer system to maintain homeostasis. The buffer system works via reabsorption and secretion of bicarbonate ions (HCO_3^-) in a nephron, in the presence of hydrogen ions within the plasma. There are many pathologies, including renal disease, which may contribute to metabolic acidosis or alkalosis. Metabolic acidosis occurs when bicarbonate ions are low, causing a corresponding reduction in blood pH. A sodium bicarbonate infusion may be administered to increase the blood pH to a normal range (Mulligan, 2013), however there is insufficient evidence that this is beneficial (Lawn et al., 2005), while one small study found an association between sodium bicarbonate administration in extremely preterm infants with an increased risk of IVH and death (Berg et al., 2010). A metabolic alkalosis occurs when bicarbonate levels are raised, causing a corresponding rise in pH.

The correlation of respiratory and metabolic components and resulting changes observable on blood gases is further explored in chapter 12, table 12.2.

The mechanisms of acid-base-balance are described in detail on the website, see web-based companion for chapter 10.

ACUTE RENAL INJURY

Acute renal injury (ARI) is characterised by a sudden decline in GFR. This leads to an accumulation of creatinine waste products, disturbed fluid balance and dysfunctional electrolyte homeostasis. Clinically, a reduced urine output (**oliguria** <0.5mL/kg/hour), hypertension, evidence of fluid overload or dehydration, and possible seizure activity, are red-flag signs suggestive of ARI. Neonatal susceptibility to ARI increases with the presence of factors inherently specific to the primitive renal physiology, including perinatal hypoxic-ischaemic events, prolonged resuscitation and acidosis, congenital malformations, episodes of hypotension, sepsis, and nephrotoxic medication exposure (Jetton and Askenazi, 2012). The pathophysiology of kidney disease as applicable to the preterm infant can be seen in figure 16.1.

Investigations

If ARI is suspected, the clinical history must be reviewed. As part of an examination, the bladder should then be palpated to eliminate acute urinary retention, which is not uncommon after asphyxial insults or in infants on morphine infusions. Assessment of the circulation, blood pressure, capillary refill time and core–periphery temperature gap must also be undertaken to evaluate the adequacy of renal perfusion. A renal ultrasound scan to identify the kidneys and urinary tract anatomy is advisable. Paired blood and urinalysis may assist in establishing the diagnosis of ARI. Measurement of fractional excretion of sodium (Fe_{Na}) is said to be the best indicator to distinguish between pre-renal and established renal failure. This is calculated from the sodium and creatinine concentrations of serum and spot urine samples:

$$\frac{Urine\ sodium}{Serum\ sodium} \times \frac{Serum\ creatinine}{Urine\ creatinine} \times 100$$

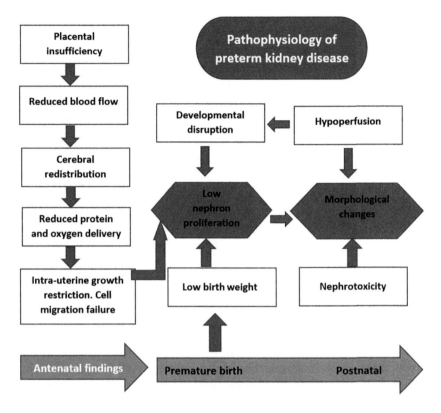

Figure 16.1 Pathophysiology of preterm kidney disease

In low perfusion states, sodium and water will be conserved and the Fe_{Na} will be less than 2.5%. However, if tubular damage is causing oliguria, the Fe_{Na} will be greater than 2.5%. These values are only pertinent to the term population, as in the very LBW population, Fe_{Na} can be up to 15% due to kidney immaturity, so that this test is unreliable in these infants. Provided there is no evidence of circulatory overload, the response to a fluid challenge may be helpful. This consists of administering 10–20mL/kg of 0.9% sodium chloride over 1–2 hours, followed by a single dose of furosemide on completion of the infusion. If the infant responds with an increase in urine output, a diagnosis of pre-renal failure is likely, and further management should be directed towards maintaining adequacy of renal perfusion. Indices for renal disease from a urinalysis can be seen in table 16.8.

Furosemide may be given as a single dose of up to 5mg/kg (Paediatric Formulary Committee, 2018). If the fluid challenge does not elicit a diuresis, fluid intake should be reduced as outlined below. As the half-life of furosemide is up to 8 hours in term infants and 24 hours in preterm babies, repeated high doses cannot be advocated due to its potential **ototoxic** and nephrotoxic effects (Moghal and Shenoy, 2008).

TABLE 16.8 INDICES OF RENAL FAILURE IN INFANTS

	Pre-renal failure	Established renal failure
Urine sodium	Low (<10mmol/L)	High (>20mmol/l)
Urine urea	High	Low
Urine creatinine	High	Low
Urine specific gravity	High (>1025)	Low (approx. 1010)
Urine osmolality	High (>500mOsm/kg)	Low (approx. 300mOsm/kg)
Fractional Na$^+$ excretion	Low (<1%)	High (>2.5–3.0%)
Urea: plasma creatinine	High (>40)	Low

Management of ARI

The aim of managing ARI is to maintain homeostasis by externally compensating for dysfunctional renal function, which is achieved by correcting fluid and electrolyte imbalances and reversing acidosis (Ottonello et al., 2014). All nephrotoxic drugs should be stopped. The adjusting of dose schedules of all renally excreted drugs also needs consideration, with drug assays guiding the adjustments. Fluids should be calculated as insensible losses plus urine output, and any gastrointestinal losses. Furosemide may be given in doses up to 5mg/kg. Loop diuretics are used for their simultaneous renal protective function, through redistribution of renal blood flow and their ability to inhibit fluid overload (Pandey et al., 2017). Low-dose dopamine at 2mcg/kg/minute may aid renal perfusion, thus improving urinary output and serum creatinine levels. Acidosis may require treatment with sodium bicarbonate 4.2%. Hyperphosphataemia associated with ARI, if persistent, may require oral calcium carbonate 8-hourly to bind intestinal phosphate (Paediatric Formulary Committee, 2018). Symptomatic hypocalcaemia may be treated with infusion of calcium gluconate 10% at 0.5–1mmol/kg per 24 hours. Management of persistent or intrinsic failure should include twice-daily measurement of body weight and regular serum electrolyte, urea and creatinine assessment.

If the condition is not improving with conservative management and there is severe fluid overload, metabolic acidosis, hyperkalaemia, electrolyte disturbances with uraemic central nervous system depression, dialysis should be considered (Sinha et al., 2017). In this case, consultation with a paediatric nephrologist must be sought.

The Neonatal Kidney Collaborative was formed in 2014 to advance the study of acute renal disease in vulnerable neonates (Selewski et al., 2015). It was previously assumed if infants and children survived ARI, long-term sequelae were unlikely. A study by Mammen et al. (2012), reported that 10% of children in paediatric intensive care with ARI had reduced GFR for up to 3 years later, and around 50% had risk factors for chronic renal disease. Irreversible kidney disease requiring dialysis is rare in the neonate. Although the need for dialysis is relatively rare, there is a very high incidence of co-morbidity, and this affects survival, which for those on dialysis is about 80% at 5 years (Rees, 2017). Peritoneal dialysis (PD) is generally regarded as the optimal dialysis modality for neonates. PD allows for the slow removal of fluid and solutes while avoiding hemodynamic instability and is a relatively safe, simple and effective procedure. Nursing management of an infant undergoing PD is focused upon prevention of complications of the procedure. These are peritonitis, fluid overload or dehydration, thermal instability and respiratory compromise during dwelling time. To prevent these from occurring, aseptic non-touch technique for IV therapy must be adopted (Loveday et al., 2014; RCN, 2016; NICE, 2017). The drained PD fluid should be observed for **turbidity**, and additionally sampled daily and sent for culture and sensitivity. Fastidious attention must be paid to fluid balance recording of cycle volumes both in and out, to establish whether the infant is in a positive or negative balance state. The circuitry should be well secured and supported, and not subject to kinking, which may impede flow either in or out. PD fluid should be warmed using a blood warmer set at 37°C, so that dramatic cooling does not occur from cold dialysate being instilled.

Impairment of the infant's respiratory status can occur during cycles due to increased intra-abdominal pressure causing diaphragmatic embarrassment. This can be lessened by reducing the cycle volume and nursing the infant in a pronounced head-up tilt position to reduce infra-diaphragmatic pressure.

Haemofiltration for neonates is technically challenging due to their size and access to blood vessels. While the nursing management from fluid balance, infection and temperature perspectives is not that dissimilar to the infant undergoing PD, the risk of bleeding is a major consideration in these infants. Due to the extracorporeal nature of the circuit, significant heparinisation is usually required to prevent clotting within the circuit and filter. Careful observation of the skin for petechiae and for oozing needs to be undertaken. Procedures that can create trauma to tissue, for example, oral or endotracheal suction and removal of adhesive tape, should be carried out carefully and kept to a minimum. Infants should not have intramuscular injections, and blood sampling should be undertaken via the circuit rather than venepuncture. Clotting studies should be done regularly to ascertain how much heparinisation is required. Constant observation of flow through the filter is necessary; flow ceasing abruptly suggests that the filter is blocked and needs to be changed.

CONCLUSION

Maintenance of fluid and electrolyte homeostasis has a significant role in the progress and subsequent outcome of infants. The heterogenous nature of disturbed homeostasis emphasises the importance of a multidisciplinary approach to managing these infants. Long-term consequences of preterm birth and associated fluid imbalances should be considered in this important area of nursing management (Stritzke et al., 2017), so that attention is paid as soon as the infant is born continuing during the neonatal stay. This has never been more apparent than in recent times with the management of increasingly preterm infants who, with their exquisitely fragile skin coupled with organ immaturity, make fluid and electrolyte therapy a great challenge. The burden of complexity relating to treating these infants, has been somewhat alleviated with technological advancement and physiological understanding of managing fluid disturbances. Great care and respect should be given to fluid management as part of the holistic care of infant and family. Maintaining stability and detection of potential (and real) problems in this area is another pivotal role of the nurse and should not be underestimated.

Parents should have information about this aspect of care so that they understand the rationale behind the fluid and electrolytes that are administered to their infant, in conjunction with feeding strategies, often occurring and titrated together during the course of the infant's care on the NNU.

C A S E   S T U D Y

CASE STUDIES

Case study 1: Assessment and monitoring of fluid balance

Alice has twelve months' neonatal experience; she is providing the neonatal nursing care for Fenna today. Fenna was born at 26 weeks' gestation and she is 20 hours old. Her birth weight is 750g. Her mum, Sara, has received antenatal steroids 48 hours ago due to preterm labour. Sara has been well in her pregnancy.

Currently Fenna is:

■ Ventilated but stable
■ Has lines in situ – a double lumen umbilical venous catheter, an umbilical arterial line, percutaneous long line. All the intravenous lines are patent
■ Is receiving humidity at 90%
■ Incubator temperature set at 38.5°C
■ T1 37.3°C and T2 36.8°C – temperatures are stable
■ HR 140, RR 60, BP 55/30mmHg, SaO$_2$ 93%
■ Electrolytes – Sodium 137mmol/L, potassium 3.8mmol/L, glucose 4.8mmol/L
■ Clear fluids and maintenance parenteral nutrition. Fenna is nil by mouth
■ Skin – her skin feels sticky and warm to touch
■ Activity – she is flexed and appears comfortable.

Address the questions below:

Q.1. How will you assess Fenna's fluid and electrolyte balance?
Q.2. How will you monitor her fluid intake and output and minimise her heat and water losses?
Q.3. Outline the observations you would undertake each hour.

Case study 2: The infant who is volume-depleted

Molly has just been transferred back to her referring neonatal unit after a period in another unit where she has gone for stabilisation and respiratory management on day 1 of life. She was born at 29 weeks' gestation and is now 2 weeks old. She is on PN and a small amount of enteral feed (breast milk) via a nasogastic tube and is on nasal CPAP. Her intravenous long line appears to have ceased working properly and her peripheral cannula has tissued. Her gastric aspirates are larger than previously noted and she is not tolerating her milk. On assessment, it is noted that she looks 'dry', and Molly's parents comment that she does not look right, particularly her skin colour.

Q.1. What assessment is required on Molly in relation to her fluid balance?
Q.2. How will she present if she is fluid-depleted?
Q.3. What fluid management and nursing care will Molly need?
Q.4. What advice do the parents require?

Case study 3: The infant with fluid imbalance

Ali is a term infant admitted to the neonatal unit at birth with meconium aspiration. He has been very unwell with high oxygen and ventilatory requirements and on the ward round, Ali's father comments that he looks very 'puffy' compared to the previous day. His chest X-ray shows a white appearance through both lungs, again different to previous X-rays.

Q.1. What do you think the reasons are for these observations?
Q.2. Can you explain the physiology behind this picture?
Q.3. What fluid management and nursing care will Ali need?
Q.4. How would you explain this to the parents?

For suggested answer guides to the questions posed in these case studies, please refer to the web-based companion site specific to this chapter (see URL below).

WEB-BASED RESOURCES

For further information, online resources and greater detail on the case studies featured in this chapter go to www.routledge.com/cw/nicnursing

References

Barrington, K. J., Fortin-Pellerin, E., & Pennaforte, T. (2017). Fluid restriction for treatment of preterm infants with chronic lung disease. *Cochrane Database of Systematic Reviews*, Issue 2. Art. No.: CD005389. DOI: 10.1002/14651858.CD005389.pub2

Bekhof, J., van Asperen, Y., & Brand, P. L. (2013). Usefulness of the fluid balance: A randomised controlled trial in neonates. *Journal of Paediatrics and Child Health*, 49(6), 486–492.

Bell, E. .F, & Acarregui, M. J. (2014). Restricted versus liberal water intake for preventing morbidity and mortality in preterm infants. *Cochrane Database of Systematic Reviews*, Issue 12. Art. No.: CD000503. DOI: 10.1002/14651858.CD000503.pub3

Berg, C. S., Barnette, A. R., Myers, B. J., Shimony, M. K., Barton, A. W., & Inder, T. E. (2010). Sodium bicarbonate administration and outcome in preterm infants. *The Journal of Pediatrics*, 157(4), 684–687.

Bezerra, C. T. D. M., Vaz Cunha, L. C., & Libório, A. B. (2013). Defining reduced urine output in neonatal ICU: Importance for mortality and acute kidney injury classification. *Nephrology Dialysis Transplantation*, 28(4), 901–909.

Bhatia, J. (2006). Fluid and electrolyte management in the very low birth weight neonate. *Journal of Perinatology*, 26(S1), S19.

Bischoff, A. R., Tomlinson, C., & Belik, J. (2016). Sodium intake requirements for preterm neonates: review and recommendations. *Journal of Pediatric Gastroenterology and Nutrition*, 63(6), e123–e129.

Blackburn, S. T. (2003). *Maternal, Fetal and Neonatal Physiology: A Clinical Perspective.* Philadelphia: WB Saunders.

Bolisetty, S., Legge, N., Bajuk, B., Lui, K., & New South Wales and the Australian Capital Territory Neonatal Intensive Care Units' Data Collection. (2015). Preterm infant outcomes in New South Wales and the Australian Capital Territory. *Journal of Paediatrics and Child Health*, 51(7), 713–721.

Cairns, P. (2012). Parenteral nutrition. In Rennie, J. M. (Ed.) *Rennie & Roberton's Textbook of Neonatology* (5th Edition). London: Elsevier Health Sciences.

Cheetham, T., & Schenk, D. J. (2012). Metabolic and endocrine disorders. Part 2: Endocrine disorders. In Rennie, J. M. (Ed.) *Rennie & Roberton's Textbook of Neonatology* (5th Edition). London: Elsevier Health Sciences.

Cornblath, M., Hawdon, J. M., Williams, A. F., Aynsley-Green, A., Ward-Platt, M. P., Schwartz, R., & Kalhan, S. C. (2000). Controversies regarding definition of neonatal hypoglycemia: Suggested operational thresholds. *Pediatrics*, 105(5), 1141–1145.

Diacon, A., & Bell, J. (2014). Investigating the recording and accuracy of fluid balance monitoring in critically ill patients. *Southern African Journal of Critical Care (Online)*, 30(2), 55–57.

Falakaflaki, B., Mousavinasab, S. N., & Mazloomzadeh, S. (2011). Dipstick urinalysis screening of healthy neonates. *Pediatrics & Neonatology*, 52(3), 161–164.

Fredrick, F., Sawe, H., Muze, K., Mally, D., & Majaliwa, E. (2016). A seven weeks old baby with diabetic ketoacidosis: a case report. *Clinical Case Reports*, 4(2), 147–150.

Gawlowski, Z., Aladangady, N., & Coen, P. G. (2006). Hypernatraemia in preterm infants born at less than 27 weeks gestation. *Journal of Paediatrics and Child Health*, 42(12), 771–774.

Ghandi, K. (2017). Approach to hypoglycemia in infants and children. *Translational Pediatrics*, 6(4), 408–420.

Halaby, L. P., & Steinkrauss, L. (2012). Hypoglycemia: Symptom or diagnosis? *Journal of Pediatric Nursing: Nursing Care of Children and Families*, 27(1), 97–99.

Harding, J. E., Harris, D. L., Hegarty, J. E., Alsweiler, J. M., & McKinlay, C. J. (2017). An emerging evidence base for the management of neonatal hypoglycaemia. *Early Human Development*, 104, 51–56

Harish Madhava, M. S., & Settle, P. (2009). Fluid restriction for symptomatic patent ductus arteriosus in preterm infants. *Cochrane Database of Systematic Reviews* Issue 2. Art. No.: CD007800. DOI: 10.1002/14651858.CD007800.

Hartnoll, G. (2003). Basic principles and practical steps in the management of fluid balance in the newborn. *Seminars in Fetal and Neonatal Medicine, 8*(4), 307–313.

Hartnoll, G., Betremieux, P., & Modi, N. (2001). Randomised controlled trial of postnatal sodium supplementation in infants of 25–30 weeks gestational age: effects on cardiopulmonary adaptation. *Archives of Disease in Childhood: Fetal and Neonatal Edition, 85*(1), F29–F32.

Hawdon, J. (2007). The medicolegal implications of hypoglycaemia in the newborn. *Clinical Risk, 13*(4), 135–137.

Hawdon, J. (2012). Metabolic and endocrine disorders. Part 1: Disorders of metabolic homeostasis in the neonate. In Rennie, J. M. (Ed.) *Rennie & Roberton's Textbook of Neonatology* (5th Edition). London: Elsevier Health Sciences.

Hay, W. W. Jr. (2006). Placental-fetal glucose exchange and fetal glucose metabolism. *Transactions of the American Clinical and Climatological Association, 117*, 321–339.

Haycock, G. B. (2003). Management of acute and chronic renal failure in the newborn. *Seminars in Fetal and Neonatal Medicine, 8*(4), 325–334.

Iacobelli, S., Kermorvant-Duchemin, E., Bonsante, F., Lapillonne, A., & Gouyon, J. B. (2012). Chloride balance in preterm infants during the first week of life. *International Journal of Pediatrics.* www.hindawi.com/journals/ijpedi/2012/931597/

Jetton, J. G., & Askenazi, D. J. (2012). Update on acute kidney injury in the neonate. *Current Opinion in Pediatrics, 24*(2), 191.

Joseph, C., & Gattineni, J. (2016). Proteinuria and hematuria in the neonate. *Current Opinion in Pediatrics, 28*(2), 202–208.

Kim, Y. J., Lee, J. A., Oh, S., Choi, C. W., Kim, E. K., Kim, H. S., ... & Choi, J. H. (2015). Risk factors for late-onset hyponatremia and its influence on neonatal outcomes in preterm infants. *Journal of Korean Medical Science, 30*(4), 456–462.

Lander, A. (2016). Updated guidelines for the management of fluid and electrolytes in children. *Surgery (Oxford), 34*(5), 213–216.

Lawn, C. J., Weir, F. J., & McGuire, W. (2005). Base administration or fluid bolus for preventing morbidity and mortality in preterm infants with metabolic acidosis. *Cochrane Database of Systematic Reviews*, Issue 2. Art. No.: CD003215. DOI: 10.1002/14651858.CD003215.pub2

Lindower, J. B. (2017). Water balance in the fetus and neonate. *Seminars in Fetal and Neonatal Medicine, 22*(2), 71–75.

Loveday, H. P., Wilson, J., Pratt, R. J., Golsorkhi, M., Tingle, A., Bak, A., ... & Wilcox, M. (2014). Epic3: national evidence-based guidelines for preventing healthcare-associated infections in NHS hospitals in England. *Journal of Hospital Infection, 86*, S1–S70.

Low Birth Weight and Nephron Number Working Group. (2017). The impact of kidney development on the life course: a consensus document for action. *Nephron. Clinical Practice, 136*(1), 3.

Maddock, N., & Gottstein, R. (2007). Neonatal urine output measurement by weighing nappies. Abstract presented at the meeting of the Neonatal Society, Portsmouth.

Mahoney, B. A., Smith, W. A. D., Lo, D., Tsoi, K., Tonelli, M., & Clase, C. (2005). Emergency interventions for hyperkalaemia. *Cochrane Database of Systematic Reviews*, Issue 2. Art. No.: CD003235. DOI: 10.1002/14651858.CD003235.pub2

Mammen, C., Al Abbas, A., Skippen, P., Nadel, H., Levine, D., Collet, J. P., & Matsell, D. G. (2012). Long-term risk of CKD in children surviving episodes of acute kidney injury in the intensive care unit: A prospective cohort study. *American Journal of Kidney Diseases, 59*(4), 523–530.

Mannan, M. A., Shahidulla, M., Salam, F., Alam, M. S., Hossain, M. A., & Hossain, M. (2012). Postnatal development of renal function in preterm and term neonates. *Mymensingh Medical Journal, 21*(1), 103–108.

Masilamani, K., & van der Voort, J. (2012). The management of acute hyperkalaemia in neonates and children. *Archives of Disease in Childhood, 97*(4), 376–380.

Mattson Porth, C. (2011). *Essentials of Pathophysiology* (4th Edition). Wisconsin: Wolters Kluwer.

Mobasheri, A. (2012). Glucose: an energy currency and structural precursor in articular cartilage and bone with emerging roles as an extracellular signaling molecule and metabolic regulator. *Frontiers in Endocrinology, 3*, 153.

Modi, N. (2004). Management of fluid balance in the very immature neonate. *Archives of Disease in Childhood: Fetal and Neonatal Edition, 89*(2), F108–F111.

Modi, N. (2012a). Fluid and electrolyte balance. In Rennie, J. M. (Ed.) *Rennie & Roberton's Textbook of Neonatology* (5th Edition). London: Elsevier Health Sciences.

Modi, N. (2012b). Disorders of the kidney and urinary tract. Part 1: Renal function and renal disease in the newborn. In Rennie, J. M. (Ed.) *Rennie & Roberton's Textbook of Neonatology* (5th Edition). London: Elsevier Health Sciences.

Moghal, N. E., & Shenoy, M. (2008). Furosemide and acute kidney injury in neonates. *Archives of Disease in Childhood: Fetal and Neonatal Edition, 93*(4), F313–F316.

Mulligan, M., & Point, N. (2013). Blood gas interpretation in the neonate – what do you need to know now? *Blood.* https://acutecaretesting.org/en/articles/blood-gas-interpretation-in-the-neonate

National Institute for Health and Care Excellence. (2015). *Intravenous fluid therapy in children and young people in hospital.* NICE.

National Institute for Health and Care Excellence. (2017). *Infection: Prevention and control of healthcare-associated infections in primary and community care. Quality standards CG139.* NICE.

O'Brien, F., & Walker, I. A. (2014). Fluid homeostasis in the neonate. *Pediatric Anesthesia, 24*(1), 49–59.

Oddie, S., Adappa, R., & Wyllie, J. (2004). Measurement of urine output by weighing nappies. *Archives of Disease in Childhood: Fetal and Neonatal Edition, 89*(2), F180–F181.

Ofek Shlomai, N., Reichman, B., Lerner-Geva, L., Boyko, V., Bar-Oz, B., & Collaboration with the Israel Neonatal Network. (2014). Population-based study shows improved postnatal growth in preterm very-low-birthweight infants between 1995 and 2010. *Acta Paediatrica, 103*(5), 498–503.

O'Hare, F., & Molloy, E. (2008). What is the best treatment for hyperkalaemia in the preterm infant? *Archives of Disease in Childhood, 93*(2), 174–176.

Oh, W. (2012). Fluid and electrolyte management of very low birth weight infants. *Pediatrics & Neonatology, 53*(6), 329–333.

Ottonello, G., Dessì, A., Neroni, P., Trudu, M. E., Manus, D., & Fanos, V. (2014). Acute kidney injury in neonatal age. *Journal of Pediatric and Neonatal Individualized Medicine, 3*(2), e030246.

Paediatric Formulary Committee. (2018). *BNF for Children 2018–2019.* London: BMJ Group, Pharmaceutical Press and RCPCH Publications.

Pandey, V., Kumar, D., Vijayaraghavan, P., Chaturvedi, T., & Raina, R. (2017). Non-dialytic management of acute kidney injury in newborns. *Journal of Renal Injury Prevention, 6*(1), 1–11.

Pasala, S., & Carmody, J. B. (2017). How to use … serum creatinine, cystatin C and GFR. *Archives of Disease in Childhood-Education and Practice, 102*(1), 37–43.

Petty, J. (2015). *Bedside Guide to Neonatal Care.* London: Palgrave.

Rees, L. (2017). Renal replacement therapies in neonates: issues and ethics. *Seminars in Fetal and Neonatal Medicine, 22*(2), 104–108.

Rigo, J., Pieltain, C., Christmann, V., Bonsante, F., Moltu, S., Iacobelli, S., & Marret, S. (2017). Serum magnesium levels in preterm infants are higher than adult levels: A systematic literature review and meta-analysis. *Nutrients, 9*(10), 1125.

Rocha, G., Ribeiro, O., & Guimarães, H. (2010). Fluid and electrolyte balance during the first week of life and risk of bronchopulmonary dysplasia in the preterm neonate. *Clinics, 65*(7), 663–674.

Royal College of Nursing. (2016). *Standards for Infusion Therapy* (4th Edition). London: RCN.

Saint-Faust, M., Boubred, F., & Simeoni, U. (2014). Renal development and neonatal adaptation. *American Journal of Perinatology, 31*(9), 773–780.

Sava, L., Pillai, S., More, U., & Sontakke, A. (2005). Serum calcium measurement: Total versus free (ionized) calcium. *Indian Journal of Clinical Biochemistry, 20*(2), 158–161.

Selewski, D. T., Charlton, J. R., Jetton, J. G., Guillet, R., Mhanna, M. J., Askenazi, D. J., & Kent, A. L. (2015). Neonatal acute kidney injury. *Pediatrics*, *136*(2), e463–e473.

Sinha, S., Miall, L., & Jardine, L. (2017). *Essential Neonatal Medicine (6)*. Hoboken: John Wiley & Sons.

Stafford-Smith, M. (2007). Preservation of Renal Function. In: Newman, M. F., Fleisher, L. A., & Fink, M. P. (Eds.). *Perioperative medicine: Managing for outcome*. London: Elsevier Health Sciences.

Stanley, C. A., Rozance, P. J., Thornton, P. S., De Leon, D. D., Harris, D., Haymond, M. W., ... & Sperling, M. A. (2015). Re-evaluating 'transitional neonatal hypoglycemia': Mechanism and implications for management. *The Journal of Pediatrics*, *166*(6), 1520–1525.

Stritzke, A., Thomas, S., Amin, H., Fusch, C., & Lodha, A. (2017). Renal consequences of preterm birth. *Molecular and Cellular Pediatrics*, *4*(1), 2.

Sutherland, M. R., Gubhaju, L., Moore, L., Kent, A. L., Dahlstrom, J. E., Horne, R. S., ... & Black, M. J. (2011). Accelerated maturation and abnormal morphology in the preterm neonatal kidney. *Journal of the American Society of Nephrology*, *22*(7), 1365–1374.

Vemgal, P., & Ohlsson, A. (2012). Interventions for non-oliguric hyperkalaemia in preterm neonates. *Cochrane Database of Systematic Reviews*, Issue 5. Art. No.: CD005257. DOI: 10.1002/14651858. CD005257.pub3

17 NUTRITION AND FEEDING IN THE NEONATAL UNIT

Kaye Spence and Alexandra Connolly

CONTENTS

GUIDANCE ON HOW TO ENHANCE PERSONAL LEARNING FROM THIS CHAPTER

Key points covered in this chapter

■   Nutritional requirements, assessment and monitoring of nutrition in the neonatal unit.

■   Types and methods of feeding, assessment and cue-based feeding for the infant in the neonatal unit.

■   Working with the multidisciplinary team and family when feeding the high-risk neonate.

Reflection

Reading through the chapter, you are encouraged to engage with the key points and related literature in an enquiring way. Ask these questions:

■   What are the key elements of providing optimum nutrition to the infant in the neonatal unit and beyond?

■   How would you assess the infant for readiness to feed?

■   How can you support the parents to provide nutrition and successfully feed their infant?

Implications for nursing care

■   Finally: how will this chapter enable you to consider supporting the family in feeding their infant in the neonatal unit and following discharge? Consider the implications of what you learn for your nursing care relating to feeding and nutrition.

INTRODUCTION AND BACKGROUND

Nutritional management of the preterm or sick term infant is essential for survival and an optimal outcome. Nutritional needs of the preterm infant differ from the term infant, but they also differ for each baby according to the infant's gestation, degree of growth restriction, postnatal age and accompanying disease (Ramel et al., 2014). Nurses are faced with many challenges as they aim to meet the nutritional goals of the infant in their care and at the same time decide on the most appropriate method of feeding according to the individual infant's stage of development. In the past ten years there have been changes in the approach for neonatal nutrition, and there is a growing body of evidence to support these changes (Abiramalatha et al., 2017; Quigley et al., 2018). This chapter provides an individualised approach to nutrition and feeding neonates in intensive care and supporting families in their choice for feeding. It is beyond the scope of this chapter to provide an in-depth coverage of nutritional requirements and feeding practices. These topics are readily available in a range of reference materials.

An understanding of the development and function of the gastrointestinal tract is vital to enable the reader to make an informed choice for initiating enteral feeds. The outcomes of nutrition are explored, with particular emphasis on the assessment of adequate nutrition evidenced by optimal growth and development and clinical outcomes. Challenges of feeding sick infants with reference to appropriate nutritional requirements, feeding methods and parental choices must be based on current research.

In this chapter we will present the model of best practice in supporting the journey to suck-feeding from the Speech and Language Therapist's (SALT) perspective. It is important to consider how the neonatal nurse can work collaboratively with the wider feeding team to support the infant and parents' feeding journey while enabling bonding and attachment between the baby and their family.

THE GASTROINTESTINAL SYSTEM

The gastrointestinal tract's role in ingestion, digestion and elimination is important for long-term growth and survival in infants. Development occurs *in utero*, and the tract is structurally prepared for oral feeding by 20 weeks' gestation. However, many of the functions required for successful feeding are not fully developed. Functional maturity occurs after anatomical maturity, with many functions still immature at birth, and continues to develop for many years. After birth, the newborn's gastrointestinal tract takes over from the placenta in the task of assimilation of nutrients. When the function is impaired due to disease such as infection, shock, hypoxia, or extreme prematurity, the results may be a delay in gastric emptying and intestinal peristalsis, leading to impaired digestion and absorption. The presence of early infant gut microbiome is an important regulator of many developing functions and can influence the risk for a variety of conditions such as necrotising enterocolitis (NEC). Infant feeding remains a critical determinant of the early gut microbiome, and thus, early feeding may have important long-term effects (Di Mauro et al., 2013).

Successful transition to extrauterine nutrition requires the gut to be able to function rapidly and efficiently. Two factors are important in this transition: first, the gestational age of the neonate, and second, the composition of the food the neonate receives following birth.

Differences in the physiology of the gut between term and preterm infants include delayed gastric emptying with a slower intestinal transit time. The digestive and absorptive capacities vary with the preterm gut not maturing to term levels until 34 weeks postconceptual age. Other physiological differences include higher metabolic demands and an immature metabolic and digestive and absorption system in the premature gut (Ramel et al., 2014).

Functional problems of the gastrointestinal tract may occur, which can limit the ability to achieve nutritional requirements by the enteral route. These may be due to congenital anomalies of the gastrointestinal tract such as oesophageal atresia or stenosis, pyloric stenosis, extrahepatic biliary atresia, and malformation of the small and large intestines such as gastroschisis or Hirschsprung's disease.

NUTRITIONAL REQUIREMENTS

Goals for nutritional support during the first few days of life are the maintenance of fluid status, glucose homeostasis, and normal serum electrolytes and mineral concentrations. Extremely premature infants have decreased body stores of nutrients and consequently a limited capacity to tolerate starvation, especially if coupled with metabolic demands imposed by illness (Chan et al., 2016).

Providing adequate nutrition to meet the needs of sick immature preterm infants as well as the growing premature and healthy term infants provides a challenge for the neonatal team (table 17.1). An important goal is to ensure that the neurodevelopmental outcomes are not compromised by inadequate nutrition during hospitalisation (Ramel et al., 2014; Belfort and Ehrenkranz, 2017). Requirements vary and are influenced by both prenatal factors such as intrauterine growth restriction and postnatal illnesses such as sepsis, stress, surgery and chronic lung disease. With increases in the metabolic rate because of neonatal conditions and diseases, a rapid mobilisation of energy and protein stores is required to meet the demand.

Nutrition is complex, and there is a pattern of optimal intake of multiple nutrients, including energy, amino acids and micronutrients, all in balance with metabolic capacity of the infant (Chan et al., 2016). An individualised approach to nutritional requirements ensures that the underlying condition and stage of illness as well as growth trends are considered for each infant to enable adequate growth. Nutrients can have a metabolic cost during an acute illness in neonates, especially premature infants, as each additional calorie increases oxygen consumption when not stored or used for growth, thereby increasing the metabolic load (Ramel et al., 2014). The focus is on nutritional assessment to determine the need, as this is the responsibility of all clinicians, medical and nursing, in the neonatal unit (NNU). When caring for infants in intensive or special care, nurses should aim to promote energy conservation and growth by implementing practices such as minimal handling, maintaining a neutral thermal environment and providing developmentally supportive strategies to reduce stress (White-Traut et al., 2015). Including neurodevelopment as an outcome measure is vitally important when considering nutrition in the NNU.

TABLE 17.1 IMPACT OF ILLNESS ON NUTRITIONAL REQUIREMENTS

Brain	Uses 60% of total body metabolic requirements
	Need for increased glucose increases energy requirements
	Seizures increase requirements by 30%
Heart	Uses a high metabolic rate
	Increase in oxygen consumption
	Increase energy demand by 30%
	Cyanotic heart disease increased iron and calcium requirements
Intrauterine growth restriction (IUGR)	Increase in metabolic rate
	Increase in energy expenditure
	Decrease in fat absorption
	Decrease in iron stores
	Compromised protein status
Small for gestational age (SGA)	Deficiency in protein metabolism
	Decrease in urea excretion
Chronic lung disease (CLD)	Increase in energy expenditure by 15%
	Diuretics increase alkalosis, increase sodium requirements
	Compromised bone health
Sepsis	Protein catabolism
	Increase in energy requirements
Stress	Protein breakdown
Necrotising enterocolitis (NEC)/ short bowel	Decrease in zinc
	Poor growth

(adapted from Ramel et al., 2014)

NUTRITIONAL ASSESSMENT

The most effective method of determining whether nutritional goals have been achieved is growth, both short and long term. This may be assessed by measurement of weight, length, head circumference and skin fold thickness. The pattern of growth rate may influence the management of the infant and their length of stay in the NNU. For graduates of intensive care, it is important to ensure that their dietary management is appropriate, as it may influence long-term growth, neurological development and subsequent illnesses such as allergies (Ramel et al., 2014). Suboptimal nutrition during sensitive stages in early brain development may have long-term effects on cognitive function, and avoidance of undernutrition in sick preterm infants is important to optimise neurodevelopmental outcomes (Belfort and Ehrenkranz, 2017).

Recommendations for target growth rates have varied from 15–20g/kg/day, and rates have been plotted on growth charts with expected percentage trends. There are various

TABLE 17.2 RECOMMENDED 5 STEPS TO IMPROVE GROWTH IN PRETERM INFANTS BETWEEN BIRTH AND HOSPITAL DISCHARGE

Step 1	Audit to identify the severity/nature of problem in a given unit. A. Timing, after NNU admission, of introduction of PN as well as the composition of the solution(s). B. Transition from PN to enteral nutrition, a time when PN is reduced on a ml-to-ml basis as enteral volume is increased. Because nutrient density is greater with PN than enteral feeds, actual intake, for example, protein, may decrease. C. Nutritional management during 'nil by mouth' episodes, a time when feeds are stopped because of 'concern' and PN and/or enteral nutrition may not be restarted in a timely fashion.
Step 2	The introduction of a standardised feeding protocol that is evidence-based and monitored on a regular basis.
Step 3	Individualised nutritional care, with particular attention to: A. Accurate measurements of body weight and CHL. B. Use of standardised deviation or ZSs to monitor growth.
Step 4	The establishment of a nutritional support team that supports/monitors all aspects of nutritional care in the special care baby unit.
Step 5	A repeat audit 3–6 months after the introduction of the feeding protocol.

(adapted from Cooke, 2016)

charts currently used in practice to help determine a neonate's nutritional status. Charts that are suitable for the appropriate clinical, demographic, ethnic and socioeconomic similarities of the population should be used, as growth patterns vary according to the population under review. The use of intrauterine or extrauterine growth charts may not always be suitable, as almost 40% of preterm infants are small for gestational age, and up to 50% of preterm labours are associated with placental insufficiency. The use of Z-scores has been recommended to compare the growth between birth weight and discharge weight as a more suitable method of measuring growth in an individual infant (Cooke, 2016). Table 17.2 outlines recommended steps to improve growth between birth and hospital discharge in the preterm infant. Linked to this, table 17.3 then identifies the evidence in pertaining to the various interventions in relation to a variety of indices/outcome measures.

MONITORING GROWTH IN NEONATES

Accuracy/precision of anthropometric measures are crucial in 'tailoring' intake to meet needs, that is, ensuring weight and linear growth at a minimum parallel to growth *in utero* (Cooke, 2016). Adequate nutrition can be estimated by measuring the infant's body weight, length and head circumference. Postnatal head growth is a strong predictor of early

TABLE 17.3 EVIDENCE FOR EFFECTS OF NUTRITIONAL STRATEGIES ON GROWTH AND NEURODEVELOPMENTAL OUTCOMES IN VLBW INFANTS

	Weight gain and/or linear growth	Head growth	Neurodevelopmental outcomes
Fortified preterm vs. term formula	positive	positive	positive
Modifications to preterm formula	positive	none	negative
Higher protein	none	none	positive/none
Long chain polyunsaturated fatty acids	none	none	little
Bile salt-stimulated lipase	negative	negative	positive
Human milk vs. formula	positive	positive	positive
Human milk fortification vs. formula	positive	positive	little
Adjuncts to human milk fortifier	positive	positive	little
Added proteins	none	none	positive
Human milk cream	positive	none	none
Maternal DHA[a] supplement during lactation	none	none	none
Parental nutrition (early vs. late)			
Iron supplementation			

(adapted from Belfort and Ehrenkranz, 2017)
a Docosahexaenoic acid (omega-3 fatty acid)

developmental outcome in LBW infants, and insufficient calories provided for small for gestational age (SGA) infants beyond the first two weeks of life may result in failure to initiate catch-up head growth (Tan et al., 2008). The ponderal index, which is a calculation of body weight and length, gives an indication of the quality of the growth by relating body weight to the overall length. Length and head circumference are important to measure, as they are indices of skeletal and organ growth, whereas weight may change due to fluid balance changes and fat deposition. Growth is not linear and is characterised by growth spurts and stagnation, making the interpretation of daily weights difficult. However, these measures can be inaccurate, and care needs to be taken to ensure consistency and skill in taking these measurements for them to be meaningful.

The practicalities of weighing a baby in NNU can be a source of concern for nurses caring for these infants. The reliability of weighing sick ventilated infants has not been evaluated, and the possible harms of weighing the infant need to be balanced against the accuracy of the technique. The use of in-bed scales has not been adequately tested as a reliable method for assessing growth in sick and/or small infants who are ventilated. However, to provide a good estimate of the trends in the infant's weight, the procedure of weighing needs to be meticulous. The time an infant is weighed needs to be considered with reference to the enteral intake, defecation and urination (Cooke, 2016). The baby should be weighed at the same time of day, using the same scales, and the weight checked by two persons. The accuracy of the scales should be evaluated regularly. A documented unit policy on the procedure may be beneficial in achieving some consistency, especially in intensive care, as the infant may have splints, drains and multiple lines to consider in the total weight.

Regular measurements of head circumference will provide information to inconsistent growth. There needs to be a uniform approach to the measurement, such as placing the tape measure around the widest part of the head (maximal occipital-frontal diameter), and this should be performed by a nurse or doctor who makes a minimum of two reproducible measurements. Measurements of length by the crown-to-heel length (CHL) method using an infantometer is the most accurate determination of length. The infant's clothes and nappy are removed, and the infant placed supine on a flat base covered with thin cloth with the head held against the headboard by an assistant. The measurer holds and applies gentle pressure to both knees to straighten the legs, while the assistant ensures the hips and shoulders are aligned at right angles to the long axis of the body, with the spine not arched. The measurer then slides the foot board along the base until flat against the soles of both feet, and records the measurement to the nearest complete millimetre (mm). Once recorded, the measurer and assistant switch roles and repeat this procedure, thereby acquiring a pair of independently obtained CHL measurements (Ismail et al., 2016).

The nutrients required to maintain growth and improve neurodevelopmental outcomes are many, and there is an expansive body of evidence for various strategies both for enteral and parenteral routes of administration. Current evidence supports the use of preterm formula or fortified human milk rather than standard (term) formula as a nutritional strategy for neurodevelopmental benefits (Belfort and Ehrenkranz 2017).

PARENTERAL NUTRITION

The administration of nutrients using the vascular system has been in clinical practice for more than 30 years. Parenteral nutrition (PN) is used to fill the gap between the time of birth and the establishment of full volume enteral feeds for very LBW infants as well as those who are unable to have enteral feeds due to congenital or acquired abnormalities of the gastrointestinal tract or following surgery in the newborn period. PN may be used as a supplement to enteral nutrition, or it may be used exclusively. It may be administered using a variety of routes, the most popular being via a peripherally inserted central catheter (PICC).

The use of PN in the NNU is widespread, however there is limited evidence as to the benefits on the long-term neurodevelopmental outcomes (Uthaya and Modi, 2014). It has been recommended that there should be consistency across NNUs in the delivery and management of PN, as well as a set of measurable outcomes, including neurodevelopmental aspects, to ensure good-quality nutritional management (Chan et al., 2016). When PN is used in the NNU, specific care is required to ensure the complications associated with its use are avoided. Infants should be monitored regularly for their fluid intake and output, their tolerance of glucose by measuring both blood and urine glucose levels, and their tolerance of lipids by monitoring plasma turbidity, either by observing a sample of settled blood or spinning a sample of blood. If signs of turbidity persist, then a sample should be sent for analysis in the laboratory. Other complications include sepsis, metabolic disturbances and catheter-related problems. Preterm infants have poor tolerance of both glucose and fat when infused above physiological levels (Klein, 2002). Therefore, nurses need to ensure that the infusion rate remains constant and avoid the temptation to 'catch up' with volumes when the infusion has been disrupted.

The focus of early nutritional support in extremely preterm infants should be the prevention of early nutritional deficits and avoidance of the need for catch-up growth (Uthaya and Modi, 2014). Increased early enteral nutrition may reduce neurodevelopmental impairment in very preterm and/or very low birth weight (LBW) infants, but the direct relationship between neurodevelopmental outcome and nutrition remains unclear (Chan et al., 2016).

ENTERAL NUTRITION

Human milk is the preferred diet for enteral feeds. There is wide variation in the nutrient and non-nutrient content of the milks currently available. Formulas designed for preterm use differ in composition from milks designed for term infants. Human milk also varies in composition during the course of lactation, diurnally and during a breastfeed. The milk from mothers who have delivered prematurely has a different composition from that of mothers who have delivered at term, as it is higher in protein (2.4g versus 1.8g/100mL). If formula is to be used for term infants, then standard formulas based on cows' milk with a protein concentration of 13–15g/L provide the best nutritional source (Eidelman and Schanler, 2012).

Early nutrition of LBW infants can influence later neurodevelopment (Belfort and Ehrenkranz, 2017) so it remains vital that nutritional needs are met. Whereas breast milk supplies adequate nutrients to meet the nutritional demands of the term infant, the nutrient component of premature human milk provides insufficient quantities to meet the estimated needs of the premature infant. Fortification of human milk with multicomponent supplementation has been used to increase the rate of growth in very LBW infants.

Enteral nutrition often starts with early trophic feeds, however there is no evidence that early trophic feeding affects feed tolerance, growth rates or NEC (Morgan et al., 2013). In some specific conditions, early trophic feeds have been associated with shorter duration of mechanical ventilation, a trend towards more stable postoperative haemodynamics, less fluid overload, and earlier postoperative feeding tolerance in infants undergoing open cardiac surgery (Toms et al., 2015). It remains a widespread practice with the aim to prime the gut in readiness for full enteral feeds. Box 17.1 outlines the various strategies for enteral feeding.

The various routes of administering enteral nutrition all have associated adverse events. It remains the responsibility of the neonatal nurse to provide expert and vigilant care when caring for a neonate on tube feeds. Assessing tolerance of feeds when a tube

BOX 17.1 STRATEGIES OF ADMINISTERING ENTERAL FEEDS

Gastric tube route

Preterm/ low birth weight infants too immature or unwell to suck-feed can receive their milk through a feeding tube passed via either the nose or the mouth.

Neonates are obligate nose breathers, thus nasogastric tubes can obstruct the nasal passage and compromise breathing.

Tubes placed via the nose may be more stable and less prone to displace than tubes passed via the mouth.

No evidence to support one route over the other, so it remains up to clinician preference based on the assessment of the individual infant (Watson and McGuire, 2013a).

Checking for correct placement is vital to avoid aspiration, and safety notices have been issued to avoid adverse events occurring (National Patient Safety Agency, 2011).

Various methods of measurement have found to be inaccurate, so caution is required when inserting and securing gastric tubes (Cirgin Ellett et al., 2011).

Continuous vs. intermittent bolus tube feeding

Milk feeds can be given via oro-/nasogastric tube either intermittently, typically over 10–20 minutes every two or three hours, or continuously, using an infusion pump.

Bolus-fed neonates tolerate feeds better and gain weight faster.

Neonates on continuous feeds have been shown to take longer to reach full enteral feeds, but there is no difference in days to discharge, somatic growth and incidence of NEC (Premji and Chessell, 2011).

Gastrostomy tube feeds

This route is used when longer-term enteral feeding is indicated.

Feeds maybe administered either as a bolus over 15–20 minutes, or continuously using an enteral feeding pump.

Transpyloric tube feeds

A transpyloric tube (TPT) allows for feeding directly into the jejunum. TPTs are difficult to place and maintain in position.

Feeding straight into the jejunum can cause dumping syndrome due to the rapid delivery of a hyperosmolar feed, therefore feeds are always delivered continuously in small volumes

Transpyloric feeding is associated with more adverse events without any evidence of benefits over gastric feeding (Watson and McGuire, 2013b).

is in situ remains a challenge, and many practices of measuring and managing residuals (aspirates) vary across institutions and individual clinicians. There is insufficient evidence that the routine use of gastric residuals can assist in the diagnosis of feeding intolerance (Parker et al., 2015).

Transitioning from tube to suck-feeds requires assessment of the ability of the individual infant based on their underlying disease, level of maturity and measures of tolerance.

SUCK FEEDING ON THE NEONATAL UNIT

Feeding is one of the first interactions between the mother and her healthy term baby. For the breastfeeding mother, this is her primary role in the postnatal period and well beyond. While feeding, the mother has her first opportunity to get to know her baby, interact and communicate. She learns how her baby expresses contentment and distress, and how she as a mother responds to this. The father's role in initiation of breastfeeding and continuation post discharge is now more widely recognised (Sherriff et al., 2014). Most mothers of healthy term babies find establishing feeding in the early weeks challenging, exhausting and confusing. However, they are more than likely in the comfort of their own homes with some degree of support. It is in this environment that the feeding relationship begins to develop. Often the baby needs to get to know just one caregiver, sometimes both parents and in other families a few close relatives. Each person has time to get to know the new addition and the baby has time to get to know them.

The feeding journey for the baby on the NNU and their parents is often a very different experience – for some, the neonatal environment can be one of maternal separation, long periods without suck-feeding, an environment with potentially loud sounds from machines and unfamiliar voices, sometimes harsh lighting, necessary yet painful interventions, noxious smells and tastes and intrusive procedures to the face and mouth (Jadcherla et al., 2010). Multiple caregivers instead of just one or two, each with their own way of interpreting and responding to the baby's cues, results in stressful and unpredictable early feeding experiences.

Others whose babies may be born at a later gestational age or with fewer complications still may face the overwhelming introduction to motherhood and suck-feeding seperated from the support of their home environment. An insight into the experiences the new parent and infant faces on the unit and how this may impact the journey to suck feeding is integral for any member of the neonatal team and will enable sensitive conversations and more mindful interactions to take place.

As neonatal professionals supporting babies and their families, our understanding of suck-feeding has evolved over the last 30 years. The complexity of this fundamental neurodevelopmental skill is now better understood (Jadcherla et al., 2010), and the vulnerability of the neonatal population more widely accepted. Most significantly, the impact of prematurity and the quality the environment, of early interactions and experiences (including those that occur during feeding) on later neurodevelopmental outcomes in all NNU graduates is well documented (Als and Gilkerson, 1997; Als, 2004; Moore et al., 2012;

Coughlin, 2014). More evidence is being highlighted, which demonstrates the risk of later psychiatric morbidities in adolescence and adulthood in our preterm population (Lindström et al., 2009; Lai and Huang, 2011). What we, the neonatal team do in the early stages of the infant's life, has a long-lasting effect on both their individual developmental trajectory and the mental health of the baby and their family.

Models of neonatal care have shifted and there have been a number of initiatives introduced to support best practice. Best practice For example, Baby Friendly (Unicef, 2019), and other models of care that prioritise family-centred and family-integrated care models (O'Brien et al., 2015; 2018). Developmental care ethos and practice is promoted (Als, 2004). Despite these changes, the practice of suck-feeding continues to vary widely among NNUs.

Overwhelmingly, the focus continues to be on the volume consumed and weight gained rather than the quality of the feed and the parent–infant relationship (Thoyre, 2000). Successful discharge from the NNU continues to prioritise weight gain and adequate suck-feeding. NNU graduates are often discharged from the unit feeding well enough, but are not yet skilled feeders (Shaker, 2016), resulting in up to 40% of the ex-preterm population experiencing ongoing feeding difficulties (Thoyre et al., 2005). Prolonged suck-feeding difficulties impact bonding and increase maternal stress long after discharge (Thoyre, 2000). The increasing medical costs from enteral feeding and the interventions needed to support children with feeding difficulties places demands on both acute and community settings.

THE NEONATAL MULTIDISCIPLINARY FEEDING TEAM

The number of professionals supporting suck-feeding on the NNU has increased (see figure 17.1). Where the nursing and medical teams would once act in isolation, now a team of therapists and health professionals are able to contribute to the overall care and support of the newborn baby and their family, each adding their own unique perspective on the baby's developmental feeding strengths and needs. The collective aim is to provide age-appropriate neuroprotective care. There is much variation in the makeup of each unit's individual feeding team depending on the level of the NNU, the needs of the infant, and the resources available to the unit. The parents are at the heart of the team. Within the context of family-centred care, the neonatal team should be providing a supportive environment for families to enable them to take the primary role in the care of their baby including suck-feeding once this commences. When it is not possible for the parent to be present, the neonatal nurse will adopt this role.

An understanding of how the nurse and SALT work together to support suck-feeding and how their roles differ will enable effective multidisciplinary working and for timely referrals to be made (Table 17.4). Many neonatal SALTs have taken a dual qualification to specialise as a lactation consultant.

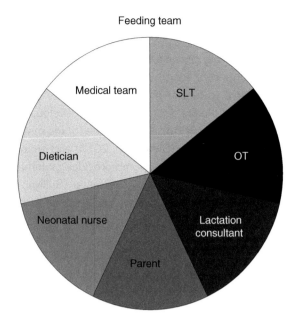

Figure 17.1 Members of the neonatal feeding team

TABLE 17.4 ROLES OF NEONATAL NURSE AND NEONATAL SPEECH AND LANGUAGE THERAPIST

Neonatal nurse	Speech and Language Therapist
Responsible for feeding all babies in their care	Only responsible for babies referred to SALT. (Unless unit uses a referral by gestational age).
Involved with babies who follow typical feeding milestones and babies who have identified feeding and/or swallowing difficulties	Involved with babies who do not follow the typical feeding course.
Identifies babies who are having difficulties with feeding and/or swallowing that cannot be managed in isolation	Identifies babies who are at risk of feeding and/ or swallowing difficulties and communication difficulties (Royal College of Speech & Language Therapists, 2019).
Informally screens feeding of each infant in their care at each feed	Provides assessment of feeding, swallowing and communication difficulties and supports safe and positive oral feeding.
Follows recommendations made by the SALT	Provides individualised therapeutic care plans for each infant and family.
Supports Developmental Care practices as part of the wider multidisciplinary team	Supports Developmental Care practices as part of the wider multidisciplinary team.

THE SENSORY EXPERIENCES OF THE NEONATE

Each baby is born with genetically predetermined processes for feeding such as sucking, rooting, swallowing and hunger. *In utero*, the baby is exposed to multiple positive sensory experiences, which serve to further prepare the baby for suck-feeding at birth. The chemosensory system is one of the first foetal systems to develop, enabling *in utero* opportunities for taste and smell (Browne 2008). A preference for the mother's amniotic fluid and mother's odour is present by 28 weeks (Blackburn, 2013) and enables later odour identification and attachment (Browne, 2008). The womb provides maternal proximity, and a preference for the mother's voice is seen in the third trimester (Sullivan et al., 2011). Feeding reflexes such as swallow develop at 10–14 weeks' gestation, while sucking emerges around 18–30 weeks' gestation. Flexion supports hands to mouth to aid the practice of sucking and swallowing. Any disruption in this journey, such as premature birth or maternal separation due to medical complications, can affect the development of these skills and has the potential to alter feeding experiences throughout childhood.

READINESS TO SUCK-FEED

Historically, decisions on when to initiate and advance suck-feeds were based on gestational age and weight. It is now recognised that this is not a reliable indication of readiness to feed (Holloway, 2014). Feeding readiness cues and maturational competence provide more crucial information in guiding the neonatal nurse as to when to initiate suck-feeds (Coughlin, 2014) (see table 17.5).

For the preterm or medically complex infant, achieving the prerequisite skills necessary for suck-feeding readiness can take time and subsequently many infants, particularly extremely preterm infants or babies requiring surgical intervention, may face long periods of parenteral or enteral feeding before suck-feeding is introduced. The infant requires

TABLE 17.5 ACTIVITIES TO ENCOURAGE FEEDING READINESS

Activity	Feeding cues
Skin-to-skin/gentle handling just before feed	Wakefulness before feeds/ability to maintain quiet awake state (Harding et al., 2014; 2018; Pickler et al., 2006; McCain, 1997; 2003)
Skin-to-skin just before enteral feed	Rooting (opening their mouth to searching for the breast with) or rubbing their face on the bedding/head turning (Browne and Ross, 2011)
Mouth care/non-nutritive sucking	Increased tongue movements/increased sucking (Browne and Ross, 2011)

respiratory and physiological stability, neuromotor maturation and behavioural state regulation at rest before being able to fully engage with suck-feeding (Ludwig and Waitzman, 2007; Kish, 2013; Harding et al., 2018).

Respiratory stability is a necessary component of successful suck-feeding. There are currently no standardised guidelines regarding the safety of suck-feeding while receiving non-invasive ventilation, and subsequently clinical practice varies across NNUs. Ferrara et al. (2017) suggest that suck-feeding should not take place while the infant is receiving continuous positive airway pressure (CPAP) due to an increased risk of laryngeal penetration and aspiration in the context of an altered pharyngeal swallow. Concerns exist regarding missed developmental windows for the initiation of suck-feeding for infants who require long-term CPAP, however, a larger body of evidence is needed to inform clinicians. Suck feeding while infants receive high flow nasal cannula oxygen also presents challenges, as data refuting or supporting its use is limited.

An ability to maintain an alert state (behavioural organisation) is an indicator of maturity and readiness to feed. Studies found that awake behaviour dominated in the successful feeders, leading to the conclusion that awake and quiet behaviours represent optimal feeding states (Pickler et al., 2006; Griffith et al., 2017; Harding et al., 2018). Recognising behavioural states, particularly a quiet alert state that indicates readiness to interact and subsequently feed (Brazelton et al., 1995), is a necessary skill for the caregiver. The SALT or Occupational Therapist (OT) can support the nurse to feel more confident in recognising behavioural states. Once achieved, the infant is understandably better able to demonstrate hunger cues.

Postmenstrual age (PMA) continues to play a significant role in decision-making to ensure safe and stress-free feeding is achieved, but it should not be used in isolation. Whereas breastfeeding was once thought to be a difficult skill for the preterm infant to achieve, it is now known to place less physiological stress on the infant and can therefore be introduced at an earlier age. Nyqvist et al. (2017) found infants as young as 29 weeks PMA supported in skin-to-skin contact were able to demonstrate feeding readiness cues such as rooting, and were able to demonstrate emerging oral skills such as an areolar grasp with short suck-bursts. Infants in this study were able to achieve exclusive breastfeeding between 32 and 38 weeks.

Bottle-feeding, where the flow and sometimes pace is determined by the teat and bottle used and caregiver, requires maturation of suck-swallow-breathe-cycles not present until 34–36 weeks (Kish, 2013; Pickler et al., 2015). Even at 36 weeks PMA, the infant will require supportive interventions to achieve safe and positive oral feeding (Sables-Baus et al., 2013). Infants with more significant respiratory compromise will experience greater physiological stress if they are challenged with coordinating their suck-swallow-breathe coordination too soon (Gewolb and Vice, 2006). As standard practice, parents should be supported to recognise feeding cues, so they can more easily identify them.

As there are no standardized, internationally recognised guidelines for clinicians initiating suck feeds, decision-making still varies significantly. This results in a trial and error approach to suck-feeding in an already vulnerable population (Pickler et al., 2006; 2015).

ASSESSMENT OF FEEDING

The infant who demonstrates readiness to suck-feed must also be able to maintain autonomic, behavioural and motor stability when faced with the demand of milk flow while breast- or bottle-feeding. An awareness of the behavioural, biological and environmental factors that contribute to the success of suck-feeding will enable the neonatal nurse to provide positive suck-feeding experiences, avoiding unnecessary physiological stress (Harding et al., 2016).

Using the principles of developmental care, the neonatal nurse assesses each baby in his or her care. The infant's individual behavioural cues are observed during daily cares and the environment and interactions adapted accordingly, to enhance the infant's strengths and self-regulation capacities (Als and McAnulty, 2011). These principles apply to suck-feeding, and observations made during breast- or bottle-feeds can act as an indicator of a baby's current neurological ability (Shaker, 2013), informing the team of the infant's general progress and their place on their unique developmental timeline. Where a baby shows signs of the risk of swallowing difficulty (dysphagia), has a condition which is associated with a risk of dysphagia or refuses the bottle (oral aversion) that are not reduced by the use of supportive strategies, the SALT will assess suck feeding further. This will involve carrying out an oral motor assessment and swallow evaluation to assess the potential risk of aspiration. The SALT will work alongside the parents and neonatal nurse to support understanding and identification of engagement and disengagement cues during suck-feeding whilst recommending appropriate strategies to implement.

COORDINATION OF SUCKING, SWALLOWING AND BREATHING

Oral motor control and coordination of the suck-swallow-breathe sequence are the foundations of safe and efficient oral feeding (Lau, 2016). Oral motor control consists of the functional use of the lips, tongue, jaw, and hard and soft palate, all of which are involved in sucking.

Sucking

Sucking comprises compression and suction. Suction is absent in the immature suck patterns of the preterm infant and is replaced with an arrhythmic expression pattern. This can be used to feed with a bottle, but not feed efficiently, and often leads to fatigue. The breastfeeding infant requires both compression and suction and subsequently may need further assessment if difficulties with the latch arise (Wolff, 1968). Anatomical abnormalities of the oral cavity as seen with cleft palate or micrognathia can impact feeding efficiency. Babies with neurological impairment such as hypoxic-ischaemic encephalopathy or neuromuscular conditions such as spinal muscular atrophy may experience hyper or hypotonia which can also affect strength of suck and intraoral pressure needed for suction.

Swallowing

Swallowing is seen *in utero* as early as 10 weeks' gestation. Polyhydramnios may be one of the first indicators of swallowing difficulty when identified in early gestation. The swallow consists of three stages in the infant (oral, pharyngeal and oesophageal). Aspiration (when material moves below the level of the vocal cords into the lungs) occurs if airway protection is incomplete or does not occur in a timely manner. Dysfunction at any of these three stages may impact swallow safety and efficiency.

Breathing

Breathing stops momentarily to protect the airway during each swallow; this is known as swallow apnoea. Catch up breathes to compensate for the reduction in respiration during the sucking bursts occur in the pauses. Where respiratory compromise is present, particularly in infants with bronchopulmonary dysplasia, the repetitive interruptions to breathing in their already challenged respiratory systems can compromise their breathing resulting in insufficient opportunities to recover their breathing when feeding. This results in less oxygen exchange in the lungs and subsequent desaturations. Reduced intake and fatigue are also common clinical indicators associated with demand of feeding being too great for the infant. Preterm infants also find this skill particularly challenging, and difficulties with endurance during suck-feeds may manifest because of the increased cardiorespiratory demands from the work of feeding.

TRANSITION FROM TUBE TO SUCK-FEEDS

Various factors can affect the transition to suck-feeding (see table 17.6), such as gestational age at the time of birth, birth weight, and the length of time spent on ventilation, with the number of days on oxygen being the strongest predictor of bottle-feeding initiation and feeding ability (Bier et al., 1993). Infants of less than 28 weeks' gestation face significant delays with respect to initiation and progression of both enteral and suck-feeds, with an increased length of stay (Jadcherla et al., 2010). Neonates with cardiac or respiratory morbidities are at increased risk of delayed attainment of full suck-feeds.

An awareness of the typical development of these integral feeding milestones, and how this may vary according to prematurity and/or contributing co-morbidities is essential to promoting safe and positive oral feeding.

One in ten preterm infants was diagnosed with gastro-oesophageal reflux in a study conducted across 33 NNUs in the United States (Jadcherla et al., 2010). If not identified and managed, the presence of gastro-oesophageal reflux can prolong transition to suck-feeds, subsequently increasing the length of stay (up to 29.9 days) (Jadcherla et al., 2010). It can be distressing for the infant, mother and caregiver trying to establish suck-feeds, affecting the parent–infant feeding relationship.

TABLE 17.6 POTENTIAL RISK FACTORS FOR FEEDING DIFFICULTIES IN NEONATES

Risk factor	Associated conditions	Potential impact
Prematurity	Extreme prematurity, very low birth weight	Immature neurodevelopment, requirement for ventilation, immature gut.
Neurological	Hypoxic-ischaemic encephalopathy (stages II and III), intraventricular haemorrhage (grades III and IV), periventricular haemorrhage	Absent or weak suck, poor latch. Hyper/hypotonia.
Respiratory	Long periods of intubation, Continuous positive airway pressure (CPAP), High flow or low flow nasal cannula oxygen Chronic lung disease Respiratory distress syndrome (RDS)	Endurance difficulties – fatigue. Gastro-oesophageal reflux disease GORD.
Cardiac	Congenital abnormalities	Endurance difficulties, increased risk of aspiration post Patent ductus arteriosus (PDA) ligation if recurrent laryngeal nerve is damaged during surgery.
ENT	Cleft lip or palate, laryngeal cleft Laryngomalacia Tracheo-oesophageal fistula (TOF) Micrognathia	Latch affected. Reduced intraoral pressure with cleft palate impacts milk transfer/efficiency. Potential respiration compromise affecting suck, swallow, breath synchrony. Risk of aspiration with laryngeal cleft, TOF.
Gastrointestinal	Necrotising enterocolitis (NEC) Oesophageal Atresia, Gastro-oesophageal reflux (GOR)	Long periods of nil orally if surgery required. Tolerance issues. GORD associated with oral aversion.
Genetic	Trisomy 21, Pierre-Robin sequence, Neuromuscular conditions, e.g. spinal muscular atrophy	Individual to each condition.

Practices are often based on empirical opinion. The role gut dysmotility plays on swallow function as well as pleasure in feeding and later oral aversion is now widely acknowledged and emphasises the importance of both non-medical and medical management of gastro-oesophageal reflux in the preterm population.

Non-nutritive sucking (NNS) is a supportive intervention which can be used by parents or nurses to support the transition from tube to suck-feeds. It refers to sucking on an empty breast or dry pacifier. It should be offered prior to attempting sucking feeds to encourage a quiet awake state, or during tube feeds when infants are alert or restless, to support digestion.

Benefits of non-nutritive sucking

■ NNS has a positive impact on transition from tube to oral feeding and the time from the start of suck-feeding to full oral feeds (Foster et al., 2016)

■ Reduction of the length of hospital stay (Foster et al., 2016)

■ NNS as an intervention to support parents to read their baby's early communication cues could potentially reduce the length of stay on the unit (Harding et al., 2014).

CUE-BASED FEEDING

The many long-term neurodevelopmental and medical benefits of breastfeeding are internationally recognised (Lubbe, 2018), however, establishing breastfeeding and sustaining this post discharge continues to be a challenge for the parents and members of the neonatal team on the unit. For a large number of infants, bottle-feeding to some degree will be part of their suck-feeding plan upon discharge. It is therefore necessary for the caregiver to be equipped with knowledge of supportive strategies to improve the feeding experience and decrease physiological stress on the infant's often vulnerable systems. The team should encourage and support the parent to be present for as many feeds as possible, as the primary caregiver, to enable the development of bonding and attachment through the feeding relationship and develop parental confidence. Supportive caregiver interventions can be seen in box 17.2.

Breastfeeding is by nature infant-driven and cue-based. Latching and sucking occur if optimal behavioural organisation is achieved and oral skills are mature and intact. If the infant is not able to move to a quiet alert state they will not be able to latch and feed. If the pace is too fast or they are uncomfortable, they will pull off the breast.

Bottle-feeding has the potential to override these sometimes subtle cues of engagement and disengagement. Confusion arises from the belief that caregiving practices carried out with healthy term babies can be used with the vulnerable neonatal population. Bottle-feeding practices continue to vary between clinicians and institutions. In a traditional model

---

BOX 17.2 SUPPORTIVE CAREGIVER INTERVENTIONS FOR SAFE AND POSITIVE BOTTLE-FEEDING

■ Modifying flow rate using slow flow teats

■ Providing elevated side-lying position

■ Co-regulated pacing

■ Behavioural state support

■ Supportive swaddling.

TABLE 17.7 SIGNS OF STRESS DURING INFANT FEEDING

Autonomic	Motor	State
Respiratory rate	Limbs tensed or extended	Sudden loss of alertness
Heart rate	Jerky movements	Sudden fuss or cry
SpO₂ levels (desaturations)	Flaccidity of trunk, neck, face, extremities	Sudden onset of sleepiness
Colour change	Arching	Frowns, grimaces
Hiccoughs	Variable tone	Sudden fatigue or weak state
Vomiting	Tongue extensions	Irritability
		Shift to hyperalert, panicked or worried face

of practice, a daily schedule of suck-feeds is ordered by the physician, who aims to gradually wean the infant off enteral tube feeds and onto suck-feeds until they are able to consume enough calories orally to grow. Feeds are time-scheduled every 2, 3 or 4 hours in isolation of the infant's ability to achieve a quiet alert state or demonstrate hunger signs (Browne and Ross, 2011). This 'volume-driven' approach prioritises completed feed volumes. The infant who feeds faster is viewed as a skilled feeder, or the caregiver who 'gets' the baby to complete the bottle is viewed as more experienced. When using this approach, stress signs (see table 17.7) are often overlooked.

Using a volume-driven approach does not consider the infant's individual signs of feeding readiness at each feed (see table 17.7). Every feeding experience is different for the baby, and mastering optimal feeding skills is prolonged as each new caregiver brings their own experience and outlook on the baby's feed. When nursing documentation does not include information about the quality of the feed and which supportive methods facilitate safe and positive feeding, learning to suck-feed is protracted, increasing the length of stay (Ludwig and Waitzman, 2007).

Internationally, the feeding culture on the NNU is changing direction, and many units are moving towards more individualised cue-based feeding, responsive to the infant's needs in line with other developmentally supportive practices. Using a cue-based approach, suck-feeds are offered when the baby demonstrates feeding readiness rather than at specific times as per the prescribed schedule. A Cochrane review of responsive feeding versus scheduled feeds concluded that responsive feeding may support a faster transition to full oral feeds, however more randomised controlled trials are needed (Watson and McGuire, 2016).

The barriers to a cue-based approach, involving care planned according to the infant's needs rather than a set routine, are well known. This can be challenging for the nurse working on a unit where staffing levels are stretched, or for the nurse who has followed a

TABLE 17.8 VOLUME-DRIVEN STRATEGIES WITH ALTERNATIVE CUE-BASED RATIONALE

Problem	Volume-driven strategy	Alternative rationale
Baby is asleep at time of feed	Removing blanket and feeding unswaddled	Baby is not demonstrating feeding readiness.
Baby is not completing bottles	Increasing flow rate	Baby is demonstrating they are not developmentally ready for full bottle-feeds.
Baby falls asleep while bottle-feeding	Prodding, jiggling the teat to initiate more sucking	Baby does not yet have the stamina to maintain an awake state during suck-feeds or suck-feeds are overwhelming causing the baby to 'shut down'.
Baby is losing milk from the mouth	Chin/cheek support	Baby is unable to manage flow. Providing this type of support may increase aspiration risk.
Baby is slow to take the bottle	Putting infant's head/neck back	Feeding is too challenging for this baby. He or she may not have the skill or is not developmentally ready.

(adapted from Shaker, 1999; 2013; 2016)

a See the SOFFI (Ross, 2011) for suggested supportive interventions

routine-led feeding practice for most of her career as a neonatal nurse. Equally, challenges can be met for the newly qualified nurse by colleagues who take a more traditional stance. Many units choose to follow a volume-driven approach due to concerns about compromising weight gain or increasing the length of stay. Studies carried out by units applying a more cue-based, infant-driven approach have demonstrated that using a clinical pathway (Kirk et al., 2007) or tool (Ludwig, 2007) to guide this process resulted in earlier attainment of full oral feeding and improved weight gain (Kirk et al., 2007).

The advantages of parents becoming the primary feeder on the NNU using a cue-based approach are well documented. By encouraging parents to take a key role in suck-feeding, they are better able to understand and respond to their baby's cues (White and Parnell, 2013). This helps them to understand that feeding is a process and will be individual to their baby. It enables the parents to have more realistic expectations of their baby's feeding journey, something which remains difficult in a unit that adopts the more traditional approach.

Responsive feeding is a term used within the Unicef UK Baby Friendly Initiative standards, which can be applied to both breast- and bottle-feeding, and should not be confused with cue-based feeding practice. It promotes a parental focus on the cues of the baby rather than scheduled feeds, it concentrates on a shared recognition that the act of feeding provides love, interaction and opportunities to communicate, as well as nutrition.

CONCLUSION

Understanding the nutritional requirements and feeding challenges for neonates in the NNU remains an integral part of the role of the neonatal nurse and feeding team. Growth is a measure of outcome and is thought to have a direct impact on healthy neurodevelopment. It is important to remember that the quality of the experience to establish oral feeds and sustained growth is the important goal for the neonates, family and healthcare professional.

CASE STUDY

CASE STUDIES

Case study 1: Nutrition management for a preterm infant

Joseph was born at 26 weeks' gestation. He was the first child of a young married couple. At birth, Joseph breathed spontaneously and required minimal resuscitation. He was transferred to the NICU. His birth weight was 780g. An arterial blood gas and chest X-ray indicated respiratory distress syndrome and he was intubated, received surfactant and was ventilated. Joseph required assisted ventilation for the first two days then he was extubated and placed on CPAP. He was nursed in a double-walled incubator and was requiring supplemental oxygen of 25%. His weight at 2 weeks of age when plotted on the growth chart was less than the 3rd centile.

Joseph's mother was with him each day and was expressing good volumes of milk. She was keen to be able to eventually breastfeed. Her concern was for his future and that he would develop normally.

Q.1. What would be the most appropriate method to supply Joseph's nutritional requirements for the first week of his life?

Q.2. Which are the risk factors that may impact on Joseph commencing enteral feeds?

Q.3. Once Joseph was to commence enteral feeds, what method would be appropriate for him?

Q.4. How would you reliably assess the outcome of Joseph's nutritional goals?

Q.5. What are some strategies you could implement to improve Joseph's growth?

Case study 2: Support for successful breastfeeding in the neonatal unit

Olga, mother of Francesca born at 26 weeks' gestation, struggled to express her breast milk in the early days of her baby's life. After a significant amount of support and advice from various people and sources, she finally managed to produce enough breast milk to store in readiness for when Francesca started to feed enterally.

Q.1. What advice and support do you think was given to Olga to enable her to eventually produce and express sufficient qualities of breast milk?
Later when Francesca's condition had improved, and she was 7 weeks old, Francesca strongly wanted to breastfeed her baby. However, again, she required assistance to do this successfully.

Q.2. Which members of the neonatal multidisciplinary team would be required to assist her?

Q.3. How would Francesca's readiness to feed be assessed?

Q.4. How would this feeding assessment be integrated with the principles of developmental care outlined in chapter 5?

Case study 3: The very low birth weight infant

Tommy is a 36-week gestation baby who is very low birth weight; his weight is under the 3rd centile and this was due to placental problems during pregnancy leading to poor foetal growth. He required enteral feeding by nasogastric tube as well as orally when he was admitted to the neonatal unit as he lost a significant amount of weight in the first few days after delivery and had a very low blood sugar. His mum was not well and was in intensive care with pre-eclampsia, so breast milk was not available. A later problem presenting was severe reflux which impacted on the time taken to reach an adequate weight and tolerate full feeding requirements.

Q.1. Why was it important that Tommy was enterally fed so early?

Q.2. Can you identify key strategies you would employ in this situation to ensure adequate nutrition and feeding tolerance, in line with both management of his growth restriction and poor weight gain, and later the gastroesophageal reflux?

For suggested answer guides to the questions posed in these case studies, please refer to the web-based companion site specific to this chapter (see URL below).

WEB-BASED RESOURCES

For further information, online resources and greater detail on the case studies featured in this chapter go to www.routledge.com/cw/nicnursing

References

Abiramalatha, T., Thomas, N., Gupta, V., Viswanathan, A., & McGuire, W. (2017). High versus standard volume enteral feeds to promote growth in preterm or low birth weight infants. *Cochrane Database of Systematic Reviews*, Issue 9. Art. No.: CD012413. DOI: 10.1002/14651858.CD012413.pub2

Als, H., Duffy, F. et al. (2004). Early Experience alters brain function and structure. *Pediatrics, 113*(4), 846–857.

Als, H., & Gilkerson, L. (1997). The role of relationship-based developmentally supportive newborn intensive care in strengthening outcome of preterm infants. In *Seminars in Perinatology, 21*(3), 178–180.

Als, H., & McAnulty, B. (2011). The newborn individualized developmental care and assessment program (NIDCAP) with kangaroo mother care (KMC): Comprehensive care for preterm infants. *Current Women's Health Reviews*, 7(3), 288–301.

Belfort, M. B., & Ehrenkranz, R. A. (2017). Neurodevelopmental outcomes and nutritional strategies in very low birth weight infants. In *Seminars in Fetal and Neonatal Medicine, 22*(1), 42–48.

Bier, J. A. B., Ferguson, A., Cho, C., Oh, W., & Vohr, B. R. (1993). The oral motor development of low-birth-weight infants who underwent orotracheal intubation during the neonatal period. *American Journal of Diseases of Children, 147*(8), 858–862.

Blackburn, S. T. (2013). *Maternal, fetal, & neonatal physiology: A clinical perspective.* Maryland Heights: Elsevier Saunders.

Brazelton, T. B., Brazelton, T. B., & Nugent, J. K. (1995). *Neonatal behavioral assessment scale* (No. 137). Cambridge University Press.

Browne, J. V. (2008). Chemosensory development in the fetus and newborn. *Newborn and Infant Nursing Reviews*, 8(4), 180–186.

Browne, J. V., & Ross, E. S. (2011). Eating as a neurodevelopmental process for high-risk newborns. *Clinics in Perinatology, 38*(4), 731–743.

Chan, S. H., Johnson, M. J., Leaf, A. A., & Vollmer, B. (2016). Nutrition and neurodevelopmental outcomes in preterm infants: A systematic review. *Acta Paediatrica, 105*(6), 587–599.

Cirgin Ellett, M. L., Cohen, M. D., Perkins, S. M., Smith, C. E., Lane, K. A., & Austin, J. K. (2011). Predicting the insertion length for gastric tube placement in neonates. *Journal of Obstetric, Gynecologic, & Neonatal Nursing, 40*(4), 412–421.

Cooke, R. J. (2016). Improving growth in preterm infants during initial hospital stay: principles into practice. *Archives of Disease in Childhood: Fetal and Neonatal Edition, 101*(4), F366–F370.

Coughlin, M. (2014). *Transformative nursing in the NICU: Trauma-informed age-appropriate care.* New York: Springer Publishing Company.

Di Mauro, A., Neu, J., Riezzo, G., Raimondi, F., Martinelli, D., Francavilla, R., & Indrio, F. (2013). Gastrointestinal function development and microbiota. *Italian Journal of Pediatrics, 39*(1), 15.

Eidelman, A. I., & Schanler, R. J. (2012). Breastfeeding and the use of human milk. *Pediatrics* 129(3), e827–841.

Ferrara, L., Bidiwala, A., Sher, I., Pirzada, M., Barlev, D., Islam, S., ... & Hanna, N. (2017). Effect of nasal continuous positive airway pressure on the pharyngeal swallow in neonates. *Journal of Perinatology, 37*(4), 398.

Foster, J. P., Psaila, K., & Patterson, T. (2016). Non-nutritive sucking for increasing physiologic sta-bility and nutrition in preterm infants. *Cochrane Database of Systematic Reviews*, Issue 10. Art. No.: CD001071. DOI: 10.1002/14651858.CD001071.pub3

Gewolb, I. H., & Vice, F. L. (2006). Maturational changes in the rhythms, patterning, and coordination of res-piration and swallow during feeding in preterm and term infants. *Developmental Medicine and Child Neurology*, *48*(7), 589–594

Griffith, T., Rankin, K., & White-Traut, R. (2017). The relationship between behavioral states and oral feeding efficiency in preterm infants. *Advances in Neonatal Care: Official Journal of the National Association of Neonatal Nurses*, *17*(1), E12–E19.

Harding, C., Frank, L., Van Someren, V., Hilari, K., & Botting, N. (2014). How does non-nutritive sucking support infant feeding? *Infant Behavior and Development*, *37*(4), 457–464.

Harding, C., Bowden, C., Lima, L. & Levington, A. (2016). How do we determine oral readiness in infants? *Infant*, *12*(1), 10–12.

Harding, C., Mynard, A., & Hills, E. (2018). Identification of premature infant states in relation to introducing oral feeding. *Journal of Neonatal Nursing*, *24*(2), 104–110.

Holloway, E. M. (2014). The dynamic process of assessing infant feeding readiness. *Newborn and Infant Nursing Reviews*, *14*(3), 119–123.

Ismail, L. C., Puglia, F. A., Ohuma, E. O., Ash, S. T., Bishop, D. C., Carew, R. M., … & Chumlea, W. C. (2016). Precision of recumbent crown-heel length when using an infantometer. *BMC Pediatrics*, *16*(1), 186.

Jadcherla, S. R., Wang, M., Vijayapal, A. S., & Leuthner, S. R. (2010). Impact of prematurity and co-morbidities on feeding milestones in neonates: A retrospective study. *Journal of Perinatology*, *30*(3), 201.

Kirk, A. T., Alder, S. C., & King, J. D. (2007). Cue-based oral feeding clinical pathway results in earlier attainment of full oral feeding in premature infants. *Journal of Perinatology*, *27*(9), 572–578.

Kish, M. Z. (2013). Oral feeding readiness in preterm infants: A concept analysis. *Advances in Neonatal Care*, *13*(4), 230–237.

Klein, C. J. (2002). Nutrient requirements for preterm infant formulas. *The Journal of Nutrition*, *132*(6), 1395S–1577S.

Lai, M. C., & Huang, L. T. (2011). Effects of early life stress on neuroendocrine and neurobehavior: mechanisms and implications. *Pediatrics & Neonatology*, *52*(3), 122–129.

Lau, C. (2016). Development of infant oral feeding skills: What do we know? *The American Journal of Clinical Nutrition*, *103*(2), 616S–621S. DOI:10.3945/ajcn.115.109603

Lubbe, W. (2018). Clinicians guide for cue-based transition to oral feeding in preterm infants: An easy-to-use clinical guide. *Journal of Evaluation in Clinical Practice*, *24*(1) 80b88. DOI:10.1111/jep.12721

Ludwig, S. M. (2007). Oral feeding and the late preterm infant. *Newborn and Infant Nursing Reviews*, *7*(2), 72–75.

Lindström, K., Lindblad, F., & Hjern, A. (2009). Psychiatric morbidity in adolescents and young adults born preterm: a Swedish national cohort study. *Pediatrics*, *123*(1), e47–e53.

Ludwig, S. M., & Waitzman, K. A. (2007). Changing feeding documentation to reflect infant-driven feeding practice. *Newborn and Infant Nursing Reviews*, *7*(3), 155–160.

McCain, G. (1997). Behavioral state activity during nipple feedings for preterm infants. *Neonatal Network*, *16*(5), 43–47.

McCain, G. (2003). An evidence-based guideline for introducing oral feeding to healthy preterm infants. *Neonatal Network*, *22*(5), 45–50.

Moore, T., Hennessy, E. M., Myles, J., Johnson, S. J., Draper, E. S., Costeloe, K. L., & Marlow, N. (2012). Neurological and developmental outcome in extremely preterm children born in England in 1995 and 2006: the EPICure studies. *BMJ*, *345*, e7961.

Morgan, J., Bombell, S., & McGuire, W. (2013). Early trophic feeding versus enteral fasting for very pre-term or very low birth weight infants. *Cochrane Database of Systematic Reviews*, Issue 3. Art. No.: CD000504. DOI: 10.1002/14651858.CD000504.pub4

National Patient Safety Agency. (2011). *Reducing the harm caused by misplaced nasogastric feeding tubes in adults, children and infants*. NPSA.

Novak, D. A. (1996). Gastroesophageal reflux in the preterm infant. *Clinics in Perinatology, 23*(2), 305–320.

Nyqvist, K. H., Rosenblad, A., Volgsten, H., Funkquist, E. L., & Mattsson, E. (2017). Early skin-to-skin contact between healthy late preterm infants and their parents: an observational cohort study. *PeerJ, 5*, e3949. doi:10.7717/peerj.3949

O'Brien, K., Bracht, M., Robson, K., Xiang, Y. Y., Mirea, L., Cruz, M., ... & Narvey, M. (2015). Evaluation of the Family Integrated Care model of neonatal intensive care: a cluster randomized controlled trial in Canada and Australia. *BMC Pediatrics, 15*(1), 210.

O'Brien, K., Robson, K., Bracht, M., et al. (2018). Effectiveness of Family Integrated Care in neonatal intensive care units on infant and parent outcomes: a multicentre, multinational, cluster-randomised controlled trial. Lancet; *Child Adolesc Health, 2*, 245–254.

Parker, L., Torrazza, R. M., Li, Y., Talaga, E., Shuster, J., & Neu, J. (2015). Aspiration and Evaluation of Gastric Residuals in the Neonatal Intensive Care Unit. *The Journal of Perinatal & Neonatal Nursing, 29*(1), 51–59.

Pickler, R. H., Best, A. M., Reyna, B. A., Gutcher, G., & Wetzel, P. A. (2006). Predictors of nutritive sucking in preterm infants. *Journal of Perinatology, 26*(11), 693.

Pickler, R. H., Reyna, B. A., Wetzel, P. A., & Lewis, M. (2015). Effect of four approaches to oral feeding progression on clinical outcomes in preterm infants. *Nursing Research and Practice*, Article ID 716828, http://dx.doi.org/10.1155/2015/716828

Premji, S. S., & Chessell, L. (2011). Continuous nasogastric milk feeding versus intermittent bolus milk feeding for premature infants less than 1500 grams. *Cochrane Database of Systematic Reviews*, Issue 11. Art. No.: CD001819. DOI: 10.1002/14651858.CD001819.pub2

Quigley, M., Embleton, N. D., & McGuire, W. (2018). Formula versus donor breast milk for feeding preterm or low birth weight infants. *Cochrane Database of Systematic Reviews*, Issue 6. Art. No.: CD002971. DOI: 10.1002/14651858.CD002971.pub4

Ramel, S. E., Brown, L. D., & Georgieff, M. K. (2014). The impact of neonatal illness on nutritional requirements: One size does not fit all. *Current Pediatrics Reports, 2*(4), 248–254.

Royal College of Speech and Language Therapists. (2019). *Neonatal Care Overview*. Retrieved from www.rcslt.org/clinical_resources/neonatal_care/overview

Sables-Baus, S., DeSanto, K., Henderson, S., et al. (2013). Infant-Directed Oral Feeding for Premature and Critically Ill Hospitalized Infants: Guideline for Practice. Chicago, IL: National Association of Neonatal Nurses.

Shaker, C. S. (1999). Nipple feeding preterm infants: An individualized, developmentally supportive approach. *Neonatal Network, 18*(3), 15–22.

Shaker, C. S. (2013). Cue-based feeding in the NICU: Using the infant's communication as a guide. *Neonatal Network, 32*(6), 404–408.

Shaker, C. S. (2016). Supporting Parents feeding their Preemies [Webinar]. In *Catherine Shaker Swallowing and Feeding Seminars*. Retrieved from https://shaker4swallowingandfeeding.com/2016/04/14/shaker-webinar-parents-feeding-preemies-its-not-just-about-intake/

Sherriff, N., Hall, V., & Panton, C. (2014). Engaging and supporting fathers to promote breast feeding: A concept analysis. Midwifery, 30(6), 667–677.

Sullivan, R., Perry, R., Sloan, A., Kleinhaus, K., & Burtchen, N. (2011). Infant bonding and attachment to the caregiver: Insights from basic and clinical science. *Clinics in Perinatology, 38*(4), 643–655.

Tan, M., Abernethy, L., & Cooke, R. (2008). Improving head growth in preterm infants – A randomised controlled trial II: MRI and developmental outcomes in the first year. *Archives of Disease in Childhood: Fetal and Neonatal Edition, 93*(5), F342–F346.

Thoyre, S. M. (2000). Mothers' ideas about their role in feeding their high-risk infants. *Journal of Obstetric, Gynecologic, & Neonatal Nursing, 29*(6), 613–624.

Thoyre, S. M., Shaker, C. S., & Pridham, K. F. (2005). The early feeding skills assessment for preterm infants. *Neonatal Network, 24*(3), 7–16.

Toms, R., Jackson, K. W., Dabal, R. J., Reebals, C. H., & Alten, J. A. (2015). Preoperative trophic feeds in neonates with hypoplastic left heart syndrome. *Congenital Heart Disease, 10*(1), 36–42.

Unicef. (2019). The Baby Friendly Initiative. Retrieved from www.unicef.org.uk/babyfriendly/

Uthaya, S., & Modi, N. (2014). Practical preterm parenteral nutrition: systematic literature review and recommendations for practice. *Early Human Development, 90*(11), 747–753.

Watson, J., & McGuire, W. (2013a). Nasal versus oral route for placing feeding tubes in preterm or low birth weight infants. *Cochrane Database of Systematic Reviews*, Issue 2. Art. No.: CD003952. DOI: 10.1002/14651858.CD003952.pub3

Watson, J., & McGuire, W. (2013b). Transpyloric versus gastric tube feeding for preterm infants. *Cochrane Database of Systematic Reviews*, Issue 2. Art. No.: CD003487. DOI: 10.1002/14651858. CD003487.pub3

Watson, J., & McGuire, W. (2016). Responsive versus scheduled feeding for preterm infants. *Cochrane Database of Systematic Reviews*, Issue 8. Art. No.: CD005255. DOI: 10.1002/14651858. CD005255.pub5

White, A., & Parnell, K. (2013). The transition from tube to full oral feeding (breast or bottle): A cue-based developmental approach. *Journal of Neonatal Nursing, 19*(4), 189–197.

White-Traut, R. C., Rankin, K. M., Yoder, J. C., Liu, L., Vasa, R., Geraldo, V., & Norr, K. F. (2015). Influence of H-HOPE intervention for premature infants on growth, feeding progression and length of stay during initial hospitalization. *Journal of Perinatology, 35*(8), 636–641.

Wolff, P. H. (1968). The serial organization of sucking in the young infant. *Pediatrics, 42*(6), 943–956.

18 NEONATAL INFECTION

Lisa Kaiser

CONTENTS

GUIDANCE ON HOW TO ENHANCE PERSONAL LEARNING FROM THIS CHAPTER

Key points covered in this chapter

■ The nature of immunity and how this predisposes the high-risk neonate to infection.

■ The types and presentations of infection in the neonatal period.

■ The signs and symptoms of infection and the nurse's role in recognising and managing it in the neonatal unit.

Reflection

Reading through the chapter, you are encouraged to engage with the key points and related literature in an enquiring way. Ask these questions:

■ Have you seen infection presenting in the neonates in your care, and what challenges does this pose for the infant and family?

■ What are the current evidence base and guidelines relating to neonatal infection?

■   What are the key nursing care responsibilities in relation to infection control in the neonatal unit?

Implications for nursing care

■   Finally: how will this chapter enable you to consider the implications of what you learn for your nursing care relating to neonatal infection, assessment and nursing care.

INTRODUCTION AND BACKGROUND

Infection is an important cause of mortality and morbidity in the newborn period. The incidence of early onset neonatal infection is said to have dramatically declined over the past 10 years, due to increased use of antenatal antibiotics and more effective management of premature rupture of membranes (Bedford Russell and Isaacs, 2012), however, there has been an increase in late onset infection. This increase is due, in part, to the improved survival of extremely low birth weight (ELBW) infants, who are especially susceptible due to their immunological incompetence, long stay in hospital and prolonged administration of parenteral nutrition (Camacho-Gonzalez et al., 2013; Dong and Speer, 2015). Particularly late onset infection has associated cost implications and may result in poor neurodevelopmental outcomes of affected infants (Legeay et al., 2015). This chapter will review the current information regarding neonatal susceptibility to, and acquisition of infection, the organisms commonly implicated and investigation and treatment modalities. It should serve to increase the neonatal nurse's ability to detect and manage the infected infant.

IMMUNITY

The human immune system consists of innate (natural) and acquired (adaptive) immunity, which work in conjunction but via different mechanisms (see table 18.1).

Innate immunity

This is less specific than acquired immunity, and present from birth. It acts via three main mechanisms:

■   *Surface barriers* such as the skin and mucous membranes; additional protection of stomach acid.

■ *White blood cell (WBC) system:* The different components of the WBC system tackle invaders either by ***phagocytosis*** or by triggering an inflammatory response.

■ *Granulocytes*, named for the granules contained in their cytoplasm, consist of *neutrophils, eosinophils* and *basophils*.

Neutrophils Approximately one trillion neutrophils are produced by the bone marrow each day, but this can increase up to tenfold in stress or infection. Their production is regulated by granulocyte colony-stimulating factor (G-CSF) and granulocyte-macrophage colony-stimulating factor (GM-CSF). Usually the neutrophil only leaves the bone marrow once mature, but in infection the presence of immature neutrophils may be noticed, and this is referred to as a 'left shift'. The function of a neutrophil are the engulfment and destruction of pathogens and other solid particles (known as *phagocytosis* – see figure 18.1).

Eosinophils are raised in allergic reactions and parasitic infections. Their granules are lysosomes, which contain hydrolytic enzymes.

Basophils contain large amounts of granules in their cytoplasm. These release compounds important in the inflammatory response cascade, which is designed to bring phagocytic cells to an area of tissue injury/infection, and to isolate it from the rest of the body by reducing venous and lymphatic return. Basophils furthermore have receptors for certain immunoglobulins and aspects of the complement system (part of the immune system which facilitates the function of phagocytic cells and antibodies).

Mast cells are filled with basophil granules and thus have the same characteristics, but unlike basophils, are found outside the circulation in body tissues. Mononuclear cells, as their name suggests, have a single nucleus rather than granules in their cytoplasm, and consist of *monocytes* and ***lymphocytes***. The latter however play a more prominent part in the acquired aspect of immunity and are discussed below.

TABLE 18.1 TYPES OF IMMUNITY

Innate immunity	Acquired immunity
■ Present from birth	
■ Not antigen-specific	■ Antigen-specific
■ Same response to repeated exposure	■ Enhanced response to subsequent exposure
■ Has no memory	■ Has memory
■ Uses cellular and molecular components	■ Uses cellular and **humoral** components
■ Works in conjunction with acquired immunity	■ Works in conjunction with innate immunity

(adapted from Delves and Roitt, 2000a)

Monocytes originate from the bone marrow and subsequently migrate to various organs and tissues to mature into *macrophages*, another type of phagocytic cells.

■ *Molecular components* of the innate immune system include the complement system, acute-phase proteins (such as C-reactive protein), and cytokines (e.g. interleukin, **interferon**, tumour necrosis factor α). These compounds may be found in saliva, tears, sweat, serum, and some cells and tissues. Their function is to attach to foreign organisms and facilitate their recognition and destruction via phagocytosis (Delves and Roitt, 2000a).

Acquired immunity

Acquired immunity is antigen-specific and thus results from exposure to a pathogen. It functions through two main mechanisms:

■ *Humoral immunity* The body develops circulating antibodies (immunoglobulins) which contribute to the elimination of pathogens through aggregation of targets, **opsonisation** ('labelling') for removal by phagocytes, activation of the complement system, or direct neutralisation of some viruses or toxins. Only immunoglobulin G (IgG) antibodies can cross the placenta and protect the foetus, so that their presence indicates an antenatally acquired infection – for example, cytomegalovirus (CMV) infection. IgM antibodies on the other hand, as 'first responders' to an antigen, would signify an infection contracted after birth.

■ ***Cell-mediated immunity*** This aspect of acquired immunity consists of mature lymphocytes. a subgroup of the mononuclear WBC system.

　　■ Lymphocytes become active only after interaction with an antigen, when they differentiate into effector cells which act to eliminate/inactivate the invader. Lymphocytes originate from the bone marrow, are carried to peripheral tissues by the blood, and can be divided into three functional subgroups, which mature in different organs: **T-Cells**, **B-Cells** and Natural Killer (NK) or Null Cells (see table 18.2; Delves and Roitt 2000b).

TABLE 18.2 LYMPHOCYTE SUBGROUPS

T-cells	B-cells	Natural killer (NK) or null cells
■ Maturation in the thymus ■ Protection against infections caused by intracellular bacteria, viruses and fungi ■ Immune response regulation ('Surveillance')	■ Maturation in the bone marrow ■ Protection against bacterial infections ■ Production of immunoglobulins (antibodies) when stimulated	■ Originate from bone marrow ■ Protection against viral infections and attack of abnormal (cancerous) cells ■ Not specific like T- and B-cells

(adapted from Delves and Roitt, 2000b)

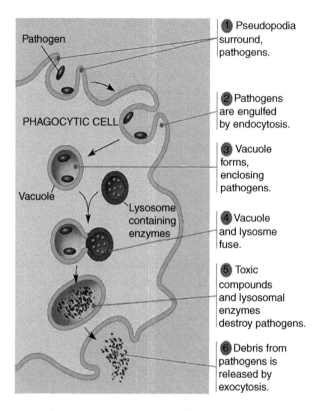

Figure 18.1 Phagocytosis (Source: Creative Commons)

Immunity in the neonate

The neonatal immune system, while complete, is not mature at birth with qualitative and quantitative insufficiencies (see table 18.3), having to develop a full immune response to every encountered pathogen. Preterm infants have not yet benefited from passively acquired immunity – this is mediated through placental transfer of IgG antibodies, which predominantly occurs in the third trimester. Furthermore, in both term and preterm infants, first-line barriers (mucosal immunity) are ineffective. It is not yet fully understood how quickly maturation of the immune system occurs in the postnatal period (Holt and Jones, 2000).

NEONATAL INFECTION

Significant mortality and morbidity is associated with neonatal infection, particularly in the preterm and low birth weight (LBW) population (Stoll et al., 2004; Cailes et al., 2018a). A term often used interchangeably with infection, 'sepsis', is a rare but serious complication

TABLE 18.3 NEONATAL IMMUNITY

Immunity aspect	Neonate	Consequence
Non-specific immunity	Phagocytes functional but less effective migration to infection site	Slow response to infection
Specific immunity	Develops during foetal life, but T- and B-cells are immature Low number of 'surveillance' T-cells Poor cytokine production of T-cells Very low levels of immunoglobulins (IgG antibodies virtually absent in extremely preterm infants)	Inefficient primary immune response, which means increased susceptibility to infection

(adapted from Holt and Jones, 2000)

defined as life-threatening organ dysfunction due to a dysregulated host response to infection (National Institute for Health and Care Excellence (NICE), 2016). Without quick treatment, sepsis can lead to serious complications including, in the worst instance, organ failure and potential risk of death. Infections causing sepsis, meningitis, or pneumonia contributed directly to around 0·6 million neonatal deaths worldwide in 2016, and indirectly to many more, through resultant preterm birth and neonatal encephalopathy (Seale and Agarwal, 2018).

In several countries across the world, surveillance networks have been set up to document the incidence of neonatal infections, associated pathogens and their resistance patterns. Among their objectives are the comparison and optimisation of clinical practice and antibiotic regimes (Cailes et al., 2015). In the UK 30 neonatal units (NNUs) throughout the country have been contributing data on neonatal sepsis to the Neonatal Infection Surveillance Network (NeonIN) since 2004. Their evidence shows an infection incidence of 2.9/1000 live births (LB) and 23.5/1000 NNU admissions (Cailes et al., 2018a). These figures are similar to data from the United States of America (USA) and Australasia (Isaacs et al., 1995; Shane et al., 2017) but considerably lower than those reported from developing countries, where the rates of neonatal infection can be as high as 170/1000 LB (Thaver and Zaidi, 2009).

Infection in the neonate is typically described as early onset sepsis (EOS) or late onset sepsis (LOS). Depending on definition, EOS occurs within 48–72 hours of life, and its mode of acquisition is described as 'vertical'; i.e. transplacental or ascending vaginal infection.

LOS arises after 48–72 hours from birth and is most commonly a 'horizontal' or healthcare-acquired (nosocomial) infection (Bedford Russell and Isaacs, 2012).

> ## BOX 18.1 RISK FACTORS FOR EOS
>
> - Invasive group B streptococcal infection in a previous baby
> - Maternal group B streptococcal colonisation, bacteriuria or infection in the current pregnancy
> - Pre-labour rupture of membranes
> - Preterm birth following spontaneous labour (before 37 weeks' gestation)
> - Suspected or confirmed rupture of membranes for more than 18 hours in a preterm birth
> - Intrapartum fever higher than 38°C, or confirmed or suspected chorioamnionitis.
>
> (adapted from NICE, 2014)

Early onset sepsis

The overall incidence of EOS in the UK has been decreasing over the past decade. Nearly half of all infants affected were born >37 weeks and weighed >2500g. The pathogens most commonly associated with EOS are Group B streptococcus (GBS; 43%) and *Escherichia coli* (18%; Cailes et al., 2018a). *Listeria monocytogenes* infection, while very rare, will also usually present in the early postnatal period (Okike et al., 2013).

Risk factors associated with EOS are outlined in box 18.1.

PATHOGENS IN EARLY ONSET INFECTION

- *S. agalactiae*, more commonly referred to as GBS, colonises the bowel flora of 20–40% of adults, including pregnant women. Carriers can be identified via rectal and vaginal swabs or urine samples. The Royal College of Obstetricians and Gynaecologists (RCOG) has produced a guideline with the aim of preventing GBS EOS by offering antibiotic prophylaxis in labour to any woman who is a known GBS carrier, who had a previous baby with GBS infection, or who goes into preterm labour (Hughes et al., 2017; Williams, 2018). Routine screening for GBS is not advocated in the UK due to a lack of evidence that it would be beneficial (UK National Screening Committee, 2008). In the USA and Australasia, the introduction of universal screening guidelines has shown a subsequent decrease of GBS disease, unlike in the UK (Daley et al., 2004; Camacho-Gonzalez et al., 2013; Bedford Russell and Kumar, 2015), where there has more recently been a rise in its incidence (O'Sullivan et al., 2016; Hughes et al., 2017).

    GBS infection, which most frequently presents as congenital pneumonia or bacteraemia, can also manifest as meningitis or focal infections, and is associated with a mortality of around 10% (Heath et al., 2004). Most infants with GBS disease will display signs of infection within 12 hours of life, which is why this is recommended as a min-imum observation period for infants born to GBS-colonised mothers (NICE, 2014).

■   *E. coli* is one of the family of gram-negative (see figure 18.2) *Enterobacteriaceae*, which can survive under both aerobic and anaerobic conditions and predominantly reside in the gut. Gram-negative infections result in high morbidity and mortality in newborn infants (Kortsalioudaki et al., 2014). There are increasing cases of *E.coli* known to produce extended-spectrum β-lactamases (ESBL), enzymes which can deactivate antibiotics from the penicillin and cephalosporin groups, making their treatment a potential challenge (Bedford Russell and Isaacs, 2012).

■   *L. monocytogenes* is transmitted through certain foods, particularly dairy products and some meat varieties, and predominantly affects pregnant women and their babies (Farber and Peterkin, 1991). When early pregnancy is affected, this is highly associated with spontaneous abortion or poor prognosis for the surviving infant. In later pregnancy, listeriosis can result in foetal death and preterm birth (50%). Meconium-stained liquor is present in 75% of cases and should arouse suspicion especially in preterm infants (Okike et al., 2013). The majority of *L. monocytogenes* infections are transplacentally or perinatally acquired, and thus present early and similarly to GBS with pneumonia, bacteraemia, meningitis and focal infections, with a mortality rate of over 50%. A later onset of listeriosis more commonly presents with meningitis and is fatal in approximately 25% of cases (Bedford Russell and Isaacs, 2012; Okike et al., 2013).

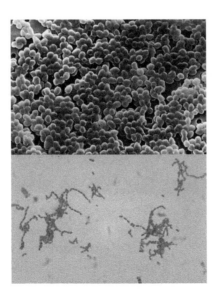

Figure 18.2 Gram-positive and gram-negative organisms (Source: Creative Commons)

TREATMENT OF EARLY ONSET INFECTION

Because of their susceptibility to perinatally and nosocomially acquired infection, newborn infants are often empirically prescribed antibiotics for presumed sepsis pending culture results to avoid acute deterioration. It has been suggested that as many as 95% of all infants treated for suspected sepsis ultimately had no biochemical or microbiological evidence of this (Luck et al., 2003). Initially, broad-spectrum cover is prescribed, which is usually dependent on local policies and the unit flora, changing to specific antibiotics when dictated by the culture and sensitivity results. While this is accepted as the most appropriate and safe practice for the infant, administration of broad-spectrum agents for empirical treatment of presumed sepsis is highly implicated in antimicrobial resistance, which is an increasing problem worldwide. In the UK, Antimicrobial Stewardship Programmes are aiming to address this issue. These suggest after broad-spectrum cover has been commenced, focusing antibiotic treatment to the narrowest spectrum possible, ensuring appropriate route of administration and dose, and limiting the duration to the shortest necessary course (NICE, 2015; Public Health England, 2015). In line with these principles, NICE (2014) has devised a guideline to inform decisions about the treatment of EOS (see table 18.4), though antibiotic regimens may vary in different NNUs.

The recommendation is that antibiotics should be stopped at the earliest opportunity (usually 36 hours) once negative blood cultures have been obtained. A 7-day course is suggested for infants with positive blood cultures or with a strong suspicion of infection, and a minimum of 14 days' treatment for proven meningitis (NICE, 2014).

PENICILLINS

These antimicrobials belong to the group of β-lactam antibiotics, which have bactericidal action by interfering with the synthesis of the bacterial cell wall. They are safe to use in neonates. Some pathogens, particularly some gram-negative bacteria and *Staphylococcus aureus* have evolved resistance to penicillin antibiotics by producing β-lactamases.

TABLE 18.4 ANTIBIOTICS FOR PREVENTION AND TREATMENT OF EOS

Antibiotic	Clinical Scenario
Benzylpenicillin and Gentamicin	Suspected EOS, GBS meningitis
Cefotaxime and Gentamicin	Gram-negative bacteraemia
Cefotaxime	Gram-negative meningitis
Amoxicillin and Cefotaxime	Meningitis, pathogen unknown or gram-positive
Amoxicillin and Gentamicin	Listeria bacteraemia/meningitis

(adapted from NICE, 2014)

- *Benzylpenicillin*, also known as penicillin G, has good efficacy in a number of gram-positive bacterial infections, including GBS, and is thus among the antibiotics of choice for EOS. While there is poor cerebrospinal fluid (CSF) penetration under normal circumstances, higher permeability of inflamed meninges and its good effectiveness mean a combination of benzylpenicillin and gentamicin is recommended for the treatment of GBS meningitis.

- *Amoxicillin* and *ampicillin,* compared to other antibiotics from the penicillin group, have an extended spectrum of action and are thus effective against some gram-negative bacteria, such as *Enterococci* and *E. coli.* Amoxicillin or ampicillin constitute the antibiotic of choice in the treatment of *L. monocytogenes.* Of note, there is a higher association with *candida* infections secondary to antimicrobial therapy compared to other penicillins (Isaacs, 2014).

AMINOGLYCOSIDE ANTIBIOTICS

Antimicrobials from the aminoglycoside group have both bactericidal action, by damaging the bacterial cell membrane, and bacteriostatic (inhibition of bacterial reproduction) action. Their potential to have nephrotoxic and ototoxic effects necessitate drug level monitoring. Extended dosing frequency was suggested to reduce the likelihood of toxic trough levels (Rao et al., 2006).

- *Gentamicin* is effective against a number of gram-negative pathogens such as *Pseudomonas aeruginosa* and microbes from the *Enterobacteriaceae*, but also coagulase-negative staphylococci (CoNS) and *S. aureus*, so that it is commonly used in LOS as well as EOS. In the context of EOS, it is useful in the treatment of listeriosis, and has a synergistic effect in combination with benzylpenicillin against GBS (Isaacs, 2014).

CEPHALOSPORINS

Cephalosporin antibiotics belong to the group of β-lactam antimicrobials and are thus bactericidal. They provide good cover against gram-positive and gram-negative organisms and are not affected by the β-lactamases produced by staphylococci. These antibiotics are used both in EOS and LOS. Cephalosporins are classified into 'generations'; each generation has undergone modification to be more stable to β-lactamases (Isaacs, 2014).

- *Cefotaxime* is a third-generation cephalosporin, and effective in a number of organisms affecting neonates, apart from *Pseudomonas* and *Listeria*. It has good CSF penetration, but problems associated with its use include the occurrence of secondary fungal infections (Cotten et al., 2006), and the emergence of pathogens producing ESBL (Isaacs, 2014).

Late onset infection

Improved survival rates of extremely preterm and very LBW (VLBW) infants have led to an increase in LOS incidence (Camacho-Gonzalez et al., 2013). The strong association between low gestational age (GA) and birth weight with LOS is supported by NeonIN findings that over 90% of cases in the UK occur in infants of <32 weeks GA (Cailes et al., 2018a). Factors apart from prematurity and immunological immaturity predisposing to LOS are prolonged hospitalisation, resulting in exposure to a multitude of hospital staff, nosocomial pathogens and potentially contaminated equipment, missed opportunities for early enteral breast milk administration and protracted use of parenteral nutrition, which necessitates the presence of indwelling central venous catheters (CVC), and other invasive apparatus, such as endotracheal tubes (Dong and Speer, 2015; Legeay et al., 2015; Shane et al., 2017). It follows that a significant role in the management of LOS may be preventative strategies, and indeed the introduction of such is thought to have resulted in a decreasing trend of LOS (Cailes et al., 2018a).

PREVENTION OF LATE ONSET INFECTION

- *Early introduction of breast milk* Development of normal gut flora is impaired in infants admitted to the NNU, due to exposure to both broad-spectrum antibiotics and a range of bacteria with the potential of pathogenicity (Schwiertz et al., 2003; Cotten et al., 2009; Greenwood et al., 2014). It has been demonstrated that commencing early trophic feeds of breast milk has a positive impact on evolving neonatal gut flora, with a protective effect from necrotising enterocolitis (NEC) as well as sepsis (Rønnestad et al., 2005). In keeping with this, the effect of probiotic administration on reduction of LOS has been studied (The ProPrems Study) but not shown to make a significant difference (Jacobs et al., 2013).
- *CVC care* The recognition of an association between increased incidence of LOS and the presence of a CVC has led to a number of attempts to reduce CVC-related infection (Shane et al., 2017). Trials investigating the impact of prophylactic antibiotics with CVCs (Inglis and Davies, 2005; Inglis et al., 2007; Jardine et al., 2008), antimicrobial dressings (Lai et al., 2016) and early vs. expectant removal of CVCs (Gordon et al., 2017) among others have not yet shown any significant difference in the incidence of LOS compared to controls. It appears that the most effective strategies in the reduction of CVC-associated infection remain care bundles involving aspects such as hand hygiene, barrier precautions and adequate catheter care, such as the Matching Michigan programme (Bion et al., 2013; Smulders et al., 2013).
- *Immuno-supportive treatment* With the awareness that the neonatal immune system is immature, several methods of supportive therapy have been examined, but none have demonstrated any benefit in the treatment or prevention of LOS. These include the administration of intravenous immunoglobulin (The INIS Study) and GM-CSF (The PROGRAMS Study; Carr et al., 2009; INIS Collaborative Group, 2011).

PATHOGENS IN LATE ONSET INFECTION

■ *Gram-positive pathogens*
   ■ *Coagulase-negative Staphylococci (CoNS)* This group of pathogens (see box 18.2) frequently colonises the skin and mucous membranes, and invasive CoNS infections are predominantly nosocomially acquired, though vertical transmission is possible (Legeay et al., 2015; Cailes et al., 2018a).

BOX 18.2 CONS CAUSING NEONATAL SEPSIS

S. epidermidis

S. haemolyticus

S. hominis

S. warneri

S. saprophyticus

S. capitis

S. cohnii

(adapted from Isaacs, 2014)

Some CoNS have the ability to produce a biofilm, which has a protective effect against antimicrobials and immune defences, but also allows the pathogen to adhere to or even penetrate intravenous catheters (Isaacs, 2014).

According to NeonIN data, CoNS infections constitute over 50% of LOS cases, and predominantly occur in the extremely preterm, VLBW population. CoNS mostly cause bloodstream infections (Cailes et al., 2018a). High antimicrobial resistance to flucloxacillin and other penicillins has been reported in the UK, while at present there is still good sensitivity to vancomycin (Kent et al., 2014). Definitive diagnosis of CoNS bacteraemia can be challenging, as contamination of blood cultures can trigger a falsely positive result (Dong and Speer, 2015; Isaacs, 2014).

■ *S. aureus* This staphylococcus can cause EOS, but was associated with 31% of gram-positive LOS cases in UK NNUs (Cailes et al., 2018a). It can lead to a variety of presentations, including bacteraemia, soft tissue infections such as staphylococcal scalded skin syndrome and omphalitis, pneumonia, meningitis, endocarditis and osteomyelitis. Initially susceptible to penicillin antimicrobials, treatment can be a potential challenge, as *S. aureus* strains have evolved increasing virulence and resistance, such as methicillin resistance (Isaacs, 2014). Recent UK data showed that nearly half of all methicillin-resistant *S. aureus* (MRSA) infections among the paediatric population occurred in NNU residents (Johnson et al., 2010).

■ *Enterococci* Two of the *Enterococcus* species are commonly associated with neonatal infection, *E. faecalis* and *E. faecium*. These normally reside in the intestine, but when translocated can cause EOS or LOS, which may present as bacteraemia or meningitis, and are often associated with acute clinical deterioration (Isaacs, 2014).

■ *Gram-negative pathogens* Infections produced by gram-negative bacteria (see table 18.5) make up 45% of LOS, remain a significant cause of mortality and are associated with prolonged hospital stay and adverse neurodevelopmental outcomes in the neonatal population (Anthony et al., 2013; Cailes et al., 2018a).

   Gram-negative pathogens are mostly associated with bacteraemia, but also meningitis and pneumonia. They contain endotoxins which, when released, can result in septic shock (Isaacs, 2014). Many produce ESBL, and resistance is much more an issue among this group of pathogens compared to those commonly associated with EOS (Kent et al., 2016; Cailes et al., 2018b).

■ *Fungi* A number of risk factors predispose neonates to invasive fungal infections; among these are prolonged use of CVCs and parenteral nutrition (particularly its lipid aspect), prolonged ventilation, fungal colonisation, use of antacids, but particularly extreme prematurity and the use of broad-spectrum antibiotics (Cotten et al., 2006; Benjamin et al., 2010; Isaacs, 2014). 10% of LOS is caused by fungi, mostly of the *Candida spp.* (Cailes et al., 2018a). Because invasive fungal infection is associated with significant mortality and poor neurodevelopmental outcome, antifungal prophylaxis is advocated by some and has shown to significantly reduce the incidence of fungal sepsis but has not improved mortality (Austin et al., 2015; Cleminson et al.,

TABLE 18.5 GRAM-NEGATIVE PATHOGENS CAUSING NEONATAL SEPSIS AND THEIR TRANSMISSION PATHWAYS

Pathogen	Naturally occurring	Transmission
E. coli Klebsiella spp. Enterobacter spp. Citrobacter spp. Salmonella spp. Morganella morganii	Gut colonisation	Translocation
Neisseria spp.	Mucosal colonisation	Translocation
Pseudomonas aeruginosa Acinetobacter Serratia marescens	Water reservoirs	Healthcare staff

(adapted from Issacs, 2014; Kent et al., 2014; 2016)

2015). However, the threat of resistance has led others to favour a cautious approach, limiting the use of antifungal agents only to cases of confirmed fungal sepsis, or a prophylactic approach only in NNUs where there is a high incidence of invasive fungal infection (Chapman, 2007; Benjamin et al., 2010; Bedford Russell and Isaacs, 2012). Treatment of invasive fungal sepsis should continue until 14–21 days after clearance of cultures. A number of antifungal agents are available:

- *Fluconazole* is fungistatic, and frequently used for systemic prophylaxis. Problems with resistance have been observed. One of its advantages is that it can be administered orally.
- *Amphotericin B* is a fungicidal agent, and its use has been associated with reversible renal failure in the neonatal population. Resistance is rarely seen, and it is preferable particularly if fluconazole was used prophylactically.
- *Flucytosine* is seldom used due to rapid development of resistance.
- *Echinocandins:* The latest class of antifungal agents has not been adequately researched in the neonatal population; resistance is rarely seen (Chapman, 2007; Hsieh et al., 2012).

TREATMENT OF BACTERIAL LATE ONSET INFECTION

- *Penicillins*
  - *Flucloxacillin* belongs to the group of anti-staphylococcal penicillins which are very effective against *S. aureus*, but not most CoNS, *Enterococci* and enteric gram-negative bacteria (Isaacs, 2014). In UK NNUs, flucloxacillin in combination with gentamicin often constitutes first-line antibiotic choice in suspected LOS, which provides good coverage of many causative organisms except CoNS (Vergnano et al., 2011).
  - *Piperacillin with Tazobactam* Piperacillin alone has good activity against *Pseudomonas aeruginosa* and *Enterococci*, but does not provide coverage for organisms producing β-lactamases or ESBL. It has therefore been combined with tazobactam, which is a β-lactamase inhibitor (Isaacs, 2014).
- *Cephalosporins* see p. 475. Some UK units use a combination of amoxicillin and cefotaxime for LOS (Vergnano et al., 2011).
- *Aminoglycosides* see p. 475.
- *Glycopeptide antibiotics* Due to their effectiveness against CoNS, which are the most common causative organisms of LOS, glycopeptide antimicrobials are among the most frequently used antibiotics in the treatment of LOS. Their spectrum of activity means they are bactericidal only to *Enterococci*, and otherwise have bacteriostatic action.
  - *Vancomycin* was predominantly developed for the treatment of staphylococcal infections and remains important in infections secondary to MRSA. Issues

associated with drug reactions ('Red Man Syndrome'), ototoxicity and nephro-toxicity are circumvented with considerations around administration, such as infusion over 30–60 minutes or continuously, and drug level monitoring (Avent et al., 2013; Isaacs, 2014). However, emergence of vancomycin-resistant enterococci (VRE) and MRSA means empiric use of vancomycin should be avoided, and its usage limited to infants who are seriously ill, particularly in the presence of a CVC (Vergnano et al., 2011; Cailes et al., 2015).

- *Teicoplanin* may be considered a good alternative to vancomycin, as it provides coverage of a similar spectrum of pathogens but is not as nephrotoxic and has not been associated with the 'Red Man Syndrome'.

- *Metronidazole* has excellent activity against gram-negative bacteria and should be used if there is a high index of suspicion for NEC.

- *Meropenem* is part of the broad-spectrum Carbapenem antimicrobials, which provide excellent cover for many gram-positive and gram-negative pathogens. Meropenem has good CSF penetration.

  Carbapenems are strongly associated with emerging resistance among a multitude of pathogens, including those producing metallo-β-lactamase for which there is hardly any effective antimicrobial treatment. Therefore, empiric treatment with meropenem should be avoided (Isaacs, 2014).

Viral infections

A number of viruses can affect infants in the neonatal period. These are mostly vertically transmitted, though postnatal infection can also occur. Those most likely to be encountered in the UK are briefly discussed in this section, which is by no means exhaustive.

THE TORCH GROUP OF VIRAL INFECTIONS

The acronym TORCH stands for **T**oxoplasma, **O**ther (usually chickenpox), **R**ubella, **C**ytomegalovirus and **H**erpes. The presentation associated with each virus varies, but common signs seen in affected infants are growth restriction, a petechial rash, jaundice, hepatosplenomegaly and sometimes thrombocytopaenia. Some infections can be associated with severe systemic illness.

- *Toxoplasmosis* Maternal infection usually occurs as a result of exposure to cat faeces and can be silent or accompanied by mild flu-like symptoms. If the infection is transmitted to the foetus (usually transplacentally), outcomes are generally poor with a mortality of approximately 25%, or deafness, congenital cataracts, intracranial calcifications and hydrocephalus.

- *Chickenpox (Varicella zoster)* This virus is part of the herpesvirus family and may be antenatally, perinatally or postnatally acquired. Depending on disease onset, varicella can result in devastating systemic illness. Based on maternal onset of the illness, treatment is with zoster immunoglobulin +/− systemic aciclovir. Precautions to avoid the spread of this highly contagious disease need to be taken.
- *Rubella* The incidence of rubella is now extremely low thanks to routine vaccination. Transmission to the foetus occurs transplacentally, frequently results in abortion and is associated with multiple congenital anomalies, particularly if it occurs before the third trimester of pregnancy. Apart from the common signs named above, these can include congenital cataracts or glaucoma, sensorineural deafness, microcephaly and developmental delay. There is no treatment other than supportive management. Like with chickenpox, barrier precautions need to be considered.
- *Cytomegalovirus (CMV)* Maternal infection can be primary or recurrent, with more serious implications for the foetus in primary infection. Apart from growth restriction, jaundice and thrombocytopaenia, CMV infection may otherwise be silent in the neonate, and if untreated can lead to progressive sensorineural hearing loss.

  Acquisition can be postnatal as well as vertical, for example through CMV-positive breast milk (Bedford Russell and Isaacs, 2012). Treatment is with ganciclovir or valganciclovir (Gandhi et al., 2010).
- *Herpes simplex (HSV)* Transmission of HSV can be transplacentally (rarely), perinatally via passage through an infected birth canal, or postnatally, nosocomially or from family members. Illness severity varies from superficial skin lesions only to disseminated systemic/central nervous system disease requiring intensive care, and its onset can be delayed (day 10–14). Treatment is with systemic aciclovir (Bedford Russell and Isaacs, 2012; Isaacs, 2014). Preventative obstetric practices such as maternal oral aciclovir prophylaxis late in pregnancy and delivery via elective caesarean section seek to eliminate perinatal transmission of HSV (Foley et al., 2014).

HUMAN IMMUNODEFICIENCY VIRUS

The most common route of Human Immunodeficiency Virus (HIV) infection in infants is through mother-to-child-transmission. Based on this, the World Health Organization (WHO) regularly publishes evidence-based guidelines on the management of HIV-positive pregnant women. The most recent version of this suggests that women receive antiretroviral prophylaxis only during the high-risk period for their child, i.e. during pregnancy, perinatally and while breastfeeding, rather than lifelong (WHO, 2010). In the UK, the recommendation remains that HIV-positive women should not breastfeed, in order to minimise the risk of transmission (Taylor et al., 2011).

SIGNS OF NEONATAL INFECTION

The neonatal nurse, with expert clinical skills and judgement, is pivotal in the early recognition of sepsis. It is imperative that sepsis is pre-empted or detected as early as possible, as the recognised inadequacies of the immune system response, and its inability to contain micro-organisms may lead to rapid proliferation and dissemination of pathogens leading to overwhelming septicaemia or meningitis or, at worst, death.

Respiratory signs

Infants presenting with tachypnoea, grunting, recession and apnoea may have early onset congenital infection or respiratory distress syndrome. It is impossible to differentiate these conditions clinically or even following chest radiography, as the chest X-ray reveals similar findings in both cases (Bedford Russell and Isaacs, 2012). More recently, the introduction of pulse oximetry screening in some UK hospitals has enabled early detection of sepsis or pneumonia even in asymptomatic infants (Ewer et al., 2011; Thangaratinam et al., 2012)

The respiratory symptoms associated with GBS infection are due, in part, to the organism-mediated release of the vasoactive agent thromboxane A_2, which causes severe pulmonary vascular constriction. This, combined with the infant's reduced WBC ability to eliminate the organism, leads to rapid dissemination of the disease process and profound generalised cardiorespiratory instability. Late onset sepsis and meningitis may manifest with increased ventilatory requirements or respiratory signs due to central effects on the respiratory centre leading to tachypnoea or apnoea (Bedford Russell and Isaacs, 2012; Isaacs, 2014).

Thermal signs

Temperature instability, after environmental factors have been eliminated, may be an early indicator of infection. Preterm infants are more likely to display subnormal temperatures in response to infection, while most infants found to be febrile are term infants. In proven LOS, approximately half of the babies are hyperthermic, one-third are normothermic and 15% have hypothermia (Isaacs, 2014). The further the deviation from the normal range, be it high or low, the more significant the finding. A widening toe:core temperature gap (>1.5°C) may also occur as the peripheral perfusion of the infant reduces in response to sepsis.

Cardiovascular signs

Cardiovascular changes of tachycardia, hypotension and prolonged capillary refill times (CRT) may indicate sepsis. A heart rate of greater than 160bpm is often present in early sepsis (Bedford Russell and Isaacs, 2012). Abnormal CRT may occur due to compromised cardiac output or peripheral vasoconstriction.

Skin signs

A variety of skin anomalies may be present in neonatal sepsis and must be differentiated from non-infectious causes. Jaundice may be physiological or occurring as a result of pathological haemolysis. The presence of generalised pallor or mottling (cutis marmorata) warrant careful evaluation of the infant's universal wellbeing. A petechial rash is cause for serious concern, as it may result from congenital viral infection or disseminated intravascular coagulation, a devastating late sign of sepsis. Umbilical erythema, with or without malodorous purulent discharge, is a sign of omphalitis, which is now predominantly a problem in developing countries but requires antimicrobial treatment if it occurs, as it can be associated with systemic deterioration. Depending on the causative organism, rashes and skin lesions can have characteristic appearances (Bedford Russell and Isaacs, 2012; Isaacs, 2014).

Gastrointestinal signs

Gastrointestinal signs of distension and ileus are a common and important sign of sepsis and need to be differentiated from intestinal obstruction or NEC, all of which may present similarly with poor feed tolerance and bile-stained gastric aspirates. The latter may be early signs of sepsis in an infant who has previously been enterally fed. Blood sugar instability may also be an early sign, with hyperglycaemia requiring insulin therapy (Isaacs, 2014; NICE, 2014).

Neurological signs

Lethargy, irritability or 'not handling' well occurs in approximately half of the number of infants with sepsis and should always be further investigated. Meningitis may be heralded by increasing irritability, alterations in consciousness, poor tone and tremors, with up to 75% of infants having some seizure activity (Klein and Marcy, 1995).

INVESTIGATIONS

If the decision for antibiotic treatment has been made based on a baby's risk factors for infection or clinical concerns, a number of investigations, generally known as a septic screen (see table 18.6), have to be carried out before therapy is instigated. These will subsequently guide antibiotic choice and duration of treatment as well as aid prognosis of the illness course (NICE, 2014).

TABLE 18.6 INVESTIGATIONS PRIOR TO COMMENCING ANTIBIOTIC TREATMENT

'Partial septic screen'	'Full septic screen'
■ Blood culture	■ Blood culture
■ Full blood count (FBC)	■ Full blood count (FBC)
■ CRP	■ CRP
	■ Lumbar puncture
	■ Chest X-ray
	■ Urine culture
	■ (Skin lesion/eye swabs if indicated)

(adapted from NICE, 2014)

Microbiology

BLOOD CULTURE

Despite ongoing evaluations of alternative methods, blood culture remains the gold standard diagnostic tool for neonatal sepsis. This should be obtained as soon as possible once infection is suspected. Appropriate skin preparation helps reduce false positive results, and for the same reason sampling from pre-existing intravenous devices should be avoided, as they are frequently colonised with CoNS (Buttery, 2002). In the absence of other abnormal results and if there are no ongoing clinical concerns, the suggestion is that negative blood culture results after 36 hours should lead to cessation of antibiotic treatment (NICE, 2014).

CSF CULTURE AND ANALYSIS

As infants with meningitis have been known to have negative blood cultures, a lumbar puncture to obtain CSF cultures is necessary if meningitis is suspected. If the infant is clinically unstable or has low platelet count, the procedure may need to be deferred until it is deemed that it will be tolerated from a cardiorespiratory perspective, or until after a platelet transfusion, but should not be omitted if the index of suspicion is high. Microscopy and biochemical evaluation of the CSF will identify white cell count (WCC) as well as protein and glucose. Elevated WCC and protein levels, and low glucose levels as compared with a simultaneously obtained plasma sample, are suggestive of meningitis (Heath et al., 2003; Bedford Russell and Isaacs, 2012).

URINE CULTURE

Urinary tract infections (UTI) are predominantly late onset infections, so that routine urine culture in suspected EOS is not recommended (NICE, 2014). The collection method of urine cultures is of importance: 'bag specimens' will only exclude a UTI if clear, but not be of diagnostic value in a true UTI due to high contamination rates. Collection via suprapubic aspiration (SPA) or catheterisation are preferable; it has been suggested that catheterisation is more often successful and less painful than SPA (Isaacs, 2014).

SURFACE SWABS, GASTRIC ASPIRATE AND ENDOTRACHEAL ASPIRATE

Cultures from these sites will identify colonisation, which is not necessarily an indication of invasive infection. Management and antimicrobial therapy therefore need to be guided by other investigations and the baby's clinical status rather than these results alone (Bedford Russell and Isaacs, 2012).

Cell count

- *White cell count (WCC)* This has been suggested to be of limited value in the diagnosis of infection, as the normal range is wide, dependent on gestational and postnatal age, and can be raised in conditions other than sepsis, such as hypoxic-ischaemic encephalopathy (HIE) and neonatal seizures.
- *Neutrophil count* A low neutrophil count in early postnatal life is only rarely associated with infection and more often due to causes such as growth restriction or pregnancy-induced hypertension and pre-eclampsia. However, after the first three days of life, neutropaenia is more indicative of sepsis or NEC.

    An abnormal I:T (immature:total neutrophil) ratio and evidence of toxic granulation on the blood film are reasonably sensitive indicators of infection.
- *Platelets* Neonates can be thrombocytopaenic for the same non-infective reasons they can be neutropaenic, or due to HIE in early life. Infective causes of thrombocytopaenia include congenital or acquired viral as well as bacterial infections. As with neutrophil count, a trend over time may be more useful than the absolute value (Bedford Russell and Isaacs, 2012; Isaacs, 2014).

Biochemistry

- *C-reactive protein (CRP)* Measurement of the CRP is recommended when antibiotic therapy is commenced, with elevated levels being indicative of sepsis (NICE, 2014). CRP levels also rise in NEC, meconium aspiration, HIE and following surgery. Whether it is a sensitive enough predictor for sepsis in isolation is debatable, but its value in monitoring the course of infection and infant response to therapy is recognised, as its level should return to normal in less than 2–7 days if the stimulus to its production has been removed (Yoxall et al., 1996; Bedford Russell and Isaacs, 2012).
- *Procalcitonin* This infection marker has superseded CRP measurements in some UK hospitals, and there is evidence that it is more sensitive with the ability to differentiate bacterial from viral infections and non-infective causes of raised inflammatory

markers (Simon et al., 2004; van Rossum et al., 2004). At present procalcitonin is still recommended as an adjunct rather than a replacement of CRP measurements (Madhu et al., 2008).

■ *Cytokines* There is some suggestion that measurements of TNF-α and Interleukin 6 may be useful in the diagnosis of neonatal sepsis, but as yet these have not been widely adopted in clinical practice (Bedford Russell and Isaacs, 2012).

Radiology

A chest X-ray should be performed in infants with suspected sepsis, particularly if respiratory signs of infection are present. Depending on clinical presentation, an abdominal X-ray should furthermore be considered, which may be helpful in the exclusion of NEC or other surgical causes of clinical abdominal concerns (Bedford Russell and Isaacs, 2012).

THE NURSE'S ROLE IN NEONATAL INFECTION

Due to the potential complications of neonatal infection, it is imperative that neonatal nurses are able to identify potential risk factors and recognise the signs of infection in the infant as early as possible, so that appropriate management is undertaken, and complications are avoided. Rapid clinical deterioration sometimes found in neonatal infection makes, as discussed previously, the immediate detection of early sepsis signs very important. In this aspect, the neonatal nurse, as the infant's advocate in partnership with the parents, is excellently placed to pick up on subtle clinical and behavioural changes and communicate these to the medical members of the multidisciplinary team. However, the prevention of infection must be among the first concerns in providing neonatal care, and in this the neonatal nurse's role is essential.

The prevention of CVC-related LOS has been broadly discussed in relation to reducing sepsis rates through the introduction of care bundles. More specifically, thorough CVC care is predominantly the responsibility of the nurse caring for the infant with indwelling lines, and good practice in this area has been associated with a reduction in infection rates. This consists of regular review of the insertion site as well as the ongoing need for the line and, if deemed no longer required, its prompt removal, and furthermore aseptic techniques when manipulation of the catheter hub is necessary (Bion et al., 2013; Legeay, 2015).

A further infection issue on the NNU is ventilator-associated pneumonia (VAP), which can be caused by micro-organisms colonising the endotracheal tube or ventilator circuits, oro- or nasopharyngeal secretions and gastric contents, which can be aspirated, but may also be transmitted through the hands of healthcare professionals.

The risk for VAP increases in direct relation to the duration of invasive ventilation, so that early extubation remains the most effective precautionary approach. However, where this is not possible, a number of preventative strategies aside from good hand hygiene have been suggested. These advocate the use of endotracheal suction only when this is clinically indicated, minimal interference with the ventilator circuit, i.e. a change of this only when it is visibly contaminated or not functioning, and slightly elevated positioning to prevent aspiration of colonised secretions (Cooper and Haut, 2013; Cernada et al., 2014). The importance of mindful positioning has furthermore been highlighted in a study which found infants who had been predominantly nursed supine to be significantly more likely to be colonised with potentially pathogenic micro-organisms compared to those nursed in lateral positions (Aly et al., 2008). The cornerstone of infection prevention, however, remains good hand hygiene, which the expert neonatal nurse does not only practice, but also promotes by fulfilling monitoring and educational functions among the multidisciplinary team, parents and visitors (Legeay et al., 2015).

CONCLUSION

Not only is neonatal infection a considerable cause of mortality in this population, but significant morbidity with adverse neurodevelopmental outcomes in survivors has been described. This, alongside increasing issues around antimicrobial resistance, highlights the neonatal nurse's crucial role in the prevention of infection. Other important aspects of good nursing care include the identification of early, often soft signs of infection, and thus instigation of investigations and timely treatment, as well as caring for the septic, potentially unstable neonate and providing support to his or her family.

CASE STUDIES

Case study 1: Early onset infection in a term neonate

Esme is a term baby born vaginally to a second-time mother after 42 hours' rupture of the membranes. She was admitted to the NNU as she developed severe respiratory distress in the delivery room and commenced on CPAP, requiring 35–40% oxygen to maintain normal saturations. She continues to have significant subcostal recession and is noted to be grunting, which worsens with handling.

Following admission, Esme was started on benzylpenicillin and gentamicin following a partial septic screen, and she is NBM on IV fluids.

Esme's chest X-ray shows bilateral 'ground glass' consolidation.

After 2 hours her blood gases still show a respiratory acidosis, her oxygen requirements are climbing, and her work of breathing is worsening. Her blood results show a raised WCC, and her initial CRP is 27mg/L.

CASE STUDY

C
A
S
E

S
T
U
D
Y

Q.1.   What is Esme's diagnosis likely to be? Can you think of a pathogen which typically presents like this?

Q.2.   Do you think Esme's condition is likely to improve over the next few hours?

Q.3.   What other supportive treatment may be required in this case?

Q.4.   Which other investigations may need to be considered here?

Case study 2: The extremely preterm NICU resident

Harry is a 39-day-old baby born at 24^{+6} weeks. He now weighs 984grams. He is currently stable on Optiflow 6L in 28–34% and on a combination of nasogastric feeds of maternal breast milk and TPN through a CVC to aid his growth. This was inserted when he was a week old.

Q.1.   What measures can you take to help prevent Harry developing CVC-related infection?

Q.2.   Which changes in his observations would make you concerned that he may be septic?

Q.3.   Is there anything you would like to discuss with the medical team on Harry's ward round this morning?

Case study 3: Unexpected admission from the postnatal ward

Baby Tariq, a term baby boy, is admitted to the NNU from the postnatal ward at 2 hours of age following an episode of becoming cyanosed. On assessment, the midwife heard respiratory grunting and his breathing rate had become more rapid, with his colour looking pale and mottled.

Q.1.   What do you think is going on here and what risk factors would you need to consider in relation to his birth, delivery and details about his mother's health?

Q.2.   What nursing assessment would he require?

Q.3.   What would you explain to the parents and how would they be supported at this time?

For suggested answer guides to the questions posed in these case studies, please refer to the web-based companion site specific to this chapter (see URL below).

WEB-BASED RESOURCES

For further information, online resources and greater detail on the case studies featured in this chapter go to www.routledge.com/cw/nicnursing

References

Aly, H., Badawy, M., El-Kholy, A., Nabil, R., & Mohamed, A. (2008). Randomized, controlled trial on tracheal colonization of ventilated infants: Can gravity prevent ventilator-associated pneumonia? *Pediatrics*, *122*(4), 770–774.

Anthony, M., Bedford Russell, A., Cooper, T., Fry, C., Heath, P. T., Kennea, N., … & Wilson, P. (2013). Managing and preventing outbreaks of Gram-negative infections in UK neonatal units. *Archives of Disease in Childhood: Fetal and Neonatal Edition*, *98*(6), F549–F553.

Austin, N., Cleminson, J., Darlow, B. A., & McGuire, W. (2015). Prophylactic oral/topical non-absorbed antifungal agents to prevent invasive fungal infection in very low birth weight infants. *Cochrane Database of Systematic Reviews*, Issue 10. Art. No.: CD003478. DOI: 10.1002/14651858. CD003478.pub5

Avent, M. L., Vaska, V. L., Rogers, B. A., Cheng, A. C., Van Hal, S. J., Holmes, N. E., … & Paterson, D. L. (2013). Vancomycin therapeutics and monitoring: a contemporary approach. *Internal Medicine Journal*, *43*(2), 110–119.

Bedford Russell, A. R., & Isaacs, D. (2012). Neonatal infection. Part 2: Infection in the newborn. In Rennie, J. M. (Ed.) *Rennie & Roberton's Textbook of Neonatology* (5th Edition). London: Elsevier Health Sciences.

Bedford Russell, A. R., & Kumar, R. (2015). Early onset neonatal sepsis: Diagnostic dilemmas and practical management. *Archives of Disease in Childhood: Fetal and Neonatal Edition*, *100*(4), F350–F354.

Benjamin Jr, D. K., Stoll, B. J., Gantz, M. G., Walsh, M. C., Sánchez, P. J., Das, A., … & Walsh, T. J. (2010). Neonatal candidiasis: Epidemiology, risk factors, and clinical judgment. *Pediatrics*, *126*(4), e865.

Bion, J., Richardson, A., Hibbert, P., Beer, J., Abrusci, T., McCutcheon, M., … & Patten, M. (2013). 'Matching Michigan': A 2-year stepped interventional programme to minimise central venous catheter-blood stream infections in intensive care units in England. *British Medical Journal Quality & Safety*, *22*(2), 110–123.

Buttery, J. P. (2002). Blood cultures in newborns and children: Optimising an everyday test. *Archives of Disease in Childhood: Fetal and Neonatal Edition*, *87*(1), F25–F28.

Cailes, B., Vergnano, S., Kortsalioudaki, C., Heath, P., & Sharland, M. (2015). The current and future roles of neonatal infection surveillance programmes in combating antimicrobial resistance. *Early Human Development*, *91*(11), 613–618.

Cailes, B., Kortsalioudaki, C., Buttery, J., Pattnayak, S., Greenough, A., Matthes, J., … & Heath, P. T. (2018a). Epidemiology of UK neonatal infections: The neonIN infection surveillance network. *Archives of Disease in Childhood: Fetal and Neonatal Edition*, *103*(6), F547–F553.

Cailes, B., Kortsalioudaki, C., Buttery, J., Pattnayak, S., Greenough, A., Matthes, J., … & Heath, P. T. (2018b). Antimicrobial resistance in UK neonatal units: Neonin infection surveillance network. *Archives of Disease in Childhood: Fetal and Neonatal Edition*, *103*(5), F474–F478.

Camacho-Gonzalez, A., Spearman, P. W., & Stoll, B. J. (2013). Neonatal infectious diseases: Evaluation of neonatal sepsis. *Pediatric Clinics of North America*, *60*(2), 367.

Carr, R., Brocklehurst, P., Doré, C. J., & Modi, N. (2009). Granulocyte-macrophage colony stimulating factor administered as prophylaxis for reduction of sepsis in extremely preterm, small for gestational age neonates (the PROGRAMS trial): A single-blind, multicentre, randomised controlled trial. *The Lancet*, *373*(9659), 226–233.

Cernada, M., Brugada, M., Golombek, S., & Vento, M. (2014). Ventilator-associated pneumonia in neonatal patients: an update. *Neonatology, 105*(2), 98–107.

Chapman, R. L. (2007). Prevention and treatment of Candida infections in neonates. *Seminars in Fetal and Neonatal Medicine, 31*(1), 39–46.

Cleminson, J., Austin, N., & McGuire, W. (2015). Prophylactic systemic antifungal agents to prevent mortality and morbidity in very low birth weight infants. *Cochrane Database of Systematic Reviews*, Issue 10. Art. No.: CD003850. DOI: 10.1002/14651858.CD003850.pub5

Cooper, V. B., & Haut, C. (2013). Preventing ventilator-associated pneumonia in children: An evidence-based protocol. *Critical Care Nurse, 33*(3), 21–29.

Cotten, C. M., McDonald, S., Stoll, B., Goldberg, R. N., Poole, K., & Benjamin, D. K. (2006). The association of third-generation cephalosporin use and invasive candidiasis in extremely low birth-weight infants. *Pediatrics, 118*(2), 717–722.

Cotten, C. M., Taylor, S., Stoll, B., Goldberg, R. N., Hansen, N. I., Sánchez, P. J., … & Benjamin Jr, D. K. (2009). Prolonged duration of initial empirical antibiotic treatment is associated with increased rates of necrotizing enterocolitis and death for extremely low birth weight infants. *Pediatrics, 123*(1), 58.

Daley, A. J., Isaacs, D., & Australasian Study Group for Neonatal Infections. (2004). Ten-year study on the effect of intrapartum antibiotic prophylaxis on early onset group B streptococcal and Escherichia coli neonatal sepsis in Australasia. *The Pediatric Infectious Disease Journal, 23*(7), 630–634.

Delves, P. J., & Roitt, I. M. (2000a). The immune system. First of two parts. *New England Journal of Medicine, 343*(1), 37–49.

Delves, P. J., & Roitt, I. M. (2000b). The Immune System. Second of two parts. *New England Journal of Medicine, 343*(2), 108–117.

Dong, Y., & Speer, C. P. (2015). Late-onset neonatal sepsis: Recent developments. *Archives of Disease in Childhood: Fetal and Neonatal Edition, 100*(3), F257–F263.

Ewer, A. K., Middleton, L. J., Furmston, A. T., Bhoyar, A., Daniels, J. P., Thangaratinam, S., … & PulseOx Study Group. (2011). Pulse oximetry screening for congenital heart defects in newborn infants (PulseOx): A test accuracy study. *The Lancet, 378*(9793), 785–794.

Farber, J. M., & Peterkin, P. I. (1991). Listeria monocytogenes, a food-borne pathogen. *Microbiology and Molecular Biology Reviews, 55*(3), 476–511.

Foley, E., Clarke, E., Beckett, V.A., Harrison, S., Pillai, A., FitzGerald, M., Owen, P., Low-Beer, N., & Patel, R. (2014). *Royal College of Obstetricians and Gynaecologists Management of Genital Herpes in Pregnancy*. Retrieved from www.rcog.org.uk/en/guidelines-research-services/guidelines/genital-herpes/

Gandhi, R. S., Fernandez-Alvarez, J. R., & Rabe, H. (2010). Management of congenital cytomegalovirus infection: an evidence-based approach. *Acta Paediatrica, 99*(4), 509–515.

Gordon, A., Greenhalgh, M., & McGuire, W. (2017). Early planned removal of umbilical venous catheters to prevent infection in newborn infants. *Cochrane Database of Systematic Reviews*, Issue 10. Art. No.: CD012142. DOI: 10.1002/14651858.CD012142.pub2

Greenwood, C., Morrow, A. L., Lagomarcino, A. J., Altaye, M., Taft, D. H., Yu, Z., … & Schibler, K. R. (2014). Early empiric antibiotic use in preterm infants is associated with lower bacterial diversity and higher relative abundance of Enterobacter. *The Journal of Pediatrics, 165*(1), 23–29.

Heath, P. T., Yusoff, N. N., & Baker, C. J. (2003). Neonatal meningitis. *Archives of Disease in Childhood: Fetal and Neonatal Edition, 88*(3), F173–F178.

Heath, P. T., Balfour, G., Weisner, A. M., Efstratiou, A., Lamagni, T. L., Tighe, H., … & McCartney, A. C. (2004). Group B streptococcal disease in UK and Irish infants younger than 90 days. *The Lancet, 363*(9405), 292–294.

Holt, P. G., & Jones, C. A. (2000). The development of the immune system during pregnancy and early life. *Allergy, 55*(8), 688–697.

Hsieh, E., Smith, P. B., Jacqz-Aigrain, E., Kaguelidou, F., Cohen-Wolkowiez, M., Manzoni, P., & Benjamin Jr, D. K. (2012). Neonatal fungal infections: When to treat? *Early Human Development*, *88*, S6–S10.

Hughes, R. G., Brocklehurst, P., Steer, P. J., Heath, P., & Stenson, B. M. on behalf of the Royal College of Obstetricians and Gynaecologists (2017). Prevention of Early-onset Neonatal Group B Streptococcal Disease. Green-top Guideline No. 36. *British Journal of Obstetrics and Gynaecology*, *124*(12), e280–305.

Inglis, G. D. T., & Davies, M. W. (2005). Prophylactic antibiotics to reduce morbidity and mortality in neonates with umbilical venous catheters. *Cochrane Database of Systematic Reviews*, Issue 4. Art. No.: CD005251. DOI: 10.1002/14651858.CD005251.pub2

Inglis, G. D. T., Jardine, L. A., & Davies, M. W. (2007). Prophylactic antibiotics to reduce morbidity and mortality in neonates with umbilical artery catheters. *Cochrane Database of Systematic Reviews*, Issue 4. Art. No.: CD004697. DOI: 10.1002/14651858.CD004697.pub3

INIS Collaborative Group. (2011). Treatment of neonatal sepsis with intravenous immune globulin. *New England Journal of Medicine*, *365*(13), 1201–1211.

Isaacs, D., Barfield, C. P., Grimwood, K., McPhee, A. J., Minutillo, C., & Tudehope, D. I. (1995). Systemic bacterial and fungal infections in infants in Australian neonatal units. *Medical Journal of Australia*, *162*(4), 198–201.

Isaacs, D. (2014). *Evidence-Based Neonatal Infections*. Chichester: Wiley & Sons.

Jacobs, S. E., Tobin, J. M., Opie, G. F., Donath, S., Tabrizi, S. N., Pirotta, M., … & Garland, S. M. (2013). Probiotic effects on late-onset sepsis in very preterm infants: a randomized controlled trial. *Pediatrics*, *132*(6), 1055–1062.

Jardine, L. A., Inglis, G. D. T., & Davies, M. W. (2008). Prophylactic systemic antibiotics to reduce morbidity and mortality in neonates with central venous catheters. *Cochrane Database of Systematic Reviews*, Issue 1. Art. No.: CD006179. DOI: 10.1002/14651858.CD006179.pub2

Johnson, A. P., Sharland, M., Goodall, C. M., Blackburn, R., Kearns, A. M., Gilbert, R., … & Cookson, B. (2010). Enhanced surveillance of methicillin-resistant Staphylococcus aureus (MRSA) bacteraemia in children in the UK and Ireland. *Archives of Disease in Childhood*, *95*(10), 781–785.

Kent, A., Kortsalioudaki, C., Watts, T., Satodia, P., Kennea, N., Embleton, N., Clarke, P., Chang, J., Geethanath, R., Scorrer, T., & Heath, P. T. on behalf of the neonIN network (2014). Coagulase-Negative Staphylococcal Infections in UK Neonatal Units (NNUs) *Archives of Disease In Childhood Fetal Neonatal Edition*, *99* (Suppl 2), A56.

Kent, A., Kortsalioudaki, C., Monahan, I. M., Bielicki, J., Planche, T. D., Heath, P. T., & Sharland, M. (2016). Neonatal gram-negative infections, antibiotic susceptibility and clinical outcome: An observational study. *Archives of Disease in Childhood: Fetal and Neonatal Edition*, *101*(6), F507–F512.

Klein, J. O., & Marcy, S. M. (1995). Bacterial sepsis and meningitis. In Remington, J. S., & Klein, J. O. (Eds.) *Infectious Diseases of the Fetus and Newborn*. Philadelphia: WB Saunders.

Kortsalioudaki, C., Kent, A., Kennea, N., Clarke, P., Watts, T., Embleton, N., Satodia, P., Scorrer, T., Chang, J., Geethanath, R., & Heath, P. T. (2014). Epidemiology and antibiotic susceptibility of gram-negative (GN) neonatal infections over 10 years: Data from the neonIN infection surveillance network. *Archives of Disease in Childhood*, *99* (Suppl 2), A440.

Lai, N., Taylor, J. E., Tan, K., Choo, Y., Ahmad Kamar, A., & Muhamad, N. (2016). Antimicrobial dressings for the prevention of catheter-related infections in newborn infants with central venous catheters. *Cochrane Database of Systematic Reviews*, Issue 3. Art. No.: CD011082. DOI: 10.1002/14651858.CD011082.pub2

Legeay, C., Bourigault, C., Lepelletier, D., & Zahar, J. R. (2015). Prevention of healthcare-associated infections in neonates: Room for improvement. *Journal of Hospital Infection*, *89*(4), 319–323.

Luck, S., Torny, M., d'Agapeyeff, K., Pitt, A., Heath, P., Breathnach, A., & Russell, A. B. (2003). Estimated early-onset group B streptococcal neonatal disease. *The Lancet*, *361*(9373), 1953–1954.

Madhu, R., Agarwal, R., Ofoegbu, B., Guy, M., & Vail, A. (2008). Procalcitonin is a useful additional marker in late-onset neonatal sepsis. *Archives of Disease in Childhood: Fetal Neonatal Edition, 93* (Suppl 1), Fa31.

National Institute for Health and Care Excellence. (2014). *Antibiotics for early-onset neonatal infection. NICE clinical guideline 149.* NICE.

National Institute for Health and Care Excellence. (2015). *Antimicrobial stewardship: Systems and processes for effective antimicrobial medicine use. NICE Guideline 15.* NICE.

National Institute for Health and Care Excellence. (2016). *Sepsis: Recognition, diagnosis and early management.* NICE.

O'Sullivan, C., Lamagni, T., Efstratiou, A., Patel, D., Cunney, R., Meehan, M., ... & Davies, E. (2016). P3 Group B Streptococcal (GBS) disease in UK and Irish infants younger than 90 days, 2014–2015. *Archives of Disease in Childhood.* 101:A2.

Okike, I. O., Lamont, R. F., & Heath, P. T. (2013). Do we really need to worry about Listeria in newborn infants? *The Pediatric Infectious Disease Journal, 32*(4), 405–406.

Public Health England. (2015). *Start Smart – Then Focus. Antimicrobial Stewardship Toolkit for English Hospitals.* Public Health England.

Rao, S. C., Srinivasjois, R., & Moon, K. (2011). One dose per day compared to multiple doses per day of gentamicin for treatment of suspected or proven sepsis in neonates. *Cochrane Database of Systematic Reviews*, Issue 11. Art. No.: CD005091. DOI: 10.1002/14651858.CD005091.pub3

Rønnestad, A., Abrahamsen, T. G., Medbo, S., Reigstad, H., Lossius, K., Kaaresen, P. I., ... & Markestad, T. (2005). Late-onset septicemia in a Norwegian national cohort of extremely premature infants receiving very early full human milk feeding. *Pediatrics-English Edition, 115*(3), e269.

Schwiertz, A., Gruhl, B., Löbnitz, M., Michel, P., Radke, M., & Blaut, M. (2003). Development of the intestinal bacterial composition in hospitalized preterm infants in comparison with breast-fed, full-term infants. *Pediatric Research, 54*(3), 393.

Seale, A. C., & Agarwal, R. (2018). Improving management of neonatal infections. *The Lancet, 392*(10142), 100–102.

Shane, A. L., Sánchez, P. J., & Stoll, B.J. (2017). Neonatal sepsis. *The Lancet, 390*, 1770–1780.

Simon, L., Gauvin, F., Amre, D. K., Saint-Louis, P., & Lacroix, J. (2004). Serum procalcitonin and C-reactive protein levels as markers of bacterial infection: A systematic review and meta-analysis. *Clinical Infectious Diseases, 39*(2), 206–217.

Smulders, C. A., van Gestel, J. P., & Bos, A. P. (2013). Are central line bundles and ventilator bundles effective in critically ill neonates and children? *Intensive Care Medicine, 39*(8), 1352–1358.

Stoll, B. J., Hansen, N. I., Adams-Chapman, I., Fanaroff, A. A., Hintz, S. R., Vohr, B., ... & National Institute of Child Health and Human Development Neonatal Research Network. (2004). Neurodevelopmental and growth impairment among extremely low-birth-weight infants with neonatal infection. *Journal of the American Medical Association, 292*(19), 2357–2365.

Taylor, G. P., Anderson, J., Clayden, P., Gazzard, B. G., Fortin, J., Kennedy, J., ... & Tookey, P. A. (2011). British HIV Association and Children's HIV Association position statement on infant feeding in the UK 2011. *HIV Medicine, 12*(7), 389–393.

Thangaratinam, S., Brown, K., Zamora, J., Khan, K. S., & Ewer, A. K. (2012). Pulse oximetry screening for critical congenital heart defects in asymptomatic newborn babies: A systematic review and meta-analysis. *The Lancet, 379*(9835), 2459–2464.

Thaver, D., & Zaidi, A. K. (2009). Burden of neonatal infections in developing countries: A review of evidence from community-based studies. *The Pediatric Infectious Disease Journal, 28*(1), S3–S9.

UK National Screening Committee. (2008). *Group B Streptococcus: The UK NSC Policy on Group B Streptococcus Screening in Pregnancy.* London: NSC.

van Rossum, A. M. C., Wulkan, R. W., & Oudesluys-Murphy, A. M. (2004). Procalcitonin as an early marker of infection in neonates and children. *The Lancet Infectious Diseases, 4*(10), 620–630.

Vergnano, S., Menson, E., Kennea, N., Embleton, N., Russell, A. B., Watts, T., ... & Heath, P. T. (2011). Neonatal infections in England: The NeonIN surveillance network. *Archives of Disease in Childhood: Fetal and Neonatal Edition, 96*(1), F9–F14.

Williams, M. (2018). RCOG guidance: Early-onset neonatal GBS disease. *Prescriber*, *29*(1), 34–36.

World Health Organization. (2010). *Antiretroviral drugs for treating pregnant women and preventing HIV infection in infants: Recommendations for a public health approach-2010 version*. World Health Organization.

Yoxall, C. W., Isherwood, D. M., & Weindling, A. M. (1996). The neonatal infection screen. *Current Paediatrics*, *6*(1), 16–20.

PART 4

PRACTICES AND PROCEDURES IN NEONATAL CARE

Practices and procedures in neonatal care: The parent voice

She had to be transferred out to another bigger unit many miles away from our home. Seeing her leave in the ambulance was terrifying … Thankfully, she got there and we finally arrived there, too, but it was hard being so far away and being separated from our other children.

However, we knew she had to be transferred because of the surgery – it didn't seem possible that she would cope with having an operation being so tiny and vulnerable. But it was a matter of life or death.

She pulled through and, miraculously, got better after her surgery … she fought so hard and showed us how strong she is … stronger than us. We felt exhausted, drained … trying to deal with all the uncertainty.

Voice of a father of a 24-week gestation baby, Anna (pseudonym) who spent 10 weeks in neonatal care.

Adapted from Petty et al., 2019a; 2019b

See chapter 4 reference list for full citations.

19 MEDICATION PRACTICE IN THE NEONATAL UNIT

Karen Hoover

CONTENTS

GUIDANCE ON HOW TO ENHANCE PERSONAL LEARNING FROM THIS CHAPTER

Key points covered in this chapter

- Neonatal pharmacokinetics impacting on medication practice.
- The nurse's role in all important aspects of neonatal drug administration.
- The factors for consideration in relation to minimising risk and ensuring safety in neonates who require drugs.

Reflection

Reading through the chapter, you are encouraged to engage with the key points and related literature in an enquiring way. Ask these questions:

- Do you understand your role in relation to safe drug administration for infants in neonatal care?
- What are neonatal-specific considerations in this area of practice?
- Are you aware of the latest guidance relating to neonatal drugs and administration?

Implications for nursing care

- Finally: consider the implications of what you learn for your nursing care relating to neonatal medication practice.

INTRODUCTION AND BACKGROUND

The aim of medication therapy in the newborn is to administer a given drug at a given dose to achieve a desired therapeutic effect, with the minimum risk of toxicity (Pauwels and Allegaert, 2016). However, this is a complex issue, as neonates are a very diverse group comprising wide gestational and postnatal age and weight ranges, requiring individualised dosing with drugs lacking data for the neonatal population. There is great variability in how drugs act in this population with maturational changes and illness as well as modern interventions such as therapeutic hypothermia (TH) impacting on the effects of a given drug. The risks of toxicity are high, as demonstrated by numerous historical examples, and medication error remains a major concern. However, drug therapy is vital to contribute to improved neonatal outcomes (Allegaert and Van Den Anker, 2014), and decisions about appropriate drugs should be tailored to the specific needs of neonates (Smits et al., 2017). This chapter will provide a concise summary of the above issues, relating them to how, as neonatal nurses, we can improve care and reduce risks by being aware of the impact of medications in these vulnerable patients.

PHARMACOKINETICS

Effective and safe drug administration in neonates should be based on current knowledge of the physiological characteristics of the infant and the pharmacokinetics (PK) of a given drug (Allegaert et al., 2014). Pharmacokinetics relates to the movement of drugs into the body, and a drug's effect is determined by its absorption, distribution, metabolism and excretion (ADME) (De Wildt et al., 2014). These components, outlined in table 19.1, are all influenced by maturational differences as age-related changes in drug metabolism impact a drug's effect, with the greatest effects being seen in the neonatal period (Choonara and Sammons, 2014).

Absorption of drugs

Absorption is the movement of the drug from its administration site to the bloodstream, and the route of administration determines how available the drug is to the circulation (bioavailability). Intravenous (IV) drugs require no absorption and have 100% bioavailability (Johnson, 2011). Enteral absorption is determined by gastric pH and rate of gastric emptying (Bennett, 2014). At birth babies have a gastric pH that is near neutral and immature acid secretion (Skinner, 2011) which results in decreased absorption of weakly acidic drugs such as phenobarbital. However, it allows increased absorption of other acidic drugs such as penicillin and ampicillin. With increasing maturity and postnatal age, gastric pH decreases (Bennett, 2014). The delayed gastric emptying in neonates allows more extensive absorption of some drugs because of diffusion through the stomach wall, but drugs

TABLE 19.1 NEONATAL PHARMACOKINETICS

Pharmacokinetic component	Neonatal considerations
Absorption of drugs	*Decreased absorption*: Oral route: Increased gastric pH decreases bioavailability Intramuscular route: Decreased muscle mass results in variable absorption *Increased absorption*: Transdermal route: ■ Increased permeability ■ Increased surface area to weight
Distributions of drugs	*Increased total body water*: Increased volume of distribution for water soluble drugs *Decreased fat*: Increased plasma concentration for fat-soluble drugs *Decreased plasma proteins and binding ability*: Increased plasma concentration of free drug *Increased permeability of blood–brain barrier*: Increased uptake of unbound drugs to brain
Metabolism of drugs	*Decreased phase 1 and 2 hepatic enzymes*: Decreased biotransformation of drugs This is exacerbated by: ■ Prematurity ■ Serious illness ■ Genetic variation ■ Interventions, i.e. therapeutic hypothermia
Excretion of drugs	*Decreased glomerular filtration rate and tubular excretion*: ■ Decreased excretion of water soluble drugs ■ Increased half -life for most drugs This is exacerbated by: ■ Prematurity ■ Serious illness ■ Aminoglycosides

normally absorbed through the small intestine will have a delayed onset, although human milk increases gastric transit time (Skinner, 2011). Delayed gastric emptying is most apparent in preterm infants, those on high caloric feeds and in severe illness (Anderson, 2017).

Oral drugs such as propranolol, morphine and midazolam are absorbed in the small intestine after first being metabolised in the liver resulting in a drug with less predictable effects (Johnson, 2011). Decreased secretion of bile acids and the lack of flora in the gut at birth reduces fat absorption, so fat-soluble drugs such as vitamins are affected (Johnson, 2011). These factors result in a slow time to peak level of orally administered drugs, and these effects are more pronounced in the most immature (Bennett, 2014).

Distribution of drugs

Distribution is the movement of the drug from the intravascular space to the extravascular compartments where it can be utilised (Johnson, 2011).

VOLUME OF DISTRIBUTION

The volume in which the drug is distributed in the body is called the volume of distribution (V_D), and it depends on the amount of body water and fat components (Choonara and Sammons, 2014). Babies have a higher proportion of total body water than children or adults; 80% at birth vs. 60% in adults (Kearns et al., 2003), with preterm infants having up to 85% (Skinner, 2011). Because of this, neonates need higher doses per kg of weight for water-soluble drugs such as gentamicin, which is widely distributed throughout the body (i.e. has a large V_D) compared to older children. The proportion of body water decreases rapidly over the first week, therefore the dose of water-soluble drugs, must be decreased to prevent toxicity (Bennett, 2014). The percentage of fat in neonates is much less than in adults, with a term baby having around 12% body fat, but a 1.5kg baby only 3%. Therefore, drugs which rely on redistribution to fat, such as fentanyl, will have a prolonged and higher plasma concentration (Anderson, 2017).

HALF-LIFE

Half-life ($t_{1/2}$) is the period required for a drug's concentration in the body to be reduced by half; therefore, it will depend on how quickly the drug is eliminated. The concept of half-life can be demonstrated by the drug adenosine, which is used for supraventricular tachycardia (SVT): this has a half-life of less than 10 seconds. This means it must be given very quickly, before it is inactivated. It should therefore be administered IV via an upper limb, so it reaches the site of action – the sino-atrial node, where it exerts its effect by slowing conduction to the atrioventricular node (Ainsworth, 2015). Other drugs including dobutamine, dopamine, and noradrenaline have half-lives around 5–10 minutes and need to be given by continuous infusion. In contrast, phenobarbital has a half-life of 2–4 days in newborns (Ainsworth, 2015), and caffeine has an even longer half-life of 2.5–6 days (Ainsworth, 2015). With such long half-lives, these drugs are prescribed once daily. Therefore, the longer the half-life, the longer the drug takes to be eliminated and the less often it needs to be given (Johnson, 2011).

The changes in drug dosing with increasing postnatal age and improving renal function reflects the changes in half-life, and this can be demonstrated by the commonly used antibiotic cefotaxime. At birth the half-life of the drug is 2–6 hours, the half-life being inversely related to gestational age. It is recommended the drug be given 12-hourly in the first 6 days, then 8-hourly between 7 and 20 days, then 6–8-hourly after this (Paediatric Formulary Committee, 2018).

STEADY STATE

Administration of a large first dose (loading dose) results in steady state being rapidly reached, where the amount of the drug administered in each new dose equals the amount eliminated since the last dose. Generally, steady state is reached in around 5 half-lives of the drug (Johnson, 2011). In drugs with long half-lives such as caffeine and phenobarbital, the loading dose ensures that the desired effect is achieved more rapidly.

BLOOD–BRAIN BARRIER

The blood–brain barrier (BBB) mediates the transport of nutrients into, and toxic metabolites out of, the central nervous system (CNS). However, the BBB is more permeable in neonates compared to adults, and integrity is reduced further by severe illness (Anderson, 2017). This immaturity results in faster morphine uptake into the CNS and may be responsible for the increased sensitivity of the neonate to morphine (Anderson, 2017).

PLASMA PROTEIN BINDING

The binding of drugs to proteins within the vascular department also determines how the drug is distributed throughout the body. Unbound drugs are able to exert their effect, whereas drugs bound to proteins cannot (Johnson, 2011). However, plasma proteins such as albumin are decreased in neonates, and they have less binding ability compared to adults (Kearns et al., 2003). This lower protein binding of drugs means there is greater free drug concentration and therefore greater drug effects (Anderson, 2017). Protein-bound drugs can displace bilirubin from albumin, potentially increasing the risk of bilirubin-induced neurotoxicity (kernicterus), as unbound bilirubin crosses the BBB (Amin and Wang, 2018). For example, in 1956, neonates who received sulphonamide antibiotics had a higher incidence of kernicterus, and it was later found that this was due to the marked ability of these drugs to displace bilirubin from albumin (McIntyre and Choonara, 2004).

Preterm infants below 30 weeks' gestation are at higher risk of kernicterus at lower concentrations of bilirubin than term babies, because they have a decreased ability to bind bilirubin as well as lower albumin levels (Amin and Wang, 2018). Ibuprofen displaces bilirubin from albumin, but clinically significant displacement in preterm infants is unlikely if used at the recommended dosage and the serum albumin level is normal. Intralipids can also displace bilirubin, and evidence suggests that intake should be limited in babies under 28 weeks in the first week of life when unconjugated levels of bilirubin are high (Amin, 2016). Routine measurements of albumin levels in preterm infants below 34 weeks with elevated unconjugated bilirubin levels and consideration of treatment at lower bilirubin levels when other risk factors for bilirubin displacement, such as hypoxia, acidosis or sepsis are also present, have been recommended (Amin, 2016).

Metabolism of drugs

The liver is the main organ of metabolism of drugs. Metabolism occurs through hepatic enzymes transforming drugs to a water-soluble form for excretion in the urine or to render the drug inactive or weaker (Johnson, 2011). Hepatic enzymes metabolise drugs via phase 1 or phase 2 reactions, with both involving a variety of metabolic pathways. These all mature at different rates (Choonara and Sammons, 2014).

PHASE 1 REACTIONS

Phase 1 reactions are important for the metabolic transformation (biotransformation) of most drugs, and alter the structure of the drug by a variety of chemical reactions (Skinner, 2011). An important group of enzymes involved in phase 1 reactions include the **cytochrome** P450 (CYP450) system, which is made up of a number of enzymes, although not all are present at birth, and their activity is reduced compared to adults (Kearns et al., 2003). Individual enzymes mature at different rates, and the most important – CYP3A4 isoenzyme – metabolises more than 50% of all drugs. Its activity is very low in neonates and does not reach adult levels until a month of age (Choonara and Sammons, 2014). For example, clearance of midazolam is prolonged particularly in the preterm infant because of reduced CYP3A4 activity (Anderson, 2017). Some drugs, such as the antibiotic erythromycin, inhibit individual CYP enzymes, while others, including phenobarbital, dexamethasone and phenytoin, induce multiple enzymes (De Wildt et al., 2014). Reduced phase 1 enzymes can also have paradoxical effects as demonstrated by the metabolism of paracetamol. Paracetamol normally breaks down to the toxic metabolite NAPQ1 which is excreted but will cause hepatotoxicity if produced in large amounts. Neonates, however, are less prone to liver toxicity from paracetamol overdose than older children and adults, because they have reduced levels of the phase 1 enzyme necessary to convert paracetamol to NAPQ1 (Anderson, 2017).

PHASE 2 REACTIONS

Phase 2 reactions convert lipid-soluble drugs to water-soluble compounds by conjugation (attachment) of the drug to a molecule, enabling it to be excreted by the kidneys. Phase 2 reactions mature slowly, with only 50% activity at birth, and reach adult levels around 2 years (Bennett, 2014). Examples of the implications of this immaturity are demonstrated by a number of drugs. In the 1950s, the antimicrobial chloramphenicol was commonly used, until several babies presented with cardiovascular collapse and the so-called 'grey baby syndrome'. This was due to toxic levels of the drug because of a lack of a phase 2 enzyme, which normally metabolises chloramphenicol (McIntyre and Choonara, 2004). The phase 2 pathway that converts morphine to its metabolites is also reduced in neonates, so clearance is lower, and the risk of toxicity is increased. There is a rapid increase in metabolism from 27 weeks' gestation, necessitating a correspondent increase in the dose to maintain sedation (Kearns et al., 2003).

OTHER FACTORS THAT AFFECT DRUG METABOLISM

Genetic variation in genes involved in drug metabolism may result in increased or decreased drug metabolism (Hawcutt et al., 2013). Certain genetic mutations have been linked to sensitivity to ototoxic aminoglycosides, and these individuals are at high risk of bilateral deafness if treated with aminoglycosides, even when therapeutic blood levels are normal (Jing et al., 2015). CYP enzyme activity is reduced by serious illness, and this can decrease elimination of some drugs, resulting in accumulation and possible toxicity (Wildschutt et al., 2013). Many drugs metabolised by liver enzymes are temperature-dependent, therefore TH can lead to a lack of action for some drugs and accumulation of others. Drug metabolism changes during re-warming, when drugs that have been dormant in peripheral tissues, such as fentanyl, are recirculated, resulting in increased serum concentrations and the risk of toxicity (Wildschutt et al., 2013).

The delayed clearance of some drugs has been seen with increased intra-abdominal pressure after exomphalos repair for example, and this is thought to be due to reduced hepatic blood flow from regions of CYP450 activity (Anderson, 2017).

Excretion of dugs

The major pathway for drug excretion is the kidney. However, this is dependent on glomerular filtration rate (GFR), which is the rate at which blood is filtered through the kidney. GFR is around 30% of adult levels in the newborn and even lower in preterm infants (Skinner, 2011). GFR is also reduced by serious illness and the use of drugs such as ibuprofen. It increases over the first few weeks of life and reaches 50% of adult levels at 3 months, but takes longer in extremely preterm babies (Anderson, 2017). Nephron development is not complete until around 36 weeks postconceptional age (Bennett, 2014) and kidney tubules are also immature. Therefore, the half-life of many drugs is prolonged, as they require longer to be eliminated. Thus dosing intervals of drugs with high renal clearance, such as gentamicin, must reflect the changes in GFR and tubular maturity that occur with increasing gestational and postnatal age (Kearns et al., 2003). Hypothermia induces vasoconstriction, which reduces GFR and therefore elimination of drugs requiring renal clearance. Since neonates requiring TH often already have renal impairment, dosages for drugs excreted via the kidney will require adjustment to prevent toxicity (Bijleveld et al., 2016). Other drugs with decreased clearance during TH include phenobarbital, which requires doses to be adjusted according to serum levels (Zanelli et al., 2011).

ROUTES OF DRUG ADMINISTRATION

Buccal

Drugs are absorbed through the buccal membrane in neonates, but this results in uneven absorption and inability to control the dosage (Johnson, 2011). One drug that is very effective via this route is glucose gel, a quick-acting carbohydrate for the treatment of hypo-glycaemia. It is massaged into the cheek's mucosa and absorbed rapidly through the buccal membrane into the systemic circulation (Harris et al., 2013).

Oral

Oral drugs once absorbed pass through the portal system and are metabolised in the liver before they reach the systemic circulation to exert their effects. This mechanism is called 'first pass metabolism'; most oral drugs undergo this. However, if this is extensive, the drug will have a lower concentration in the blood and therefore lower bioavailability (Bennett, 2014). Oral drugs have poor bioavailability in the newborn. Caffeine is an exception as it is completely absorbed orally with almost no first pass metabolism (Shrestha and Jawa, 2017). Oral drugs are drawn up using enteral syringes and then administered into the mouth slowly while waiting for the baby to swallow, or via a gastric tube. The practical problems associated with oral administration in newborns include vomiting after a dose and residual volumes of the drug remaining in gastric tubes if these are not fully flushed (Bennett, 2014).

Inhalation

Inhaled budesonide, a corticosteroid, for the prevention of bronchopulmonary dysplasia (BPD) in extremely preterm newborns, has become more popular in recent years. However, a Cochrane review found no evidence that budesonide reduced BPD compared to systemic steroids, although there were fewer adverse effects (Shah et al., 2017). Numerous factors such as equipment used affect drug delivery into the lungs, and the amount of aerosol delivered can be less than 14% (Ainsworth, 2015).

Intratracheal

The classic example of an intratracheally administered drug is pulmonary surfactant. Surfactants include beractant (Survanta®) or poractant alfa (Curosurf®), and are used for preterm infants with surfactant-deficient lung disease (respiratory distress syndrome), and in those with meconium aspiration where surfactant is inactivated. In recent times, non-invasive techniques of surfactant administration have been incorporated in neonatal care. With the INSURE (**In**tubation – **Sur**factant – **E**xtubation) method, the baby is intubated, usually after a small dose of morphine or fentanyl, and the dose injected into the endotracheal tube (ETT), followed by extubation. The tube used to inject the drug should not protrude beyond the end of the ETT, or only one lung will receive the surfactant. The newer technique of inserting a fine-bore tube through the vocal cords to administer surfactant while the baby remains on non-invasive respiratory support is known as LISA (Less Invasive Surfactant Administration). In this scenario, surfactant is injected directly via the catheter which is then removed. Sedation is not always given with this technique (Niemarkt et al., 2017).

Percutaneous

Percutaneous absorption of a drug is related to surface area and the thickness of the stratum corneum (Tayman et al., 2011). Neonates, and in particular extremely preterm infants have a high surface area to weight ratio and a thinner stratum corneum compared to older children and adults. This results in greater absorption through the skin into the systemic circulation and can result in toxicity. For example, the use of hexachlorophene in baby bathing products resulted in neurotoxicity and death in a number of babies in France and the United States in the 1970s (McIntyre and Choonara, 2004). In the modern era, there is concern that the use of iodine-containing skin cleansing solutions may cause hypothyroidism in babies of less than 32 weeks, yet it remains in use (Aitken and Williams, 2014). Chlorhexidine skin disinfection prior to umbilical and central line placement in newborns under 32 weeks has been shown to result in chlorhexidine in the bloodstream of neonates, of which the long-term effects are not known. The other main risk is skin damage from contact dermatitis and burns (Chapman et al., 2012; Neri et al., 2017).

An example of topical administration that does work well is tetracaine gel (Ametop 4%), a local anaesthetic. The entire contents of the tube (1.5g) is applied to the skin 30 minutes prior to a procedure such as cannulation or lumbar puncture and an occlusive dressing applied. The gel should only be applied to a small area of skin (around 5cm by 5cm, and it must be wiped off before the procedure (Ainsworth, 2015).

Subcutaneous

This is rarely used in neonates due to the lack of subcutaneous tissue and variable perfusion (Johnson, 2011).

Intramuscular

This is used less commonly in neonates because they have little muscle mass and a poorer blood supply to muscle, so absorption is unpredictable with variable times to onset of action and peak concentrations (Bennett, 2014). However, this slow absorption is ideal for vitamin K administration, as it provides slow release over a few months, protecting the baby from haemorrhagic disease of the newborn (Bennett, 2014). Vaccines are now given via the intramuscular (IM) route, as there is less tissue injury than in subcutaneous administration, and IM injection induces an immune response (Ainsworth, 2015). However, this route of administration should not be used in babies who have a risk of bleeding i.e. those with thrombocytopaenia (Ainsworth, 2015). The only safe site for IM administration in neonates is the anterior aspect of the quadriceps muscle, as the buttocks do not have enough muscle mass. The needle should be inserted well into the muscle and the plunger withdrawn to ensure a blood vessel has not been entered (Ainsworth, 2015).

Intravenous

Although IV administration eliminates variables associated with other routes, the infusion of a drug via a lower limb vein or a low umbilical venous catheter can result in reduction of the active drug entering the circulation, because it is metabolised as it passes through the liver (Johnson, 2011). Other factors such as in-line filters can also affect IV delivery of a drug. These filters remove bacteria and endotoxins, but a drug can be adsorbed by the filter and delivery prevented until the filter is saturated. This is a well-known effect with insulin, where a filter should not be used (Sherwin et al., 2014). Insulin can also adsorb to the IV tubing, so this needs to be primed with the insulin infusion solution to allow total adsorption into the lining. This is particularly important when the syringe and line are being changed, as the initial response determines the infusion rate, but inadequate preparation of a replacement set could destabilise the glucose level (Ainsworth, 2015).

Intraosseous

The intraosseous (IO) route provides access to the systemic circulation via the bone marrow and can be used if access via an IV line or umbilical vein is not possible. The onset of action of drugs is the same as for those administered IV, and any drug or fluid which can be given IV can be administered via this route, including blood products. A dedicated IO needle is inserted into the upper tibia (see figure 19.1), and correct placement is confirmed by aspiration of marrow (Ellemunter, 1999). Other needles can be used, and there is an example of an 18-gauge butterfly needle placed in an oedematous preterm infant (Lake and Emmerson, 2003). Complications include osteomyelitis, bone fracture and extravasation, and the needle should be removed as soon as IV access is obtained (Ellemunter, 1999).

Rectal

Rectal absorption is variable in neonates, and the enhanced expulsion reflex can make administration difficult (Skinner, 2011). Suppositories are often cut in half or even quarters, and as drug content is not evenly distributed in a suppository, the actual dose delivered will not be accurate (Ainsworth, 2015).

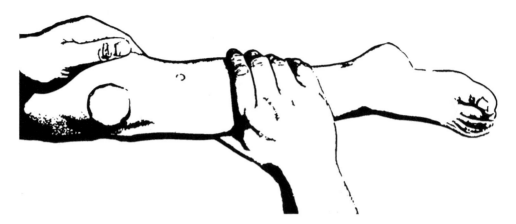

Figure 19.1 Site of intraosseous needle insertion (Source: Creative Commons)

THERAPEUTIC DRUG MONITORING

This is necessary for drugs with a narrow therapeutic index, where the range between the therapeutic and toxic dose (i.e. where the drug is effective but not toxic) is narrow. The result is then used to adjust dosage intervals (Pauwells and Allegeart, 2016). Drugs that may be encountered in the neonatal unit (NNU) which require drug monitoring include gentamicin, vancomycin, phenobarbital and digoxin. Peak (post-dose) levels are evaluated to monitor the efficacy of a drug, and are taken *after* the dose is given. Trough (pre-dose) levels on the other hand are used to avoid toxicity from drug accumulation, and are the levels of the drug in the body *before* the drug dose is administered. The most common drug monitored in neonates is the antibiotic gentamicin, and toxicity is related to trough levels (Pauwels and Allegaert, 2016). If the trough level is high, the drug dosing interval should be extended (Paediatric Formulary Committee, 2018).

Drug toxicity

Neonates experience additional side effects of drugs due to direct toxicity on immature and developing organs. There are numerous historical examples of drugs that proved to be toxic in neonates. These include the use of benzyl alcohol as an antibacterial in sodium chloride ampoules for IV use in the 1980s, resulting in the death of 10 preterm babies in the USA, and an IV formulation of vitamin E, used in 1984 to potentially prevent retinopathy of pre-maturity, was withdrawn after 38 neonates died. The deaths were thought to be related to the emulsifier used to make the vitamin E soluble (McIntyre and Choonara, 2004). Postnatal corticosteroids were introduced in the 1980s to prevent and treat BPD and they were targeted to preterm babies who could not be weaned off the ventilator. However, in the late

1990s their use fell out of favour after it was found that they doubled the risk of cerebral palsy, and subsequently decisions for their administration were made cautiously, after obtaining parental consent (Broad and Maxwell, 2017). However, the neonatal specialty has remained interested in corticosteroids as a means to prevent BPD, and it is thought that low-dose treatment regimens may be reasonably safe with regard to adverse neurodevelopmental outcomes compared to historically used dosing regimes (Zeng et al., 2018).

DRUGS AND BREASTFEEDING

All medications enter breast milk to some degree, although in small amounts, and most are considered to be compatible with breastfeeding. However, there is a lack of data regarding the risks of adverse effects in infants. The presence and concentration of drug compounds in breast milk depends upon factors such as how much of it binds to plasma proteins, and how soluble it is in lipids. Highly lipid-soluble drugs such as diazepam and phenobarbital penetrate milk, as do low molecular weight drugs such as alcohol and amphetamines. The dose the baby receives depends upon the amount excreted into breast milk, the volume of milk ingested and how fast the infant eliminates the substance (Berlin and Van Den Anker, 2013).

However, there are reports of clinical toxicity from some medications, particularly opioids. Koren et al., 2006 described a case where a 13-day-old breastfed baby died of morphine poisoning. The mother was taking codeine regularly for episiotomy pain, and when the baby became sleepy and was not feeding well, she froze the breast milk, which was later found to contain high levels of morphine. Codeine is metabolised to morphine via the CYP450 pathway, and some individuals are ultra-rapid metabolisers, as this mother was found to be. Therefore, it is advised that codeine should be avoided in breastfeeding mothers considering that the frequency of ultra-metabolisers is common, particularly in individuals of African descent (Koren et al., 2006). For mothers on methadone for narcotic addiction, there is evidence that babies may benefit from breastfeeding by having less severe withdrawal symptoms than babies on formula (Berlin and Van Den Anker, 2013). The British National Formulary (BNF) for Children identifies drugs for breastfeeding mothers which should be used with caution or are contraindicated, and this and other breastfeeding references, of which many are available online, should be consulted when offering advice to a breastfeeding mother.

UNLICENSED MEDICINES

Many studies have shown that neonates, in particular preterm babies, receive medications unlicensed (their use has not been approved for the indication which it is administered for), or off-label (the indication has been approved, but not for the age, dose, frequency or route used). Unlicensed or off-label drugs are associated with significant medication errors (Conroy, 2011). However, they are used in most infants below 32 weeks' gestation (Kieran et al., 2014).

The use of unlicensed drugs is exemplified by those used for suspected gastro-oesophageal reflux (GOR). Gastric acidity is a major defence mechanism against infection, so the use of **histamine** receptor blockers (H_2 blockers) such as ranitidine, which reduce stomach acidity in preterm babies with GOR, have been shown to increase the risk of necrotising enterocolitis (NEC; Cotten and Malcolm, 2013). Proton pump inhibitors (PPIs) such as omeprazole also decrease gastric acid secretion and pose similar risks as ranitidine (De Bruyne and Ito, 2018). Cisapride is a **prokinetic** agent which was widely used for neonatal GOR in the 1980s to early 1990s. It was withdrawn in 2000 after multiple reports of arrhythmias in children (Collins and Sondheimer, 2008). Since then the prokinetic drug domperidone has been widely used; however, it was reported in 2008 that, like cisapride, it prolonged the QT interval, resulting in a risk of arrhythmias (Djeddi et al., 2008). Yet, a recent review of the management of GOR in NNUs in the UK showed that the use of these unlicensed drugs is still widespread, with 53% using ranitidine, 23% PPIs and 22% domperidone (Rossor et al., 2018).

MEDICATION ERRORS

Medication use in neonates is more complex than in any other group due to differences in weight, gestational and postnatal age requiring individualised, dosing and their physical size and immaturity of body systems leaving a narrow margin of safety for error (Krzyaniak and Bajorek, 2016). Table 19.2 outlines medication errors in the NNU. The widespread use of unlicensed and off-label medications and limited access to neonatal-specific formulations also increase the risk of error, which can have serious consequences in such small, immature patients (Conroy, 2011). A review of 20 articles on medication errors throughout the age spectrum found that up to 60% of incidents involved administration errors by nurses, with the most common being incorrect preparation, dilution, administration time, and administration of an extra dose. 47% of administration errors involved at least tenfold overdoses. One of the studies found that 31% of IV medications prescribed for neonates were at doses of less than one-tenth of a vial, increasing the risk from ten- to a hundred-fold dosing errors. Medicines most commonly associated with dosing errors included IV formulations of morphine, furosemide, gentamicin, insulin and benzylpenicillin (Krzyaniak and Bajorek, 2016).

The dead space of a syringe and needle may be sufficient to overdose a very small baby, as was found in the case of a neonate who developed arrhythmias due to a digoxin overdose. This was accounted for by the drug contained in the dead space of a 1mL syringe; the diluent was drawn up into the same syringe as the drug itself, which meant the baby received four times the amount of the drug prescribed (Bhambhani et al., 2005).

TABLE 19.2 MEDICATION ERRORS IN THE NEONATAL UNIT

Type of error	Clinician involved	Causes of error
Prescribing	Prescriber	Wrong administration route Wrong unit, i.e. grams instead of milligrams Incorrect placement of decimal point
Transcription	Prescriber	Wrong weight Wrong dosage Wrong unit, i.e. grams instead of milligrams
Dispensing	Pharmacists	Wrong labelling of drug Incorrect calculation or dose Incorrect dilution Delayed dispensing time
Administration	Nursing staff	Incorrect administration time Incorrect preparation and dilution Patient misidentification Administering additional dose of drug
Monitoring	Medical and nursing staff	Incorrect interpretation of laboratory results Omission of therapeutic drug monitoring Missing symptoms of adverse events

Therefore, it is recommended to inject a drug directly into its diluent, so that the excess drug remains in the hub.

Administering drugs via the wrong route used to be a common problem because of identical Luer Lok® connections in both peripheral and central lines and enteral feeding tubes, with reports of serious adverse effects. For example, a case report from Germany described a 6-week-old baby who was inadvertently given 5mL breast milk via an IV line (Döring et al., 2014). The baby became unwell immediately, but responded to oxygen and IV antibiotics. Such wrong route errors were more prevalent in the UK before the introduction of specifically designed enteral lines and syringes fitted with connectors which were no longer compatible with intravenous lines (National Patient Safety Agency, 2007). Other errors include administration to the wrong patient, the incidence of which one review found to be as high as 25%, mainly due to similar or identical names, and confusion with babies of multiple births. One cause noted for this was that identification bracelets on wrists and ankles were often removed in order to place IV lines or to take blood samples, and then not replaced, leading to risk of misidentification (Krzyaniak and Bajorek, 2016).

Preventing medication errors

Medication errors are unavoidable but can be minimised by specific interventions. Electronic prescribing eliminates errors due to illegible handwriting and the rewriting of prescription charts. It also provides an audit trail of the prescriber and who administered the medicine. However, there is little evidence that administration errors can be reduced (Caldwell and Power, 2012). The single most effective measure in reducing medication errors particularly in high-risk areas such as neonatal intensive care is the involvement of a clinical pharmacist (Krzyaniak and Bajorek, 2016). Pharmacists' activities included reviewing prescription charts, providing advice on medication on ward rounds and implementing educational activities for staff. However, administration errors are unlikely to be affected greatly by pharmacist intervention. Educational intervention programmes provide practical teaching sessions for nurses covering medication preparation and administration, and one study showed this to result in a significant reduction of error rate from 49–31% (Chedoe et al., 2012). However, the authors acknowledged other methods are needed to improve medication safety further.

An innovative intervention to improve medication safety in the NNU is providing simulated clinical scenarios for the preparation and administration of IV medications to neonates. This was seen as a risk-free approach to learning, furthermore integrating teamworking skills that were transferable to the clinical working environment. These simulation sessions, using drugs with a high risk of potential error associated with preparation and administration, such as adrenaline and dobutamine, resulted in a significant reduction in the number of administration errors (Kirk and Cookson, 2013).

NON-MEDICAL PRESCRIBING

Nurse independent prescribers (NIP) or non-medical prescribers (NMP) are able, after an appropriate educational programme, to prescribe any medicine for any medical condition, including the administration of scheduled and controlled drugs. However, they must work within their own level of professional competence and expertise (Paediatric Formulary Committee, 2018).

In neonatology, NIPs are usually Advanced Neonatal Nurse Practitioners who often work autonomously in either a medical or nursing role, or a combination of both. Their ability to prescribe has had demonstrable positive effects on the quality of patient care (Carey et al., 2009).

CONCLUSION

The use of medications in the NNU is complicated by the wide range of birth weights and gestational ages, and the immaturity of body systems. Maturational development, disease and therapeutic interventions add to the complexity of medication management in this diverse group of patients. The lack of pharmacological research in neonates has resulted in extensive use of unlicensed and off-label drugs, which increase the risks of adverse events. Administering medications to neonates is a high-risk task for nurses, and medication errors are most common in this group of patients. However, the increasing focus on prevention has led to interventions that should help to ensure a safer process in providing medications for newborns.

CASE STUDIES

Case study 1: The preterm infant who has become unwell

Jonathan is a 25^{+2}-week baby who is now 3 weeks old. He has developed signs of NEC and has been prescribed cefotaxime 6-hourly, and metronidazole IV as a loading dose, followed by a maintenance dose after 24 hours.

Q.1. Why is cefotaxime prescribed 6-hourly for this baby?
Q.2. How often would you expect it to be prescribed in a 1-day-old baby?
Q.3. Why does metronidazole need a loading dose and why is the next dose not given for 24 hours?
Q.4. What drugs would you consider for pain and stress management in line with any non-pharmacological strategies?

Jonathan becomes increasingly unwell and is intubated and ventilated, then is started on dopamine and dobutamine infusions for hypotension.

Q.5. Why are some drugs given by continuous infusion?
Q.6. What factors predispose this baby to medication errors?
Q.7. What are the potential side effects of inotropes such as dopamine and dobutamine?

After a period of stabilisation, Jonathan improves and at the age of 5 weeks is being weaned from ventilation requirements. He is commenced on caffeine as part of this management.

Q.8. Why is caffeine given to the infant?

Case study 2: Medication during therapeutic hypothermia

Caroline is a 2-day-old term baby undergoing TH for hypoxic-ischaemic encephalopathy (HIE). She was commenced gentamicin after birth but has now developed renal failure. She is also receiving phenobarbital, a morphine infusion, and a dopamine infusion.

CASE STUDY

C
A
S
E

S
T
U
D
Y

Q.1. How are the medications Caroline is on affected by TH?
Q.2. Does the gentamicin dosage need amending and why?
Q.3. What are the potential side effects of morphine and phenobarbitone?

Case study 3: The late preterm infant with multiple issues

A new mother of a 35-week gestation baby girl called Petra who is admitted to the neonatal unit with a low blood sugar and jaundice, wants to breastfeed but is concerned about medication she is taking. The infant also develops an eye infection and thrush around the nappy area.

Q.1. What advice would you give to mum about breastfeeding, eye and skin care, and how would this baby be managed?

For suggested answer guides to the questions posed in these case studies, please refer to the web-based companion site specific to this chapter (see URL below).

WEB-BASED RESOURCES

For further information, online resources and greater detail on the case studies featured in this chapter go to www.routledge.com/cw/nicnursing

References

Ainsworth, S. B. (Ed.). (2015). *Neonatal Formulary 7: Drug use in pregnancy and the first year of life.* (7th Edition). Chichester: John Wiley & Sons.

Aitken, J., & Williams, F. L. (2014). A systematic review of thyroid dysfunction in preterm neonates exposed to topical iodine. *Archives of Disease in Childhood: Fetal and Neonatal Edition, 99*(1), F21–F28.

Allegaert, K., & Van Den Anker, J. N. (2014). Clinical pharmacology in neonates: Small size, huge variability. *Neonatology, 105*(4), 344–349.

Allegaert, K., Van De Velde, M., & Van Den Anker, J. (2014). Neonatal clinical pharmacology. *Pediatric Anesthesia, 24*(1), 30–38.

Amin, S. B. (2016). Bilirubin binding capacity in the preterm neonate. *Clinics in Perinatology, 43*(2), 241–257.

Amin, S. B., & Wang, H. (2018). Bilirubin albumin binding and unbound unconjugated hyperbilirubinemia in premature infants. *The Journal of Pediatrics, 192*, 47–52.

Anderson B, J. (2017). Neonatal pharmacology. *Anaesthesia and Intensive Care Medicine, 18*(2), 68–74.

Bennett, S. (2014). Pharmacology in neonatal care: Prescribing considerations. *Nurse Prescribing, 12*(2), 87–92.

Berlin Jr, C. M., & Van Den Anker, I. N. (2013). Safety during breastfeeding: Drugs, foods, environmental chemicals, and maternal infections. *Seminars in Fetal and Neonatal Medicine, 18*(1), 13–18.

Bhambhani, V., Beri, R. S., & Puliyel, J. M. (2005). Inadvertent overdosing of neonates as a result of the dead space of the syringe hub and needle. *Archives of Disease in Childhood: Fetal and Neonatal Edition*, *90*(5), F444–F445.

Bijleveld, Y. A., De Haan, T. R., Van Der Lee, H. J., Groenendaal, F., Dijk, P. H., Van Heijst, A., … & Zonnenberg, I. A. (2016). Altered gentamicin pharmacokinetics in term neonates undergoing controlled hypothermia. *British Journal of Clinical Pharmacology*, *81*(6), 1067–1077.

Broad, S. R., & Maxwell, N. C. (2017). Steroids on the neonatal unit. *Paediatrics and Child Health*, *27*(1), 9–13.

Caldwell, N. A., & Power, B. (2012). The pros and cons of electronic prescribing for children. *Archives of Disease in Childhood*, *97*(2), 124–128.

Carey, N., Stenner, K., & Courtenay, M. (2009). Adopting the prescribing role in practice: Exploring nurses' views in a specialist children's hospital. *Paediatric Nursing*, *21*(9), 25.

Chapman, A. K., Aucott, S. W., & Milstone, A. M. (2012). Safety of chlorhexidine gluconate used for skin antisepsis in the preterm infant. *Journal of Perinatology*, *32*(1), 4.

Chedoe, I., Molendijk, H., Hospes, W., Van den Heuvel, E. R., & Taxis, K. (2012). The effect of a multifaceted educational intervention on medication preparation and administration errors in neonatal intensive care. *Archives of Disease in Childhood: Fetal and Neonatal Edition*, *97*(6), F449–F455.

Choonara, I., & Sammons, H. (2014). Paediatric clinical pharmacology in the UK. *Archives of Disease in Childhood*, *99*(12), 1143–1146.

Collins, K. K., & Sondheimer, J. M. (2008). Domperidone-induced QT prolongation: add another drug to the list. *The Journal of Pediatrics*, *153*(5), 596–598.

Conroy, S. (2011). Association between licence status and medication errors. *Archives of Disease in Childhood*, *96*(3), 305–306.

Cotten, C. M., & Malcolm, W. F. (2013). Ranitidine use is associated with increased morbidity and mortality in very low birthweight infants. *British Medical Journal Evidence-Based Medicine*, *18*(1), 36–37.

De Bruyne, P., & Ito, S. (2018). Toxicity of long-term use of proton pump inhibitors in children. *Archives of Disease in Childhood*, *103*(1), 78–82.

De Wildt, S. N., Tibboel, D., & Leeder, J. S. (2014). Drug metabolism for the paediatrician. *Archives of Disease in Childhood*, *99*(12), 1137–1142.

Djeddi, D., Kongolo, G., Lefaix, C., Mounard, J., & Léké, A. (2008). Effect of domperidone on QT interval in neonates. *The Journal of Pediatrics*, *153*(5), 663–666.

Döring, M., Brenner, B., Handgretinger, R., Hofbeck, M., & Kerst, G. (2014). Inadvertent intravenous administration of maternal breast milk in a six-week-old infant: A case report and review of the literature. *BMC Research Notes*, *7*(1), 17.

Ellemunter, H., Simma, B., Trawöger, R., & Maurer, H. (1999). Intraosseous lines in preterm and full term neonates. *Archives of Disease in Childhood: Fetal and Neonatal Edition*, *80*(1), F74–F75.

Harris, D. L., Weston, P. J., Signal, M., Chase, J. G., & Harding, J. E. (2013). Dextrose gel for neonatal hypoglycaemia (the Sugar Babies Study): A randomised, double-blind, placebo-controlled trial. *The Lancet*, *382*(9910), 2077–2083.

Hawcutt, D. B., Thompson, B., Smyth, R. L., & Pirmohamed, M. (2013). Paediatric pharmacogenomics: an overview. *Archives of Disease in Childhood*, *98*(3), 232–237.

Jing, W., Zongjie, H., Denggang, F., Na, H., Bin, Z., Aifen, Z., … & Ring, B. Z. (2015). Mitochondrial mutations associated with aminoglycoside ototoxicity and hearing loss susceptibility identified by meta-analysis. *Journal of Medical Genetics*, *52*(2), 95–103.

Johnson, P. J. (2011). Neonatal pharmacology – pharmacokinetics. *Neonatal Network, 30*(1), 54–61.

Kearns, G. L., Abdel-Rahman, S. M., Alander, S. W., Blowey, D. L., Leeder, J. S., & Kauffman, R. E. (2003). Developmental pharmacology—drug disposition, action, and therapy in infants and children. *New England Journal of Medicine*, *349*(12), 1157–1167.

Kieran, E. A., O'Callaghan, N., & O'Donnell, C. P. (2014). Unlicensed and off-label drug use in an Irish neonatal intensive care unit: A prospective cohort study. *Acta Paediatrica*, *103*(4), e139–e142.

Kirk, S., & Cookson, J. (2013). Reflecting on intravenous drug administration: towards safer practice. *Infant*, *9*(5), 166–169.

Koren, G., Cairns, J., Chitayat, D., Gaedigk, A., & Leeder, S. J. (2006). Pharmacogenetics of morphine poisoning in a breastfed neonate of a codeine-prescribed mother. *The Lancet*, *368*(9536), 704.

Krzyzaniak, N., & Bajorek, B. (2016). Medication safety in neonatal care: A review of medication errors among neonates. *Therapeutic Advances in Drug Safety*, *7*(3), 102–119.

Lake, W., & Emmerson, A. J. B. (2003). Use of a butterfly as an intraosseous needle in an oedematous preterm infant. *Archives of Disease in Childhood: Fetal and Neonatal Edition*, *88*(5), F409–F409.

McIntyre, J., & Choonara, I. (2004). Drug toxicity in the neonate. *Neonatology*, *86*(4), 218–221.

National Patient Safety Agency. (2007). Promoting safer measurement and administration of liquid medicines via oral and other enteral routes. *Patient Safety Alert.*, *19*, 1–12.

Neri, I., Ravaioli, G. M., Faldella, G., Capretti, M. G., Arcuri, S., & Patrizi, A. (2017). Chlorhexidine-induced chemical burns in very low birth weight infants. *The Journal of Pediatrics*, *191*, 262–265.

Niemarkt, H. J., Hütten, M. C., & Kramer, B. W. (2017). Surfactant for respiratory distress syndrome: New ideas on a familiar drug with innovative applications. *Neonatology*, *111*(4), 408–414.

Paediatric Formulary Committee. (2018). *BNF for Children 2018–2019.* London: BMJ Group, Pharmaceutical Press and RCPCH Publications.

Pauwels, S., & Allegaert, K. (2016). Therapeutic drug monitoring in neonates. *Archives of Disease in Childhood*, *101*(4), 377–381.

Rossor, T., Andradi, G., Bhat, R., & Greenough, A. (2018). Investigation and management of gastro-oesophageal reflux in United Kingdom neonatal intensive care units. Acta Paediatrica, *107*(1), 48–51.

Shah, V. S., Ohlsson, A., Halliday, H. L., & Dunn, M. (2017). Early administration of inhaled corticosteroids for preventing chronic lung disease in very low birth weight preterm neonates. *Cochrane Database of Systematic Reviews*, Issue 1. Art. No.: CD001969. DOI: 10.1002/14651858.CD001969.pub4

Sherwin, C. M., Medlicott, N. J., Reith, D. M., & Broadbent, R. S. (2014). Intravenous drug delivery in neonates: lessons learnt. *Archives of Disease in Childhood*, *99*(6), 590–594.

Shrestha, B., & Jawa, G. (2017). Caffeine citrate – Is it a silver bullet in neonatology? *Pediatrics & Neonatology*, *58*(5), 391–397.

Skinner, A. V. (2011). Neonatal pharmacology. *Anaesthesia & Intensive Care Medicine*, *12*(3), 79–84.

Smits, A., Van Den Anker, J. N., & Allegaert, K. (2017). Clinical pharmacology of analgosedatives in neonates: Ways to improve their safe and effective use. *Journal of Pharmacy and Pharmacology*, *69*(4), 350–360.

Tayman, C., Rayyan, M., & Allegaert, K. (2011). Neonatal pharmacology: Extensive interindividual variability despite limited size. *The Journal of Pediatric Pharmacology and Therapeutics*, *16*(3), 170–184.

Wildschut, E. D., De Wildt, S. N., Mâthot, R. A., Reiss, I. K. M., Tibboel, D., & Van Den Anker, J. (2013). Effect of hypothermia and extracorporeal life support on drug disposition in neonates. *Seminars in Fetal and Neonatal Medicine*, *18*(1), 23–27.

Zanelli, S., Buck, M., & Fairchild, K. (2011). Physiologic and pharmacologic considerations for hypothermia therapy in neonates. *Journal of Perinatology*, *31*(6), 377.

Zeng, L., Tian, J., Song, F., Li, W., Jiang, L., Gui, G., … & Mu, D. (2018). Corticosteroids for the prevention of bronchopulmonary dysplasia in preterm infants: a network meta-analysis. *Archives of Disease in Childhood: Fetal and Neonatal Edition*, *103*(6), F506–F511.

20 NEONATAL ANAESTHESIA

Liam Brennan and Louise Oduro-Dominah

CONTENTS

GUIDANCE ON HOW TO ENHANCE PERSONAL LEARNING FROM THIS CHAPTER

Key points covered in this chapter

■ Assessment and management of infants who require anaesthesia, preoperatively, intraoperatively and postoperatively.

■ An overview of anaesthetic procedures and equipment used in neonatal care.

■ The important role of monitoring any infant who requires anaesthesia including the nurses' responsibilities.

Reflection

Reading through the chapter, you are encouraged to engage with the key points and related literature in an enquiring way. Ask these questions:

■ Have you observed or cared for infants who have required anaesthesia – why did they require it?

■ How should infants and parents be prepared in line with the potential risks of anaesthesia?

■ How should infants be managed throughout the whole anaesthetic period including pre-, intra- and postoperative phases?

Implications for nursing care

■ Finally: how will this chapter enable you to consider best practice in caring for the high-risk infant requiring anaesthesia? Consider the implications of what you learn for your nursing care relating to safe practice of infant and family in this area.

INTRODUCTION AND BACKGROUND

The demand for neonatal anaesthesia continues to grow due to the increased survival of premature infants born in the UK and elsewhere in the world annually, along with developments in surgical techniques for conditions previously considered inoperable. The neonatal anaesthetist needs to have technical skills, specialist knowledge and be thoroughly acquainted with the differing patterns of disease present in the neonatal age group. This is especially important due to the marked differences in anatomy, physiology and pharmacology of neonates compared with older children and adults. Perioperative complications are more common in infancy (Weiss et al., 2016) compared to older age groups; the perioperative period being defined as around or at the time of surgery. This includes preoperative, intraoperative and postoperative phases. Meticulous attention to all aspects of perioperative care is essential to ensure optimum outcomes in this vulnerable group (Ivanova and Pittaway, 2014), and best possible perioperative care for all children and their parents should be the goal of neonatal anaesthetic care (Weiss et al., 2015). The aim of this chapter is to enhance the neonatal nurse's knowledge and understanding of anaesthesia, so that he or she can provide the best possible care for vulnerable patients in the perioperative period along with their families at this stressful time.

PHYSIOLOGICAL DIFFERENCES BETWEEN INFANTS AND ADULTS: PERIOPERATIVE IMPLICATIONS

Several key anatomical differences influence management of the infant airway:

- Relatively large head with prominent occiput
- Small facial structures and oral cavity
- Narrow nasal passages contributing to increased airway resistance
- Proportionally large tongue with limited mobility within small oropharynx (Schmidt et al., 2014).

A baby also has a different body composition to that of adults, with higher water and lower fat content. There is a proportionally higher cardiac output, more permeable blood–brain barrier and immature renal systems and liver. All these factors are rapidly changing in the early days of life, as are the body composition and the growing and maturing organ systems. This 'creates complex, rapidly changing pharmacokinetics and pharmaco-dynamics' (King and Booker, 2004 as cited in McGregor, 2017, p. 78), so that it is less predictable how neonates and infants metabolise anaesthetic drugs (McGregor, 2017). In all, these points emphasise the vulnerability of the neonatal population in relation to anaesthesia.

PREOPERATIVE ASSESSMENT

All infants in neonatal care should be carefully assessed preoperatively by a suitably experienced paediatric anaesthetist, with emphasis on detecting and optimising, whenever possible, the problems below. Neonatal nurses also need to familiarise themselves with these specific issues to ensure they contribute to optimum care for anaesthesia and surgery.

Problems of prematurity affecting anaesthesia

PULMONARY DISEASE

The incidence of respiratory distress syndrome (RDS) and associated chronic lung disease increases with decreasing gestational age at birth, with infants of less than 32 weeks' gestation being at particular risk. Occasionally it is necessary to perform urgent surgery on an infant during the initial respiratory illness. Many of these infants will require either oxygen therapy or ventilatory assistance, increasingly in the form of continuous positive airway pressure (CPAP) as opposed to mechanical ventilation. Careful note should be made of pre-existing ventilatory settings, since minor ventilatory changes perioperatively can result in serious sequelae such as pneumothorax and pulmonary hypertensive crises. Even after minor surgery, infants with a lesser degrees of RDS may also require a period of post-operative ventilation.

Ex-premature infants with chronic lung disease may require particular attention, as they are prone to bronchoconstriction, although the current aim to protect these infants' airways by preventing intubation and giving CPAP means this may be less likely (Wain, 2003; Greenough et al., 2008).

CARDIOVASCULAR DISEASE

There is an increasing incidence of patent ductus arteriosus (PDA) with decreasing birth weight and with decreasing gestational age, with an incidence of 70% in preterm infants born at 25 weeks' gestation (Dagle et al., 2009). Clinical features include a **dynamic praecordium**, a systolic murmur and signs of congestive cardiac failure. A significant PDA – that is one associated with heart failure and/or pulmonary oedema – should be treated before surgery for other conditions. This may not always be possible, as the gut hypoperfusion associated with a PDA increases the risk of necrotising enterocolitis (NEC), and thus the need for emergency laparotomy.

Persistent pulmonary hypertension results from constriction of the pulmonary vascular bed causing a delay or reversal of the transition from foetal to adult circulation. It most frequently occurs in response to acidosis, hypoxaemia or hypotension; all common in the sick surgical neonate (Friesen and Williams, 2008). The result is a right-to-left shunt of blood at atrial and ductal level, leading to worsening hypoxaemia and acidosis. Attempts should be made to reduce pulmonary vascular resistance before surgery by treating the underlying causes and by using pulmonary vasodilators if necessary.

GLYCAEMIC CONTROL

Carbohydrate reserves in all neonates are low but preterm infants have particularly poor stocks because glycogen is not stored significantly until the third trimester (Rao et al., 2013). Hypoglycaemia is therefore likely to accompany any significant period of preoperative starvation and must be avoided. In preterm infants normoglycaemia is maintained by commencing an intravenous (IV) glucose infusion at the beginning of the starvation period if enterally fed or by continuing parental nutrition if the gut is being rested.

THERMOREGULATION

The ability of neonates to maintain a normal core temperature is limited by a large surface area to volume ratio, immature sweating, poor insulation (due to less body fat) and a high basal metabolic rate, with preterm infants being at greatest risk of developing hypothermia (Ibrahim and Yoxall, 2009). The range of ambient temperatures over which the core temperature of the infant is maintained at between 36.7 and 37.3°C while metabolic heat production is kept at a minimum is known as the neutral thermal environment (Hackman, 2001).

Associated congenital/chromosomal anomalies

Surgery in the neonatal period is frequently for the correction of congenital anomalies. Many of these may be associated with other abnormalities, which should be actively sought preoperatively. The following sections look at those anomalies of particular relevance to the anaesthetist.

CONGENITAL HEART DISEASE

Some cardiac abnormalities may not present until several days or even weeks after birth, with symptoms often arising following closure of the ductus arteriosus. A high index of suspicion is therefore necessary, particularly if a heart murmur is detected on clinical examination and there are accompanying signs of cardiorespiratory impairment. Important considerations in an infant with congenital heart disease include the direction of any intracardiac shunt, the presence of cyanosis or cardiac failure, the dependence of the circulation on flow through the ductus arteriosus and drug therapy. The infant's condition should be optimised before surgery in conjunction with neonatologists and paediatric cardiologists if necessary, with consideration given to transferring the baby to a specialist cardiac unit (White and Peyton, 2011).

AIRWAY ABNORMALITIES

A number of different conditions can make airway management and tracheal intubation difficult. Down's syndrome remains one of the most frequently occurring congenital syndromes. Common associated airway abnormalities include upper cervical spine instability, subglottic narrowing, and a large tongue. The presence of a cleft lip and palate or of a more severe facial abnormality such as Pierre-Robin sequence (see figure 20.1), Treacher-Collins

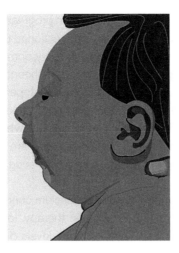

Figure 20.1 Profile view of an infant with Pierre-Robin sequence

syndrome, Goldenhar syndrome, or the presence of cystic hygroma may also present major airway management challenges for the anaesthetist and neonatologist (Infosino, 2002).

FAMILIAL ANAESTHETIC PROBLEMS

Most neonates will be undergoing their first anaesthetic. A history of any familial anaesthetic complications – particularly the development of malignant hyperpyrexia or suxamethonium apnoea – should therefore be sought by the anaesthetist.

PREOPERATIVE INVESTIGATIONS AND PREPARATION

Investigations

The need for preoperative investigations will depend on the age and clinical condition of the baby and the nature of the proposed surgery.

- *Weight* An accurate weight preoperatively is essential in order to calculate appropriate drug doses, fluid volumes and ventilatory parameters.
- *Haemoglobin* The haemoglobin (Hb) concentration should be measured in all infants, except healthy term babies undergoing minor surgery. The Hb at birth varies with gestational age, with a normal value of 145g/L at 28 weeks rising to 155–170g/L at term. The Hb subsequently declines, the fall being greater in preterm babies due to lower red cell survival and poorer production of red cells (Proytcheva, 2009). Transfusion practices are changing with an increasing appreciation of the risks involved, such as new variant Creutzfeld-Jacob disease. There are also questions around neurocognitive outcomes

post transfusion with a large multicentre trial in progress to examine this (ETTNO; Eicher et al., 2012). Whereas previously it was unquestioned that an Hb less than 100g/L was abnormal and should be corrected before surgery, some anaesthetists now tolerate low Hb for some surgery (Higgins et al., 2016), even though anaemia in preterm infants may be associated with an increased incidence of postoperative apnoea.

■ *Clotting studies* These should be carried out in neonates with sepsis (particularly NEC) or jaundice, and abnormalities corrected where possible preoperatively. It is important to note that the reference ranges are age-dependent and therefore appropriate haematological advice should be sought prior to initiating corrective therapy.

■ *Blood electrolytes* Serum sodium and potassium concentrations should be measured in any infant receiving IV fluids or diuretic therapy. Ionised calcium levels fall during the first week of life with a slow rise to adult levels during the second week. The fall is greatest in low birth weight (LBW) infants. Calcium levels should be checked preoperatively in any preterm or sick infant, and levels below 1.75mmol/l corrected, as severe hypocalcaemia can cause generalised hypotonia, jitteriness and seizures.

■ *Blood glucose* Blood glucose concentration should be monitored closely perioperatively and then at least four-hourly until satisfactory glucose homeostasis is achieved.

■ *Blood cross-match* This is essential if major surgery is proposed for any infant, and even for minor surgery in very LBW infants, in whom small amounts of intraoperative blood loss may be very significant. Cytomegalovirus-seronegative blood is recommended by the British Committee for Standards in Haematology Transfusion Task Force (New et al., 2016).

■ *Oxygen saturation and blood gas analysis* Oxygen saturation is easily measured non-invasively with a pulse oximeter and should be recorded in all infants preoperatively. Blood gas analysis should be performed in babies with severe cardiorespiratory disease or with sepsis and prior to any major surgery.

■ *Chest X-ray* A chest X-ray is required in babies with cardiorespiratory disease, those on mechanical ventilation, and if they have a tracheo-oesophageal fistula or a diaphragmatic hernia.

■ *Echocardiography* This should be performed preoperatively in any neonate or infant with a heart murmur, regardless of the presence or the absence of signs of cardiorespiratory impairment, and particularly children with conditions that are known to be associated with congenital heart lesions, e.g. Down's syndrome, tracheo-oesophageal fistula and exomphalos.

Preparation

The infant's condition should be optimised before surgery, with correction of fluid deficits, electrolyte, acid-base and haematological abnormalities wherever possible. In conditions

TABLE 20.1 PREOPERATIVE FASTING TIMES FOR NEONATES AND INFANTS

Type of feed	Duration of fast (hours)	
	Neonates	Infants
Clear fluid	2	0–2 (centre-dependent)
Breast milk	4	4
Formula milk	4	6
Solids	N/A	6

(adapted from Emerson et al., 1998; Frykholm et al., 2018)

associated with intestinal obstruction, a nasogastric tube should be inserted and aspirated at frequent intervals to minimise the risk of pulmonary aspiration of gastric contents. Prolonged preoperative starvation is hazardous in neonates, as they are at increased risk of hypoglycaemia. Appropriate exclusion periods for milk feeds and clear liquids are now well defined, although recently in many centres these have become even more permissive, especially for clear liquids (see table 20.1; Frykholm et al., 2018).

PREMEDICATION

- *Atropine* This drug is rarely, if ever, used as a routine premedicant now that the inhalational anaesthetic agent halothane has largely fallen out of use in UK practice. However, it should still be kept immediately available to treat **bradyarrhythmias** and excessive airway secretions (which can produce troublesome airway complications during the perioperative period). The dose is 20micrograms/kg IV or intramuscularly.
- *Sedatives* These drugs are unnecessary in the neonatal patient group in whom pre-operative anxiety is not a factor. Prolonged effects of sedative drugs may be hazardous in this age group.
- *Caffeine* IV caffeine has been shown to reduce the incidence of postoperative apnoea and bradycardia in former preterm infants and has been advocated preoperatively by some authorities (Henderson-Smart and Steer, 2001).

TRANSFER TO THE OPERATING THEATRE

Neonates should be transported to the operating theatre in a transport incubator system, with monitoring appropriate to the severity of illness. All neonatal intensive care units should have a transport incubator equipped with an appropriate ventilator and the capability to monitor oxygen saturation, electrocardiogram (ECG) and arterial blood pressure. It should also carry all drugs and equipment required for neonatal resuscitation.

THE OPERATING THEATRE ENVIRONMENT

It is essential to maintain an environment that limits heat loss and thus reduces the necessity for additional metabolic heat production. Morbidity and mortality have been shown to increase if an infant cools, with increased tendency to hypoxaemia, acidosis, coagulopathy and intraventricular haemorrhage (Laptook and Watkinson, 2008). The operating theatre should therefore be warmer than for adult surgery, with a temperature of 25°C and humidity of 50%. (Additional measures that may be taken to reduce thermal stress are discussed in the section on anaesthetic equipment.)

INTRAOPERATIVE MANAGEMENT

Induction of anaesthesia

Anaesthesia should be induced in the operating theatre to improve safety and to avoid unmonitored transfers (however brief) of the anaesthetised infant. If parents express a desire to be present at induction, their wishes should be respected. A period of pre-oxygenation in 100% oxygen is recommended prior to the induction of anaesthesia to reduce the chance of hypoxia during apnoea and intubation. The risk of hypoxia greatly outweighs the risk of oxygen toxicity at this vulnerable time for the infant. Anaesthesia may be induced using either an inhalational or intravenous agent. The choice of techniques depends on the preference of the anaesthetist, the infant's condition and the procedure to be performed. For example, airway surgery often requires the baby to be breathing spontaneously, which is often easier to achieve using an inhalational induction.

INTRAVENOUS INDUCTION

Following IV cannulation, but before giving any drugs, the baby is given 100% oxygen via a face mask. A sleep dose of an induction agent is then given. Thiopental has waned in popularity due to availability issues in the UK. Propofol is now the most frequently used induction agent in paediatric anaesthesia. Sleep doses are smaller in neonates due to increased endorphin and progesterone levels and a deficient blood–brain barrier. Following induction of anaesthesia, muscle relaxants may be given to facilitate tracheal intubation. If rapid intubation is required, for example for infants at risk of aspiration of gastric contents, either suxamethonium 2–3mg/kg or rocuronium 1.2mg/kg may be used. In other situations, muscle relaxants with a slower onset of action such as atracurium or vecuronium are commonly used. In cardiac surgery the longer-acting pancuronium is more frequently used.

INHALATION INDUCTION

This is a useful alternative to IV induction, particularly in vigorous infants and those requiring long-term access in whom IV cannulation may prove difficult. Sevoflurane is the volatile anaesthetic agent of choice for inhalational induction of anaesthesia in infants. Sleep is achieved smoothly and rapidly (within 60 seconds), and there is minimal tendency for a bradycardia to occur. Sevoflurane is added to oxygen or an equal mixture of oxygen and nitrous oxide and administered via an anaesthetic face mask in concentrations of up to 8% until the baby is deeply enough anaesthetised to tolerate IV cannulation (Disma et al., 2016). Muscle relaxants may then be administered to facilitate tracheal intubation (Martin, 2017).

Airway management

The airway may be difficult to maintain using a face mask, and inhalational anaesthetic agents produce marked respiratory depression in this age group. Hypoxaemia due to reduced lung volumes and inefficient ventilation is therefore likely to occur unless controlled ventilation is used (Disma et al., 2016). In addition, gastric dilatation occurs following assisted ventilation using a face mask. This can lead to difficulty in ventilation and increased risk of aspiration of gastric contents. During general anaesthesia for neonates, it is thus usual to intubate the trachea and use positive-pressure ventilation during all but the shortest surgical procedures and those involving inspection of the airway. The laryngeal mask airway (LMA; see figure 20.2) may be useful in the case of a difficult airway, such as Pierre-Robin syndrome, but is not otherwise used to substitute for tracheal intubation in the neonatal age group.

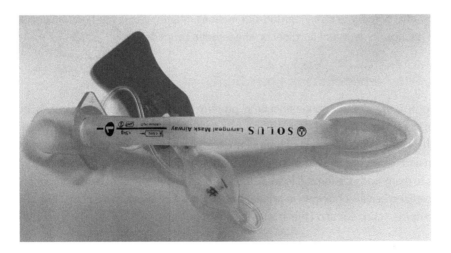

Figure 20.2 Laryngeal mask airway (Source: Louise Oduro-Dominah)

Maintenance of anaesthesia

Adequate anaesthesia during surgery has been demonstrated to reduce the infant's stress response and may improve outcome (Anand et al., 1988). However, high inspired concentrations of inhalational anaesthetics can cause severe cardiovascular depression in young children. In addition, more recently there have been concerns raised about potential adverse neurodevelopmental effects beyond infancy (Chiao and Zuo, 2014; Flick et al., 2014; Lee et al., 2015). Consequently, a 'balanced' technique is usually favoured, combining a low concentration of inhalational anaesthetic in nitrous oxide and oxygen or an air–oxygen mixture to ensure that the infant is anaesthetised. This is combined with muscle relaxants and adequate analgesia. Ventilation is maintained intraoperatively, either manually or via a mechanical ventilator. In 2016, the Food and Drug Administration issued a warning about the potential deleterious effects of anaesthesia on the developing brain. The warning was due to data from animal and *in vitro* research. The results from the General Anesthesia vs. Spinal Anesthesia (GAS) study (Davidson et al., 2016) and the Pediatric Anesthesia and Neurodevelopment Assessment (PANDA) study (Sun et al., 2016) have not found significant undesirable effects. In addition, the Mayo Anesthesia Safety in Kids (MASK) study (Warner et al., 2018) found that anaesthesia exposure before the age of 3 years was not associated with deficits in the primary outcome of general intelligence. However, they also suggest that multiple, but not single, exposures are associated with a pattern of changes in specific neuropsychological domains that is associated with behavioural and learning difficulties. The consensus is that general anaesthesia in the infant age group should be avoided for treatment of conditions that can safely be delayed until the child is older. However, as non-essential surgery is rarely carried out in small infants, this issue has resulted in no significant change to neonatal surgical or anaesthetic practice.

Oxygen and retinopathy of prematurity

The use of oxygen during anaesthesia in preterm neonates should be carefully controlled. Preterm babies are at risk of developing retinopathy of prematurity if blood oxygen levels are too high, even for short periods of time (Finer and Leone, 2009). Hyperoxia causes vasoconstriction and allows the release of angiogenic substances and oxygen free radicals which may be toxic to many body systems. It is wise, therefore, to limit the inspired oxygen concentration to give a partial pressure of oxygen in arterial blood (PaO_2) of between 7 and 10 kPa. The lowest inspired oxygen concentration that maintains an oxygen saturation of 90–94% should be used.

EMERGENCE FROM ANAESTHESIA AND EXTUBATION

If extubation is anticipated, the inhaled anaesthetic should be discontinued shortly before completion of surgery. When the surgical drapes are removed, the infant should be kept warm. The effects of muscle relaxants should be reversed completely, and ventilation maintained with an air–oxygen mixture until the infant awakens and re-establishes spontaneous ventilation. The nose and mouth should be cleared of secretions and the nasogastric tube aspirated and removed if not required postoperatively. Extubation should only take place once the infant is fully awake and breathing regularly and adequately. After extubation, oxygen should continue to be delivered via a face mask due to the potential for postoperative hypoventilation.

ANALGESIA

Historically, postoperative paediatric analgesia was poorly managed. Neonates in particular were assumed to be incapable of perceiving pain and were seldom given adequate post-operative analgesia. However, advances in neonatal neurobiology have prompted a reconsideration of this approach. There is now no doubt that even the most premature infants respond to noxious stimuli, with well-developed physiological and behavioural responses (Bellieni, 2012). The modern view is that all infants must receive appropriate pain relief after surgery. Most of the methods of pain control used in adults can be modified for neonatal use; a multimodal regimen using paracetamol, local anaesthesia and opioids is central to this approach.

Opioids

The term 'opioid' is used to describe a group of drugs which act at specific receptors in the central nervous system resulting in profound analgesia. The most commonly used drugs in neonatal anaesthesia are morphine and fentanyl, while the intraoperative use of ultra-short-acting remifentanil is increasing. Opioids must be used cautiously in neonates because immature metabolic pathways, particularly in the liver, may result in very unpredictable or prolonged responses to these drugs (Kearns et al., 2003). The most major concern is the risk of opioid-induced respiratory depression. If the neonate is to receive respiratory support postoperatively, then morphine or fentanyl can be used quite safely. Indeed, many paediatric anaesthetists would plan to electively ventilate a neonate after major surgery that necessitated ongoing opioid analgesia. Whether ventilated or breathing spontaneously, all neonates who have received opioids must be managed in a high dependency environment, with continuous pulse oximetry and apnoea monitoring being mandatory (Bell and Homer, 2015).

■ *Morphine* This has a longer duration of action and greater potency in neonates than in older children and adults (Hall and Anand, 2014). This is mainly because of immature hepatic function resulting in delayed metabolism of opioid drugs. It should therefore be given less frequently and in a smaller dose. If postoperative ventilation is planned, then up to 50micrograms/kg may be given intraoperatively. Postoperatively, up to 20micrograms/kg of morphine per hour may be used by continuous IV infusion, but most neonates are kept pain-free by 5–10mcg/kg per hour (Paediatric Formulary Committee, 2018). Morphine should be used with extreme caution in neonates who are breathing spontaneously after surgery. Many authorities avoid morphine in this situation, or limit the infusion to 5micrograms/kg per hour (Sale et al., 2012).

- *Fentanyl* This synthetic opioid is useful in neonates with haemodynamic instability, particularly those with pulmonary vascular problems. It is a much more potent drug than morphine but has a shorter duration of action after a single bolus dose. After prolonged infusions, however, the drug will accumulate, resulting in excessive sedation, hypoventilation and risk of apnoeic episodes. For intraoperative use during major neonatal surgery, up to 10micrograms/kg is commonly used, necessitating postoperative respiratory support. Larger doses may be used but can potentially induce chest rigidity, particularly in preterm infants (Fahnenstich et al., 2000).

- *Remifentanil* This newer synthetic opioid is useful when profound analgesia is required intraoperatively but ongoing analgesia will be provided by other means. With both a rapid onset and an ultra-short half-life it is readily titrated to changes in levels of surgical stimulus, and is thus especially useful in neonates with haemodynamic instability. It is given by infusion at doses up to 0.25micrograms/kg/minute; the dose is limited by potential for chest wall rigidity. However, unlike fentanyl, remifentanil will not accumulate even in renal or liver failure (Ainsworth, 2015).

Paracetamol

Paracetamol has been safely used in preterm and term babies and is a useful adjunct to opioid analgesia and nerve blockade after both major and minor surgery. Its analgesic effects are due to the inhibition of prostaglandin synthesis in the central nervous system. Single doses given orally or IV can achieve therapeutic serum concentrations and may be repeated, but rectally a loading dose is required, followed by further doses at intervals if adequate serum levels are to be achieved (Anderson et al., 2002). Total dose should not exceed 30–60mg/kg per 24-hour period. Doses should be further reduced in neonates with evidence of impaired hepatic function, particularly those with significant jaundice (Ainsworth, 2015).

Non-steroidal anti-inflammatory drugs

These drugs are not recommended in the neonatal period as they can interfere with platelet function and hence blood clotting mechanisms, and can furthermore compromise renal function.

Local anaesthesia

Local anaesthetic techniques are invaluable in neonates, reducing or avoiding the need for opioids with their attendant risks in this high-risk group. All of the local anaesthetic techniques utilised in adults are feasible in neonates. The free (biologically active) fraction of local anaesthetic drugs is higher than that in older infants due to a reduced concentration of plasma-binding proteins; doses should thus be adjusted accordingly (Sale et al., 2012). Levobupivacaine is the most commonly used drug, for which the dose should not exceed 2mg/kg. Levobupivacaine is considered safer than bupivacaine because of its lower potential to cause cardiac arrhythmias in overdose or when inadvertently injected into a blood vessel (Burlacu and Buggy, 2008).

Wound infiltration

Wound infiltration is a simple and safe method of providing postoperative analgesia. It has been found to be effective following pyloromyotomy (Walker, 2014) and is a useful alternative to ilio-inguinal nerve block for inguinal herniotomy. The opportunity to use this valuable technique in neonatal surgery should never be neglected; there is, however, no current evidence indicating that this reduces postoperative analgesia requirements (Leelanukrom et al., 2012).

Peripheral nerve blocks

A wide range of peripheral nerve blocks are potentially applicable to neonatal surgery, but in practice only a few are commonly utilised. They are generally used in conjunction with general anaesthesia and can provide very effective, long-lasting postoperative analgesia. Dorsal penile nerve block is very useful for penile surgery, especially circumcision, and has in fact been used as the sole anaesthetic technique for this procedure (Teunkens et al., 2018). Blockade of the ilio-inguinal nerve provides very effective analgesia after groin surgery, particularly inguinal herniotomy (Ahmad and Greenaway, 2018). An increase in availability and advances in ultrasound technology have allowed these blocks to be performed with greater accuracy and have facilitated other blocks such as transversus abdominus plane blocks to be performed on neonates. Ultrasound is also being used to confirm catheter placement for some neuro-axial blocks.

Central (neuro-axial) blocks

Local anaesthetic drugs introduced into the epidural or subarachnoid space can produce anaesthesia and analgesia of the lower limbs, abdomen and even thorax depending on the technique and the dose and volume of local anaesthetic used. Such techniques are becoming increasingly popular in neonates, as they allow major surgery to be undertaken under very light or even without general anaesthesia (Walker and Yaksh, 2012). In addition, they provide excellent postoperative analgesia, eliminating or reducing the need for opioid analgesia and thus potentially avoiding mechanical ventilation after surgery.

Caudal epidural anaesthesia

Single-shot caudal anaesthesia is suitable for all surgical procedures below the umbilicus, and is mainly indicated in neonates for inguinal herniotomy, lower limb surgery and genito-urinary surgery (figure 20.3). It is a very simple technique and major complications are rare. Continuous caudal epidural anaesthesia involves the insertion of a catheter into the caudal space, often under ultrasound guidance. The catheter may be threaded in a **cephalad** (towards the head) direction to a lumbar or thoracic level. An infusion of local anaesthetic can then be used to provide analgesia following major abdominal and thoracic surgery (Maitra et al., 2014).

Lumbar and thoracic epidural anaesthesia

Lumbar and thoracic epidural blockade is less popular than the caudal block because it is technically more difficult to perform, needs specially designed equipment and has the potential for more serious complications. These complications include inadvertent total spinal anaesthesia or IV injection of local anaesthetic, with the potential for convulsions and profound cardiovascular collapse. Other rare complications include epidural haema-toma or abscess. The UK national paediatric epidural audit revealed 96 complications

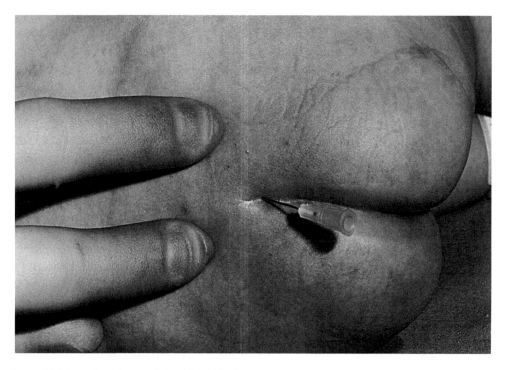

Figure 20.3 Insertion of a caudal epidural block

out of 10,633 epidurals performed during a five-year period; of these, only five were classed as serious, and only one child had lasting effects 12 months later (Llewellyn and Moriarty, 2007).

The haemodynamic instability commonly seen with epidural anaesthesia in adult practice (especially hypotension due to sympathetic nervous system blockade) is very unusual in the infant age group. This has been attributed to incomplete maturation of the sympathetic nervous system in the newborn resulting in very low levels of basal vascular tone. Epidural analgesia is now being increasingly used to provide excellent analgesia after abdominal and thoracic surgery. Though it is difficult to assess accurately the level of sensory block in a neonate, an adequate level can be assumed if the infant appears comfortable, while an excessively high block may be associated with an increased incidence of bradycardia or respiratory impairment.

Spinal anaesthesia

Spinal anaesthesia involves performing a lumbar puncture followed by injection of local anaesthetic into the subarachnoid space. It is technically easier than an epidural, has a rapid onset and provides complete motor and sensory blockade. The main disadvantages are a short and variable duration of action, which is rarely more than one hour. Spinal blockade is a useful technique for inguinal herniotomy in ex-preterm neonates where it is associated with a lower incidence of postoperative bradycardia and desaturation than following general anaesthesia (Whiteside and Wildsmith, 2005). It may also be used in combination with epidural anaesthesia for major abdominal surgery.

FLUID THERAPY

Fluid administration during surgery must take into account the maintenance requirements of the infant, the loss of fluid from sequestration and evaporation, and blood loss (Cunliffe, 2007). The goal of intraoperative fluid replacement is to maintain cardiovascular stability and organ perfusion, though caution should be taken to prevent fluid overload as this could potentially cause cardiac failure secondary to the reopening of a PDA.

Maintenance fluids

The fluid deficit generated during the fasting period should be replaced during surgery in addition to ongoing maintenance requirements (Cunliffe, 2007). Opinions vary as to the best intravenous fluid to use, with much debate surrounding the problem of hyponatraemia caused or exacerbated by overzealous perioperative administration of hypotonic fluids (Paut and Lacroix, 2006). The most recent guidelines from the National Institute for Health and Care Excellence (NICE) on fluid therapy in children recommend the use of isotonic fluids making solutions such as 4% with 0.18% sodium chloride virtually obsolete (NICE, 2015). In UK practice, very premature infants would generally be maintained on 10% glucose solutions with sodium supplements guided by serum sodium levels. 5% glucose with 0.45% sodium chloride and more recently 5% glucose with 0.9% saline are in general use for older infants. However, the hormonal stress response to surgery usually raises blood glucose concentrations in neonates (Yuki et al., 2017) and hyperglycaemia may occur with glucose-containing fluids. Hyper- and hypoglycaemia are hazardous for the neonatal brain, and so intravenous fluid therapy should always be guided by regular blood glucose monitoring.

Replacement of fluid lost by evaporation/sequestration

During surgery, water is lost by evaporation from the operative site and protein-rich fluid is sequestered in the surrounding tissues as a result of surgical trauma, depleting the intravascular fluid volume. In infants, these fluid losses during abdominal surgery are estimated to be between 6 and 10mL/kg per hour, 4–7mL/kg per hour in thoracic surgery, and only 1–2mL/kg per hour in superficial procedures (including neurosurgery; Cunliffe, 2007). This should be replaced by Hartmann's solution or 0.9% sodium chloride.

Replacement of blood loss

The preoperative Hb concentration and blood loss perioperatively will determine whether blood loss is replaced by blood or nonsanguinous fluid. The estimated blood volume (EBV) should be calculated (90mL/kg for a preterm baby, 85mL/kg for a term baby). The maximal allowable blood loss (ABL) can then be calculated from the formula:

$$ABL = \frac{EBV \times initial\ Hb - lowest\ acceptable\ Hb}{initial\ Hb}$$

The lowest acceptable Hb will depend on clinical circumstances. Blood loss can be determined by accurate weighing of surgical swabs and noting suction losses, and replaced with a colloid or crystalloid solution until the maximal ABL is reached. Thereafter, blood should be used. There is no evidence to show that colloid solutions are superior to crystalloids in the treatment of hypotension in neonates (So et al., 1997). There is also some evidence to suggest that the physiological response to sepsis and surgery enhances the rate at which colloids are extravasated into the interstitial space. The most commonly used colloid in neonates is still 4.5% human albumin solution, although controversy regarding its safety has led to the increased use of other synthetic colloids, including Gelofusine® and Haemaccel®, although these may be associated with an increased risk of anaphylaxis. Synthetic starches are no longer recommended due to their association with renal failure and an increase in mortality (European Medicines Agency, 2013). Replacement of clotting factors by the use of fresh frozen plasma (FFP) should commence earlier rather than later due to the relatively deficient clotting systems in neonates. Platelet infusions may be required in cases of massive blood transfusion or severe sepsis.

Assessment of the adequacy of volume replacement can be gauged clinically. Changes in pulse and blood pressure are both unreliable guides to hypovolaemia in neonates. Assessment of the peripheral circulation gives far more information: capillary refill time should be rapid (less than two seconds) and extremities should be pink and warm. Prolonged refill time and increased core–peripheral temperature gradient are important clinical signs, suggesting volume depletion (Ussat et al., 2015). Measurement of urine output and central venous pressure may also provide useful information, particularly during prolonged surgery or where large blood and fluid losses are anticipated. Arterial or venous lactate measurement, which is a marker of tissue perfusion, may also be useful in guiding fluid therapy.

ANAESTHETIC EQUIPMENT

Neonatal anaesthesia requires specialised equipment. All equipment should be thoroughly checked before commencing any anaesthetic.

Airway equipment

Many of the items of equipment required for airway maintenance are available in a variety of sizes to suit all infants. It is not always possible to predict which will be appropriate, so a full range should be immediately available for every case.

- *Face masks* Face masks should have a low dead space to prevent rebreathing of expired gases. Several types are available: Nowadays a circular cushioned rim-type face mask is used which many anaesthetists (and neonatal intensive care staff) find easier to manipulate in small infants (see figure 20.4). For slightly larger babies a more tapered mask may be preferred. Care must be taken that the mask is not covering the baby's eyes, as there is a risk of causing corneal abrasions.
- *Oropharyngeal airways* Difficulties maintaining the airway in an anaesthetised neonate may be lessened if an oropharyngeal airway is used, but will be increased if one of an incorrect size is chosen. Too small an airway may fail to overcome airway obstruction

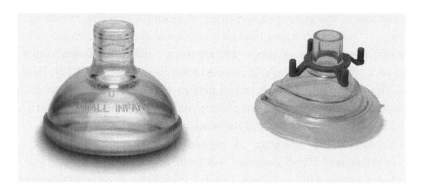

Figure 20.4 Anaesthetic face masks (Source: Intersurgical)

due to the tongue falling backwards, whereas too large an airway may produce airway obstruction itself or induce laryngospasm or vomiting in a semi-conscious baby. The size is estimated by placing the airway against the baby's chin; with the flange at the middle of the baby's lips with the tip of the airway reaching the angle of the mandible (Wyllie et al., 2016).

■ *Laryngoscope* The infant larynx lies higher and more anteriorly than in older children or adults. In addition, the **epiglottis** is large and leaf-shaped and can obscure the laryngeal inlet. The best view of the larynx is obtained by using a laryngoscope with a short, straight blade. In addition to the standard straight blades, there now exists a range of indirect video laryngoscopes available for neonatal use. These are of particular use in cases where tracheal intubation proves difficult using conventional techniques (Wyllie et al., 2016).

■ *Tracheal tubes* Historically, only uncuffed endotracheal tubes were used for neonates. More recently, with the advent of tubes with high volume low-pressure cuffs made of ultra-thin polyurethane (Microcuff™), an increasing number of paediatric anaesthetists are choosing to use a cuffed tube especially for laparoscopic and thorascopic procedures (Thomas et al., 2016). All tubes should be parallel-sided, radio-opaque and marked at 1cm intervals from the tip. Each tube is sized according to the internal diameter. The approximate sizes and lengths of tracheal tubes according to the weight of the infant are shown in table 20.2. Microcuff™ tubes are not recommended for babies below 3kg (Thomas et al., 2016). Plain tubes are suitable for most procedures and can be used via the oral or nasal route, though 'south-facing' preformed RAE™ oral tubes are popular for orofacial and neurosurgery and 'north-facing' preformed RAE™ oral tubes are often used for other procedures because they are easy to secure in position and are less likely to kink (figure 20.5).

■ *Other equipment* In addition to the equipment mentioned above, small Magill forceps should be available for insertion of nasal tracheal tubes or throat packs and intubation

TABLE 20.2 SIZE AND LENGTH OF TRACHEAL TUBES FOR NEONATES

Body weight (kg)	Internal diameter (mm)	External diameter (mm)	Length at lips (cm)	Length at nares (cm)
< 0.7	2.0	2.9	5.0	6.0
0.7–1	2.5	3.7	5.5	7.0
1.1–2	3.0	4.4	6.0	7.5
2.1–3	3.0	4.4	7.0	9.0
3.1–3.5	3.0	4.4	8.5	10.5
> 3.5	3.5	4.8	9.0	11.0

(adapted from Peutrell and Weir, 1996)

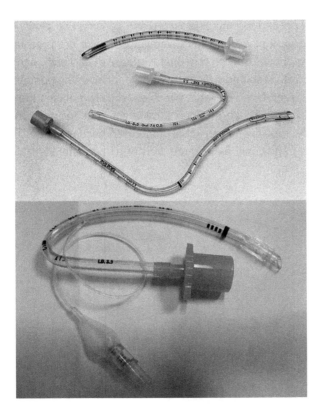

Figure 20.5 Tracheal tubes (Source of Microcuff™ tube: Louise Oduro-Dominah)

stylets narrow enough to fit through the smallest tracheal tube should be available to aid a difficult intubation. Nasal intubation is rarely performed; although the chance of tube dislodgement or kinking is lower with this route, the risk of causing troublesome sinusitis is increased.

■ *Breathing systems* The breathing system provides the means of delivering the anaesthetic gases and vapours to the patient. In a neonate, it should be lightweight, easy to assemble, present minimal resistance to breathing and have as small a dead space as possible. The most popular system in the UK is the Jackson–Rees modification of the Ayre's T-piece (figure 20.6). This can be used for spontaneous or positive-pressure ventilation. It can also be used to apply positive end-expiratory pressure (PEEP) or CPAP, manoeuvres which are essential in neonates to prevent collapse of the small airways and improve oxygenation (Wyllie et al., 2016).

■ *Ventilators* Neonates are ventilated intraoperatively either by hand or by attachment to a mechanical ventilator. Manual ventilation is popular in this patient group, as it provides the anaesthetist with a 'feel' of the compliance of the lungs. There is a danger, however, of applying too much pressure and causing pulmonary barotrauma or even a pneumothorax. T-piece occluding ventilators which are pressure-limited (including the majority of those used on a neonatal intensive care unit), can be used in the very sick neonate with respiratory disease. More popular in the operating theatre setting is the 'bag squeezer'-type ventilator, which essentially replaces the anaesthetist's hand squeezing the bag. These produce a constant flow and tidal volume unless higher pressures are required, when most become pressure-limited. For reasons already mentioned, an additional feature required of all neonatal ventilators is the facility to apply PEEP.

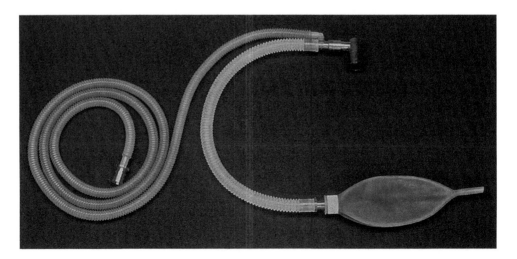

Figure 20.6 T-piece breathing system

Equipment for maintenance of body temperature

The importance of maintaining an infant's body temperature cannot be overemphasised (see chapter 11). In addition to a warm operating theatre, several supportive measures are available.

■ *Warming mattresses* These are essential to reduce conductive heat loss through a cold operating table. The surface temperature should not exceed 39°C to prevent skin burns. An alternative is the hot air mattress, which surrounds the infant in a microclimate of warm air (Blum and Cote, 2009). Body temperature must be monitored whenever active warming is used, to avoid hyperthermia.

■ *Humidifiers* Humidification of inspired anaesthetic gases reduces evaporative heat loss from the respiratory tract and may be either active or passive. Active humidification requires a water bath with careful temperature control. This method is commonly used in the neonatal intensive care unit. Passive humidifiers are devices with a high surface area that allow an exchange of heat and moisture from exhalation to inhalation. They are included in the anaesthetic breathing system in close proximity to the tracheal tube. They have been shown to be as efficient as a heated humidifier when used in ventilated neonates over a six-hour period (McNulty and Eyre, 2015).

■ *Other methods* All fluids administered should be warmed to 37°C. In addition, the infant can be wrapped in cotton wool, aluminium foil or plastic sheets (such as food grade plastic wrap) to prevent radiant and convective heat loss. Particular attention should be paid to the head, which is relatively larger in neonates and exposes a big surface area for heat loss.

Equipment for intravenous fluid administration

■ *Intravenous cannulae* For reliable venous access, an over-the-needle, plastic cannula should be used. These are available in sizes as small as 26G. For all but the most minor surgical procedures, most neonatal anaesthetists would ensure that there are two functioning IV cannulae in situ.

■ *Fluid administration sets* The small volume of infusate required by neonates makes syringe pumps and other sorts of infusion devices preferable for the administration of maintenance fluids. They should have a volume limiter and a pressure alarm. Administration of fluid boluses, including colloid and blood products, is most easily achieved manually by a syringe attached via a three-way tap, provided care is taken not to introduce any bubbles, which could traverse the still-patent foramen ovale, causing systemic air emboli. This is particularly the case if nitrous oxide is used during the anaesthetic as this gas will cause expansion of any air bubbles and exacerbate the potential for embolisation.

ANAESTHETIC MONITORING

Although there is no substitute for the continuous presence of a well-trained anaesthetist, there is evidence to suggest that intraoperative adverse events can be avoided by physiological monitoring of the neonate (Chandrashekhar et al., 2015). The monitoring modalities which should be used as a minimum in any baby undergoing surgery are discussed in the following sections.

Cardiovascular monitoring

■ *Electrocardiography* Cardiac output in neonates is rate-dependent. Bradycardia leads to a fall in cardiac output and hypotension, whereas tachycardia may be a sign of hypovolaemia, pain or inadequate anaesthesia. Although a very useful monitor, the ECG does not give any indication of the adequacy of vital organ perfusion.
■ *Blood pressure* The oscillometric method and Doppler method of non-invasive blood pressure (BP) measurement are most commonly used in neonatal practice. The oscillometric method measures mean BP accurately and derives systolic and diastolic pressure using a computer algorithm. It is a reliable method in neonates provided the correct cuff size is used (cuff width to arm circumference ratio should be approximately 0.5; Takci et al., 2012). The Doppler method uses an arm cuff and an ultrasonic transducer. This is placed over the radial or brachial artery and detects changes in vessel wall movement to record systolic and diastolic BP. Invasive arterial pressure should be measured via a catheter inserted into the umbilical artery or a peripheral artery when rapid fluid shifts, particularly large blood losses or sudden haemodynamic changes, are anticipated (for example, during cardiac surgery). Indwelling arterial access also allows blood gases and other parameters such as blood glucose and haematocrit to be easily monitored during major and prolonged surgery. Limb perfusion must be closely monitored when arterial catheters are in situ.
■ *Praecordial and oesophageal stethoscope* A praecordial stethoscope is a device secured over the left sternal border. An oesophageal stethoscope is a soft catheter with holes in its distal end positioned in the mid-oesophagus. Both allow continuous monitoring of heart and breath sounds, though they do not give accurate information about the adequacy of cardiac output or pulmonary ventilation. Neither of these devices is in common use in contemporary UK practice.

Respiratory monitoring

■ *Pulse oximetry* Pulse oximetry is essential in the monitoring of neonates. It provides continuous, non-invasive beat-to-beat monitoring of oxygen saturation and heart rate. Positioned in neonates over the lateral border of the foot or **medial** border of the hand, it also provides information about peripheral perfusion and therefore cardiac output and volume status. Limitations of pulse oximetry are interference from diathermy and motion. It does not accurately detect hyperoxia and may be inaccurate at oxygen saturations below 75% (Nitzan et al., 2014).

■ *Capnography* A capnograph measures the change in carbon dioxide (CO_2) with each breath by sampling expired gas. In healthy neonates the end-tidal CO_2 concentration closely approximates arterial PCO_2. The value of end-tidal CO_2 is influenced not only by arterial PCO_2 but also by cardiac output and ventilation. It is, therefore, a useful monitor of cardiovascular status in addition to the adequacy of ventilation, including inadvertent disconnection from mechanical ventilation.

Temperature monitoring

Temperature should be monitored in all neonates undergoing surgery. Core temperature can be estimated at several sites, including oesophagus, rectum, tympanic membrane or nasopharynx. Oesophageal probes are the most convenient. Skin temperature should also be measured, because the gradient between core and peripheral temperature gives a useful indication of the adequacy of cardiac output (Sessler, 2008).

POSTOPERATIVE CARE

All small infants require close observation and monitoring in the postoperative period. This may be in a high dependency area or in an intensive care unit, depending on the prematurity of the infant, the surgical condition and other coexisting medical problems. As with all postoperative patients, adequate analgesia must be provided; this may be achieved by several methods which have already been described. Fluid administration should be tailored to the needs of the infant, and measures taken to maintain body and peripheral temperature (Lee et al., 2008). There are certain postoperative problems that are encountered far more frequently in infants. These include apnoeic episodes, post-extubation stridor and respiratory insufficiency requiring ventilatory support.

Postoperative apnoeas

The neonate, particularly the preterm infant, breathes irregularly. Periodic respiration in which breathing and apnoea alternate is common; however, cessation of breathing for longer than 15 seconds (or less if associated with bradycardia or desaturation) is significant and abnormal. Neonates are prone to develop apnoeas following general anaesthesia, the risk rising with increasing prematurity and with the use of intraoperative opioids (Walther-Larsen and Rasmussen, 2006). Regional anaesthesia without sedation reduces the risk significantly. High-dose caffeine (10mg/kg IV) may also be protective, although this is not common practice in the child managed postoperatively on a neonatal intensive care unit. Most apnoeas can be treated successfully with stimulation and oxygen. Rarely, CPAP or mechanical ventilation is necessary if apnoeic episodes are recurrent in the postoperative period. Apnoea monitoring is recommended for infants especially if managed on a ward postoperatively (Kurth and Coté, 2015).

Post-extubation stridor

Stridor may rarely occur, either immediately or within a few hours of tracheal extubation. It is usually due to subglottic oedema caused by trauma exerted on the tracheal mucosa by an incorrectly sized tracheal tube. The risk is greatest if there is no leak around an uncuffed tracheal tube following insertion, if the tube moves within the trachea during surgery and if multiple intubation attempts were necessary (Infosino, 2002). Possible therapies include the provision of CPAP via nasal prongs, inhalation of nebulised adrenaline, or IV dexamethasone (Couser et al., 1992; Davis and Henderson-Smart, 2001). If reintubation is required, a smaller tracheal tube should be used (Infosino, 2002), and an audible gas leak around the tube should be present before it is subsequently removed.

Assessing the need for postoperative ventilation

A key issue in early postoperative management is the increased need for postoperative ventilatory support. Both pre- and postoperative factors are important in assessing the need for postoperative ventilation.

■ *Preoperative factors* Ventilatory drive is immature in neonates and puts the premature infant at increased risk of postoperative apnoeas; for the term infant this risk applies up to 46 weeks' postconceptional age, and for the ex-premature infant for as long as 60 weeks' postconceptional age. Infants who have had repeated problems with apnoeic spells are more likely to require respiratory support postoperatively. In addition, common problems of prematurity, such as RDS and PDA affect the efficiency of pulmonary gas exchange and make postoperative respiratory support more likely (Rocha et al., 2018). Other pre-existing problems such as congenital heart disease and airway problems such as laryngomalacia ('floppy larynx') make postoperative respiratory insufficiency more likely.

■ *Postoperative factors* Respiratory insufficiency is likely to occur following a prolonged anaesthetic due to the residual effects of anaesthetic and analgesic drugs (particularly opioids) on ventilatory drive. Abdominal distension following abdominal surgery may compromise diaphragmatic function and therefore effective spontaneous ventilation. Other factors, including hypothermia, acidosis and anaemia, may also be indications for a period of postoperative ventilation.

Signs of respiratory distress

The assessment of postoperative respiratory distress is largely clinical. A respiratory rate of greater than 60 breaths per minute should alert the anaesthetist to the possibility of respiratory insufficiency, particularly if associated with signs of increased work of breathing demonstrated by grunting respiration, nasal flaring and the presence of subcostal, intercostal and substernal recession. Restlessness, irritability, apnoeic episodes or failure to regain consciousness may also reflect hypoxaemia or hypercapnia.

Any suspicion of postoperative respiratory insufficiency should prompt blood gas and acid-base analysis. Other investigations, including chest radiography, may be indicated, but if there is any suggestion that ventilatory support is required on clinical grounds, this should be instituted without delay. This may initially be by bag and mask ventilation, and subsequently nasal CPAP or reintubation and mechanical ventilation.

THE NURSE'S ROLE IN ANAESTHESIA IN NEONATAL CARE

Neonatal nurses working in the surgical field play a critical role in monitoring and assessment before and after any anaesthetic; therefore, they should have a sound understanding of the principles of anaesthesia, particularly in relation to the effects of agents used, to enable them to identify abnormal signs and symptoms in the infant. In turn, this will assist an understanding of how to effectively manage any adverse reaction in conjunction with the multidisciplinary team. Nurses are present at the cot side on a 24-hour basis, and so are in a unique position to identify any observable changes in a baby.

In addition, during any procedure, the neonatal nurse has various key responsibilities, which can be seen in box 20.1.

BOX 20.1 THE NURSE'S ROLE IN NEONATAL ANAESTHESIA

Monitor: Monitoring of vital signs before anaesthetic is important to provide baseline values before any drugs or procedures are carried out.

Alert: Assistance must be sought immediately if any adverse reactions to anaesthetic drugs/analgesics/sedatives are suspected – e.g. bradycardia, apnoea, changes to blood pressure and circulation, muscle paralysis/twitching and malignant hyperthermia.

Prepare: In neonatal unit-based intubation events, neonatal nurses are involved in preparing emergency equipment and drugs.

Act: If any interventions are required, be ready to assist colleagues.

Document: The history of events should be recorded and documented in line with the regulatory body guidance (Nursing and Midwifery Council, 2018).

Report: Should an adverse reaction be suspected, it must be reported.

(adapted from Cowley, 2013)

Finally, one of the key roles of the neonatal nurse in relation to anaesthesia is preparation and support of the parents. Parents and care providers alike should be aware of the potential risks involved in this area of practice, and families should be fully informed about all stages. Parents must be able to ask questions (Weiss et al., 2016) and the neonatal nurse should be able to offer information and reinforce that given by the anaesthetist during the preoperative and postoperative phases of the surgical intervention.

CONCLUSION

Many full-term neonates undergo anaesthesia and surgery uneventfully. Problems are most frequently encountered in sick and premature infants, particularly if cardiorespiratory insufficiency is present preoperatively. Care of these infants requires a multidisciplinary approach by skilled personnel. The importance of communication between the anaesthetist and the neonatal nursing and medical team cannot be overemphasised and is essential if the best possible outcome is to be achieved.

CASE STUDY

CASE STUDIES

Case study 1: The infant with congenital diaphragmatic hernia

Leo is a term infant who has suffered a respiratory arrest soon after delivery. There is a suspected diagnosis of congenital diaphragmatic hernia due to his scaphoid abdomen and worsening respiratory distress.

Q.1. What is the nurse's role in intubating and ventilating this infant for further management on the neonatal unit?

Q.2. What preoperative preparation will this infant and his parents require and who will be involved in this?

Q.3. What specific information will the parents need about the pending anaesthesia for their baby?

Case study 2: The preterm infant with a patent ductus arteriosus

Annie, a preterm infant (born at 25 weeks), returned from theatre 2 hours ago to the neonatal unit following surgery to ligate a patent ductus arteriosus. She is ventilated, and it is noted that she is tachycardic with minimal spontaneous respiratory effort. Her blood gas shows a mixed acidosis.

Q.1. What are the possible reasons for these observations?

Q.2. What intraoperative information would be useful in managing this infant?

Q.3 What do you need to explain to the parents?

Case study 3: The premature infant undergoing bowel surgery

Holly is a 5-week-old infant who was born at 26 weeks' gestation. She required ventilation for 20 days and is still receiving nasal CPAP. Over the past 48 hours her condition has deteriorated with abdominal distension, increasing oxygen requirements and deranged blood clotting indices. She has a diagnosis of necrotising enterocolitis and now requires a laparotomy at the regional paediatric surgical centre 40 miles away.

Q.1. What additional ventilatory support is likely to be required for transport of this infant?

Q.2. What blood products will need to be ordered prior to her going to theatre?

Q.3. What are the challenges for the anaesthetist and the nursing team in the intraoperative management of this case?

Q.4. Is any special monitoring and nursing care required in the postoperative period?

Q.5. What assessment and methods may be used to provide adequate pain relief in the postoperative period?

For suggested answer guides to the questions posed in these case studies, please refer to the web-based companion site specific to this chapter (see URL below).

WEB-BASED RESOURCES

For further information, online resources and greater detail on the case studies featured in this chapter go to www.routledge.com/cw/nicnursing

References

Ahmad, N., & Greenaway, S. (2018). Anaesthesia for inguinal hernia repair in the newborn or ex-premature infant. *BJA Education. 18*(7), 211–217.

Ainsworth, S. B. (Ed.). (2015). *Neonatal Formulary 7: Drug use in pregnancy and the first year of life.* (7th Edition). Chichester: John Wiley & Sons.

Anand, K. J., Sippell, W. G., Schofield, N. M., & Aynsley-Green, A. (1988). Does halothane anaesthesia decrease the metabolic and endocrine stress responses of newborn infants undergoing operation? *British Medical Journal (Clinical Research Edition)*, *296*(6623), 668–672.

Anderson, B. J., van Lingen, R. A., Hansen, T. G., Lin, Y. C., & Holford, N. H. (2002). Acetaminophen Developmental Pharmacokinetics in Premature Neonates and Infants: A Pooled Population Analysis. *Anesthesiology: The Journal of the American Society of Anesthesiologists*, *96*(6), 1336–1345.

Bell, G., & Homer, R. (2015). Equipment in paediatric anaesthesia. *Update in Anaesthesia*. *30*(1),13–22.

Bellieni, C. V. (2012). Pain assessment in human fetus and infants. *The AAPS Journal*, *14*(3), 456–461.

Blum, R., & Cote, C. (2009). Pediatric equipment. In Blum, R., & Cote, C. (Eds.) *A Practice of Anaesthesia for Infants and Children*. Philadelphia: Saunders Elsevier.

Burlacu, C. L., & Buggy, D. J. (2008). Update on local anesthetics: Focus on levobupivacaine. *Therapeutics and Clinical Risk Management*, *4*(2), 381.

Chandrashekhar, S., Davis, L., & Challands, J. (2015). Anaesthesia for neonatal emergency laparotomy. *BJA Education*, *15*(4), 194–198.

Chiao, S., & Zuo, Z. (2014). A double-edged sword: Volatile anesthetic effects on the neonatal brain. *Brain Sciences*, *4*(2), 273–294.

Couser, R. J., Ferrara, T. B., Falde, B., Johnson, K., Schilling, C. G., & Hoekstra, R. E. (1992). Effectiveness of dexamethasone in preventing extubation failure in preterm infants at increased risk for airway edema. *The Journal of Pediatrics*, *121*(4), 591–596.

Cowley S. (2013). The nurse's role in a suxamethonium-based neonatal rapid sequence intubation. *Infant*. *9*(6): 207–11.

Cunliffe, M. (2007). *APA Consensus Guideline on Perioperative Fluid Management in Children*. London: Association of Paediatric Anaesthetists.

Dagle, J. M., Lepp, N. T., Cooper, M. E., Schaa, K. L., Kelsey, K. J., Orr, K. L., ... & Marazita, M. L. (2009). Determination of genetic predisposition to patent ductus arteriosus in preterm infants. *Pediatrics*, *123*(4), 1116.

Davidson, A. J., Disma, N., De Graaff, J. C., Withington, D. E., Dorris, L., Bell, G., ... & Hardy, P. (2016). Neurodevelopmental outcome at 2 years of age after general anaesthesia and awake-regional anaesthesia in infancy (GAS): An international multicentre, randomised controlled trial. *The Lancet*, *387*(10015), 239–250.

Davis, P. G., & Henderson-Smart, D. J. (2001). Intravenous dexamethasone for extubation of newborn infants. *Cochrane Database of Systematic Reviews*, Issue 4. Art. No.: CD000308. DOI: 10.1002/14651858.CD000308

Disma, N., Mameli, L. Bonfiglio, R., Zanaboni, C., & Tuo, P. (2016). Neonatal Anesthesia. In Buonocore, G., Bracci, R., & Weindling, M. *Neonatology*. New York: Springer Publishing Company.

Eicher, C., Seitz, G., Bevot, A., Moll, M., Goelz, R., Arand, J., ... & Lacaze-Masmonteil, T. (2012). The 'Effects of transfusion thresholds on neurocognitive outcome of extremely low birth-weight infants (ETTNO)'study: Background, aims, and study protocol. *Neonatology*, *101*(4), 301–305.

Emerson, B. M., Wrigley, S. R., & Newton, M. (1998). Pre-operative fasting for paediatric anaesthesia: A survey of current practice. *Anaesthesia*, *53*(4), 326–330.

European Medicines Agency (2013). *Assessment report for solutions containing hydroxyethyl starch EMA/66764/2013*. www.ema.europa.eu/en/documents/referral/hydroxyethyl-starch-article-31-referral-prac-assessment-report_en.pdf.

Fahnenstich, H., Steffan, J., Kau, N., & Bartmann, P. (2000). Fentanyl-induced chest wall rigidity and laryngospasm in preterm and term infants. *Critical Care Medicine*, *28*(3), 836–839.

Finer, N., & Leone, T. (2009). Oxygen saturation monitoring for the preterm infant: The evidence basis for current practice. *Pediatric Research*, *65*(4), 375.

Flick, R. P., Nemergut, M. E., Christensen, K., & Hansen, T. G. (2014). Anesthetic-related Neurotoxicity in the Young and Outcome Measures The Devil Is in the Details. *Anesthesiology: The Journal of the American Society of Anesthesiologists*, *120*(6), 1303–1305.

Friesen, R. H., & Williams, G. D. (2008). Anesthetic management of children with pulmonary arterial hypertension. *Pediatric Anesthesia, 18*(3), 208–216.

Frykholm, P., Schindler, E., Sümpelmann, R., Walker, R., & Weiss, M. (2018). Preoperative fasting in children: Review of existing guidelines and recent developments. *British Journal of Anaesthesia, 120*(3), 469–474.

Greenough, A., Premkumar, M., & Patel, D. (2008). Ventilatory strategies for the extremely premature infant. *Pediatric Anesthesia, 18*(5), 371–377.

Hackman, P. (2001). Recognizing and understanding the cold-stressed term infant. *Neonatal Network, 20*(8), 35–41.

Hall, R. W., & Anand, K. J. (2014). Pain management in newborns. *Clinics in Perinatology, 41*(4), 895–924.

Henderson-Smart, D. J., & Steer, P. A. (2001). Prophylactic caffeine to prevent postoperative apnoea following general anaesthesia in preterm infants. *Cochrane Database of Systematic Reviews*, Issue 4. Art. No.: CD000048. DOI: 10.1002/14651858.CD000048

Higgins, R. D., Patel, R. M., & Josephson, C. D. (2016). Preoperative anemia and neonates. *JAMA Pediatrics, 170*(9), 835–836.

Ibrahim, C. P. H., & Yoxall, C. W. (2009). Use of plastic bags to prevent hypothermia at birth in preterm infants – do they work at lower gestations? *Acta Pædiatrica, 98*(2), 256–260.

Infosino, A. (2002). Pediatric upper airway and congenital anomalies. *Anesthesiology Clinics of North America, 20*(4), 747–766.

Ivanova, I., & Pittaway, A. (2014). Principles of anaesthesia for term neonates: An updated practical guide. *Anaesthesia & Intensive Care Medicine, 15*(3), 103–106.

Kearns, G. L., Abdel-Rahman, S. M., Alander, S. W., Blowey, D. L., Leeder, J. S., & Kauffman, R. E. (2003). Developmental pharmacology–drug disposition, action, and therapy in infants and children. *New England Journal of Medicine, 349*(12), 1157–1167.

King, H., & Booker, P. D. (2004). General principles of neonatal anaesthesia. *Current Anaesthesia & Critical Care, 15*(4–5), 302–308.

Kurth, C. D., & Coté, C. J. (2015). Postoperative Apnea in Former Preterm Infants General Anesthesia or Spinal Anesthesia–Do We Have an Answer? *Anesthesiology: The Journal of the American Society of Anesthesiologists, 123*(1), 15–17.

Laptook, A. R., & Watkinson, M. (2008). Temperature management in the delivery room. *Seminars in Fetal and Neonatal Medicine, 13*(6), 383–391.

Lee, H. C., Ho, Q. T., & Rhine, W. D. (2008). A quality improvement project to improve admission temperatures in very low birth weight infants. *Journal of Perinatology, 28*(11), 754.

Lee, J. H., Zhang, J., Wei, L., & Yu, S. P. (2015). Neurodevelopmental implications of the general anesthesia in neonate and infants. *Experimental Neurology, 272*, 50–60.

Leelanukrom, R., Suraseranivongse, S., Boonrukwanich, V., & Wechwinij, S. (2012). Effect of wound infiltration with bupivacaine on postoperative analgesia in neonates and infants undergoing major abdominal surgery: A pilot randomized controlled trial. *Journal of Anesthesia, 26*(4), 541–544.

Llewellyn, N., & Moriarty, A. (2007). The national pediatric epidural audit. *Pediatric Anesthesia, 17*(6), 520–533.

McGregor, K. (2017). Principles of anaesthesia for term neonates. *Anaesthesia & Intensive Care Medicine, 18*(2), 75–78.

McNulty, G., & Eyre, L. (2015). Humidification in anaesthesia and critical care. *BJA Education, 15*(3), 131–135.

Maitra, S., Baidya, D. K., Pawar, D. K., Arora, M. K., & Khanna, P. (2014). Epidural anesthesia and analgesia in the neonate: A review of current evidences. *Journal of Anesthesia, 28*(5), 768–779.

Martin, L. D. (2017). The basic principles of anesthesia for the neonate. *Revista Colombiana de Anestesiología, 45*(1), 54–61.

New, H. V., Berryman, J., Bolton-Maggs, P. H., Cantwell, C., Chalmers, E. A., Davies, T., … & Stanworth, S. J. (2016). Guidelines on transfusion for fetuses, neonates and older children. *British Journal of Haematology, 175*(5), 784–828.

National Institute for Health and Care Excellence (2015). *Intravenous fluid therapy in children and young people in hospital.* NICE.

Nitzan, M., Romem, A., & Koppel, R. (2014). Pulse oximetry: Fundamentals and technology update. *Medical Devices (Auckland, NZ), 7*, 231.

Nursing and Midwifery Council (NMC) (2018). *Professional standards of practice and behaviour for nurses, midwives and nursing associates.* London: NMC. www.nmc.org.uk/ standards/ code/.

Paediatric Formulary Committee. (2018). *BNF for Children 2018–2019.* London: BMJ Group, Pharmaceutical Press and RCPCH Publications.

Paut, O., & Lacroix, F. (2006). Recent developments in the perioperative fluid management for the paediatric patient. *Current Opinion in Anesthesiology, 19*(3), 268–277.

Peutrell, J. M., & Weir, P. (1996) Basic principles of neonatal anaesthesia. In Hughes, D. G., Mather, S. J., & Wolf, A. R. (Eds.) *Handbook of Neonatal Anaesthesia,* London: WB Saunders.

Proytcheva, M. A. (2009). Issues in neonatal cellular analysis. *American Journal of Clinical Pathology, 131*(4), 560–573.

Rao, P. S., Shashidhar, A., & Ashok, C. (2013). In utero fuel homeostasis: Lessons for a clinician. *Indian Journal of Endocrinology and Metabolism, 17*(1), 60.

Rocha, G., Soares, P., Gonçalves, A., Silva, A. I., Almeida, D., Figueiredo, S., … & Guimarães, H. (2018). Respiratory Care for the Ventilated Neonate. *Canadian Respiratory Journal, 2018.*

Sale, S.M., Jain, A, & Meek, J. (2012). Neonatal analgesia. In Rennie, J. M. (Ed.) *Rennie & Roberton's Textbook of Neonatology.* (5th Edition). London: Elsevier Health Sciences.

Schmidt, A. R., Weiss, M., & Engelhardt, T. (2014). The paediatric airway: Basic principles and current developments. *European Journal of Anaesthesiology, 31*(6), 293–299.

Sessler, D. I. (2008). Temperature monitoring and perioperative thermoregulation. *Anesthesiology: The Journal of the American Society of Anesthesiologists, 109*(2), 318–338.

So, K. W., Fok, T. F., Ng, P. C., Wong, W. W., & Cheung, K. L. (1997). Randomised controlled trial of colloid or crystalloid in hypotensive preterm infants. *Archives of Disease in Childhood: Fetal and Neonatal Edition, 76*(1), F43–F46.

Sun, L. S., Li, G., Miller, T. L., Salorio, C., Byrne, M. W., Bellinger, D. C., … & DiMaggio, C. J. (2016). Association between a single general anesthesia exposure before age 36 months and neurocognitive outcomes in later childhood. *Jama, 315*(21), 2312–2320.

Takci, S., Yigit, S., Korkmaz, A., & Yurdakök, M. (2012). Comparison between oscillometric and invasive blood pressure measurements in critically ill premature infants. *Acta Paediatrica, 101*(2), 132–135.

Teunkens, A., Van De Velde, M., Vermeulen, K., Van Loon, P., Bogaert, G., Fieuws, S., & Rex, S. (2018). Dorsal penile nerve block for circumcision in pediatric patients: A prospective, observer-blinded, randomized controlled clinical trial for the comparison of ultrasound-guided vs landmark technique. *Pediatric Anesthesia, 28*(8), 703–709.

Thomas, R., Rao, S., & Minutillo, C. (2016). Cuffed endotracheal tubes for neonates and young infants: A comprehensive review. *Archives of Disease in Childhood: Fetal and Neonatal Edition, 101*(2), F168–F174.

Ussat, M., Vogtmann, C., Gebauer, C., Pulzer, F., Thome, U., & Knüpfer, M. (2015). The role of elevated central-peripheral temperature difference in early detection of late-onset sepsis in preterm infants. *Early Human Development, 91*(12), 677–681.

Wain, J. C. (2003). Postintubation tracheal stenosis. *Chest Surgery Clinics, 13*(2), 231–246.

Walker, S. M. (2014). Neonatal pain. *Pediatric Anesthesia, 24*(1), 39–48.

Walker, S. M., & Yaksh, T. L. (2012). Neuraxial analgesia in neonates and infants: A review of clinical and preclinical strategies for the development of safety and efficacy data. *Anesthesia and Analgesia, 115*(3), 638–62.

Walther-Larsen, S., & Rasmussen, L. S. (2006). The former preterm infant and risk of post-operative apnoea: Recommendations for management. *Acta Anaesthesiologica Scandinavica, 50*(7), 888–893.

Warner, D. O., Zaccariello, M. J., Katusic, S. K., Schroeder, D. R., Hanson, A. C., Schulte, P. J., ... & Hu, D. (2018). Neuropsychological and Behavioral Outcomes after Exposure of Young Children to Procedures Requiring General Anesthesia: The Mayo Anesthesia Safety in Kids (MASK) Study. *Anesthesiology: The Journal of the American Society of Anesthesiologists. 129*(1), 89–105.

Weiss, M., Vutskits, L., Hansen, T. G., & Engelhardt, T. (2015). Safe anesthesia for every tot–The SAFETOTS initiative. *Current Opinion in Anesthesiology, 28*(3), 302–307.

Weiss, M., Hansen, T. G., & Engelhardt, T. (2016). Ensuring safe anaesthesia for neonates, infants and young children: What really matters. *Archives of Disease in Childhood, 101*(7), 650–652.

White, M. C., & Peyton, J. M. (2011). Anaesthetic management of children with congenital heart disease for non-cardiac surgery. *Continuing Education in Anaesthesia, Critical Care & Pain, 12*(1), 17–22.

Whiteside, J. B., & Wildsmith, J. A. W. (2005). Spinal anaesthesia: an update. *Continuing Education in Anaesthesia, Critical Care & Pain, 5*(2), 37–40.

Wyllie, J., Ainsworth, S., Tinnion, R., & Hampshire, S. (2016) *Newborn Life Support* (4th Edition). London: Resuscitation Council UK.

Yuki, K., Matsunami, E., Tazawa, K., Wang, W., DiNardo, J. A., & Koutsogiannaki, S. (2017). Pediatric Perioperative Stress Responses and Anesthesia. *Translational Perioperative and Pain Medicine, 2*(1), 1–12.

21 NEONATAL SURGICAL CARE

Yvonne Cousins

CONTENTS

GUIDANCE ON HOW TO ENHANCE PERSONAL LEARNING FROM THIS CHAPTER

Key points covered in this chapter

■ An overview of surgical problems that present in the neonatal population.

■ General management and nursing care of the surgical neonate in the pre- and postoperative periods.

■ Common diagnoses, their underlying pathophysiology and clinical presentation.

Reflection

Reading through the chapter, you are encouraged to engage with the key points and related literature in an enquiring way. Ask these questions:

■ Have you been involved in the care of infants with surgical problems? What were these and the underlying causes?

■ How did these infants present?

■ How were these infants managed?

Implications for nursing care

■ Finally: how will this chapter enable you to approach the assessment, management and nursing care of neonates with surgical problems? Consider the implications of what you learn for your daily practice relating to this area.

INTRODUCTION AND BACKGROUND

Neonatal surgery has evolved rapidly over the past 50 years, its success contributing to a reduction in neonatal mortality. Sophisticated antenatal screening and foetal anomaly apperception have led to a changing pattern of operable malformations, and the delivery of a baby with an undiagnosed major structural anomaly is now rare. This chapter will cover surgical issues commonly seen in the neonatal period, providing an insight into their causes and clinical presentation. General perioperative management will be discussed, with more detailed care considerations relating to individual conditions under their respective headings.

GENERAL PRINCIPLES OF MANAGEMENT

Antenatal considerations and delivery room management

With the development of high-resolution non-invasive foetal imaging, many congenital defects are being diagnosed earlier, and with this there has been an increase in the area of foetal interventions (Graves et al., 2017). This can be seen in areas such as cleft lip and palate (Papadopulus et al., 2005), lower urinary tract obstruction (Enninga and Ruano, 2018) congenital diaphragmatic hernia (Ruano et al., 2014), congenital pulmonary airway malformation (CPAM; Wilson et al., 2006) and myelomeningocoele (Moron et al., 2018).

Antenatal diagnosis of surgically correctable malformations will allow for *in utero* transfer and planned delivery in a specialist centre. Regionalisation secures exemplary utilisation of resources and the expertise of the multidisciplinary team (MDT). The expertise of the highly specialised MDT is crucial to the perioperative care and recovery of these babies. Parents should meet with the surgeon as soon as the diagnosis is made, ideally with the support of the foetal medicine team where information about the anomaly, its short-term management and the possible long-term sequelae needs to be given. Meeting staff who will be involved in the baby's care, visiting the neonatal unit (NNU), and early receipt of specialist information booklets may help to avoid long periods of uncertainty, especially when the diagnosis is made antenatally.

Following delivery of the baby, the parents need support in dealing with the information given to them. Informed consent stating the risks, benefits and nature of the procedure will be required from the parents in order for surgery to take place. The father can only give consent if the parents are married, or if he is named on the birth certificate. Other people able to give consent include a legally appointed guardian; the local authority if the child is on a care order; or a person named in a residence order in respect of the child (Department of Health, 2009).

Multiple defects can be associated with chromosomal abnormalities. If a chromosomal anomaly is found in the foetus or neonate, the parents should be offered genetic counselling.

The timing and mode of delivery should be a joint decision between the obstetrician, the neonatal team and the surgeon. Although many conditions are managed with a natural birth, occasionally a caesarean section might be safer with an anomaly such as gross hydrocephalus. In infants with known congenital anomalies, appropriately skilled personnel should be present at the delivery. The main goal on arrival of a baby into the NNU is expedient stabilisation. Skilful assessment and management preoperatively will ensure minimal risk from anaesthesia and surgery.

Thermoregulation

Thermoregulation for the neonate, especially low birth weight infants, can be a challenge. Infants requiring surgical intervention such as laparotomy, and those with anomalies like abdominal wall defects, are going to be at increased risk of temperature instability due to heat loss from exposed viscera. Perioperatively, as discussed in chapter 20, anaesthetics inhibit non-shivering thermogenesis contributing to potential heat loss, with hypothermia reducing the metabolism of medications, and slowing the emergence from anaesthesia (Martin, 2017). Temperature instability is associated with increased metabolic demands, leading to increased oxygen consumption, which may further compromise the cardiorespiratory system and ultimately contribute to mortality and morbidity (Hodson, 2018).

Maintenance of stable temperatures can be a challenge within the operating theatre. Heat loss mechanisms and preventative measures need to be considered when transferring the neonate for surgery and during the preoperative period. The operating theatre needs to be warm to provide a neutral thermal environment, with the additional use of radiant warmers, force air heating units, heated mattresses, humidified and warm inspired gases, warm solutions for cleansing and intraoperative irrigation, and warm blood and intravenous (IV) solutions. The baby's core temperature should be maintained at 37°C with peripheral temperature maintained at 36°C; a wider toe-core gap may indicate underperfusion possibly due to hypovolaemia or infection.

Respiratory function

Assessment of respiratory function is a prerequisite for all surgical neonates, as urgent intervention may be required. Anatomical abnormalities or increasing abdominal distension may compromise ventilation, such as in the case of congenital diaphragmatic hernia, which is often associated with pulmonary hypertension due to lung hypoplasia. Additionally, some infants with surgical problems may be further compromised from surfactant deficiency or aspiration pneumonia.

Gastric decompression

Intestinal obstruction and/or sepsis predispose the infant to increased gastric secretions which may consist of bile, gastric juices or blood. Gastric decompression is necessary to avoid vomiting and aspiration pneumonia; it will also reduce splinting of the diaphragm and aid ventilation. Gastric decompression is achieved with a correctly positioned nasogastric tube (NGT) large enough to prevent blockage (8fg or greater), left on continuous open drainage with gentle intermittent aspiration as directed by the surgeon.

Circulation

Surgery can exacerbate physiological imbalances in the newborn. It is essential, therefore, to continuously assess and monitor perfusion, parenteral fluid and electrolyte requirements, and metabolic response to surgical trauma. Adequate nutrition and hydration can be provided by glucose and electrolyte solutions and/or parenteral nutrition (PN). Some infants will need fluid resuscitation preoperatively – hypovolaemia can result from continuous loss of fluid from, for example, the exposed viscera in gastroschisis and exomphalos. Losses via the NGT should be measured and may need replacement with electrolyte solutions, usually normal saline with potassium. Alterations in acid-base balance can be caused by several factors. Respiratory acidosis results from inadequate ventilation, for example, in pulmonary hypoplasia secondary to congenital diaphragmatic hernia. Metabolic acidosis can occur when bicarbonate losses are increased, or with poor tissue perfusion, tissue necrosis, infection, hypovolaemia and because of intestinal fistulas and necrotising enterocolitis (NEC).

Glycogen is a carbohydrate stored in skeletal muscle and the liver and is metabolised when blood glucose falls outside the homeostatic range (Kotoulas et al., 2006). Neonates have poor glycogen stores due to decreased availability of substrate *in utero*, and therefore need a constant glucose intake. It is essential that glucose should be administered, and the blood glucose monitored frequently, maintaining a level of 2.6–5.0mmol/L (Nicholl, 2003).

The goal of intraoperative fluid replacement is maintenance of cardiovascular stability, organ perfusion and prevention of fluid overload. The main factors influencing postoperative fluid balance include: intraoperative fluid overload, mechanical ventilation leading to relaxation and fluid retention, the neonate's tendency to hyponatraemia, intraoperative stress (hyperglycaemic tendency), third space losses into the interstitium and gut, and inappropriate antidiuretic hormone (ADH) secretion.

Fluid and electrolyte balance is dependent upon fulfilling the maintenance requirements (insensible water losses, urine and stool), the correction of ongoing losses, and the replacement of deficit losses due to fluid compartment shifts (third space losses). Fluid compartment shifts can be difficult to determine and depend on response to replacement. The neonatal nurse's role, through observations of alterations in heart rate, urine output, capillary refill, blood pressure, and core-to-peripheral temperature difference, is crucial with regard to this. Laboratory tests form the mainstay of assessment: serum urea and electrolytes, plasma osmolality, urine electrolytes and specific gravity and blood gas analysis.

The stimulus of surgery and mechanical ventilation lead to increased aldosterone and ADH secretion resulting in water and sodium retention. Therefore, postoperative fluids will be restricted to two-thirds of the previous requirement, with further restriction being a possibility.

A neonate's blood volume is approximately 80mL/kg body weight. A 2kg infant, therefore, has a circulating volume equivalent to the average loss during minor adult surgery. A full blood count, urea and electrolytes, should be obtained preoperatively, and the need for a coagulation profile discussed with the surgeon and anaesthetist. Any requirements should be treated accordingly, and necessary blood products made available for surgery. The neonate should have received vitamin K in the first few hours of life.

Appropriate vascular access will depend upon the nature of the surgery. However, for major surgery at least two intravenous lines will be needed, including a central venous line. This is necessary to provide inotropic support, and for prolonged venous access in the provision of PN. Arterial access should always be made available for major surgery.

Pharmacological support

There is a risk of sepsis whenever surgery is performed. However, with the rise of antibiotic resistant organisms, prophylactic antibiotic therapy needs to be continually reviewed with regard to its duration and effectiveness (Llewelyn et al., 2017). Inotropes are often necessary to improve cardiac function, thus improving organ perfusion. Pain relief is an important consideration both pre- and postoperatively. Cellular damage, particularly in cases of NEC, release pain-producing substances, augmenting the perception of pain (Brophy, 2007). Intubation and ventilation are usually necessary for the facilitation of adequate pain relief, as neonates are sensitive to the respiratory depressant effects of opiates. Effective analgesia via an epidural catheter can be provided without depressing respiration, providing toxic doses of regional bupivacaine are avoided (Reynolds, 2005). Recently, the use of wound catheters with an infusion of local anaesthetic, such as levobupivacaine, have started to be used in neonates. There is limited data available concerning their use, however, adequate wound healing, low pain scores and a reduced need for opioids have been observed in the neonatal population (Krylborn et al., 2015).

Postoperative considerations

Management in the postoperative period mirrors the preoperative care in aiming to achieve and maintain physiological stability, but in addition the factors listed in box 21.1 need careful consideration.

BOX 21.1 GENERAL CONSIDERATIONS FOLLOWING MAJOR SURGERY

- Do not leave the operating theatre until the baby is stable and a complete handover has taken place. A doctor/nurse practitioner and nurse should be in attendance on the return journey to the NNU.
- Optimise sedation, analgesia and muscle relaxants (if required) for the return journey.
- Check baby's temperature and use additional heat aids as required for transfer.

On arrival back to NNU

- Before returning the baby to the incubator and connecting to the ventilator, check settings of both.
- Ensure ventilator settings are still appropriate when reconnecting. Check airway and position of endotracheal tube. Check blood gas and adjust ventilation accordingly.
- Reconnect all monitor leads and record hourly:
  - blood pressure
  - SpO_2
  - transcutaneous pO_2/pCO_2 (as indicated)
  - skin temperature – peripheral and core.
- Check infusion sites, then reconnect fluids.
- Adjust maintenance and arterial line fluids. Take into consideration any fluids given intraoperatively. Check surgical instructions regarding maintenance fluids.
- Aspirate NGT according to surgical instructions and leave on free drainage. Record accurately and commence NG replacement of losses if necessary.
- Take a blood glucose level, monitor according to results.
- Organise a chest X-ray if the baby was intubated in theatre, if there is a chest drain in situ, and following diaphragmatic hernia repair.
- Record urinary output – attach urine bag, weigh nappies or measure catheter output – expect 1mL/kg/hour after the first 24 hours.
- Check biochemical and haematological status.
- Position baby as comfortably as possible, developmentally appropriate, while responding to specific requirements of surgery.
- Assess, administer and evaluate pain relief.
- Carefully observe wounds, stomas etc., recording any losses, and replacing as prescribed.
- Consult surgical instructions for care of any drains.
- Ensure parents are informed of the outcome of surgery and of the postoperative management plan
- Encourage parental involvement in care as possible.

MOST COMMONLY ENCOUNTERED CONGENITAL DISORDERS

Oesophageal atresia and tracheo-oesophageal fistula

The oesophagus and trachea have a common embryological origin. Initially they are fused, but a septal separation occurs by week 6 – where this is not the case, this results in fistula formation. The oesophagus should re-canalise and become patent by week 10; failure to do this leads to atresia (Merei et al., 1997). Thus tracheo-oesophageal fistula (TOF) and oesophageal atresia (OA) can occur as separate entities, but more frequently occur concurrently (see figure 21.1).

Associated anatomical features include a hypertrophied proximal oesophageal pouch – a result of foetal swallowing of amniotic fluid. If the pouch is not hypertrophied, a fistula should be suspected. 50–60% of neonates with TOF/OA are thought to have coexisting anomalies (Lee and Meeker, 2018), VACTERL (**V**ertebral defects – **A**norectal

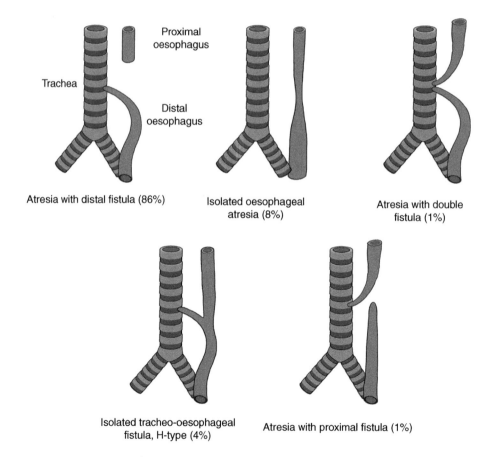

Figure 21.1 Types of fistula (Source: Jarrick Harris)

malformations – **C**ardiac defects – TOF/OA – **R**enal abnormalities – **L**imb abnormalities) association being the most common (Beasley, 2016).

Antenatal diagnosis is challenging and maternal polyhydramnios may or may not be present (Bradshaw et al., 2016). The anomaly may be diagnosed by ultrasound, where the inability to demonstrate a foetal stomach in the presence of normal or increased amniotic fluid is highly suggestive of OA. However, if there is no antenatal diagnosis, symptoms will present in the early postnatal hours. The neonate will cough and choke on excessive saliva in the oropharynx and upper respiratory tract. If enteral feeds are offered, the oesophageal pouch will fill, followed by regurgitation. Gastric contents can also reflux from the stomach through the fistula into the respiratory tract, presenting a danger of aspiration and pneumonitis. The abdomen will rapidly distend as the intestines fill with air.

Foetal magnetic resonance imaging (MRI) has been suggested to be of value in confirming the diagnosis when there is antenatal suspicion of OA (Hochart et al., 2015). The diagnosis of a proximal atresia is usually confirmed by passing a radio-opaque tube size 8–10fg through a nostril until resistance is felt, and by X-ray of the neck, chest and abdomen. The tube will sit in the oesophageal pouch or be coiled, if too small a tube is used. If there has been any suggestion of a possible fistula or atresia on the foetal ultrasound scan, an attempt at passing a tube should be made soon after birth to confirm diagnosis. Although infants with an H-type fistula may have early signs of respiratory distress, aggravated by feeding orally, the diagnosis is not often confirmed in the early neonatal period, and may not be diagnosed until adulthood (Suen, 2018).

If known antenatally, these neonates should be positioned with the head elevated at 45° or prone from birth, to prevent aspiration pneumonia. A double lumen Replogle tube (Replogle, 1963) placed in the upper pouch and connected to low-pressure continuous suction will minimise this risk (see figure 21.2). Continuous observation, monitoring and

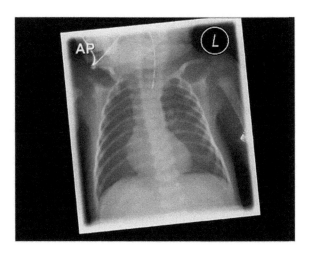

Figure 21.2 Replogle tube arrested in proximal oesophageal pouch (Source: Iain Yardley)

meticulous care of the Replogle tube are paramount to ensure this does not block with thick, tenacious secretions.

Endotracheal intubation is not usually necessary; indeed, with a distal fistula it is possible to rupture the stomach with mechanical ventilation. An echocardiogram should take place prior to surgery, to identify any associated cardiac anomalies. In particular, the position of the aortic arch needs to be identified to exclude a right-sided arch, as the OA/TOF repair via a thoracotomy is usually on the infant's right side. Other investigations to identify associated anomalies including ultrasound scans, such as renal and spinal, can be undertaken once the baby is stable postoperatively.

The timing of the repair to the fistula and the establishment of oesophageal continuity, depends on the width of the oesophageal gap. Fistulae are usually repaired within hours of birth, with ideally end-to-end primary **anastomosis** of the oesophagus performed at the same time. More recently, repairs have been made via less invasive thoracoscopy, although controversy exists over whether this is preferable to open surgery (Davenport et al., 2015).

A 'long gap' OA has traditionally been defined as a gap length equivalent of 3 or more vertebral bodies (Lal et al., 2017), however, it has been suggested that any OA that has no intra-abdominal air should be considered a long gap (van der Zee et al., 2017). This requires staged surgery allowing time for growth of the oesophagus (Spitz, 2007). A delayed repair necessitates formation of a gastrostomy to allow for milk feeding. Currently, cervical oesophagostomies are rarely used and not advocated, as they can increase the difficulty of repair (van der Zee et al., 2017). 'Sham feeding' is a technique by which any milk the baby obtains through oral feeding is simultaneously removed via a Replogle tube, and subsequently administered via a gastrostomy. This should be employed while awaiting corrective surgery to maintain the sucking reflex (Golonka and Hayashi, 2008). Although the ideal oesophagus is the patient's own and every effort should be made towards oesophageal preservation, sometimes the gap never shortens to an operable length and it is necessary to perform a jejunal, gastric or colonic interposition. However, this is a huge undertaking with potential serious complications, and should only be considered if the condition is irremediable (van der Zee et al., 2017).

The need for postoperative ventilatory support not only depends on the infant's respiratory status, but also the difficulty of the initial repair. If the anastomosis is under tension, muscle relaxants will be required, and the baby nursed with the neck flexed for several days while healing takes place. A chest drain may have been inserted depending on the surgical approach.

A transanastomotic tube (TAT) will be in situ to minimise the potential for oesophageal stenosis and allow for early enteral feeding postoperatively. It is essential that the TAT is securely fixed and labelled, as unplanned removal can delay enteral feeding, and replacement of the TAT can seriously damage the surgical site.

- Anastomotic stricture
- Gastro-oesophageal reflux
- Anastomotic leak
- **Tracheomalacia**
- Injured laryngeal nerve
- Disordered peristalsis.

Feeding difficulties and vomiting, which may last for years, especially following tight repairs, are common and often relate to oesophageal strictures (Paran et al., 2007). The causes of strictures are multifactorial and include tension, reflux and anastomotic leaks. Frequent oesophageal dilatations may be necessary to enable normal eating and swallowing. Gastro-oesophageal reflux is one of the most common long-term problems, and is thought to be due to disordered oesophageal motility and the presence of a small-volume stomach. Treatment may involve non-invasive measures such as positioning, thickened feeds, and prophylactic anti-reflux medication. However, recent studies have cast doubt over the efficacy of these medications and highlighted additional risks in their use with the low birth weight infant (Miyake et al., 2018).

An anastomotic leak can present as a tension pneumothorax, sepsis, mediastinitis, and, if a chest drain is in situ, frothy saliva (Lee and Meeker, 2018). A minor leak will heal spontaneously, while a major leak will necessitate a chest drain, antibiotics, or re-anastomosis. If a primary anastomosis has been performed, a contrast swallow may be requested to check for an anastomotic leak. However, this is an area of debate as it has been reported that routine contrast studies rarely detect a leak (Burge et al., 2013).

Tracheomalacia can be serious enough to progress to respiratory distress and causes the characteristic 'TOF cough' or 'seal bark' (Lee and Meeker, 2018). Severe cases may require aortopexy – fixation of the aorta to the sternum to maintain an adequate tracheal lumen. Recurrent fistulas may occur and should be suspected in the child who develops frequent respiratory infections, with gagging, cyanosis and apnoea. Parents should be given detailed information and advice about the long-term problems they may encounter. It may be useful to put them in contact with families of other children with OA/TOF, and/or local support groups.

Early diagnosis, improved surgical techniques, and sophisticated intensive care have positively influenced survival. Prognosis is, however, significantly altered in association with other anomalies.

Intestinal obstruction

Signs of obstruction include bile-stained vomiting, abdominal distension, large gastric aspirates, and delay or failure to pass meconium. Intestinal obstruction may be congenital and mechanical e.g. due to stenosis (incomplete obstruction), atresias, or webs within

TABLE 21.1 CAUSES OF INTESTINAL OBSTRUCTION

Upper	Lower
Duodenal atresia	Low small bowel atresia
High small bowel atresia	Meconium ileus
Malrotation with volvulus	Hirschsprung's disease

the gastrointestinal (GI) tract; or functional e.g. meconium ileus. Antenatal diagnosis of intestinal obstruction is usually identified on ultrasound scan during the second to third trimester. The more distal the obstruction, the later in gestational age the diagnosis is usually made, and the higher the likelihood of other anomalies being present. Foetal MRIs are now available, which can provide additional, more detailed information about the location of an obstruction, the presence of additional anomalies, and anomalies previously difficult to identify, such as anorectal malformation (Lau et al., 2017).

There are three common causes of obstruction in the upper part of the GI tract, and three in the lower part (table 21.1) An abdominal X-ray may highlight the position of the obstruction, with the possible assistance of additional imaging studies such as contrast studies and MRI scans.

In general, the lower down the small intestine the defect, the later the presentation after birth. Irrespective of the cause, if obstruction is suspected, a size 8fg–10fg NGT should be passed, aspirated regularly and left on free drainage. This will decompress the gut and prevent aspiration of GI contents. Intravenous therapy should be commenced, and fluid and electrolyte imbalances corrected.

DUODENAL OBSTRUCTION

The duodenum begins its development in the fourth week of gestation. Epithelial proliferation is so abundant that at five to six weeks there is temporary duodenal occlusion, and its failure to become recanalised by the end of the embryonic period (nine weeks) results in an obstruction. This obstruction varies from a simple membranous obstruction (duodenal stenosis) to a complete gap with two separate blind ends (duodenal atresia). Occasionally the pancreas surrounds the circumference of the duodenum (annular pancreas). Duodenal obstruction is characterised by the 'double bubble' sign on antenatal ultrasound scan. Approximately 50% of patients with duodenal atresias have associated anomalies (vertebral, gastrointestinal, cardiac and renal anomalies), with up to 40% having Trisomy 21 (Jones et al., 2009).

Vomiting as the most common symptom of complete atresia is usually present on the first day of life, and commonly bilious, as 80% of the obstructions are in the post-ampullary region. The high level of obstruction reduces the likelihood of abdominal distension.

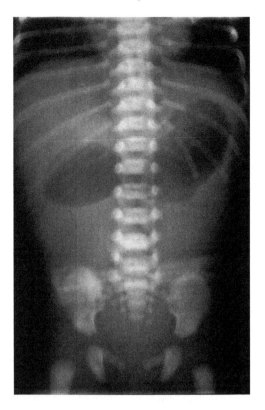

Figure 21.3 'Double bubble' indicating duodenal obstruction

Meconium may be passed in the first 24 hours, followed by constipation. An X-ray shows high intestinal obstruction with the classic 'double bubble' – fluid in the lower part of the stomach and the duodenum proximal to the obstruction (figure 21.3).

The principle of the repair (duodenoduodenostomy) is the same for both anomalies, as it is not possible to remove the web, the bile duct often opening onto it. This may be performed in a side-to-side or a diamond-shaped fashion (Karrer and Potter, 2009). Postoperatively, the baby may have a TAT in place to facilitate feeding depending on surgeon preference. Large amounts of gastric aspirate may be present due to the dilated proximal duodenum at the time of repair. These should gradually reduce over time and not necessarily delay establishment of enteral feeds.

SMALL BOWEL ATRESIA AND COLONIC ATRESIA

Jejuno-ileal and colonic atresias are thought to be due to a localised intrauterine vascular accident with ischaemic necrosis of the bowel and subsequent reabsorption of the affected segment (Rode and Millar, 2006). Antenatal diagnosis may have been made by ultrasound scan, or it may present with bilious vomiting shortly after birth. With a more distal atresia the

TABLE 21.2 TYPES OF JEJUNAL-ILEAL ATRESIAS

Type I	Mucosa and submucosa form a web
Type II	Bowel not joined, connected by fibrous cord
Type IIIa	No cord, V-shaped mesenteric defect, bowel variably shortened
Type IIIb	Large mesenteric defect, bowel significantly shortened. Also known as Christmas Tree or Apple Peel deformity due to appearance
Type IV	Multiple atresias of any combination, appearing as a string of sausages

(adapted from Jones et al., 2009)

vomiting may present later. Abdominal X-rays may show dilated loops of bowel suggestive of an atresia (table 21.2), and a contrast enema may identify a microcolon, indicative of a distal obstruction.

Colonic atresias are the least common and are classified in the same way as the small intestine atresias. At surgery, intestinal continuity is restored with an end-to-end/end-to-side anastomosis, and any malrotation corrected. A staged approach may be taken with the formation of a defunctioning stoma. Once appropriate, gradual weaning from parenteral to enteral feeding can take place. Prognosis will depend upon the remaining functional bowel, and any associated anomalies. Insufficient bowel length either as a result of the primary insult, excessive removal of residual bowel, or postoperative complications can lead to short gut syndrome.

MALROTATION WITH VOLVULUS

Development of the midgut results in rapid growth and physiological umbilical herniation during the sixth week of gestation. At 10 to 11 weeks, the gut begins a 270-degree counter-clockwise rotation around the superior mesenteric artery. The bowel destined to be the caecum re-enters the abdomen descending to the right iliac fossa, where fixation followed by closure of the abdomen occurs around the twelfth week (Bass et al., 1998). The duodenum with the duodenojejunal flexure (DJF) in the midline or to its left, and the proximal colon, are attached to the posterior abdominal wall. The small bowel is suspended posteriorly by **mesenteries** which carry blood, lymphatic vessels and nerves, and extends from the DJF to the ileocaecal region.

Normally the mesentery has a broad base and cannot undergo **torsion**. Malrotation occurs when development is halted, and the caecum ends up adjacent to the duodenum. The mesenteries fail to become normally fixated, so the small intestines are suspended by a narrow stalk, which can twist into a volvulus, causing an obstruction. All bilious vomiting in the otherwise healthy term baby should arouse the suspicion of volvulus. An upper GI contrast study can confirm the diagnosis by showing the position of the DJF. Unless surgery is carried out promptly, the volvulus continues to twist a few more degrees, the superior mesenteric artery becomes kinked and the midgut becomes infarcted, leading to necrosis.

Surgery involves untwisting the volvulus as soon as possible. Frequently Ladd's bands are found between the caecum and the peritoneum causing further obstruction by compressing the duodenum. These are divided, and the gut is mobilised and returned to the abdomen with the caecum on the left and the duodenum on the right, broadening the base of the mesentery, preventing the tendency to further twisting. Malrotation is thus changed into non-rotation (Ladd's procedure). An appendicectomy may be performed at the same time to minimise the future risk of a missed diagnosis of appendicitis, due to the position of the appendix now on the left. However, recently there has been a move away from doing this, so that the parents need to be made aware of this future potential diagnostic difficulty. Adhesive obstruction, short bowel syndrome and recurrent volvulus are considered to be common complications (Hebra and Miller, 2010).

MECONIUM ILEUS

Meconium is a dark mucilaginous material that is a mixture of secretions of the maturing intestinal glands, ingested amniotic fluid and the debris of proliferative epithelial cells. It begins to fill the lower ileum and colon late in the fourth month of gestation and continues until the time of birth. Meconium ileus is caused by abnormal meconium blocking the terminal ileum (Yoo et al., 2002) and occurs in approximately 20% of patients diagnosed with cystic fibrosis (Sathe and Houwen, 2017). The neonate with meconium ileus will need to be further investigated to determine the diagnosis of cystic fibrosis.

At birth, the infant usually has abdominal distension and is vomiting bile. On examination, loops of gut may be visible or palpable, and meconium plugs may be passed following rectal examination. The abdominal X-ray shows dilated loops of bowel with a soap-bubble appearance of the bowel contents. Differential diagnosis includes Hirschsprung's disease and meconium plug syndrome. Perforation and meconium peritonitis may occur but providing there is no evidence of this and the infant is stable, this obstruction can often be relieved with the hydroscopic action of a hyperosmolar enema. Adequate intravenous hydration is essential to avoid hypovolaemia, which could lead to shock. If enemas fail to relieve the obstruction or are contraindicated, surgery may be necessary. At laparotomy an incision is made into the bowel just above the obstruction and the abnormal meconium is washed out. A temporary de-functioning stoma may be formed.

HIRSCHSPRUNG'S DISEASE

Hirschsprung's disease (HD) is characterised by an absence of enteric ganglion cells in the submucosa of the distal bowel. These first appear in the developing oesophagus at five weeks and migrate down to the anorectal junction by 12 weeks. Their absence is attributed to the failure of migration, and the earlier the arrest of migration, the longer the affected segment of bowel. The **aganglionic** segment always includes the rectum, with the total colon affected in 8% of cases (Puri, 1996). The aganglionic segment is collapsed and non-peristaltic, causing functional intestinal obstruction. HD is the most common congenital bowel motility disorder, presenting in the first few days of life (Chhabra and Kenny, 2016). The neonate presents with signs of distal intestinal obstruction: abdominal distension, bile-stained vomiting and delay or failure to pass meconium. On abdominal X-ray, the normal bowel appears as a megacolon with dilated small bowel proximal to the agangliosis. When gentle rectal examination is performed, the rectal wall always appears tight and resists further probing. This may cause the explosive passage of meconium and flatus followed by normal bowel movements for a few days before signs of obstruction recur. Hirschsprung's enterocolitis – indicated by the presence of foul-smelling diarrhoea, abdominal distension, bile vomiting and potential perforation – may occur and, if undiagnosed, can be fatal. The diagnosis of HD is confirmed with suction biopsies of the colorectal mucosa. A staged approach to surgery is taken. Regular rectal washouts with warm saline are commenced in order to evacuate the meconium and decompress the bowel. If this is successful, the parents will need to be taught the procedure in order to perform it at home. It is imperative that they understand the risks of not performing the washouts effectively, and the signs and symptoms of enterocolitis. If regular rectal washouts are ineffective, a stoma is fashioned at the most distal part of the normal innervation to decompress the bowel, while allowing the neonate to grow. Surgery involves resection of the aganglionic bowel and a 'pull-through' procedure. Depending on the length of bowel affected, outcomes can be poor with episodes of enterocolitis, continence issues or constipation, and the need for a long-term colostomy (Chhabra and Kenny, 2016). There is ongoing research with regard to stem cell therapy in HD; this has the potential to generate new nerves capable of stimulating gut motility (Tam et al., 2017).

MECONIUM PLUG SYNDROME

A distal obstruction is caused by firm meconium remaining in the colon (DeWayne et al., 2009) The baby will present with signs of obstruction. Any condition causing dysmotility will predispose the baby to this. Treatment will be the same as that for meconium ileus.

ANORECTAL MALFORMATIONS

Anorectal malformations (ARM) result from anomalous development of the urorectal septum, causing incomplete separation into urogenital and anorectal sections, and an aberrant anal orifice (Moore and Persaud, 2003). They present with a spectrum of defects – from minor malformations requiring minimal treatment, to a very sick infant with intestinal obstruction and complex life-threatening defects (Pena, 1996). Anomalies of the upper urinary tract, cardiovascular system and sacrum are associated, as are atresias of the gastrointestinal tract. Therefore, due to the high association with other anomalies, screening tools such as echocardiograms, renal and spinal ultrasound scans need to be undertaken.

Complementary MRI studies are now providing valuable, reliable evaluation of ARM preoperatively (Madhusmita et al., 2018). Lesions are classified depending on whether the rectum ends superior or inferior to the puborectalis sling (see figure 21.4 Types of ARM). High lesions present as anorectal agenesis or rectal atresia, frequently associated with recto-urethral, -vestibular or -vaginal fistulae. Alternatively, low lesions are classified as anal agenesis, stenosis or an imperforate anus (which may be just a thin membrane through which meconium can be excreted). Low lesions are associated with anocutaneous fistulae, and in girls, an ectopic stenotic anus. Low lesions require division of fistula or anoplasty, and may need frequent subsequent anal dilatations, but the prospects of long-term faecal continence are good. If the fistula can be dilated, the parents can be taught to perform this once or twice a day, as directed by the surgeon.

High lesions require formation of a stoma, anorectoplasty at several months of age, followed by anal dilatations and subsequent closure of stoma. Continence may remain a long-term problem. Urinary tract infections are common, especially with high lesions, and therefore, these babies are often given long-term prophylactic antibiotics.

Cloaca in females, where the bladder, rectum and genitalia have remained as one channel, represents a spectrum of defects. Depending on the ARM present, surgery required can vary significantly. Complex cloaca with a common channel longer than 3cm should be treated by a specialised team dedicated to these malformations (Bischoff, 2016). A team approach involving surgeons, urologists, nephrologists, gynaecologists, clinical nurse specialists, and psychologists, will be needed in the long-term care of these children.

Congenital diaphragmatic hernia

During embryological development the thoracic and abdominal portions of the body cavity move freely until the diaphragm develops to separate them (Jesudason et al., 2000). Congenital diaphragmatic hernia (CDH) results from defective fusion of the pleuroperitoneal membrane when the intestines return at 9–10 weeks to the abdomen from the umbilical cord and allows the abdominal viscera to slip into the thorax. It usually occurs on the left side (80%), through the posterior foramen of Bochdalek, but can also occur near the **xiphisternum** through the foramen of Morgagni, or on the right. The resultant abnormal lung development leads to pulmonary hypoplasia, and pulmonary hypertension, which determine the mortality and morbidity. The mortality rate is difficult to establish with estimates between 50% and greater than 80% in specialist centres as reported in the UK (National Perinatal Epidemiology Unit (NPEU), 2014). Associated anomalies occur in 50%: chromosomal disorders and syndromes, cardiac defects, neural tube defects, skeletal anomalies, intestinal atresias and renal anomalies (Kleinman and Wilson, 2009).

Antenatal diagnosis can be made by ultrasound scan as early as 12 weeks. For some neonates, however, it may not have been detected, so that they will present with respiratory distress soon after delivery. Some children may be asymptomatic and not diagnosed

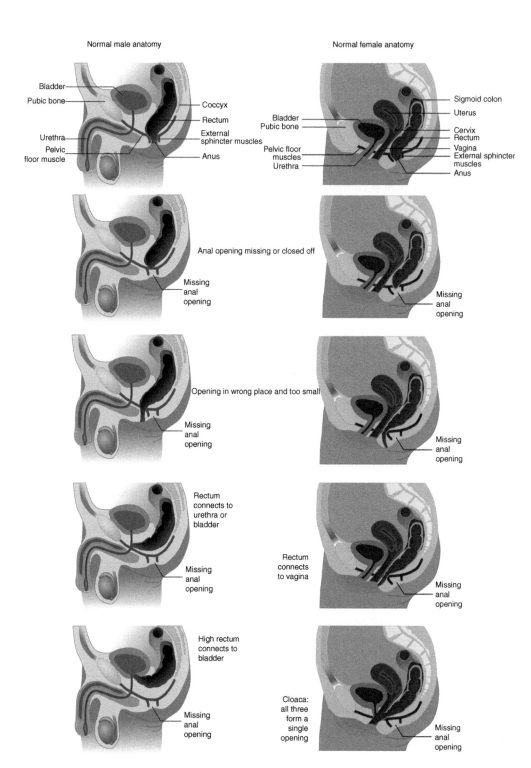

Figure 21.4 Types of ARM (Source: Jarrick Harris)

until later in infancy or childhood. The severity of CDH can be estimated using observed-to-expected lung-head ratios by ultrasound, and total foetal lung volumes by MRI (The Canadian Congenital Diaphragmatic Hernia (TCCDH) Collaborative, 2018). Foetal intervention employing techniques to occlude the trachea, thereby trapping fluid and stimulating growth, are currently being offered in some centres. However, the outcomes for this are still being debated (Ruano et al., 2014).

Clinical presentation includes a scaphoid abdomen with increased chest diameter, a shift in the trachea and cardiac impulse, and decreased breath sounds – but with bowel sounds in the chest on the ipsilateral side. Radiologically, there is bowel in the thorax and an absent diaphragm (figure 21.5). Malrotation may coexist. The main differential diagnosis is congenital pulmonary airway malformation (CPAM). Management is aimed at correcting the abnormality antenatally (rare) or ameliorating its devastating effects by preventing pulmonary hypertension postnatally. Debate persists regarding the efficacy of foetal endoscopic tracheal occlusion (FETO), but it continues to be offered at some centres (Ruano et al., 2014).

At delivery, it is important to avoid mask ventilation; if air is forced into the GI tract in the thorax, ventilation will be further compromised. GI decompression with a large bore

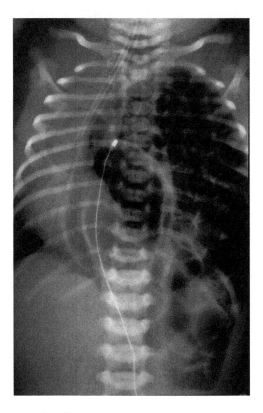

Figure 21.5 X-ray appearance of CDH

NGT on continuous drainage with intermittent aspiration is of the utmost importance. Early intubation to maintain adequate oxygenation is necessary with high frequency oscillatory ventilation (HFOV) used as required. HFOV maintains lung volume, permits adequate gaseous exchange with small tidal volumes, and has been shown to recruit collapsed alveoli. Exogenous surfactant may be of value (Steinhorn and Porta, 1997). Sedation, pain control and neuromuscular blockade may need to be provided. Arterial access is crucial for determination of blood gas values. Intravenous access is a priority to maintain adequate perfusion, although fluid restriction may be necessary. These infants do not tolerate positive fluid balance; increased circulatory volume could lead to pulmonary oedema, worsening the respiratory status. Haemodynamic support with administration of crystalloids, inotropic agents, and hydrocortisone to treat poor perfusion, to maintain urine output above 1mL/kg/hr, and maintain blood pressure within normal range, may all be required (TCCDH Collaborative, 2018). Life support in the form of extracorporeal membrane oxygenation (ECMO) may need to be considered in the management of the resulting pulmonary hypertension, although the role of ECMO remains debatable. An echocardiogram should be performed to define the intracardiac anatomy, assess pulmonary vascular resistance, and left and right ventricular function. A delayed approach to surgical repair allows for adequate preoperative stabilisation and has been shown to decrease mortality and morbidity. Surgery involves reduction of the viscera and repair of the defect through a subcostal incision. For those defects not amenable to primary repair, a synthetic patch will be used.

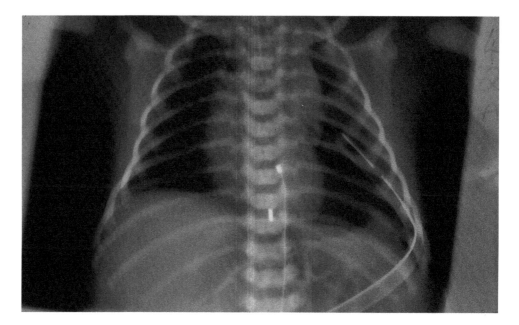

Figure 21.6 Chest radiograph following surgical repair of diaphragmatic hernia

Initial postoperative care is not significantly different from preoperative management: the goal is still to avoid pulmonary hypertension and associated shunting. Ventilatory support can be weaned once the infant is stable with normalised blood gases. Pain control should be assessed, implemented and evaluated. Nutritional requirements will be provided by PN until the GI tract has recovered from the effects of surgery, analgesia and paralysis.

Long-term complications include respiratory insufficiency, gastro-oesophageal reflux, failure to thrive, neurodevelopmental delay, behavioural problems, hearing loss, hernia recurrence and orthopaedic deformities (Takayasu et al., 2017). Long-term follow-up provided for by a multidisciplinary team is essential in view of these associated long-term morbidities. Diaphragmatic **eventration**, where there is thinning of the diaphragmatic leaflets can occur as a separate entity, or occasionally after thoracic surgery, and requires plication (Kleinman and Wilson, 2009).

Abdominal wall defects

GASTROSCHISIS AND EXOMPHALOS

Gastroschisis and exomphalos are the most common congenital abdominal wall defects. The incidence of gastroschisis appears to be rising globally, while the incidence of exomphalos has remained stable (Kong et al., 2016). The embryology of normal abdominal wall closure, and the sequence of events leading to umbilical and para-umbilical defects, are speculative. The most popular description of exomphalos is a developmental arrest resulting in failure of the midgut to return to the abdominal cavity. The amount of herniated intestine varies from a small umbilical hernia-like lesion, to a large anomaly containing the entire midgut and liver. Unless ruptured, it is covered with a sac consisting of peritoneum and amnion, the umbilical cord emerging from the caudal part. Eviscerated bowel in exomphalos is usually normal in appearance.

Gastroschisis is thought to be due to incomplete closure of the lateral abdominal folds, leading to a defect in or near the median plane of the ventral wall leading to protrusion of the intra-abdominal viscera. Other hypotheses include '*amniotic membrane rupture at the insertion of the cord, abnormal apoptotic patterns during regression of the right umbilical vein, or vascular damage to the base of the umbilicus*' (Prefumo and Izzi, 2014, pp. 391–392). There is no membrane covering the herniated bowel, and the cord is intact. The eviscerated bowel is often foreshortened, inflamed, thickened and matted with serosal peel. Clinical research suggests that this damage is caused by prolonged exposure to urine in the amniotic fluid, and/or progressive constriction on the intestine and its blood supply by the umbilical ring (Simmons and Georgeson, 1996).

Occasionally the defect may close around the viscera causing intestinal atresia and ischaemia or midgut infarction. This is known as a closing gastroschisis and often lethal (Houben et al., 2009). Accurate antenatal diagnosis can be made as early as 12 weeks of gestation, as an exomphalos in its sac is distinguishable from gastroschisis. Gastroschisis is seen in most cases to the right of the insertion of the umbilical cord. Anomalies associated with gastroschisis are thought to be around 10%, whereas with exomphalos there is a much higher association of chromosomal and genetic abnormalities (Prefumo and Izzi, 2014). Pentralogy of Cantrell, Beckwith–Wiedemann syndrome and OEIS (**O**mphalocele – **E**xstrophy of the cloaca – **I**mperforate anus – **S**pinal defects) complex are widely discussed associated syndromes.

There remains much debate surrounding the issues of early versus late delivery, and caesarean section versus vaginal delivery for these infants. However, gastroschisis is associated with a risk of intrauterine death and consequently many centres offer induction of labour at 37 weeks. Some authors feel there is no evidence that the mode of delivery improves the final outcome, with infants with unsuspected exomphalos being delivered vaginally with the sac intact (Prefumo and Izzi, 2014).

Large amounts of heat may be lost from the exposed bowel in gastroschisis, or through the amnion covering the exomphalos. The lesion should be immediately covered with cling film to protect it from trauma, contamination, and to prevent traction on the mesentery. This also allows for easier observation of the viscera and keeps the lesion covered with the infant's own body fluids. A large bore NGT left on free drainage will decompress the gut and prevent aspiration. Respiratory distress should be managed as necessary, and all infants should have chest and abdominal X-rays to evaluate the lungs, heart, diaphragm, the air pattern in the bowel and the position of the NGT. Antibiotics may be considered. Significant protein and insensible fluid losses from the abnormal bowel in gastroschisis are unavoidable and should be supplemented parenterally. Perfusion and blood pressure should be carefully monitored to ensure stability and prevent hypotension. As there is an association between exomphalos and Beckwith–Wiedemann syndrome (Pettenati et al., 1986), blood sugar levels need to be monitored. Surgery is not always necessary, and while primary closure is preferred, the intestines may be encased within a silo or an entire closure undertaken on the NNU. Mechanical ventilation with muscle relaxation may be required to aid the closure process. If a silo is used, it may remain in place for a period of 5 to 7 days, during which time the surgeons will gradually reduce the silo until full closure can take place. Pain control needs to be assessed, implemented and evaluated, and careful observation of the colour of the bowel within the silo is crucial.

Following any adjustments to the silo and immediately post closure, observations should be made for potential increased intra-abdominal pressure due to inferior vena cava compression resulting in increasing respiratory requirements, haemodynamic compromise, cyanotic lower extremities, decreased perfusion, decreased urinary output and metabolic acidosis. Surgical decompression may be required (Martin and Fishman, 2009).

There will be decreased gastric motility and/or prolonged ileus which will delay enteral feeds. Therefore, central line insertion for the administration of PN is usually necessary. The commencement and time for tolerating full enteral feeds can vary significantly, the median time to achieving this being about 21 days. Necrotising enterocolitis (NEC) poses a considerable risk and therefore breast milk should be promoted, or a partly hydrolysed formula milk used if breast milk is unavailable. This can be a very challenging time with the feeding regime subject to frequent change due to dysmotility issues.

Following delivery with exomphalos, the priority is protecting the sac from rupture and infection. A large exomphalos containing centrally herniated liver poses challenges – the most significant being space limitations of the abdominal cavity, and hypotension as well as respiratory distress from diaphragmatic splinting. In addition, the liver may exert pressure on the vena cava creating acute hepatic vascular outflow obstruction and renal compromise (Skarsgard and Barth, 1997). If primary closure is not feasible, the defect may be left to develop an eschar (covering of slough) with the final repair at a later date. Historically, various drying agents (povidone-iodine, silver sulfadiazine) have been used, until recently, when medical grade honey dressings have been used with good effect and less risk of toxicity. Granulation, epithelialisation and contraction of the sac size occur, allowing for reconstruction of the abdominal wall some months later. Enteral feeding does not normally pose as much of a challenge as with gastroschisis.

The prognosis of infants with gastroschisis is favourable if the defect can be closed. However, ischaemic changes in the wall of the damaged intestine in gastroschisis may cause absorption and motility disturbances for some infants (Simmons and Georgeson, 1996), and bowel-related morbidity associated with intestinal atresia, perforation, stenosis or volvulus in complex gastroschisis is high (Prefumo and Izzi, 2014). Mortality is usually due to short gut syndrome, or complications of long-term PN. Pulmonary hypoplasia leading to respiratory insufficiency and the need for prolonged ventilation is seen in the larger exomphalos defects. Prognosis of exomphalos is dependent on the severity of associated anomalies (Watanabe et al., 2017).

UMBILICAL HERNIA

This is due to a protrusion of a loop of bowel through the **linea alba** into a patent umbilicus. Unlike exomphalos, it is covered by subcutaneous tissue and skin. It is usually less than 2cm in diameter and distends during straining and crying. It is relatively common; complications are rare and include incarceration (where it cannot be returned to the abdominal cavity) and spontaneous rupture (Martin and Fishman, 2009). The deficit will often close spontaneously, otherwise is generally repaired by the age of 5 years (Zens et al., 2017).

INGUINAL HERNIA

An inguinal hernia develops, often bilaterally, due to the **processus vaginalis** remaining patent after birth (Tovar, 2003). It is one of the most common surgical conditions in infancy; the incidence increasing rapidly in preterm and small for gestational age infants (Johnstone, 1994), presumably precipitated by respiratory effort and artificial ventilation. It is more common in males, often associated with undescended testes (Moore and Persaud, 2003), and can be secondary to increased abdominal pressure with NEC and tight gastroschisis/exomphalos repairs.

Presentation is a swelling in the groin, extending to the scrotum or the labia, and may only be visible while the infant is crying, feeding or straining to pass stool. The hernia can usually be reduced initially by gentle pressure, when it will return to the abdomen with a characteristic 'gurgle' (Johnstone, 1994). There is significant variability between hospitals with regard to timing of repair: while it remains reducible and asymptomatic, most centres delay definitive surgery until the preterm infant is ready for discharge. However, delayed repair has been associated with incarceration, and early repair with a higher rate of reoperation (Sulkowski et al., 2015). Inguinal herniotomy consists of reduction of the contents into the abdomen, reconstruction of the posterior wall of the inguinal canal, ligation of the hernial sac and return of the testes to the scrotum (Wright, 1994).

Bowel ischaemia and ovarian or testicular atrophy can occur due to incarceration. Abdominal X-ray will show bowel, fluid levels and abdominal gas within the hernia. The infant should be nursed with the buttocks elevated until a surgical opinion can be sought. If the hernia strangulates, laparotomy and repair will be required. Resection and anastomosis may be necessary if the affected bowel is non-viable.

HYDROCOELE

Occasionally the abdominal end of the processus vaginalis remains open but is too small to permit herniation of the intestine. Peritoneal fluid passes into it and forms a hydrocoele – a painless collection of fluid around the testicle, presenting as a soft, non-tender, translucent swelling. Hydrocoeles are very common, usually resolve spontaneously, and are of no significance unless they become very large and tense, when a surgical opinion should be sought, to avert torsion of the testes. Hydrocoele is sometimes difficult to differentiate from an incarcerated hernia; a rectal examination will exclude the latter (Puri and Surana 1996). More commonly hydrocoeles can be identified through transillumination of the scrotum (Zderic and Lambert, 2012).

MOST COMMONLY ENCOUNTERED ACQUIRED DISORDERS

Necrotising enterocolitis

NEC is a gastrointestinal inflammatory disease of unknown aetiology, with a multifactorial pathophysiology, associated with high mortality and morbidity. Particularly at risk are those babies born prematurely (before 32 weeks), and/or of low birth weight (less than 1500g). Severe NEC leading to laparotomy, death or both affects 3.2% of babies born before 32weeks' gestational age (Battersby et al., 2017). There appears to be a complex relationship between mucosal injury, infection and hyperosmolar enteral feeds.

Mucosal injury Hypoxia and systemic hypotension lead to sparing of the vital organs at the expense of the gut, which is vulnerable to underperfusion and ischaemic damage. Factors associated with hypoxic stress include prolonged rupture of membranes, placental abruption, low Apgar scores, respiratory distress syndrome and apnoea. Left-to-right shunting through a patent ductus arteriosus compromises blood flow to the gut, and the presence of umbilical catheters is also implicated.

Microbial infection There is little evidence that infection is the cause of NEC, but it is an important factor in the pathogenesis. Damaged or immature epithelium may lead to a leaky mucosal barrier allowing hydrogen- and toxin-producing micro-organisms to invade the gut wall, with decreased levels of immunoglobulin G contributing to the mucosal damage (Hebra and Ross, 1996).

Enteral feeds Debate remains over optimum timing of introducing milk feeds, rates of advancement, the use of fortifiers and the use of probiotics, with limited evidence other than the use of human milk, to support interventions to prevent NEC (McGuire et al., 2015).

NEC can affect any part of the GI tract, but those most frequently affected are the terminal ileum and the splenic flexure. The clinical findings of NEC are seen in Bell's Classification (table 21.3) which can be a useful tool in predicting outcome.

Abdominal X-ray can confirm the diagnosis, showing distended loops of oedematous bowel and pneumatosis intestinalis (the presence of gas within the bowel wall). Serial films may reveal fixed, distended loops of bowel and progressive ascites. In the presence of perforation, **pneumoperitoneum** and gas in the portal vein may occur. Treatment for mild to moderate NEC is with antibiotics, intravenous nutrition and the suspension of enteral feeds

TABLE 21.3 *MODIFIED BELL'S CLASSIFICATION*

Stage	Clinical findings	X-ray findings	GI findings
IA	Apnoea and bradycardia, temperature instability	Normal or bowel dilatation indicative of mild ileus	Increased gastric aspirates, vomiting, mild abdominal distension
IB	As above	As above	Bright red blood from rectum
IIA	As above	Bowel dilatation indicative of ileus, pneumatosis	Grossly bloody stools, prominent abdominal distension, absent bowel sounds
IIB	Mild metabolic acidosis and mild thrombocytopaenia	Widespread pneumatosis, ascites, portal venous gas	Abdominal wall oedema, tenderness, palpable bowel loops
IIIA	Mixed acidosis, oliguria, hypotension, coagulopathy	Definite ascites, no free air	Generalised peritonitis, abdominal wall oedema, erythema and induration
IIIB	Shock, deteriorating laboratory values and vital signs	Pneumoperitoneum	Same as stage IIIA

(adapted from Reisinger et al., 2014)

with NG decompression for up to 10 days. Sicker infants may require platelet transfusion, supplemental oxygen, analgesia and, in severe cases, full respiratory support, inotropes, fluid resuscitation and blood transfusion, with operative intervention as a lifesaving measure.

Surgery is required when there is perforation or continued clinical deterioration. Laparotomy with surgery aims to preserve the maximum length of intestine while removing the source of sepsis. The affected gut may be just an isolated perforation, or a much larger area which is dilated and discoloured (see figure 21.7), with denuded areas of mucosa, but still viable. Alternatively, there may be patchy, necrotic or totally disintegrated areas. If resection and anastomosis of the gut are not possible, formation of one or more stomas will be necessary. The timing of subsequent stoma closure remains controversial, however, recent reports have suggested that there is no difference between different timings with regard to impact on outcome (Zani et al., 2017).

Postoperatively, the stoma should be observed closely for deterioration in perfusion. Initially, a non-adherent dressing may be used, but when the stoma begins to function, a suitably sized bag should be applied, preserving skin integrity. There is a risk of recurrence of NEC, strictures, and rarely the formation of fistulae. Malabsorption, failure to thrive and weight loss can be a problem postoperatively, and short gut syndrome may follow extensive resection. Despite improved prognosis, the aggressive form of the disease has not decreased and is still associated with significant rates of morbidity and mortality (Eaton, 2017).

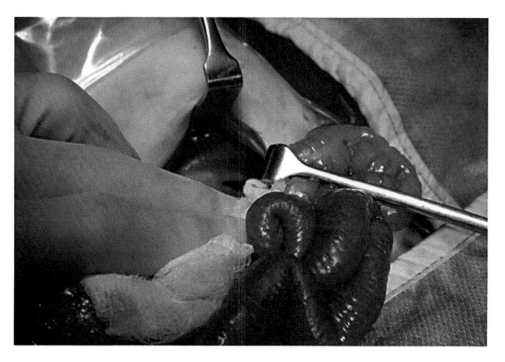

Figure 21.7 Ischaemic bowel identified at laparotomy (Source: Iain Yardley)

Spontaneous bowel perforation

Spontaneous intestinal perforation (SIP) is diagnosed at laparotomy, where an isolated focal perforation is seen with the surrounding tissue of normal appearance. The ileum is the most commonly affected part of the bowel. Due to its similarities in clinical presentation, it can be confused with NEC. There are multiple associated factors including patent ductus arteriosus, intraventricular haemorrhage, indometacin administration, and antenatal corticosteroids. Babies with SIP tend to have lower birth weights and may be less likely to develop severe illness. Mortality is noted to be significantly lower than that of NEC (Fisher et al., 2014).

MISCELLANEOUS DISORDERS

Cystic hygroma

The foetal lymphatic system develops at around five weeks' gestation. Cystic hygroma is a type of lymphangioma resulting from failure of the establishment of lymphatic drainage leading to pathological accumulations of fluid close to large veins and lymphatic ducts. They consist of a collection of fluid-filled cysts of variable size, which can continue to enlarge due to lymph accumulation. 75% are located in the neck, 20% in the axilla, 2% in retroperitoneum and intra-abdominal organs, 2% in limbs and bones, and 1% in the mediastinum. They are associated with chromosomal abnormalities, hydrops foetalis and other major malformations. Cystic hygromas are usually identified on antenatal ultrasound, with MRI providing a more accurate assessment of size and infiltration. Due to the common location in the neck, they place the foetus at risk of airway obstruction at delivery. In this situation an *ex utero* intrapartum treatment (EXIT) may be considered where the foetus is partially delivered, while placental circulation is maintained, allowing for respiratory procedures to take place to secure the airway (Butler et al., 2017).

Following delivery, if they are causing functional problems surgery may take place, or sclerotherapy – pharmacological treatment of abnormal vessels, causing them to involute. However, they are subject to local recurrence. Hygromas are benign, so although every effort should be made to excise the cyst completely, no major nerves or vessels should be sacrificed.

Teratoma

Teratomas are neoplasms containing derivatives of one or more of the embryonic germ layers. In neonates they are usually benign and can occur anywhere in the body, commonly in the sacro-coccygeal area, followed by the anterior mediastinum (Lakhoo, 2010). They may be identified by antenatal ultrasound scan and are associated with a raised alpha-fetoprotein level. A planned caesarean section will avoid dystocia, rupture or haemorrhage, as some are highly vascular. These lesions should be protected following delivery, to prevent erosion of the surface. With those at risk of respiratory distress, an EXIT procedure may be required. Complete excision is required, and delayed surgery is only feasible in unstable patients.

Ovarian cyst

Ovarian cysts in foetuses and neonates are relatively common and identified on antenatal ultrasound scan. They are thought to occur due to excessive stimulation of the foetal ovary by the placental and maternal hormones (Manjiri et al., 2017). While many will regress, complications include haemorrhage, rupture, torsion, as well as vascular, urinary tract and intestinal obstruction. They should be followed up postnatally with an ultrasound scan, and large or complex cysts should be laparoscopically removed (Manjiri et al., 2017).

Testicular torsion

Testicular torsion commonly occurs antenatally (Azmy, 1994). The neonatal testis may be prone to torsion because of its extreme mobility within the scrotum. On examination, the scrotum is non-translucent, swollen, firm, and discoloured. Ultrasound scan with Doppler may be used to confirm diagnosis. The management is controversial and variable, however, immediate surgery is required (Bandarkar and Blask, 2018).

Biliary atresia

Biliary atresia occurs due to failure of recanalisation of biliary ducts, or liver infection in late foetal life. The diagnosis is usually made from the recognition of prolonged jaundice in the first few weeks of life, followed by the development of pale stools and hepatomegaly. Haematological studies are mandatory for an overall evaluation. Once suspected, surgical intervention is necessary for a definitive diagnosis (intraoperative cholangiogram) and therapy (Kasai portoenterostomy; Schwarz, 2017).

Congenital pulmonary airway malformation

CPAM was previously known as congenital cystic adenomatoid malformation (CCAM) and is a developmental malformation of the lower respiratory tract. It accounts for 95% of antenatally diagnosed congenital cystic lung diseases (David et al., 2016). Management includes serial antenatal ultrasound scans with the consideration of additional MRI. Many will regress in the third trimester; however, some lesions will progress to cause hydrops foetalis, a major prognostic factor. Antenatal management includes administration of steroids and minimally invasive procedures, such as drainage via a thoraco-amniotic shunt to alleviate the mass effect. Postnatally, surgery is recommended if the baby is symptomatic, however management of asymptomatic CPAM remains contentious (David et al., 2016).

CONCLUSION

Improvements in diagnostic approaches, neonatal care, operative techniques, anaesthetic management, and collaborative care between the foetal medicine, surgical and neonatal teams, have all led to increased survival for infants with surgical problems. However, controversies regarding optimal management remain in many areas of the field; foetal interventions particularly require careful assessment of risks and benefits to mother and baby. At present, the reduction of associated morbidities, and an evaluation of long-term quality of life remain areas in need of further research and optimisation of practice.

CASE STUDIES

Case study 1: The deteriorating preterm infant

Alex is now 1 week old following delivery at 28 weeks' gestation weighing 1.2kg. He is currently receiving full enteral feeds of expressed breast milk at 180mL/kg/day. You notice on your shift that he is having frequent apnoeas and bradycardias associated with colour changes, and his mother expresses concerns that he is not himself.

On assessment Alex is lethargic, pale and vomits his recent feed, which is slightly green in colour.

Q.1. What are your immediate actions?

Alex's condition quickly deteriorates, and he needs to go to theatre as he has a perforation near the terminal ileum.

Q.2. How can you optimise his condition in preparation for theatre?

It is now four weeks since Alex had his operation, during which he required partial bowel resection and formation of an ileostomy. He is receiving breast milk feeds at 150mL/kg/day but is not gaining weight.

Q.3. What is your management strategy?
Q.4. What are the potential future risks?

Case study 2: The term infant with delayed passage of meconium

Harry is admitted with a history of not having passed meconium since birth (30 hours ago). He also has a distended, tense abdomen.

Q.1. What do you do?
Q.2. What investigations will be required and at what stage will they take place?
Q.3. What could the diagnosis be?

Following rectal suction biopsy, Harry is diagnosed with Hirschsprung's disease.

Q.4. What specific information and support do the parents need?

Case study 3: The term baby with bile-stained vomiting

Poppy was born at term and has been admitted from the postnatal ward with a history of bile-stained vomiting.

Q.1. What do you do?
Q.2. Her mother is very anxious – what explanations would you give her, what can she expect to happen next?
Q.3. What information do you need?
Q.4. What investigations are required?
Q.5. Is this considered to be a surgical emergency? Why?

For suggested answer guides to the questions posed in these case studies, please refer to the web-based companion site specific to this chapter (see URL below).

WEB-BASED RESOURCES

For further information, online resources and greater detail on the case studies featured in this chapter go to www.routledge.com/cw/nicnursing

References

Azmy, A. A. F. (1994). Acute penile and scrotal conditions. In Raine, P., & Azmy, A. A. F. (Eds.) *Surgical Emergencies in Children*. Oxford: Butterworth-Heinemann.

Bandarkar, A. N., & Blask, A. R. (2018). Testicular torsion with preserved flow: Key sonographic features and value-added approach to diagnosis. *Pediatric Adiology*, *48*(5), 735–744. DOI:10.1007/s00247-018-4093-0

Bass, K. D., Rothenberg, S. S., & Chang, J. H. (1998). Laparoscopic Ladd's procedure in infants with malrotation. *Journal of Pediatric Surgery*, *33*(2), 279–281.

Battersby, C., Longford, N., Mandalia, S., Costeloe, K., Modi, N., & Enterocolitis, U. N. C. N. (2017). Incidence and enteral feed antecedents of severe neonatal necrotising enterocolitis across neonatal networks in England, 2012–13: A whole-population surveillance study. *The Lancet Gastroenterology & Hepatology*, *2*(1), 43–51.

Beasley, S. (2016). Oesophageal atresia and tracheo-oesophageal fistula. *Surgery, 34*(12), 612–616.

Bischoff, A. (2016). The surgical treatment of cloaca. *Seminars in Pediatric Surgery 5*(2), 102–107.

Bradshaw, C. J., Thakkar, H., Knutzen, L., Marsh, R., Pacilli, M., Impey, L., & Lakhoo, K. (2016). Accuracy of prenatal detection of tracheoesophageal fistula and oesophageal atresia. *Journal of Pediatric Surgery, 51*(8), 1268–1272.

Brophy, K. M. (2007). Opioid analgesics and opioid antagonists. In Brophy, K. M., Scarlett-Ferguson, H., & Webber, K. *Clinical Drug Therapy for Canadian Practice*. Philadelphia, PA: Lippincott Williams & Wilkins.

Burge, D. M., Shah, K., Spark, P., Shenker, N., Pierce, M., Kurinczuk, J. J., … & British Association of Paediatric Surgeons Congenital Anomalies Surveillance System (BAPS-CASS). (2013). Contemporary management and outcomes for infants born with oesophageal atresia. *British Journal of Surgery*, *100*(4), 515–521.

Butler, C. R., Maughan, E. F., Pandya, P., & Hewitt, R. (2017). Ex utero intrapartum treatment (EXIT) for upper airway obstruction. *Current Opinion in Otolaryngology & Head and Neck Surgery, 25*(2), 119–126.

Chhabra, S., & Kenny, S. E. (2016). Hirschsprung's disease. *Surgery (Oxford), 34*(12), 628–632.

Collaborative, TCCDH. (2018). Diagnosis and management of congenital diaphragmatic hernia: a clinical practice guideline. *Canadian Medical Association Journal*, *190*(4), E103.

Davenport, M., Rothenberg, S. S., Crabbe, D. C., & Wulkan, M. L. (2015). The great debate: Open or thoracoscopic repair for oesophageal atresia or diaphragmatic hernia. *Journal of Pediatric Surgery*, *50*(2), 240–246.

David, M., Lamas-Pinheiro, R., & Henriques-Coelho, T. (2016). Prenatal and postnatal management of congenital pulmonary airway malformation. *Neonatology, 110*(2), 101–115.

Department of Health (2009) *Reference guide to consent for examination or treatment (second edition)*. London: Department of Health.

DeWayne P., Hansen, A. R., & Pruder, M. (2009) Obstruction. In Hansen, A., & Pruder, M. (Eds.) *Manual of Neonatal Surgical Intensive Care*. Connecticut: People's Medical Publishing House.

Eaton, S. (2017). Necrotizing enterocolitis symposium: Epidemiology and early diagnosis. *Journal of Pediatric Surgery*, *52*(2), 223–225.

Enninga, E. A., & Ruano, R. (2018). Fetal surgery for lower urinary tract obstruction: The importance of staging prior to intervention. *Minerva Pediatrica, 70*(3), 263–269.

Fisher, J. G., Jones, B. A., Gutierrez, I. M., Hull, M. A., Kang, K. H., Kenny, M., … & Jaksic, T. (2014). Mortality associated with laparotomy-confirmed neonatal spontaneous intestinal perforation: A prospective 5-year multicenter analysis. *Journal of Pediatric Surgery, 49*(8), 1215–1219.

Golonka, N. R., & Hayashi, A. H. (2008). Early 'sham' feeding of neonates promotes oral feeding after delayed primary repair of major congenital esophageal anomalies. *The American Journal of Surgery, 195*(5), 659–662.

Graves, C. E., Harrison, M. R., & Padilla, B. E. (2017). Minimally invasive fetal surgery. *Clinics in Perinatology, 44*(4), 729–751.

Hebra, A. & Miller, M. (2010). Intestinal Volvulus. http://emedicine.medscape.com/article/930576

Hebra, A. & Ross, A. J. (1996). Necrotising enterocolitis. In Spitzer, A. R. (Ed.) *Intensive Care of the Fetus and Neonate*. St Louis, MO: Mosby.

Hochart, V., Verpillat, P., Langlois, C., Garabedian, C., Bigot, J., Debarge, V. H., … & Avni, F. E. (2015). The contribution of fetal MR imaging to the assessment of oesophageal atresia. *European Radiology*, *25*(2), 306–314.

Hodson, W. A. (2018). Temperature regulation. In Gleason, C. A., & Juul, S. E. (Eds.) *Avery's Diseases of the Newborn* (10th Edition). Philadelphia, PA: Elsevier.

Houben, C., Davenport, M., Ade-Ajayi, N., Flack, N., & Patel, S. (2009). Closing gastroschisis: Diagnosis, management, and outcomes. *Journal of Pediatric Surgery*, *44*(2), 343–347.

Jesudason, E. C., Connell, M. G., Fernig, D. G., Lloyd, D. A., & Losty, P. D. (2000). Early lung malformations in congenital diaphragmatic hernia. *Journal of Pediatric Surgery*, *35*(1), 124–128.

Johnstone, J. M. S. (1994). Hernia in the neonate. In Freeman N. V., Burge, D. M., Griffiths, M., & Malone, P. S. J. (Eds.) *Surgery of the Newborn*. London: Churchill Livingstone.

Jones, B. A., Modi B. P., Jaksic T., Langer, M., & Garza, J. (2009). Intestinal Atresia, Stenosis and Webs. http://emedicine.medscape.com/article/940615

Karrer, F. M., & Potter, D. D. (2009). Duodenal Atresia. http://emedicine.medscape.com/article/93291

Kleinman, M. E., & Wilson, J. M. (2009). Congenital diaphragmatic hernia and diaphragmatic eventration. In Hansen, A., & Pruder, M. (Eds.) *Manual of Neonatal Surgical Intensive Care*. Connecticut: People's Medical Publishing House.

Kong, J. Y., Yeo, K. T., Abdel-Latif, M. E., Bajuk, B., Holland, A. J., Adams, S., … & Oei, J. L. (2016). Outcomes of infants with abdominal wall defects over 18 years. *Journal of Pediatric Surgery*, *51*(10), 1644–1649.

Kotoulas, O. B., Kalamidas, S. A., & Kondomerkos, D. J. (2006). Glycogen autophagy in glucose homeostasis. *Pathology-Research and Practice*, *202*(9), 631–638.

Krylborn, J., Anell-Olofsson, M. E., Bitkover, C., Lundeberg, S., Bartocci, M., Stiller, C. O., & Larsson, B. A. (2015). Plasma levels of levobupivacaine during continuous infusion via a wound catheter after major surgery in newborn infants: an observational study. *European Journal of Anaesthesiology*, *32*(12), 851–856.

Lakhoo, K. (2010). Neonatal teratomas. *Early Human Development*, *86*(10), 643–647.

Lal, D. R., Gadepalli, S. K., Downard, C. D., Ostlie, D. J., Minneci, P. C., Swedler, R. M., … & Fallat, M. E. (2017). Perioperative management and outcomes of esophageal atresia and tracheoesophageal fistula. *Journal of Pediatric Surgery*, *52*(8), 1245–1251.

Lau, P. E., Cruz, S., Cassady, C. I., Mehollin-Ray, A. R., Ruano, R., Keswani, S., … & Cass, D. L. (2017). Prenatal diagnosis and outcome of fetal gastrointestinal obstruction. *Journal of Pediatric Surgery*, *52*(5), 722–725.

Lee, S., & Meeker, T. M. (2018). Basic Knowledge of Tracheoesophageal Fistula and Esophageal Atresia. *Advances in Neonatal Care*, *18*(1), 14–21.

Llewelyn, M. J., Fitzpatrick, J. M., Darwin, E., Gorton, C., Paul, J., Peto, T. E., … & Walker, A. S. (2017). The antibiotic course has had its day. *British Medical Journal*, *358*, j3418.

McGuire, W., Young, L., & Morgan, J. (2015). Preventing necrotising enterocolitis in very preterm infants: Current evidence. *Paediatrics and Child Health*, *25*(6), 265–270.

Madhusmita, R. G. G., Mittal, M. K., & Bagga, D. (2018). Anorectal malformations: Role of MRI in preoperative evaluation. *The Indian Journal of Radiology & Imaging*, *28*(2), 187.

Manjiri, S., Padmalatha, S. K., & Shetty, J. (2017). Management of Complex Ovarian Cysts in Newborns – Our Experience. *Journal of Neonatal Surgery*, *6*(1), 3.

Martin, L. D. (2017). The basic principles of anesthesia for the neonate. *Revista Colombiana de Anestesiología*, *45*(1), 54–61.

Martin, C. R., & Fishman, S. J. (2009). Gastrointestinal disorders. Part 1: Gastroschisis. In Hansen, A., & Pruder, M. (Eds.) *Manual of Neonatal Surgical Intensive Care*. Connecticut: People's Medical Publishing House.

Merei, J. M., Farmer, P., Hasthorpe, S., Qi, B. Q., Beasley, S. W., Myers, N. A., & Hutson, J. M. (1997). Timing and embryology of esophageal atresia and tracheo-esophageal fistula. *The Anatomical Record: An Official Publication of the American Association of Anatomists*, *249*(2), 240–248.

Miyake, H., Chen, Y., Hock, A., Seo, S., Koike, Y., & Pierro, A. (2018). Are prophylactic anti-reflux medications effective after esophageal atresia repair? Systematic review and meta-analysis. *Pediatric Surgery International, 34*(5), 491–497.

Moore, K. L., & Persaud, T. V. N. (2003). *The Developing Human: Clinical Oriented Embryology* (5th Edition) Philadelphia, PA: WB Saunders.

Moron, A. F., Barbosa, M. M., Milani, H. J. F., Sarmento, S. G., Santana, E. F. M., Suriano, I. C., … & Cavalheiro, S. (2018). Perinatal outcomes after open fetal surgery for myelomeningocele repair: A retrospective cohort study. *BJOG: An International Journal of Obstetrics & Gynaecology. 125*(10), 1280–1286.

National Perinatal Epidemiology Unit (2014). *Congenital Diaphragmatic Hernia.* www.npeu.ox.ac.uk/ukoss/current-surveillance/cdh

Nicholl, R. (2003). What is the normal range of blood glucose concentrations in healthy term newborns? *Archives of Disease in Childhood, 88*(3), 238–239.

Papadopulos, N., Papadoulos, M., Kovacs, L., Zeilhofer, H., Henke, J., Boettcher, P., & Biemer, E. (2005). Foetal surgery and cleft lip and palate: current status and new perspectives. *British Journal of Plastic Surgery, 58*(5), 593–607.

Paran, T. S., Decaluwe, D., Corbally, M., & Puri, P. (2007). Long-term results of delayed primary anastomosis for pure oesophageal atresia: A 27-year follow up. *Pediatric Surgery International, 23*(7), 647–651.

Pena, A. (1996) Anorectal anomalies. In Puri, P. (Ed.) *Newborn Surgery.* Oxford: Butterworth-Heinemann

Pettenati, M. J., Haines, J. L., Higgins, R. R., Wappner, R. S., Palmer, C. G., & Weaver, D. (1986). Wiedemann-Beckwith syndrome: Presentation of clinical and cytogenetic data on 22 new cases and review of the literature. *Human Genetics, 74*(2), 143–154.

Prefumo, F., & Izzi, C. (2014). Fetal abdominal wall defects. *Best Practice & Research Clinical Obstetrics & Gynaecology, 28*(3), 391–402.

Puri, P. (1996). Hirschsprung's disease. In Puri, P. (Ed.) *Newborn Surgery.* Oxford: Butterworth-Heinemann.

Puri, P. & Surana, R. (1996). Inguinal hernia. In Puri, P. (Ed.) *Newborn Surgery.* Oxford: Butterworth-Heinemann.

Reisinger, K. W., Kramer, B. W., van Der Zee, D, Derikx, J. P. M., Buurman, W., Brouwers, H., & Van Heurn, E. (2014). Non-invasive serum amyloid A (SAA) measurement and plasma platelets for accurate prediction of surgical intervention in severe necrotising enterocolitis (NEC). *PloS One, 9*(3), e90834.

Replogle, R. L. (1963). Esophageal atresia: plastic sump catheter for drainage of the proximal pouch. *Surgery, 54*(2), 296–297.

Reynolds, F. (2005). Maximum recommended doses of local anesthetics: A constant cause of confusion. *Regional Anesthesia and Pain Medicine, 30*(3), 314–316.

Rode, H., & Millar, A. J. W. (2006). Jejunoileal atresia. In Puri, P., & Hollworth, M. (Eds.), *Pediatric Surgery, Diagnostics and Management.* New York: Springer Publishing Company.

Ruano, R., Ali, R. A., Patel, P., Cass, D., Olutoye, O., & Belfort, M. A. (2014). Fetal endoscopic tracheal occlusion for congenital diaphragmatic hernia: Indications, outcomes, and future directions. *Obstetrical & Gynecological Survey, 69*(3), 147–158.

Sathe, M., & Houwen, R. (2017). Meconium ileus in cystic fibrosis. *Journal of Cystic Fibrosis, 16*, S32–S39.

Schwarz, S. (2017). *Pediatric Biliary Atresia.* https://emedicine.medscape.com/article/927029

Simmons, M., & Georgeson, K. E. (1996). The effect of gestational age at birth on morbidity in patients with gastroschisis. *Journal of Pediatric Surgery, 31*(8), 1060–1062.

Skarsgard, E. D., & Barth, R. A. (1997). Use of doppler ultrasonography in the evaluation of liver blood flow during silo reduction of a giant omphalocele. *Journal of Pediatric Surgery, 32*(5), 733–735.

Spitz, L. (2007). Oesophageal atresia. *Orphanet Journal of Rare Diseases, 2*(1), 24.

Steinhorn, R. H., & Porta, N. F. M. (1997). *Congenital Diaphragmatic Hernia.* http://emedicine.medscape.com/article/978118

Suen, H. C. (2018). Congenital H-type tracheoesophageal fistula in adults. *Journal of Thoracic Disease, 10* (Suppl 16), S1905.

Sulkowski, J. P., Cooper, J. N., Duggan, E. M., Balci, O., Anandalwar, S. P., Blakely, M. L., … & Deans, K. J. (2015). Does timing of neonatal inguinal hernia repair affect outcomes? *Journal of Pediatric Surgery*, *50*(1), 171–176.

Takayasu, H., Masumoto, K., Jimbo, T., Sakamoto, N., Sasaki, T., Uesugi, T., … & Shinkai, T. (2017). Analysis of risk factors of long-term complications in congenital diaphragmatic hernia: A single institution's experience. *Asian Journal of Surgery*, *40*(1), 1–5.

Tam, P. K., Chung, P. H., St Peter, S. D., Gayer, C. P., Ford, H. R., Tam, G. C., … & Davenport, M. (2017). Advances in paediatric gastroenterology. *The Lancet*, *390*(10099), 1072–1082.

Tovar, J. (2003). Inguinal hernia. In Puri, P. (Ed.) *Newborn Surgery*. Oxford: Butterworth-Heinemann.

van der Zee, D. C., Bagolan, P., Faure, C., Gottrand, F., Jennings, R., Laberge, J. M., … & Teague, W. (2017). Position paper of INoEA working group on long-gap esophageal atresia: for better care. *Frontiers in Pediatrics*, *5*, 63. doi: https://doi.org/10.3389/fped.2017.00063

Watanabe, S., Suzuki, T., Hara, F., Yasui, T., Uga, N., & Naoe, A. (2017). Omphalocele and gastroschisis in newborns: over 16 years of experience from a single clinic. *Journal of Neonatal Surgery*, *6*(2), 27.

Wilson, R. D., Hedrick, H. L., Liechty, K. W., Flake, A. W., Johnson, M. P., Bebbington, M., & Adzick, N. S. (2006). Cystic adenomatoid malformation of the lung: review of genetics, prenatal diagnosis, and in utero treatment. *American Journal of Medical Genetics Part A*, *140*(2), 151–155.

Wright, J. E. (1994). Direct inguinal hernia in infancy and childhood. *Pediatric Surgery International*, *9*(3), 161–163.

Yoo, S. Y., Jung, S. H., Eom, M., Kim, I. H., & Han, A. (2002). Delayed maturation of interstitial cells of Cajal in meconium obstruction. *Journal of Pediatric Surgery*, *37*(12), 1758–1761.

Zani, A., Lauriti, G., Li, Q., & Pierro, A. (2017). The timing of stoma closure in infants with necrotizing enterocolitis: a systematic review and meta-analysis. *European Journal of Pediatric Surgery*, *27*(1), 007–011.

Zderic, S. A. & Lambert, S. M. (2012). Developmental Abnormalities of the Genitourinary System. In Gleason, C. A., & Devaskar, S. U. (Eds.) *Avery's Diseases of the Newborn* (9th Edition). Philadelphia, PA: Elsevier.

Zens, T., Nichol, P. F., Cartmill, R., & Kohler, J. E. (2017). Management of asymptomatic Pediatric umbilical hernias: a systematic review. *Journal of Pediatric Surgery*. *52*(11), 1723–1731.

22 NEONATAL TRANSPORTATION

Patrick Turton

CONTENTS

GUIDANCE ON HOW TO ENHANCE PERSONAL LEARNING FROM THIS CHAPTER

Key points covered in this chapter

- An overview of the structure and function of the neonatal transport service and team.
- The different types of neonatal transfer including clinical considerations relating to a range of different conditions.
- The safety and governance aspects surrounding transferring sick and high-risk infants.

Reflection

Reading through the chapter, you are encouraged to engage with the key points and related literature in an enquiring way. Ask these questions:

- Which infants in your care have had to be transferred, either out or in, and why?
- What considerations are required to ensure the infant is as safe and risk-free as possible when stabilising them for transfer?
- How should the family be managed and communicated with, in the event of their baby needing transfer?

> ### Implications for nursing care
>
> ■ Finally: how will this chapter enable you to consider and understand the specific issues and challenges of neonatal transport for the high-risk infant and their family? Consider the implications of what you learn for your nursing care relating to stabilisation and transfer of both infants and parents.

INTRODUCTION AND BACKGROUND

Critically ill newborn infants are a highly vulnerable and unique population who require specialised teams for stabilisation and transport to achieve optimal outcomes (Aubertin et al., 2018). There are many reasons why a neonate may need to be transferred from one unit, department, or hospital to another. Whatever the reason, however, transfers require careful preparation and planning in order to minimise potential risks to the infant and team involved (Kronforst, 2016). Having an increased awareness of the principles of safe neonatal transport will be helpful not only to staff who may be interested in working as part of a neonatal transport service, but to those who are involved in transport. This includes staff who will help prepare an infant for transport, who care for babies after they have been transferred, and who may need to transfer babies themselves. The neonatal nurse of course is an integral part of the team, and in this chapter will be considered as part of a multidisciplinary approach.

The logistic and clinical complexities of all transfers will vary, but due consideration should be given to common phases of the transport episode. These phases include:

■ Referral or request for transfer
■ Activation of the transferring team
■ Handover of patient details
■ Stabilisation and preparation for transfer
■ Arrival at receiving location
■ Handover of patient details
■ Return of transferring team to base

This chapter will aim to provide some detail and insight into preparing for and managing these phases safely and efficiently.

THE NEONATAL TRANSPORT SERVICE

In the UK, following the introduction of a centralised neonatal transfer service, response times in the transfer of sick, high-risk infants improved significantly (Kempley et al. 2007).

This resulted from the introduction of managed neonatal clinical networks in 2004 (Marlow and Gill, 2007), defining a more formal recognition of the need for established and robust neonatal transport services. Strategies to increase the numbers of extremely preterm deliveries in hospitals with neonatal intensive care units (NICUs) have seen a reduction of neonatal mortality in those populations (Gale, 2012; Marlow et al., 2014; Boland et al., 2017). Within these managed clinical networks, transport services have a key role to play in maintaining patient flow both into and out of NICUs. The requirement for neonatal transfer is acknowledged at government level. The National Health Service (NHS) Neonatal Transport Service Specification provides a framework for transport services (Department of Health, 2015), and categorises the reasons for transfer into:

- Uplift
- Resources/capacity
- Repatriation.

An uplift transfer is one where the infant is being moved to receive a level of care not available at the referring unit. For example, a 24-week gestation infant having delivered in a Special Care Unit (SCU) needs to be transferred to a NICU. It would also include an infant in a SCU needing respiratory support and transfer to a Local Neonatal Unit (LNU).

A resources/capacity transfer is one where an infant needs to be transferred due to a unit having insufficient staffing, cots or equipment, to safely provide the level of care required for the baby.

A repatriation is the transfer of an infant back to, or nearer, their booking hospital. Repatriations can be low dependency, high dependency, or intensive care transfers.

Specialist Commissioning Groups fund these transport services which are hosted by one of the NHS trusts in each Neonatal Operational Delivery Network (ODN). Some transport services operate independently of the host neonatal unit (NNU), while others are more closely integrated. The variation in these local arrangements is largely down to historic relationships between the services of each region, and the different development trajectories of the transport teams. There are currently 15 neonatal transport services covering the UK, who carry out approximately 16,000 transfers per year (UK Neonatal Transport Group (NTG), 2018). Recent years have seen teams merging with neighbouring services with the aim of providing a larger, more resilient and robust transport service for their neonatal ODNs. The NTG is made up of nursing and medical representatives from each transport service. The Neonatal Intensive Care Transport Service Specification identifies five key measures by which each transport service is benchmarked. These are:

1) Dedicated neonatal transport services transfer at least 95% of patients requiring uplift within their defined catchment area on an annual basis.
2) For time-critical transfers, the transport team mobilises towards the patient within one hour from the start of the referral call (95% of transfers annually).

3) The transport team will arrive with the patient requiring uplift and intensive care transfers within 3.5 hours of the referring call on 80% of transfers.

4) Timely collection of data as requested by the NTG/British Association of Perinatal Medicine (BAPM) dataset.

5) Publish an annual report.

Establishing a combined service requires vision, time, hard work and support from the clinical and healthcare commissioning communities. Success of the project will depend on strong clinical leadership, a dedicated, highly skilled group of professionals who share the vision, financial support, and a foundation based on quality and safety. Given the high risk nature of the activity, any new service will need to benchmark against recognised standards and key performance metrics to ensure the best care possible is provided to this most vulnerable group of patients (Hancock and Harrison, 2018).

Working on the transport team

Neonatal transport teams are composed of clinical and non-clinical team members in nursing, medical and driving roles (Chang et al., 2015). The way in which these roles are provided varies in different teams. Some teams are composed of a consultant and a transport nurse, while some teams utilise Advanced Neonatal Nurse Practitioners and transport nurses, with consultant input to enhance the team on certain transfers. Each service will have its own standard operating procedures (SOPs) to inform and support the decision-making surrounding the composition of their team (Fenton and Leslie, 2009). Following careful triage, some transfers can be safely undertaken by a nurse-led team, while others will require someone acting in the medical role with the potential addition of a transport consultant.

The nature of working in a small team means that there can be an overlap of the roles of the team members. Common tasks of transferring monitoring, transferring infusions, documentation, checking and troubleshooting equipment, and restocking equipment can be undertaken by all team members. However, there needs to be a clear understanding about the allocation and distribution of roles which considers the varying levels of skill and experience of the team members. This style of pluripotential working means that the required tasks can be achieved quickly and efficiently, as well as providing a helpful safety cross-check within the team.

Regardless of the composition of the team, there are specific training and educational needs which address the challenges of working in the transport environment (Fenton et al., 2004) in line with the essential elements of team-working outlined in box 22.1.

The challenges of working in an unfamiliar or restrictive environment under extreme pressure should not be underestimated (Royal College of Nursing (RCN), 2013). Careful preparation of the transport team can help to optimise their performance regardless of the clinical complexity of the transfer. The use of checklists, scenario training and simulation,

---

BOX 22.1 ELEMENTS OF TEAM-WORKING FOR NEONATAL TRANSPORT

■ Working effectively in small teams
■ Working in restrictive and isolated environments
■ Communicating in stressful situations
■ Develop an enhanced level of clinical assessment and decision-making
■ Independent working
■ Team/peer support and debrief.

---

and human factors training are key to building the skills of the team (Fenton et al., 2004). The development of courses such as Neonatal, Adult and Paediatric Safe Transfer and Retrieval (NAPSTaR) by the Advanced Life Support Group provide a syllabus which aims to address some of the training needs of transport team staff. Learning from strategies and approaches adopted by high reliability organisations such as the aviation, construction and nuclear industries can add another dimension to safety in healthcare (Gawande, 2010; Reason, 2016).

Equipment

Delivering a neonatal transport service means having the ability to provide a mobile intensive care unit. The transport incubator system (TIS) is generally made up of an incubator housed on a trolley with attachments for the associated intensive care equipment (see figure 22.1). There are restrictions and limitations related to equipment size and weight, and the various iterations and upgrades of equipment and therapies means that it can be difficult to maintain an up-to-date set-up.

While there are commonalities with transport equipment across different transport services, the configuration of each transport incubator system will be slightly different, often aligning with equipment already in use in the host trust and familiarity to one's own system is paramount (Fenton et al., 2004).

Designing and purchasing a TIS is expensive and must be undertaken with consideration to certain European standards (British Standards Institute, 2011). There are significant costs involved with servicing and repairing equipment, as well as the costs of developing and delivering training and competency packages to the team. This means that some teams adopt a 'one size fits all' approach, using the same TIS for all levels of transfers. However, not all infants will require high dependency or intensive level care, and so other configurations of lower dependency options using a pod and trolley system can be found.

Hospitals which might only need to undertake transports infrequently may well be better off purchasing a more rudimentary system which can easily cope with most of their

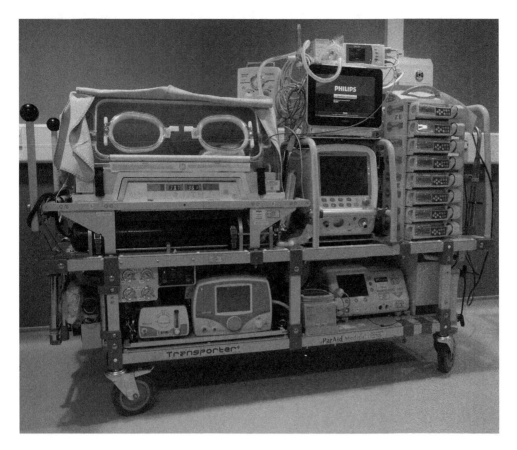

Figure 22.1 Neonatal transport incubator system

transport needs, with the option to enhance the system on the rare occasion where this is required. The benefits of some of these approaches are that they can be cheaper, lighter and therefore easier to manoeuvre, quicker to clean, and can also accommodate larger infants than can be fitted into the transport incubator. Whichever system is used, appropriate fixation of equipment to the trolley, and of the trolley to the ambulance is critical in maintaining infant and team safety in the ambulance.

As well as the TIS, the transport team will need to have a range of disposables, to cater for any interventions required. There is a constant balance between limiting the amount of equipment being carried around, with ensuring that any eventuality can be addressed *en route* if required. These will be packaged in robust and portable transport bags so that they can be safely carried between ambulance and hospital, and easily accessed if required (see figure 22.2). Compatibility of equipment around the region may vary, which means that teams are not always able to rely on using the local hospital's equipment.

The ambulance is an integral piece of equipment required for neonatal transport (Figure 22.3).

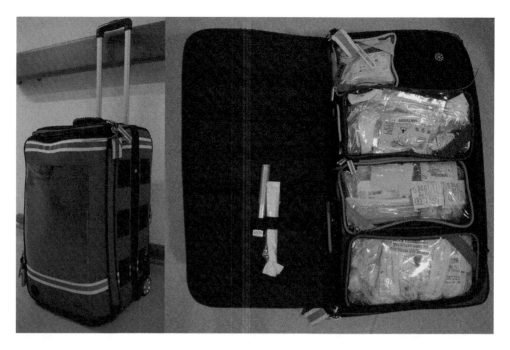

Figure 22.2 Neonatal transport pack/equipment

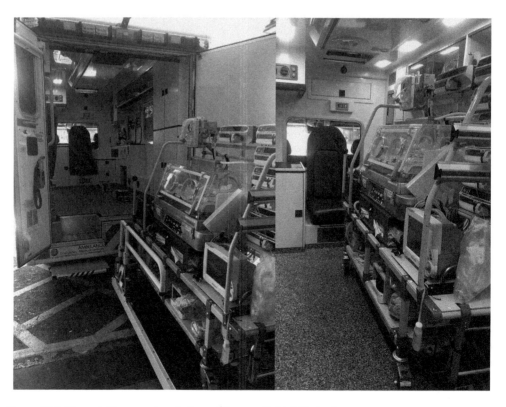

Figure 22.3 Neonatal transport ambulance (Source: Patrick Turton)

Having access to a dedicated vehicle means that the team will be aware of the layout of their vehicle, and the specific safety and manual handling constraints. The team will also be able to familiarise themselves with the storage of their equipment and supplies, so that they will be able to respond quickly and efficiently should they need to. It is also important to consider familiarity with the loading mechanisms of the vehicles, as well as the electrical and gas supply systems, so that the team can help in troubleshooting and problem-solving if required.

NEONATAL TRANSFERS NOT UNDERTAKEN BY THE TRANSPORT TEAM

There are occasions where a team other than a neonatal transport team might transfer an infant. The two likely alternatives are that the infant is transferred by a paediatric critical care transport team, if the infant is moving into a paediatric intensive care unit, or if the local team is required to transfer the infant. Examples of this are where any delay incurred waiting for the transport team to arrive will cause harm to the patient. Surgical emergencies such as volvulus or neurosurgical emergencies are two such cases where the local team may be required to transfer the patient themselves.

Transfers undertaken by the local team

There are occasions where the referring team at the local hospital will need to undertake a transfer. This may be because the principal transport service for that area is committed to another transfer. In these cases, a careful discussion must take place between the referring, transport, and specialist teams to consider the costs and benefits of waiting for the transport team to be available versus the local team moving the patient themselves. Key factors here are the underlying clinical problem, the clinical requirements of the infant at that time, and a careful triage of the transport service's current workload. These transfers place a significant burden on the local teams undertaking them. Access to the appropriate transport equipment is often difficult, and there are particular challenges with identifying an appropriately skilled team without critically depleting the staffing levels back at base.

Factors that can help reduce the stress and pressure that the transfers place on referring teams include:

■ Early communication with relevant parties to aid in decision-making
■ Local guidance (developed with support from the regional transport team) to aid a prompt and safe dispatch
■ Checklists to assist in team and equipment preparation.

Simulation and scenario training for instigating a locally delivered transfer are excellent ways to identify issues pertinent to each centre. They give hospital teams the opportunity to rehearse the process and familiarise themselves with their transport equipment.

Intra-hospital transfers

Intra-hospital transfers are another example where babies are not transferred by a specialist transport team. Even moving an infant from the delivery suite to the intensive care department requires careful planning, and transfers to operating theatre, or for radiographical imaging can provide logistical and clinical challenges. Some hospitals have these departments in different buildings, necessitating a road transfer which may well be undertaken by staff who are not experienced in neonatal transport. These teams need to ensure that they have adequate equipment available and are appropriately drilled in preparing for potential emergencies during the time off the NNU.

AEROMEDICAL TRANSFERS

In the UK, the clear majority of neonatal transfers are undertaken by road, but at times air transportation is needed depending on location and distance. Scotland has a well-established aeromedical capability, driven largely by factors such as geography and population spread, and it is increasingly accepted that helicopter (rotary wing) and aeroplane (fixed-wing) transfers have their place in UK neonatal transport provision. As the aeromedical infrastructures develop, so does the ease with which these resources can be accessed (Kempley and Ratnavel, 2012). With enhanced aeromedical training and education relating to transport physiology, aeromedical logistics and communication, some transport teams are able to offer an aeromedical response to certain transfers. Currently, transport services offering an aeromedical capability may consider a rotary wing transfer for patients requiring transfers which are predicted to last longer than two hours by road.

Fixed-wing transfers may be considered if the anticipated road journey is greater than 4 hours. This difference is due to the limited availability of airports where fixed-wing craft can land. This means that there is likely to be a significant secondary road transfer to complete the transfer to the receiving hospital, which results in additional logistical challenges. In many cases, the time-savings afforded by flying are lost due to additional planning and extended secondary road transfers required (Kempley and Ratnavel, 2012). Because of the geographical size of the UK, and distribution of centres delivering neonatal care, fixed-wing transfers are much less common than rotary wing transfers.

It is not necessarily better to have faster transport times, and this is often an assumption of air transport as a preferred method compared to road (Killion and Stein, 2009). There are a multitude of factors which will influence the decision-making regarding aeromedical transfers over and above the anticipated road transfer time (see box 22.2).

> ### BOX 22.2 FACTORS TO CONSIDER FOR DECIDING BETWEEN AIR AND ROAD TRANSFERS
>
> ■ Patient stability and other clinical flight restrictions
> ■ Requirement for/length of secondary transfer
> ■ Weather
> ■ Flight hours available
> ■ Appropriately trained/competent team available
> ■ Airframe availability
> ■ Equipment availability
> ■ Requirement of family to travel with the infant
> ■ Funding arrangements.

SAFETY DURING TRANSPORT

The transport environment is more physically restrictive and resource-poor when compared to the hospital environment, which can put the team under increased physical, intellectual and emotional demands. Promoting the safety of the team during these transport episodes is hugely important and includes a wide range of considerations. Applying principles of clinical governance and safety to transport services is challenging but requires attention (Ratnavel, 2009).

Staff should have access to personal protective equipment in the vehicles, such as gloves, aprons, goggles and hand cleaning gels, and will also need additional measures specific to the transport environment. Consideration should be given to a uniform which is comfortable and practical to allow ease of work both in the NNU as well as when unloading and loading the ambulance in all types of weather. Many teams insist upon their staff wearing protective footwear and having access to high-visibility jackets. Unloading and loading might not necessarily occur just outside the hospitals, as vehicles are at risk of breaking down or being damaged in road traffic incidents. On these occasions the transfer of equipment and possibly the patient may need to take place on the roadside where the environment is hazardous. Such instances pose multiple threats, and it will be necessary to enlist the support of other services such as the police or highways agency, to ensure the safety of the team and other road users.

Other physical challenges include the moving and handling of loads, which is made more difficult by having a small team and having to operating in a smaller restrictive environment. Some TIS weigh up to 300kg, and so extreme care must be taken when working with these loads. Feet, toes, hands and fingers are at particular risk of getting injured, as well as other musculoskeletal injuries. Heightened awareness of this through careful induction, and dynamic risk assessments using tools such as TILEO (T–task, I–individual, L–load,

E–environment, O–other factors) is important when handling the transport incubator and other transport equipment (Worksafe UK, 2019).

When loaded into the ambulance, the safety considerations continue. Ensuring the incubator is properly secured into the floor fixings is critical, which can be determined by a 'push-pull' check to confirm that the locks have engaged. The equipment bags must be secured adequately, and in such a way as to allow prompt access if required. Cupboard doors must be closed properly, so as not to swing open dangerously during the journey. The reason why these are all such important factors is that an unsecured object will become a dangerous missile in the event of an accident. A sharp change in direction or speed can cause damage to the team or their equipment.

Appropriately securing equipment also extends to making sure that all team members and passengers are wearing their seatbelts. Not only do unrestrained personnel pose a risk to themselves, they could well hurt or injure someone else in the vehicle or damage the equipment. Wind gusts, sudden braking, or swerving to avoid road debris can all make someone lose their balance while in the back of a moving vehicle. The team must remain seated and belted at all times in order to maintain a safe environment. Careful planning of the journey including anticipating potential clinical requirements and interventions is an important part of this planning. There may be rare occasions where the urgency of the situation requires the team to unsecure themselves while the vehicle is in motion. In these circumstances the driver must be made aware of the situation so that they can adjust their driving style accordingly. The driver can then find a safe place to stop for the team to deal with the ongoing needs.

Other environmental considerations that relate to ambulance safety include temperature of the vehicle, lighting, and seating arrangements. Environments that are too hot or cold can cause the team to become drowsy or nauseous, extreme or inadequate lighting can have equally distracting effects, and some people will be susceptible to travel sickness if they are sitting in a certain position. Although anyone can be affected by motion sickness, some people are more regular sufferers than others, and factors such as fatigue and hunger are likely to make it worse.

Close communication with the driving team is important in identifying the appropriate driving style to be used for each leg of the journey. Using available information such as clinical concerns of the team, the time of day, traffic volume, weather conditions, and team fatigue will help inform a team in making a safe decision. Drivers who work regularly with transport teams will often have a very good understanding of the styles appropriate to neonatal transport, but it is important to be clear about this at the start of the journey. Different teams will have different thresholds and guidance for requesting a journey under emergency conditions as opposed to normal conditions. Driving under emergency conditions has its risks, which increase when doing so for extended periods, in bad weather, when the team is fatigued, and when driving in unfamiliar areas. Working under these conditions is common in neonatal transport, so careful discussion must be held in order to mitigate the risks where identified, with judicious use of blue lights and sirens (Fenton et al., 2004).

So far in this section, the focus has been on safety inside the ambulance. It is also worth considering safety outside the vehicle, on occasions of breakdown or involvement in a road traffic incident (RTI). Transport teams should have training and guidance for decision-making should they be either first on the scene of an RTI or involved in an RTI themselves. Because the different variations on how this might manifest are numerous, it is difficult to develop a prescriptive SOP. These situations are likely to create a complicated cocktail of emotions, weighing heavily on perceived moral and professional duty, and clinical competence and confidence. Key tenets of any such guidance need to include:

■ Team safety
■ Patient safety
■ Scene safety
■ Ensuring primary team responsibilities to the patient are met.

GOVERNANCE

Central to the safety of a transport team are its governance mechanisms. To varying extents, transport services will operate within the governance structures of their host trust, with the addition of certain elements specific to transport.

A transport service will have a range of SOPs and guidelines to help standardise practice and support the staff in sometimes highly complex and challenging situations. By necessity these will be different to those adopted in the NNU, and staff working between the two specialties will need to be careful to work within the appropriate guidelines.

Documentation is key to ensuring a demonstrably safe and high-quality service. Contemporaneous note-keeping is the target as detailed in the Nursing and Midwifery Council Code, though this can be difficult to achieve in a fast-moving complex situation. Transport services will have a range of documentation to keep a record of referrals, advice calls, low dependency, high dependency and intensive care transfers, as well as documents to record the debrief and review of these transfers. Meticulous documentation of key decisions is particularly important, clearly recording the people involved in the process and the rationale discussed.

Transport services will undertake a review of the transfers carried out. This is helpful in confirming that the agreed standard of care is being given, identifying and addressing issues which arise, and in identifying issues which might not be covered in a pre-existing guideline or SOP. These might relate to equipment faults, unexpected patient deteriorations, or excessive delays due to a road traffic collision. Reviewing and reflecting on these patient-related, logistical and equipment issues is key to maintaining a proactive and high-quality service.

Each team will have their own mechanisms for capturing critical incidents, either by their Trust's platforms, or their own internal system. Whichever is used, demonstrating a robust review and governance process is important to provide evidence of working in a safety conscious manner. The NTG is building a platform for sharing specific transport-related incidents on a national level to allow for enhanced learning and development.

Other key elements related to governance include addressing team welfare and fatigue, debrief and support. Finally, adequately resourced teams to ensure safe transfer at all times are imperative in the light of previous reports highlighting that a factor causing delays in response times is staffing (Evans, 2016) which can potentially impact the infant's journey. Part of improving safety is to evaluate the workings and effectiveness of neonatal transport services. Neonatal transport teams require appropriate evaluation and assessment processes. Designing complex and detailed service standards is meaningless without having the tools to measure a service against them (Ratnavel, 2013), and this is a vital component of governance in this area (Ratnavel, 2009).

THE PATIENT JOURNEY

The patient's interaction with the transport service can be mapped and broken down into several different phases. These include referral, mobilisation of transport team, arrival of transport team and patient stabilisation, departure of transport team and 'in transit' care, arrival of team and patient at receiving unit, and departure of transport team to base unit as represented in figure 22.4 (Kempley and Ratnavel, 2012). It is worth considering that the transport episode should only be considered complete when the team and equipment are safely back at base.

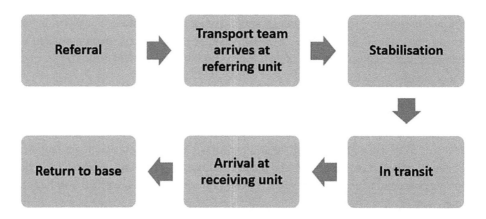

Figure 22.4 The neonatal transport journey

Referral

The patient journey starts with a referral call, which may be initially for clinical advice or a request for transfer. Many transport services offer a call conferencing facility which is an excellent way of sharing information and supporting clinical decision-making. The referring consultant, transport consultant, receiving consultant, and specialty team, as well as other members of the transport service can be included in this call which supports the development of a shared mental model of the required actions. At this time, clinical advice for stabilisation can be given, which is sometimes all that is needed. On these calls, the transport team can arrange to make contact with the referring team in an agreed timescale in order to further assess the situation (Fenton et al., 2004). On many occasions it is clear that a transfer is required, and at this stage information is sought to help triage the transfer. This allows the transport team to agree the urgency of response required, the appropriate composition of the team, and any additional specialist equipment required. At this stage the referring team still retains overall responsibility for the patient though the process of transferring responsibility from referring team, to transport team, and then on to the receiving team has started (Kempley and Ratnavel, 2012).

Transport team arrival in referring hospital

On arrival at the referring unit, the transport team and referring teams should introduce themselves. This is an important part of the process and can help improve team-working later in the transfer. It is also an important way of identifying who has been involved in the patient's care, and make sure that they are given the opportunity to add information to the handover. Every effort should be made to do a combined medical and nursing handover. This is a helpful way of ensuring a complete handover is provided and gives the referring teams an opportunity to cross-check the information being provided. At this stage the transport team is starting to take overall responsibility for the patient.

However, support and assistance from the local medical and nursing team can really help this phase of the transfer, and it is a good opportunity for local staff to be involved in delivering critical care to the infant (Fenton et al., 2004). This can help with building skills and confidence in delivering critical care, and staff often derive satisfaction from 'seeing through' this phase of the care episode.

Stabilisation is a vital component of the transport process. No matter how complex or sophisticated technological support becomes, adequate stabilisation of infants will always be a critical determinant of a successful outcome (Messner, 2011). Moreover, effective communication including handover (Wilson et al., 2017) and documentation is a very important issue: the information about the clinical condition, the priority and the procedures must be reported in the same way in the files of the referring centre, the transport team and the receiving centre (Paludetto et al., 2013).

Integral to the planning of this phase is preparing for an uneventful journey. Potential problems are identified, discussed, and actions put in place so that they do not manifest in the ambulance, or, if they do occur, the team are primed to respond promptly and effectively (Fenton et al., 2004).

In transit

As soon as the doors of the referring unit close behind the transport incubator, the transport team needs to be prepared to respond to any eventualities without the immediate support from additional staff. Fluid or drug boluses can be prepared in advance, intravenous (IV) access can be extended to allow access from the team members' seats, and some procedures such as endo-tracheal tube suctioning can be carried out prior to departure to reduce the likelihood of needing to repeat it during the journey.

Potential clinical complications which might need to be addressed, having left the referring hospital unit, include:

- Loss/blockage of airway
- Loss/blockage of IV access
- Snagging of monitoring lines/IV infusion lines/ventilator tubing
- Respiratory deterioration
- Cardiovascular deterioration
- Neurological deterioration.

Potential non-clinical complications include:

- Equipment failure
- Loss of power
- Gas supplies exhausted
- Team member becomes unwell
- Parent becomes unwell
- Deterioration in traffic/vehicle/road/weather conditions.

Arrival at receiving unit

On arrival at the receiving unit, the transport and receiving teams should again introduce themselves. It is good practice to ensure that a team handover takes place prior to moving the patient. Should there be a deterioration or problem during the transfer to the receiving cot, key details such as endotracheal tube length and IV access may be critical (Kempley and Ratnavel, 2012). It is also important to hand over and double-check infusion rates, prescriptions, and medicines which are pending, so that the receiving team have a clear picture of the clinical care requirements of the infant. This transition of care is a point of increased risk to the patient, either due to clinical deterioration, or though the incomplete handover of information. Minimising the risks to the infant can be achieved by:

■ Identifying a person who is leading this phase of the transfer
■ Keeping the area as uncluttered as possible
■ Ensuring a safety check of the receiving cot space has been carried out
■ Allocating clear roles and responsibilities
■ Planning the move and sharing this plan with the team
■ Reassessment of the patient prior to and immediately following the move.

During this phase of the transfer it is important to maintain attention in order to safely complete the task of transferring the care to the receiving team. Having arrived safely at the receiving location, the sense of relief mixed with fatigue from a long and potentially stressful transfer can contribute to errors creeping in at this stage. Pre-briefing the transport team on arrival, ensuring the use of checklists, and holding a team handover are all ways of minimising the chance of an error occurring.

Return to base

Having completed the transfer, the mission does not end until the team and equipment are all safely returned to base. Some team members may be able to 'switch off' but the driver for example still needs to be supported to complete their duties. Depending on the length of the transfer episode, the time of day, and the driving conditions, it may well be important to make sure the driver is adequately 'fed and watered' prior to departure. The journey back to base can be a useful time to hold a team debrief, which has the added benefit of providing stimulation to a fatiguing team.

Once back at base the equipment needs cleaning, checking and restocking, the paperwork needs to be checked and filed, and any incidents or issues can be highlighted for a more detailed review later.

CLINICAL CONSIDERATIONS

Greater detail of the management of specific clinical conditions can be found elsewhere in this book. However, there are times when the transport environment and process provide additional challenges to managing these conditions. While transport teams are well equipped, it is not feasible to carry every medication or piece of equipment for all eventualities. Sometimes additional subspecialty input or specialist equipment is required to refine a diagnosis and therefore assist in decisions about therapy or choice of receiving unit. An example of this could be trying to rule out a cardiac anomaly as a cause of hypoxia to ensure that the infant is transferred to an appropriate centre. At other times, certain pieces of equipment are unavailable to all transport teams, such as a ventilator which can provide high frequency oscillatory ventilation.

Extreme prematurity

In the UK, the current NHS Neonatal Service Specification outlines that infants born at certain gestations are transferred to an appropriately resourced hospital, a principle of centralisation which has been adopted in other areas of healthcare. Where possible, these infants are moved *in utero*, but there are times when this is not an option. There are particular challenges that present when transferring preterm and extremely preterm infants.

TEMPERATURE CONTROL

Maintaining the temperature of the neonate is a key tenet of neonatal care (Laptook et al., 2007). While special attention needs to be given to maintaining thermal control during all transfers, this can be particularly challenging when transferring extremely premature infants. Very low birth weight and skin integrity are two key factors making this difficult. The design of transport incubators includes being able to maintain an adequately humidified environment, though in practice controlling the patient and incubator's temperatures is often more difficult than on a NNU. This is due to environmental factors that can have a more profound impact because the baby may require multiple interventions during the stabilisation and preparation for transfer phase (Kempley and Ratnavel, 2012). The transport team should give attention to:

- Taking care to pre-warm the ambulance
- Careful planning to minimise the time to transfer infant from incubator to incubator
- Minimise the time which the transport incubator is outside the vehicle
- Ensure the incubator batteries are fully charged and plugged in
- Close (continuous) monitoring of infant temperature
- Use of thermal control adjuncts such as infant warming mattresses, hats, bubble wrap.

VITAL SIGNS MONITORING

The delicate and vulnerable skin of the extremely premature infant means that transport teams must carefully consider the balance of ensuring adequate monitoring while simultaneously protecting the integrity of the skin as much as possible. While an extremely preterm infant may not routinely have electrocardiographic (ECG) monitoring in a NNU, this may be necessary for the transport episode. These decisions should be made by the transport team caring for the infant, considering all the clinical and logistic information available. It is essential to monitor the CO_2 in ventilated infants – this may be end-tidal, although some transport services are moving to transcutaneous CO_2 monitoring.

RESPIRATORY SUPPORT

Preterm and extremely preterm infants often need a period of respiratory support immediately after birth which can include mechanical ventilation. Efforts have been made to reduce ventilator-induced lung injury and the negative side effects of mechanical ventilation resulting in a shift in respiratory support strategies. It is increasingly common for extremely preterm infants to be managed where possible using continuous positive airway pressure (CPAP) from a very early age.

When transferring these infants for centralisation, transport teams need to consider the risks involved with emergency intubation while *en route* in the ambulance with the benefits of lung protective respiratory support. Extremely premature infants are commonly transferred intubated and ventilated, though judicious use of sedation during these transfers will mean that they can be extubated and managed with non-invasive respiratory support soon after their arrival at the NICU.

THE IMPACT OF VIBRATIONS AND NOISE

Unfortunately, ambulances are noisy places where noise levels can be as high as 85–90dB. This is significantly higher than the recommended limits for a neonatal intensive care of 45dB (Almadhoob and Ohlson, 2015), and it can be difficult to reduce the noise and vibration experienced during transfer. Even the noise levels on a NNU can have negative short-term effects on the respiratory and cardiovascular systems (Wachman and Lahav, 2011), and these are likely to be enhanced in the back of an ambulance. There are limited hearing protective devices available for infants during transfer. Driving at lower speeds and careful choice of route can reduce road noise and vibrations, and extremely preterm infants are those where it is particularly important to request a smooth and steady ride (Blaxter et al., 2017).

It is also important to consider the effects of acceleration, deceleration, and cornering during a transfer. Physiologically unstable patients will have exaggerated responses to these stimuli. While it is often not possible to remove these stimuli, they can be reduced by the driving style used, and the potential complications can be discussed and prepared for in advance. There is some evidence identifying an association between an increased risk of intraventricular haemorrhage in premature infants and the need for transport (Mohammed and Aly, 2010). A more recent study (Redpath et al., 2019) identified that risk factors for serious brain injury were related to the infant's condition at birth and immediate postnatal management, not to transport factors. Research is underway looking in more detail at this, and in potential solutions to reducing the noise and vibration levels experienced during transfers. There is evidence that infants experience increased pain and discomfort during transport (Harrison and McKechnie, 2012), which is driving engineers and clinicians to look at this important element.

Surgical transfers

One common reason for transfer is the need for surgical review and input for infants with concerning abdominal signs. Necrotising enterocolitis is one such condition which can be managed medically, but often requires surgical intervention. A particular concern for the transport team is that a tense and distended abdomen can have a negative impact on the respiratory status of the infant. A significantly distended abdomen will reduce the intrathoracic volume available for lung expansion and will be painful, so that the infant is at increased risk of apnoeas. The extra handling, vehicle vibrations, and road surface issues are unfortunately likely to cause significant additional pain. Among other clinical considerations, these are two factors which may well support the decision to intubate, ventilate and sedate an infant for transfer, who may otherwise have been stable enough to observe on a NNU.

For all surgical transfers, decisions should be made by clinical collaboration between teams and, where appropriate, swift transfer provided (Ojha et al., 2017). Some examples are given now.

GASTROSCHISIS

The majority of infants with a gastroschisis will be delivered at the regional NICU with surgical services. However, transport teams must be prepared to manage and safely transfer an infant with this abdominal wall defect. Key elements here include fluid resuscitation and fluid balance, and temperature control (Ives et al., 2012). It is not unusual for infants with gastroschisis to require significant ongoing fluid resuscitation that may extend through the transport process. Ensuring that this is administered while coordinating the other elements of the transfer requires careful planning. As discussed, temperature control can be a challenge in any routine transfer, so the extra demands of maintaining normothermia in these instances requires careful attention.

Aside from managing these 'routine' elements, the key objective in these cases is that the infant arrives at the surgical centre with a pink and healthy gut. Of greatest concern is the scenario where the gut perfusion reduces which can have disastrous consequences (Prefumo and Izzi, 2014). This can be particularly difficult to manage in the transport situation as the gut will not have been put into a silo at this stage, and so accurate assessment of the gut perfusion is difficult. It is harder to observe the gut closely when in transit due to seating position, lighting, and patient positioning. These factors should be taken into account and included in a team brief before departure, with actions identified to minimise any potential risk. Close observation and documentation should be carried out before leaving the referring hospital, before driving away, and then at regular intervals during the transfer. The surgical team at the receiving hospital can be contacted for advice about managing this problem, should the basic manoeuvres not improve the perfusion of the gut. Possible outcomes are that they arrange to meet the transport team with the patient as soon as they arrive at the receiving unit, or possibly transfer the patient straight into theatre.

These transfers have the potential to evolve into an emergency situation where everything must be done to expedite the arrival at the surgical centre. In these situations, it may be necessary to deviate from standard approaches to eliminate any potential delay. Such approaches can include using bolus doses of medications, rather than making up infusions and using non-invasive blood pressure monitoring rather than waiting to obtain arterial access. These, however, are high-level, advanced clinical decisions and should be made by the most senior people available, with good communication and teamwork to achieve the desired outcome.

OESOPHAGEAL ATRESIA

Advances in antenatal ultrasonography have facilitated the early identification of surgical anomalies. This means that plans can be made for infants to be delivered at their local surgical NICU. There are, however, occasions when these anomalies are not identified or, despite knowing of their existence, the infant has to be delivered in a non-surgical unit. Sometimes the defect is only picked up postnatally when attempts to insert a nasogastric tube fail, raising suspicions of oesophageal atresia (OA), which is commonly associated with tracheo-oesophageal fistula (TOF). An isolated OA can be managed by insertion of a Replogle tube into the pouch, which can then be suctioned to prevent accumulation of secretions. The infant can then be safely transferred to the regional NICU for surgical intervention (Ives et al., 2012). However, there are increased complications for those cases where a TOF is present.

TOF can present in a variety of ways. The principal risk in these cases is aspiration of secretions or gastric contents through the fistula into the lungs. Management of these conditions are detailed in chapter 21, but there are some elements which provide a particular challenge in transport. Primary management is through insertion of a Replogle tube with continuous suction and regular flushing (Ives et al., 2012). The infant can then be assessed by the surgical team, followed by surgical repair. A small proportion of these infants can develop a requirement for respiratory support, either due to transient tachypnea of the newborn, or because of small aspirations of secretions. However, respiratory support in the form of CPAP or invasive ventilation is contraindicated, as it greatly increases the risk of aspiration. Air forced into the lungs will follow the path of least resistance, and so find its way through the fistula into the stomach and cause significant gastric distension (Ives et al., 2012). Because of this risk, the decision on how to safely transfer an infant with suspected TOF with OA, with respect to respiratory support, must be made at a senior level.

Many of these infants can be safely transferred breathing in air, with Replogle tube management. Continuous low flow suction is required, and the means to perform this will depend on the equipment available. Some portable suction units will permit low flow suction, though others may need an attenuating device to reduce the suction to an appropriate level.

CARDIAC ANOMALIES

Emergency transfers of infants with undiagnosed cardiac lesions can be high risk. Antenatal diagnosis and pulse oximetry screening to facilitate early detection may reduce this (Ismail et al., 2017). The Acute Neonatal Transfer Service (based in Cambridge) in a review of 25 infants requiring unplanned emergency transfer to cardiac centres (2.3% of total unplanned emergencies) between 2014 and 2016 found good patient outcomes while identifying aspects to be addressed in the team's education programme (Perez-Fernandez et al., 2017).

Hypoxic-ischaemic encephalopathy requiring therapeutic hypothermia

Therapeutic hypothermia (TH) has become a well-established standard of care for infants who have hypoxic-ischaemic encephalopathy (HIE; National Institute of Care Excellence, 2010). Centralisation of care has recommended that TH should be carried out in tertiary NICUs. Some LNUs and SCUs can commence active cooling using special servo-controlled equipment. This has meant that there is an increased opportunity for the infant to be safely managed to the cooling set-point while waiting for the transport team to arrive. The patient is then transferred to their regional cooling centre for ongoing treatment. The evolution of portable servo-controlled temperature regulation equipment has made this easier, and transferring infants in this way has become standard for neonatal transport teams in the UK (Johnston et al., 2012; Chaudhary et al., 2013; Torre Monmany et al., 2019).

Many LNUs and SCUs have access to cerebral function monitoring (CFM) equipment. This can help in identifying infants with deranged cerebral function resulting from their hypoxic-ischaemic event, as well as identifying subclinical and clinical seizure activity. This information is key in the decision-making for TH, and in the ongoing management of these infants. Portable CFM equipment is available, but the opportunity to record cerebral function in transport remains a challenge. The vibrations and movements while in transit can cause significant artefacts which can be unhelpful when trying to interpret the results. Consequently, it can be difficult to identify seizure activity in transit. Careful assessment of tone, as well as heart rate and blood pressure can help in establishing a baseline, from which a deviation can be identified, evaluated carefully, and, if appropriate, interventions commenced. Having the equipment available, and the CFM electrodes in situ, means that CFM could be commenced with the vehicle stationary should there be a concern about the infant's neurological status.

Another key challenge when transferring infants for TH can be the management of their respiratory support. These infants are often attempting to try and normalise their pH after the hypoxic-ischaemic event by hyperventilating to drive their blood carbon dioxide level ($PaCO_2$) down. An intubated child can still breathe above the rate at which the ventilator is set, and so cause a lower than normal $PaCO_2$. As this has been associated with adverse neurodevelopmental outcomes, ventilation of these infants needs to be cautiously managed (Robertson and Groenendaal, 2012).

Palliative care transfers

There are sadly times when a baby dies despite the attempts of the teams to resuscitate and stabilise them. There are also occasions where the clinical team may feel that the severity of injury is such that attempts to prolong life are futile, or not in the best interest of the infant (Dulkerian et al., 2011). These are particularly difficult to manage and are sometimes best dealt with by undertaking the transfer to allow more time for information gathering, and for the parents to come to terms with the tragedy. It can be a challenge for the team members who may have strong feelings about the appropriateness of these transfers, as they may be taking the infant and family away from their homes and support networks. In these instances, the team leader should make the opportunity for their colleagues to share their concerns and contribute to the decision-making process. Supportive debrief and follow-up is also key.

The area of palliative care transfers is one which is growing and gathering profile. As a result, some teams are able to offer support for these transfers as an important part of the family's experience. This might be to take the baby home or to a hospice for withdrawal of life-sustaining treatment, or to offer the infant and family the opportunity to have some shared family experiences outside the hospital environment. These transfers still require detailed planning and preparation to ensure they go smoothly.

PARENTS

It is vitally important to consider the experiences of parents whose child is being transferred (Bliss, 2016). Parents are playing a significant role in the care their baby receives in NNU (Bracht et al., 2013), and this ethos should extend to the transport environment. However, the opportunity to be involved in the actual care of the infant may be limited due to many factors. These include the emergent nature of many of these transfers, the health of the mother, as well as the pastoral needs of the partner and related family. Staff from the referring hospitals, transport teams and the receiving hospitals involved in these transfers can help to reduce the stress experienced by these families and encourage them to feel as involved and supported as possible (Mullaney et al., 2014). Family-centred care principles highlighted in chapter 4 should continue at any point in an infant's journey, including transport. Mosher (2013) refers to this skill as an 'art'.

Communication

Parents often report that the lack of control experienced during childbirth is particularly challenging, causing significant stress. This mirrors the experiences of parents on NNU, and is heightened by the need, or potential need, of transfer to a different hospital. Early and clear communication between the referring team and the parents about the possibility of transferring their baby gives them some opportunity to ask questions and prepare for this next step. A particularly important factor here is that in many cases the infant will be brought back to their booking hospital, and the parents' initial experience may well influence their behaviour when they return.

There also needs to be clear communication between the transport team and the parents/family. Simple things such as a good introduction of the team and a brief discussion of the plan can align expectations and provide timescales of the stabilisation and transfer process (Mullaney et al., 2014). Providing clinical updates and responses to therapies that have commenced, or procedures that have been undertaken, can also help to reduce anxiety. In cases where the trajectory or prognosis of the infant is poor, these early communications can help prepare the parents for what they might be facing in the hours, days, or weeks to come. As well as updating parents on the clinical state of their infant, it is also important to advise them of some of the risks of an unexpected event occurring during the transfer. Reassurance can be given that the team has the appropriate personnel, equipment and expertise necessary to deal with any unforeseen situations that might occur. Parents need to be reassured that the decision to undertake these transfers is carefully considered, and that the clinical team's opinion is that their baby will benefit from the transfer.

Another key element of communication is that between the family and the receiving team. The referring team and transport team both have a role to play in optimising this, and everything possible should be done to ensure that the first few minutes and hours at the receiving unit are as positive and supportive as possible. Parents who have become very involved in delivering their baby's care can struggle with feelings that they are relinquishing some of their control to the transport team. They can often be anxious about having to meet a new set of staff, in a new hospital, with new routines and policies, which is made more profound by the concern that the receiving team may not know all the details of their baby. Including the parents in the handover can be helpful, as can ensuring that where possible they are introduced properly to the team who will be providing ongoing care.

Travelling in the ambulance

A significant shift over the last ten years has been towards supporting parents to travel with their babies, and neonatal transport teams are encouraged to take parents with them on all transfers (Mosher, 2013). There are some caveats to when this may not be appropriate, including the parent being physically unfit to travel. Most transport teams will have local guidance about a certain time period after delivery before the mother can travel, which will extend should the mother have had a caesarean section. As well as being at risk of post-delivery complications, travelling as a passenger in an ambulance is not necessarily a comfortable experience, and the mother may well be more comfortable and rested if she travelled independently. The limitations to parental travel extend also to psychological and emotional wellbeing. The additional stress of being in the ambulance can become unbearable, and anxious parents are sometimes better advised to try to arrange alternative means of travel. A helpful family member or friend will often be very happy to help in this way. Pre-existing medical conditions may preclude safe travel.

In a significant proportion of cases, it will be entirely appropriate for a parent to travel with their baby and the transport team. In these instances, there are some important factors to consider in terms of preparing the parent for the journey. This will typically include a 'safety brief' which details what to expect, anticipated driving styles, anticipated arrival times, what to do if there is an emergency, wearing a seatbelt at all times, and looking to the transport team for guidance. Another key consideration is luggage and personal belongings. The space in the vehicles is often extremely restricted, and it is key to the safety of the team that any belongings are securely stowed. Team safety is key here, but equally so is the ability of the team to operate effectively in the event of an emergency while in the vehicle. If the vehicle is blocked up with luggage, it will make it an even more difficult environment to work in.

There are also several considerations with regard to whether the parent should travel in the front or the back of the ambulance. Some of the restrictions will relate to the configuration of the ambulance, the size of the clinical team required, and to any guidance or SOPs which the team might have. The concern that the parent may become overwhelmed with stress can have significance whether they are distracting the driver or the clinical team. It would be good practice for the team to share the responsibility of this decision, so that they can bring any relevant information forward. Any one of the team might have witnessed some unacceptable behaviour prior to departure or heard of some important information which could influence the decision.

In those cases where a parent does not travel in the ambulance, it is important to provide them with details for the receiving hospital. Information such as exactly where their baby is being cared for, parking and access information, and the best telephone number to use are hugely valuable to parents. It is also hugely important to update them on the arrival at the destination. The value of a short phone call or message to advise them of this must not be overlooked, as the journey may well have caused them significant distress (Mullaney et al., 2014).

While uplift transfers can be particularly stressful, transfers for other reasons can still be difficult for parents and families. Transfers out of a unit for capacity reasons will be putting significant distance between the baby, their family and their support networks. Careful and timely communication with the family will help them to understand the reasons behind these transfers and reduce the stress somewhat. Repatriation transfers have the advantage of tending to be of lower clinical complexity, of moving toward their booking or home hospital, and tend to be undertaken with more notice. Parents will often be aware that their baby is approaching the age or size such that they no longer require the specialist services required in their current hospital. However, despite these 'good' reasons for being transferred, parents can often be quite anxious about this transition. They will have often established close bonds with the teams looking after their baby, and with other families in the unit. They will have a good understanding of the local policies and guidelines such as times of ward round, how to access specific services such as family support and breastfeeding support, and they may have become used to doing certain tasks for their baby in a certain way. Transferring to a different NNU requires rebuilding trust and familiarity with a new team and environment, which takes time and effort and can unsettle a family significantly. Furthermore, the infant may be returning to the unit from which they were transferred when they were critically ill, and this may bring back some difficult memories for the family. The referring and transport teams are in a good position to help with this transition, preparing the parents for the transfer, and making sure the receiving team are fully aware of any potential concerns the family might have.

CONCLUSION

Over the last ten years there has been a huge change to the systems and processes involved in neonatal transport, and no doubt the evolution will continue. For political and organisational reasons some services have reconfigured to work more closely with their neighbouring neonatal or paediatric services. These models may become more widely used or promoted in the UK. In the next ten years, technological advancements will continue to support the development of specialist equipment taking into account the specific demands and requirements of transport. For example, efforts to replicate the intensive care unit environment are working to address the hostile elements of the transport environment, including the noise and vibration experienced by these infants. Improving availability of treatments in transport such as high frequency oscillatory ventilation, CFM, and phototherapy are potential areas of development. Importantly, the concept of critical care transport has become more clearly defined and is recognised by many as a specialty in itself. This may encourage further development of transport-related, post-qualification, role-specific education and training opportunities.

C A S E   S T U D Y

CASE STUDIES

These three case studies below present different infants who all require transportation for further management of their conditions. For each case study, consider the following questions:

Q.1. Can you outline the nursing considerations when stabilising these infants for transfer?

Q.2. Can you identify the potential risks relating to the actual transfer and how will these be minimised?

Q.3. What are the specific challenges for the families of these infants?

Q.4. What specific care and information do the parents need?

Q.5. What information do the receiving units needs about these infants?

Case study 1: Congenital cardiac lesion

Marcus is a term infant born with a congenital heart defect, diagnosed following a collapse on the postnatal ward in the first day of life. He requires transfer to a specialist cardiac centre which is more than 40 miles away from the current NNU. He has a duct-dependent defect. Marcus' mother is single, and the father is not present or contactable. She has her parents with her.

Case study 2: Surgical problem

Jeannie is a term infant who after delivery was found to experience problems with feeding when she went blue and encountered coughing. A nasogastric tube was passed, but this coiled back up to the mouth and an oesophageal atresia is suspected. She is currently in a level 1 SCU with no surgical care. Her parents have four other children.

Case study 3: Varying care levels in a set of twins

Aneesa and Jasmine are girl twins born at 27 weeks' gestation. There was a diagnosis of twin-to-twin transfusion during pregnancy. Aneesa is the twin who received more blood in utero and, although is experiencing some respiratory distress and a high packed cell volume, is being managed effectively and is stable. Jasmine, however, was born much smaller with a birth weight of <600g. She is very anaemic, hypovolaemic and is unstable with a high oxygen and ventilation requirement. She requires transfer to a level 3 NICU for further management. The twins' mother Meera is currently unwell with high blood pressure and remains in the postnatal ward. Father Ali is present on the NNU. The extended family is caring for their other 2 older children at home.

For suggested answer guides to the questions posed in these case studies, please refer to the web-based companion site specific to this chapter (see URL below).

WEB-BASED RESOURCES

For further information, online resources and greater detail on the case studies featured in this chapter go to www.routledge.com/cw/nicnursing

References

Almadhoob, A., & Ohlsson, A. (2015). Sound reduction management in the neonatal intensive care unit for preterm or very low birth weight infants. *Cochrane Database of Systematic Reviews*, Issue 1. Art. No.: CD010333. DOI: 10.1002/14651858.CD010333.pub2

Aubertin, C. A., Speck, G., & Redpath, S. (2018). A Dedicated Neonatal Transport Unit Pilot Program: An Innovative Partnership. *Pediatrics*, *142*(1), 492.

Blaxter, L., Yeo, M., McNally, D., Crowe, J., Henry, C., Hill, S., ... & Sharkey, D. (2017). Neonatal head and torso vibration exposure during inter-hospital transfer. *Proceedings of the Institution of Mechanical Engineers, Part H: Journal of Engineering in Medicine*, *231*(2), 99–113.

Bliss. (2016). *Transfers of premature and sick babies*. London: Bliss UK.

Boland, R. A., Davis, P. G., Dawson, J. A., & Doyle, L. W. (2017). Outcomes of infants born at 22–27 weeks' gestation in Victoria according to outborn/inborn birth status. *Archives of Disease in Childhood: Fetal and Neonatal Edition*, *102*(2), F153–F161.

Bracht, M., O'Leary, L., Lee, S. K., & O'Brien, K. (2013). Implementing family-integrated care in the NICU: A parent education and support program. *Advances in Neonatal Care*, *13*(2), 115–126.

British Standards Institute. 2011). BSEN13976-2:2011. *Rescue Systems – Transportation of incubators – Part 2: System requirements*. London: BSI Standards Publication.

Chang, A. S. M., Berry, A., Jones, L. J., & Sivasangari, S. (2015). Specialist teams for neonatal transport to neonatal intensive care units for prevention of morbidity and mortality. *Cochrane Database of Systematic Reviews*, Issue 10. Art. No.: CD007485. DOI: 10.1002/14651858.CD007485. pub2

Chaudhary, R., Farrer, K., Broster, S., McRitchie, L., & Austin, T. (2013). Active versus passive cooling during neonatal transport. *Pediatrics*, *132*(5), 841–846.

Department of Health. (2015). *Neonatal Critical Care Retrieval (Transport) Service Specification*. London: Department of Health.

Dulkerian, S. J., Douglas, W. P., & Taylor, R. M. (2011). Redirecting treatment during neonatal transport. *The Journal of Perinatal & Neonatal Nursing*, *25*(2), 111–114.

Evans, N. (2016). Understaffed transfer services may put infants' lives at risk. *Nursing Children and Young People (2014+)*, *28*(4), 8.

Fenton, A. C., Leslie, A., & Skeoch, C. H. (2004). Optimising neonatal transfer. *Archives of Disease in Childhood: Fetal and Neonatal Edition*, *89*(3), F215–F219.

Fenton, A. C., & Leslie, A. (2009). Who should staff neonatal transport teams? *Early Human Development*, *85*(8), 487–490.

Gale, C., Santhakumaran, S., Nagarajan, S., Statnikov, Y., & Modi, N. (2012). Impact of managed clinical networks on NHS specialist neonatal services in England: Population based study. *British Medical Journal*, *344*, e2105.

Gawande, A. (2010). *The Checklist Manifesto. How To Get Things Right*. India: Penguin Books.

Hancock, S., & Harrison, C. (2018). Establishing a Combined Neonatal and Paediatric Transport System From Scratch. *Current Treatment Options in Pediatrics*, *4*(1), 119–128.

Harrison, C., & McKechnie, L. (2012). How comfortable is neonatal transport? *Acta Paediatrica*, *101*(2), 143–147.

Ismail, A. Q. T., Cawsey, M., & Ewer, A. K. (2017). Newborn pulse oximetry screening in practice. *Archives of Disease in Childhood-Education and Practice*, *102*(3), 155–161.

Ives, N. K., Mieli-Vergani, G., Hadžić, N., Newell, S., Sugarman, I, Stringer, M. D., & Smyth, A. G. (2012). Gastroenterology. In Rennie, J. M. (Ed.) *Rennie & Roberton's Textbook of Neonatology* (5th Edition). London: Elsevier Health Sciences.

Johnston, E. D., Becher, J. C., Mitchell, A. P., & Stenson, B. J. (2012). Provision of servo-controlled cooling during neonatal transport. *Archives of Disease in Childhood: Fetal and Neonatal Edition*, *97*(5), F365–F367.

Kempley, S. T., Baki, Y., Hayter, G., Ratnavel, N., Cavazzoni, E., & Reyes, T. (2007). Effect of a centralised transfer service on characteristics of inter-hospital neonatal transfers. *Archives of Disease in Childhood: Fetal and Neonatal Edition*, *92*(3), F185–F188.

Kempley, S., & Ratnavel, N. (2012). Resuscitation and transport of the newborn. Part 2: Neonatal transport. In Rennie, J. M. (Ed.) *Rennie & Roberton's Textbook of Neonatology* (5th Edition). London: Elsevier Health Sciences.

Killion, C., & Stein, H. M. (2009). The impact of air ambulance transport on neonatal outcomes. *Newborn and Infant Nursing Reviews*, *9*(4), 207–211.

Kronforst, K. D., (2016). Interhospital transport of the neonatal patient. *Clinical Pediatric Emergency Medicine, 17*(2), 140–146.

Laptook, A. R., Salhab, W., & Bhaskar, B. (2007). Admission temperature of low birth weight infants: Predictors and associated morbidities. *Pediatrics, 119*(3), e643–e649.

Marlow, N., & Gill, A. B. (2007). Establishing neonatal networks: The reality. *Archives of Disease in Childhood: Fetal and Neonatal Edition*, *92*(2), F137–F142.

Marlow, N., Bennett, C., Draper, E. S., Hennessy, E. M., Morgan, A. S., & Costeloe, K. L. (2014). Perinatal outcomes for extremely preterm babies in relation to place of birth in England: The EPICure 2 study. *Archives of Disease in Childhood: Fetal and Neonatal Edition*, *99*(3), F181–F188.

Messner, H. (2011). Neonatal transport: a review of the current evidence. *Early Human Development*, (87), S77.

Mohamed, M. A., & Aly, H. (2010). Transport of premature infants is associated with increased risk for intraventricular haemorrhage. *Archives of Disease in Childhood: Fetal and Neonatal Edition*, *95*(6), F403–F407.

Mosher, S. L. (2013). The art of supporting families faced with neonatal transport. *Nursing for Women's Health*, *17*(3), 198–209.

Mullaney, D. M., Edwards, W. H., & DeGrazia, M. (2014). Family-centered care during acute neonatal transport. *Advances in Neonatal Care, 14*(5S), S16–S23.

National Institute for Health and Care Excellence (NICE). (2010). Therapeutic hypothermia with intracorporeal temperature monitoring for hypoxic perinatal brain injury: guidance. NICE.

Ojha, S., Sand, L., Ratnavel, N., Kempley, S. T., Sinha, A. K., Mohinuddin, S., … & Leslie, A. (2017). Newborn infants with bilious vomiting: A national audit of neonatal transport services. *Archives of Disease in Childhood: Fetal and Neonatal Edition*, *102*(6), F515–F518.

Paludetto, R., Di Fiore, A., Cerullo, J., Mansi, G., Van Den Heuvel, J., & Umbaldo, A. (2013). Medical–legal aspects of neonatal transport. *Early Human Development*, *89*(4), 41–2.

Perez-Fernandez, C., Broster, S., & Kelsall, W. (2017). G410 Small hearts, big risk? Service evaluation of cardiac transfers undertaken by a neonatal transport team.

Prefumo, F., & Izzi, C. (2014). Fetal abdominal wall defects. *Best Practice & Research Clinical Obstetrics & Gynaecology, 28*(3), 391–402.

Ratnavel, N. (2009). Safety and governance issues for neonatal transport services. *Early Human Development*, *85*(8), 483–486.

Ratnavel, N. (2013). Evaluating and improving neonatal transport services. *Early Human Development*, *89*(11), 851–853.

Reason, J. T. (2016). *The Human Contribution: Unsafe Acts, Accidents and Heroic Recoveries*. Oxon: Routledge.

Redpath, S., Shah, P. S., Moore, G. P., Yang, J., Toye, J., Perreault, T., & Lee, K. S. (2019). Do transport factors increase the risk of severe brain injury in outborn infants < 33 weeks gestational age? *Journal of Perinatology*, 1–9.

Robertson, N. J., & Groenendaal, F. (2012). Neurological problems in the newborn. Part 4: Hypoxic-ischaemic brain injury. In Rennie, J. M. (Ed.) *Rennie & Roberton's Textbook of Neonatology* (5th Edition). London: Elsevier Health Sciences.

Royal College of Nursing. (2013). *Nursing on the move – specialist nursing for patients requiring repatriation and retrieval*. London: Royal College of Nursing.

Torre Monmany, N., Behrsin, J., & Leslie, A. (2019). Servo-controlled cooling during neonatal transport for babies with hypoxic-ischaemic encephalopathy is practical and beneficial: Experience from a large UK neonatal transport service. *Journal of Paediatrics and Child Health*, *55*(5), 518–522.

UK Neonatal Transport Group. (2018). Neonatal Transfer Dataset 2018. http://ukntg.net/annual-reports/

Wachman, E. M., & Lahav, A. (2011). The effects of noise on preterm infants in the NICU. *Archives of Disease in Childhood: Fetal and Neonatal Edition*, *96*(4), F305–F309.

Wilson, D., Kochar, A., Whyte-Lewis, A., Whyte, H., & Lee, K. S. (2017). Evaluation of situation, background, assessment, recommendation tool during neonatal and pediatric interfacility transport. *Air Medical Journal*, *36*(4), 182–187.

Worksafe UK. (2019). What is TILE or TILEO? www.worksafe.uk.com/tile-and-other-manual-handling-acronyms/

23 EXPLORING EVIDENCE-BASED PRACTICE IN NEONATAL CARE

Marie Lindsay-Sutherland

CONTENTS

GUIDANCE ON HOW TO ENHANCE PERSONAL LEARNING FROM THIS CHAPTER

Key points covered in this chapter

■ What is evidence-based practice applied to neonatal care?
■ What are the forms of knowledge applicable to neonatal nursing practice?
■ The importance and value of an evidence-based approach to neonatal care.

Reflection

Reading through the chapter, you are encouraged to engage with the key points and related literature in an enquiring way. Ask these questions:

■ How has research generated new knowledge in neonatal care?
■ How has new knowledge and evidence influenced your own practice?
■ Can you think of any specific examples of research that has had a positive impact on infants and their families?

Implications for nursing care:

■ Finally: how will this chapter enable you to consider and understand the importance of research and evidence-based practice in neonatal care? Consider the implications of what you learn as relevant to current and future practice development.

INTRODUCTION AND BACKGROUND

This chapter builds on the knowledge base presented in the previous chapters and looks at evidence-based nursing with specific reference to the importance, relevance and application for neonatal nurses. It will establish how the concept was developed, and its transition from medical to nursing practice. It will reflect on the forms of knowledge that neonatal nurses use and the resources that are available to meet the needs of current clinical practice. It will also emphasise the importance of a critical but pragmatic approach to situations the neonatal nurse faces when caring for the neonate and their family.

WHAT IS EVIDENCE-BASED PRACTICE?

Historically, nurses relied upon experience and expert opinion to guide clinical practice. The concept of evidence-based practice (EBP) was developed to bridge the gap between scientific and theoretical knowledge, and clinical practice. Evidence-based nursing practice evolved from evidence-based medicine, which has been defined as the 'conscientious, explicit, and judicious use of current best evidence in making decisions about the care of individual patients' (Sackett et al., 1996, p. 71). Evidence-based medicine emerged from work undertaken by the Cochrane Collaboration. Cochrane sought to standardise practice and utilise resources to achieve the best outcomes for patients through the use of high-quality systematic reviews and synthesised research, and still pursues this strategy today (Cochrane, 2018). Sackett et al., (1996) sought to take up-to-date research and combine it with the patient's views and values, thus taking the concept of evidence-based medicine and transforming it into EBP as other health professionals, such as nurses, endorsed the concept (Mackey and Bassendowski, 2017).

Evidence-based nursing provided a paradigm shift from primarily practice-based care under the auspices of medical colleagues. Nurses looked to adapt the values put forward by Sackett et al. (1996) and develop a more holistic approach which would meet the growing demand for effectiveness and safety (Stevens, 2013). This approach saw nurses critically analyse research and explore its application to clinical practice, alongside clinical expertise and patient preferences, to promote healthcare transformation (Stevens, 2013; Renolen and Hjälmhult, 2015; Sadoughi et al., 2017). It was found that nurses needed to feel in control of their actions and trust the knowledge that underpins their clinical practice, and therefore often relied upon their own experience rather than research (Renolen and Hjälmhult, 2015). Stokke et al. (2014) nevertheless found a positive correlation between those nurses who valued an EBP approach to care, and those who incorporated it into their practice, but knowledge of EBP was key. However, utilising EBP is not without its obstacles for nurses. A survey of 1486 nurses found that, while 64% felt that EBP was inherent to their practice, they lacked both the skills and understanding to assess the available evidence in an appropriate manner, and the time to undertake the task (Majid et al., 2011).

In order for neonatal nurses to fully embrace an EBP approach, there needs to be a good understanding of the forms of evidence and knowledge that can be incorporated in practice. These sources of knowledge will be explored in the next section.

TYPES OF KNOWLEDGE

Knowledge derived from research

Historically, neonatal care utilised textbooks to inform practice. Nursing and medical journals provided EBP in the interim, but were impeded by publication timelines and lack of accessibility for all professionals. The advent of the internet in 1990 brought a myriad of databases by which an extensive literature review could be quickly undertaken, and changes applied to practice rapidly. This occurred alongside a considerable increase in academic output in the field of neonatal care, and nurses themselves, who sought to drive forward not just technological advances, but also work towards family-centered neonatal clinical practice.

However, it is important to appreciate the methodology and methods that underpin the evidence.

A model for the hierarchy of evidence for health professionals was developed to aid clarity in research quality (see figure 23.1). Within this model, meta-analyses, systematic reviews and national guidelines are considered the pinnacle of excellence and quality in regard to evidence for clinical practice (De Brün, 2013). The lauded gold standard, randomised controlled trials (RCT), and cohort studies are stated as intermediate quality methods, with case-controlled studies, case studies, expert opinion and patient experience forming the lowest levels of quality for evidence (De Brün, 2013).

Neonatal nurses need to balance the technical aspects of working in an intensive care area with the compassion of a caring profession, so it is important that the clinical question they need to answer is reflected in the methodologies and methods that are chosen. Also, consideration of the clinical question and therefore the most appropriate search terms will focus any database search and is the best use of limited time resources. The appropriate choice of database(s) will further focus the resulting papers for review. The Cochrane Library includes systematic reviews relating to neonatal topics, providing a good starting point for assessing the available evidence to answer a clinical question. As a large, well-resourced organisation, the Cochrane Library provides health professionals with a high-quality, reliable and valid source of information. Equally, the National Institute for Health and Care Excellence (NICE) provides guidance on neonatal topics and has published a number of guidelines, for example on early onset neonatal infection (NICE, 2012) and neonatal jaundice (NICE, 2016) to inform clinical practice and standardise treatment strategies nationally.

Other clinical databases such as AMED, Medline, Embase, CINAHL, PubMed Central and Ovid can be searched for neonatal research papers that reflect the lower methods stated in the above model (De Brün, 2013). The neonatal nurse, however, should be mindful of the risk of bias and take a critical approach when reviewing papers from these databases.

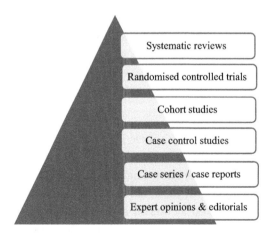

Figure 23.1 Hierarchy of evidence

Due to the constraints and ethical challenges facing the population involved, an RCT is often not practicable, so research in neonates is frequently observational. Observational study data needs to be critically analysed for its validity and applicability to clinical practice. It should also be remembered that statistically significant study results do not necessarily translate to clinically significant outcomes.

The databases will highlight articles that are published in peer-reviewed neonatal journals, such as *Journal of Neonatal Nursing*; *Archives of Diseases in Childhood – Fetal and Neonatal Edition*; *Infant*; *Journal of Perinatal & Neonatal Nursing*; and *Journal of Obstetric, Gynecologic & Neonatal Nursing*. The number of profession-specific journals evidences the growing wealth of research and publication occurring within neonatal care and neonatal nursing. Due to the accessibility of online journals, early access to articles can expedite EBP over physical formats. In addition, transferability from other professions such as education and social care should also be considered. Leach et al. (2016) in their study examining the effects of an undergraduate research programme on EBP utilisation post-qualification, stated that students found online access to databases, critique tools and full text articles useful in applying EBP to clinical practice. In addition, neonatal units (NNUs) can also increase EBP awareness with local subscriptions for staff to access both databases and printed journals during their shift (Sadoughi et al., 2017). Neonatal nurses still need to review these articles with a critical analysis approach, as peer reviewing cannot ensure good-quality results. Activities such as journal clubs can then provide a platform for the sharing of published work.

Other sources of data can be obtained from national bodies that were developed to coordinate neonatal research country-wide. In the UK, the National Neonatal Research Database (NNRD) utilises data collected from BadgerNet – a database collating details of all NNU admissions (Imperial College London, 2018). This data then informs neonatal practice, including the National Neonatal Audit Programme (NNAP), which was established in 2006 to standardise neonatal practice for the best outcomes (Royal College of Paediatrics and Child Health (RCPCH), 2017). In the United States of America (USA), there is also a collaborative neonatal research network called the National Institute of Child Health and Human Development (NICHD), which supports research that examines foetal, newborn and child health outcomes to inform practice and reduce morbidity and mortality (NICHD, 2018). The NICHD neonatal research networks were developed in 1985 and promoted the Back to Sleep campaign in the USA, supported the development of the Hib and DTaP vaccine, and researched the use of nitric oxide as a useful adjunct to conventional ventilation in the care of respiratory failure of neonates (NICHD, 2017). These databases not only provide neonatal nurses with evidence that can be applied to clinical practice, but also validate the importance of accurate and comprehensive input of data during the baby's NNU care episode.

To promote transparent research that avoids undue burden on participants and increases international collaboration, research registries have become compulsory for ongoing research studies (World Medical Association, 2013). The US National Library of Medicine oversees the ClinicalTrials.gov database (National Institutes of Health (NIH), 2019) and more recently in the UK, the University of Oxford set up the National Perinatal Epidemiology Unit (NPEU) with the remit of registering all clinical trials, not just RCTs (2018). This provides neonatal nurses who are looking to explore a clinical question with the opportunity to review the studies in progress within the topic area and consider future data that may be produced as a result.

Finally, for this section, it is important to emphasise that research can positively impact on infants and families in our care. For example, Zeitlin et al. (2016) evaluated the implementation of four evidence-based practices for the care of very preterm infants to judge their use and impact in routine clinical practice, and whether there was any influence in reducing mortality and neonatal morbidity. These practices were: delivery in a maternity unit with appropriate level of neonatal care; administration of antenatal corticosteroids; prevention of hypothermia (temperature on admission to neonatal unit ≥36°C); surfactant used within two hours of birth or early nasal continuous positive airway pressure. Evidence-based care was associated with lower in-hospital mortality or severe morbidity, or both, corresponding to an estimated 18% decrease in all deaths without an increase in severe morbidity if these interventions had been provided to all infants. More comprehensive use of EBP in perinatal medicine could result in considerable gains for very preterm infants in terms of increased survival without severe morbidity. A summary of EBP that has been shown to influence outcomes of infants and/or families is outlined below in box 23.1.

BOX 23.1 RESEARCH WHICH HAS IMPACTED NEONATAL PRACTICE

- Family integrated care
- Developmental care/Newborn Individualised Developmental Care Assessment Programme (NIDCAP)
- Parents' experiences
- Skin-to-skin care
- Pain assessment and management
- The first hour of care (Golden Hour)
- Feeding regimes
- Value of breast milk
- Thermal care (plastic bags/wraps for preterm infants)
- Non-invasive ventilation
- Surfactant therapy
- Antenatal corticosteroid and magnesium sulphate administration
- Therapeutic hypothermia for hypoxic-ischaemic encephalopathy.

Knowledge derived from clinical audit and data collection

In 1998, the NHS developed a framework for quality improvement (Scally and Donaldson, 1998). This framework stated that there were seven key components, which, with research and development, included clinical audit and clinical effectiveness. Clinical audit is a tool to assess whether care meets defined evidence-based clinical standards in neonatal care, and to evaluate any improvements for effective and quality health outcomes (Jolley, 2013; Healthcare Quality Improvement Partnership (HQIP), 2015a). HQIP are responsible for setting national clinical audits, which includes the National Maternity and Perinatal Audit (NMPA), which has been collecting data on the women and babies cared for in maternity units since April 2014 (HQIP, 2015b). The latest NMPA report estimated that data on 92% of births in England, Scotland and Wales was captured in 2015–2016 (NMPA, 2017). This report demonstrated that 1.2% of babies born within that timeframe in England, Scotland and Wales, had Apgar scores of less than 7 at 5 minutes, and that 55% of small for gestational age babies were post-mature (NMPA, 2017). This form of extensive audit provides the neonatal nurse with comprehensive national data that can be utilised in clinical practice.

Within neonatal care, the previously mentioned NNAP seeks to reduce morbidity among neonates with measures such as neonatal temperature between 36.5°C and 37.5°C in the first hour of life, the use of antenatal corticosteroids, and breast milk at discharge, which can then be audited (RCPCH, 2017). The Neonatal Data Analysis Unit (NDAU) evaluates the data from NNAP so that it can be utilised to standardise neonatal practice and assess improvements for the best neonatal outcomes (Imperial College London, 2018). NNAP data can also be used locally to benchmark against previously achieved standards of care, and to benchmark against other NNUs within the designated neonatal network. Neonatal nurses therefore have sources of clinical audit that they can utilise to inform clinical practice and support quality improvement projects.

Knowledge derived from professionals and service users

The highest levels of evidence are not always available or appropriate for the clinical question (Jolley, 2013). Qualitative studies are the best designs to understand social concepts and interactions (Anderson, 2010). Due to its design, qualitative research is an effective methodology to ascertain data about neonatal nurses within clinical practice, as well as an in-depth examination of the lived experience of the parents we interact with. It can inform practice in areas where RCTs would be inappropriate such as parents' spiritual needs around bereavement in the NNU (Sadeghi et al., 2016), or to elicit areas for improvement from the parent perspective through methods such as interview. Criticism of qualitative research relates to perceived lack of rigour, validity and generalisation of findings, along with generally small sample sizes (Choy, 2014). However, it is argued that well-conducted qualitative research can be verified as valid through approaches such as triangulation and, while not generalisable, results can be transferred to other sites (Anderson, 2010).

Mackey and Bassendowski (2017) state that EBP in nursing is not merely the utilisation of research, but the integration of scientific and tacit knowledge. Tacit knowledge has been described as implicit knowledge gained through practice and experience rather than explicit knowledge gained from scientific methods (Kothari et al., 2012). The favoured view is that tacit knowledge forms part of the continuing acquisition of knowledge, where pragmatic and situation-specific experience is integrated into clinical practice (McAdam et al., 2007). This reflects the continuum that Benner (1984) detailed in her novice to expert model.

Within the NNU, nurses develop their knowledge in clinical practice from other professionals in a variety of methods (Spence et al., 2016). This can be through mentorship, where experienced nurses provide a supportive learning relationship for student nurses; through preceptorship, where an experienced nurse acts as a learning guide to promote the professional growth of a junior nurse (Fineout-Overholt et al., 2013); and through peer review, where practice standards are measured between nurses with similar backgrounds (Jolley, 2013). Studies have shown that nurses prefer to develop clinical knowledge through peer and clinical exposure (Spence et al., 2016). An important factor in tacit knowledge is pattern recognition – an instinctive understanding of cues – which, with repeated exposure, creates high levels of expertise and has been shown to improve patient outcomes (Hill, 2010; Spence et al., 2016).

As with all knowledge, it is important that it is critically analysed for validity before applying it to practice. The use of inappropriate tacit knowledge can be obstructive to the implementation of EBP (Kothari et al., 2012). As tacit knowledge is implicit and often difficult to verbalise, it needs to be made explicit so that it can be shared. One method of achieving this is through the publication of peer-reviewed case studies and learning-in-practice experiences (Jolley, 2013). In addition, models to elicit tacit knowledge are often applied at nurse interview to assess the explicit and implicit reaction to a clinical situation (Taylor, 2007).

The Code (Nursing and Midwifery Council (NMC), 2018) requires nurses to work in partnership with patients to ensure care is delivered effectively, so that patients are empowered to share clinical decisions. Parents are a key resource for qualitative evidence regarding neonatal care, although national audits are also undertaken. Bliss is a service user advocate organisation utilising parental experiences to promote optimal baby-centred care for those neonates nursed in NNUs in the UK. Bliss undertakes surveys of parental experiences and generates reports that inform policy and national guidance for neonatal care. Members work alongside the government, commissioners and with local stakeholders to provide a user perspective for necessary resources, unit guidelines, as well as support for families in the NNUs. Bliss representatives formed part of the Neonatal Expert Advisory Group which developed national guidance including Neonatal Care in Scotland: A Quality Framework (NHS Scotland, 2013), and the All Wales National Standards for Children and Young People's Specialised Healthcare Services (Welsh Assembly Government, 2008).

Bliss' own reports are generated from the findings of the Bliss Baby Charter Audit Tool, which standardises the generalisability of the results across the UK NNUs and provides a valid method of benchmarking between units and between time points (Stewart and Masterton, 2012). Using this tool, Bliss have evidenced the financial impact of having a baby in the NNU (Bliss, 2014), the variation in resources available to parents, such as accommodation while their baby is in the NNU (Bliss, 2016a), as well as shortages in suitably qualified staff nationally (Bliss, 2016b; Bliss, 2017).

However, as well as national data on parent experience, it is important that local experience is also demonstrated and shared. This can be done through several approaches, including questionnaires such as Friends and Family, local unit questionnaires of parental experiences, thematic review of complaints and correspondence from parents and their families, and by face-to-face discussion. Integrated workshops with both service users and neonatal staff also provide valuable knowledge about the local service. The lived experience of the babies in neonatal care and their families is a valuable, enlightening and important source of evidence that neonatal nurses must synthesise into their EBP.

Renolen and Hjälmhult (2015) stated that nurses used scientific knowledge through a 'contextual balancing of knowledge'. The gap currently is not between theory and practice, it is between the application of theory to practice while remaining true to the essence of nursing. The next section will examine in greater detail how the above knowledge can be applied to practice, and the issues surrounding this utilisation.

Figure 23.2 outlines the different sources of knowledge.

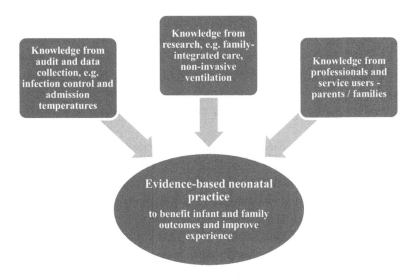

Figure 23.2 Knowledge sources for evidence-based neonatal practice

APPLICATION OF KNOWLEDGE TO PRACTICE

Empirical, scientific knowledge and EBP need to form the basis for undergraduate quali-fication and post-qualification practice. The inclusion of education on EBP is therefore an important component of student nurse programmes. Mitchell (2013), however, felt that edu-cational institutions lacked the ability to adequately undertake EBP training within their curriculum. Brooke et al. (2015) found that student nurses understood the importance of EBP and reported that they felt it would empower them in clinical practice. These student nurses also stated that it was an essential aspect of service improvement for patients and that it formed part of the development of nursing as a profession (Brooke et al., 2015). Indeed, The Code (NMC, 2018) asserts that nurses have a professional responsibility to always practice using the best available evidence and maintain the knowledge required for effective practice. A dedicated education programme on EBP for undergraduate nurses found that skills, knowledge and attitudes on EBP could be significantly improved when measured against that of those not involved in the programme (Ruzafa-Martínez et al., 2016). However, student nurses were found to experience difficulty translating academic learning about EBP to the clinical setting (Brooke et al., 2015; Cruz et al., 2016), which was further compounded by nurse preceptors not having the skills to support novice nurses with this aspect of transition (Xiaoshi, 2008; Ryan, 2016). A further study involved student nurses in a research project during their undergraduate programme, and found that this improved their adoption of EBP (André et al., 2016).

If EBP skills have not been gained during an education programme, then it can be a challenge to adopt them later. Educating neonatal nurses on EBP through mentoring strat-egies did not result in any significant improvement in their use of EBP, although they were more likely to be involved in practice changes, especially if they were younger, experienced nurses (Mariano et al., 2009). Conversely, Cruz et al. (2016) found that it was the older students who had a more positive response to EBP strategies and used it as an adjunct to experience. Student nurses on clinical placements are ideally situated to share their EBP skills with the clinical workforce and therefore promote a positive inclination towards the concept, however, this can be hindered by their lack of experience and time in the work-place (Ryan, 2016).

As a main component of clinical governance, EBP needs to be supported and applied to everyday clinical practice (Sadoughi et al., 2017). Purdy and Melwak (2009) describe the application of EBP to neonatal nursing as a 'dynamic process', one which requires ongoing assessment of effectiveness. A key aspect of this is gaining competence and confidence in literature search skills and critical analysis (André et al., 2016; Sadoughi et al., 2017). As research is more often stored and shared online, organisations need to address the barriers to adopting EBP, so that it can achieve its full potential for the benefit of babies and their families in NNUs (Sadoughi et al., 2017). Staff require protected time, accessibility and the skills to critically analyse research, and to maintain their skills against a competing clinical workload (Cruz et al., 2016; Leach et al., 2016; Ryan, 2016; Melnyk et al., 2017; Sadoughi et al., 2017). Organisation librarians could be utilised to increase literature searching and critical analysis skills through education programmes and one-to-one support of neonatal nurses (Sadoughi et al., 2017).

In addition to journals, neonatal nurses can quickly discover current innovations and changes in clinical practice through the appropriate use of social media and networking activities. Journals such as *Archives of Diseases in Childhood – Fetal and Neonatal Edition* have Twitter accounts which release snapshots of current research; neonatal conferences share tweets about interesting neonatal presentations; Twitter chats are used for discussions on neonatal care; Twitter online surveys provide a quick barometer of current issues; and many NNUs have their own accounts, which allow for sharing of innovations and improvements. Indeed, the 'Red Hat Project' that is being utilised in response to the Avoiding Term Admissions to the Neonatal Unit (ATAIN) programme, garnered support after a tweet from a neonatal unit in the Midlands about their success in reducing admissions due to hypothermia and hypoglycaemia.

Equally, other forms of social media such as Facebook, have special interest groups where nurses can network via a virtual platform and share ideas or challenges. This could be between local NNUs or between professional groups. There is, for instance, a national group for Advanced Neonatal Nurse Practitioners, and internationally, there is a group for the Association of Women's Health, Obstetric and Neonatal Nurses. Journals are also represented on this platform. While neither source can be applied to clinical practice without appropriate exploration and application of critical analysis skills, they provide an opportunity for increased awareness of neonatal practice when time resources are limited. This exposure could increase motivation to provided EBP in the busy NNU.

Other technologies include the wealth of videos and podcasts, easily accessible online, which cover the demonstration of technical skills and innovations, as well as the lived experience of parents who share stories of their time in the NNU, challenging journeys or the loss of their baby. These powerful and poignant media provide the neonatal nurse with an insight and perspective of what may be an infrequent event, and this in turn will better prepare him or her for future practice.

Away from the clinical environment, knowledge can be sourced from attendance at conferences, for example the REaSoN Neonatal Meeting, the Neonatal Nurses' Association and SIGNEC UK among others. Conferences allow knowledge, case studies and EBP to be shared via PowerPoint presentations as well as poster presentations, and the opportunity of networking with peers. Neonatal nurses can access special interest groups that share knowledge with a specific focus, such as the Linking Education and Research in Neonates (LEARN) group and the Improvement Science Research Network (ISRN). The ISRN shares knowledge gained from innovations and quality improvement efforts which can then be utilised in other settings. Equally, the NHS Improvement Maternity Neonatal Collaborative is generating local improvement knowledge to address specific national neonatal issues such as ATAIN, and this is shared via conferences, the Life Quality Improvement system and Communities of Practice.

Where research is used in clinical practice it has been linked to inquiring attitudes and job satisfaction (Fineout-Overholt et al., 2013). There are currently many national neonatal research trials being conducted through the NPEU that neonatal nurses can be involved in to increase their knowledge of the clinical research process and EBP. A link to the NPEU is provided in the web-based companion.

Ongoing education continues to be a mainstay of nursing practice (NMC, 2018). This is a key opportunity for EBP skills to be developed or enhanced. Increasing numbers of neonatal nurses are producing dissertations as part of higher awards, and publication develops the evidence base for neonatal care and highlights areas for research development.

Mitchell (2013) maintains, however, that EBP is not the remit of the individual nurse, but of the organisation the nurse works within. Strong, appropriately skilled, organisational leadership that is supportive of EBP application in the NNU is required (Xiaoshi, 2008; Ryan, 2016; Sadoughi et al., 2017). A study by Renolen and Hjälmhult (2015) found that nurses relied on their own motivation to achieve EBP, as they believed it was not a priority for managers, although the study also found that higher-grade nurses were in a position to effect more clinical implementation of scientific knowledge. The use of organisational EBP mentors and models such as the Advancing Research and Clinical Practice Through Close Collaboration (ARCC©) model have been shown to increase the organisational culture regarding the implementation of EBP into clinical practice, and have led to improved patient outcomes and staff satisfaction (Fineout-Overholt et al., 2013; Melnyk et al., 2017). However, while Mitchell (2013) believes that the EBP framework provides a cost-effective tool for organisations by controlling practice, it can detract from professional nursing values, so that a balance needs to be achieved.

CONCLUSION

Evidence-based neonatal nursing practice has evolved as the best approach to promote quality outcomes for NNU patients through the balanced integration of research, clinical experience and patient preference (Mariano et al., 2009; Purdy and Melwak, 2009; Renolen and Hjälmhult, 2015). It is an effective method of utilising limited resources and promoting safe and cost-effective practice (Leach et al., 2016). It is imperative that neonatal nurses embrace all forms of evidence in order to generate and expand upon earlier work in evidence-based nursing practice, so that the profession has a specific and independent contemporaneous basis on which to provide clinical care for the neonates and families. Bridging training is required to translate EBP education programmes to clinical practice application, and build on the appreciation, recognition and enthusiasm for EBP that student nurses demonstrate (Cruz et al., 2016). Increasing the research profile of neonatal nurses will encourage other nurses in the NNU to embrace and value the concept, as well as medical colleagues to recognise the value that this research area can offer in neonatal clinical practice. Promoting a positive EBP culture is key, and the use of EBP champions should be considered to drive forward this concept (Xiaoshi, 2008; Fineout-Overholt et al., 2013). Without cultural change, EBP will not be sustained in the clinical environment (Melnyk et al., 2017).

The Code (NMC, 2018) states that nurses should act as an advocate for the vulnerable, which would include neonates, and developing and utilising EBP is key to this process. Research is important for the neonatal population who deserve to have robust clinical care and be central to continuous quality improvement. A dedication to promoting neonatal research and improving outcomes for sick and preterm infants, and their parents, means neonatal nurses must share their knowledge and experiences through publication. This sharing allows clinical practice to be peer reviewed and objectively analysed for potential best practice in the absence of more robust research (Jolley, 2013). Neonatal nurses are therefore well placed and have the opportunity to guide healthcare transformation at multiple levels and facilitate the advancement of neonatal care through the use of EBP.

CASE STUDIES

Case study 1: Producing an evidence-based guideline

You work on a neonatal unit where parents can visit any time, but extended family can only visit at set times which are limited to one-hour periods. You are aware that a family were upset that the grandparents weren't allowed free access to their first grandchild. Staff have also expressed that it can be difficult with lots of visitors in the unit, especially when babies are very sick. You are asked to update the unit visiting guideline.

Q.1. Which sources would you use in order to provide the most evidence-based guidance?
Q.2. What are you expecting each source to add to the process?
Q.3. What obstacles do you envision occurring?
Q.4. How will you overcome these obstacles?

Case study 2: The expert vs. the novice approach

Jane is a midwifery student on her neonatal unit placement. Her mentor is an experienced neonatal nurse. They are caring for an extremely preterm infant who has redirection of care and dies shortly afterwards.

Q.1. What forms of knowledge will Jane use to provide care for the family at this time?
Q.2. What forms of knowledge will her mentor use to support the family

C
A
S
E

S
T
U
D
Y

Q.3. What forms of knowledge will her mentor use to support Jane?

Q.4. How will Jane use this experience in future practice?

Reflection

Thinking again about the above two case studies as well as the other case studies featured throughout this book:

Q.1. Is there anything different you would do, or anything you would have done differently, having now read this chapter?

Q.2. How will you apply the learning from this chapter to your practice? On your next shift? Next month? Next year?

Q.3. Are your literature searching skills up to date?

Q.4. Does your organisation provide training to improve EBP skills?

Q.5. Could you set up a journal club in your unit? Or could you support one that already exists?

Final reflection

Think about your last day or week of work on the neonatal unit.

Q.1. What forms of evidence did you use to guide your clinical practice?

Q.2. How did you know these sources were up to date and reliable?

Q.3. Was your practice evidence-based?

Q.4. Were there any areas of care that are not supported by evidence or research or that require an update in knowledge?

Finally, can you identify any area of care that requires change or one that needs to be introduced into the clinical area? What further research and enquiry is required?

For suggested answer guides to the questions posed in these case studies, please refer to the web-based companion site specific to this chapter (see URL below).

WEB-BASED RESOURCES

For further information, online resources and greater detail on the case studies featured in this chapter go to www.routledge.com/cw/nicnursing

References

Anderson, C. (2010). Presenting and evaluating qualitative research. *American Journal of Pharmaceutical Education, 74*(8), 141.

André, B., Aune, A. G., & Brænd, J. A. (2016). Embedding evidence-based practice among nursing undergraduates: results from a pilot study. *Nurse Education in Practice, 18*, 30–35.

Benner, P. (1984). *From Novice to Expert: Excellence and Power in Clinical Nursing Practice*. Menlo Park, CA: Addison-Wesley.

Bliss. (2014). *It's Not a Game: The Very Real Costs of Having a Premature or Sick Baby*. London: Bliss.

Bliss. (2016a). *Families Kept Apart: Barriers to Parents' Involvement in Their Baby's Hospital Care.* London: Bliss.

Bliss. (2016b). *Bliss Baby Report 2016: Time for Change. Wales.* London: Bliss.

Bliss. (2017). *Bliss Scotland Baby Report 2017. An Opportunity to Deliver Improvements in Neonatal Care.* London: Bliss.

Brooke, J., Hvalič-Touzery, S., & Skela-Savič, B. (2015). Student nurse perceptions on evidence-based practice and research: An exploratory research study involving students from the University of Greenwich, England and the Faculty of Health Care Jesenice, Slovenia. *Nurse Education Today, 35*(7), e6–e11.

Choy, L. T. (2014). The strengths and weaknesses of research methodology: Comparison and complimentary between qualitative and quantitative approaches. *IOSR Journal of Humanities and Social Science, 19*(4), 99–104.

Cochrane. (2018). *Strategy to 2020.* www.cochrane.org/about-us/our-strategy

Cruz, J. P., Colet, P. C., Alquwez, N., Alqubeilat, H., Bashtawi, M. A., Ahmed, E. A., & Cruz, C. P. (2016). Evidence-based practice beliefs and implementation among the Nursing Bridge Program students of a Saudi university. *International Journal of Health Sciences, 10*(3), 405–414.

De Brún, C. (2013). *Finding the Evidence. A Key Step in the Information Production Process.* The Information Standard. www.england.nhs.uk/publication/finding-the-evidence-a-key-step-in-the-information-production-process/

Fineout-Overholt, E., Levin, F., & Melnyk, B. M. (2013). Defining Mentorship for EBP. In Harriet, R., & Feldman, H. R. (Eds.). *Teaching Evidence-Based Practice in Nursing* (2nd Edition). New York: Springer Publishing Company.

Healthcare Quality Improvement Partnership. (2015a). *A Guide to Quality Improvement Methods.* London: HQIP.

Healthcare Quality Improvement Partnership. (2015b). *National Clinical Audit Programme.* London: HQIP.

Hill, K. (2010). Improving quality and patient safety by retaining nursing expertise. *Online Journal of Issues in Nursing, 15*(3). doi: 10.3912/OJIN.Vol15No03PPT03

Imperial College London. (2018). *Neonatal Data Analysis Unit.* www.imperial.ac.uk/neonatal-data-analysis-unit

Jolley, J. (2013) *Introducing Research and Evidence-based Practice for Nursing and Health Care Professionals* (2nd Ed.) London and New York: Routledge.

Kothari, A., Rudman, D., Dobbins, M., Rouse, M., Sibbald, S., & Edwards, N. (2012). The use of tacit and explicit knowledge in public health: A qualitative study. *Implementation Science, 7*(1), 20.

Leach, M. J., Hofmeyer, A., & Bobridge, A. (2016). The impact of research education on student nurse attitude, skill and uptake of evidence-based practice: A descriptive longitudinal survey. *Journal of Clinical Nursing, 25*(1–2), 194–203.

McAdam, R., Mason, B., & McCrory, J. (2007). Exploring the dichotomies within the tacit knowledge literature: Towards a process of tacit knowing in organizations. *Journal of knowledge management, 11*(2), 43–59.

Mackey, A., & Bassendowski, S. (2017). The history of evidence-based practice in nursing education and practice. *Journal of Professional Nursing, 33*(1), 51–55.

Majid, S., Foo, S., Luyt, B., Zhang, X., Theng, Y. L., Chang, Y. K., & Mokhtar, I. A. (2011). Adopting evidence-based practice in clinical decision making: Nurses' perceptions, knowledge, and barriers. *Journal of the Medical Library Association: JMLA, 99*(3), 229–236.

Mariano, K. D., Caley, L. M., Eschberger, L., Woloszyn, A., Volker, P., Leonard, M. S., & Tung, Y. (2009). Building evidence-based practice with staff nurses through mentoring. *Journal of Neonatal Nursing*, *15*(3), 81–87.

Melnyk, B. M., Fineout-Overholt, E., Giggleman, M., & Choy, K. (2017). A test of the ARCC© model improves implementation of evidence-based practice, healthcare culture, and patient outcomes. *Worldviews on Evidence-Based Nursing*, *14*(1), 5–9.

Mitchell, G. J. (2013). Implications of holding ideas of evidence-based practice in nursing. *Nursing Science Quarterly*, *26*(2), 143–151.

National Institute of Child Health and Human Development (NICHD). (2017). Inhaled Nitric Oxide Study for Respiratory Failure in Newborns (NINOS). https://clinicaltrials.gov/ct2/show/NCT00005776

National Institute of Child Health and Human Development (NICHD). (2018). Mission. www.nih.gov/about-nih/what-we-do/nih-almanac/eunice-kennedy-shriver-national-institute-child-health-human-development-nichd

National Institute for Health and Care Excellence. (2012). *Neonatal infection (early onset): antibiotics for prevention and treatment. CG149*. NICE.

National Institute for Health and Care Excellence. (2016). *Jaundice in newborn babies under 28 days. CG98*. NICE.

National Institutes of Health (NIH). (2019). About NIH. www.nih.gov/about-nih

National Perinatal Epidemiology Unit, Nuffield Department of Population Health, & University of Oxford. (2018). *NPEU*. www.npeu.ox.ac.uk/

NHS Scotland. (2013). *Neonatal Care in Scotland: A Quality Framework*. Edinburgh: NHS Scotland.

NMPA Project Team. (2017). *National Maternity and Perinatal Audit: Clinical Report 2017*. NMPA.

Nursing and Midwifery Council (NMC). (2018) *The Code. Professional Standards of Practice and Behaviour for Nurses Midwives and Nursing Associates*. www.nmc.org.uk/standards/code/

Purdy, I. B., & Melwak, M. A. (2009). Implementing evidence-based practice: A mantra for clinical change. *The Journal of Perinatal & Neonatal Nursing*, *23*(3), 263–269.

Renolen, Å., & Hjälmhult, E. (2015). Nurses experience of using scientific knowledge in clinical practice: A grounded theory study. *Scandinavian Journal of Caring Sciences*, *29*(4), 633–641.

Royal College of Paediatrics and Child Health. (2017). *Your Baby's Care. Measuring Standards and Improving Neonatal Care. A Guide to the National Neonatal Audit Programme 2017 Annual Report*. www.rcpch.ac.uk/improving-child-health/quality-improvement-and-clinical-audit/national-neonatal-audit-programme-nn-0#2016

Ruzafa-Martínez, M., López-Iborra, L., Barranco, D. A., & Ramos-Morcillo, A. J. (2016). Effectiveness of an evidence-based practice (EBP) course on the EBP competence of undergraduate nursing students: A quasi-experimental study. *Nurse Education Today*, *38*, 82–87.

Ryan, E. J. (2016). Undergraduate nursing students' attitudes and use of research and evidence-based practice – an integrative literature review. *Journal of Clinical Nursing*, *25*(11–12), 1548–1556.

Sackett, D. L., Rosenberg, W. M., Gray, J. M., Haynes, R. B., & Richardson, W. S. (1996). Evidence based medicine: What it is and what it isn't. *British Medical Journal* (Clinical Research Ed.), *312*(7023), 71–72.

Sadeghi, N., Hasanpour, M., Heidarzadeh, M., Alamolhoda, A., & Waldman, E. (2016). Spiritual needs of families with bereavement and loss of an infant in the neonatal intensive care unit: A qualitative study. *Journal of Pain and Symptom Management*, *52*(1), 35–42.

Sadoughi, F., Azadi, T., & Azadi, T. (2017). Barriers to using electronic evidence based literature in nursing practice: A systematised review. *Health Information & Libraries Journal*, *34*(3), 187–199.

Scally, G., & Donaldson, L. J. (1998). Clinical governance and the drive for quality improvement in the new NHS in England. *British Medical Journal*, *317*(7150), 61–65.

Spence, K., Sinclair, L., Morritt, M. L., & Laing, S. (2016). Knowledge and learning in speciality practice. *Journal of Neonatal Nursing*, *22*(6), 263–276.

Stevens, K. R. (2013). The impact of evidence-based practice in nursing and the next big ideas. *The Online Journal of Issues in Nursing, 18*(2), 4. doi: 10.3912/OJIN.Vol18No02Man04

Stewart, K., & Masterton, M. (2012). Bliss Baby Charter Audit Tool. *Journal of Neonatal Nursing, 18*(5), 173.

Stokke, K., Olsen, N. R., Espehaug, B., & Nortvedt, M. W. (2014). Evidence based practice beliefs and implementation among nurses: a cross-sectional study. *BMC Nursing, 13*(1), 8.

Taylor, H. (2007). Eliciting tacit knowledge using the critical decision interview method. In Jennex, E. M. (Ed.) *Knowledge Management in Modern Organizations.* IGI Global Hershey, PA and London: Idea Group Publishing..

Welsh Assembly Government. (2008). *All Wales National Standards for Children and Young People's Specialised Healthcare Services.* Cardiff: Welsh Assembly Government.

World Medical Association. (2013). *WMA Declaration of Helsinki – Ethical Principles for Medical Research Involving Human Subjects.* WMA.

Xiaoshi, L. (2008). Evidence-based practice in nursing: What is it and what is the impact of leadership and management practices on implementation? *Nursing Journal, 12*, 6–12.

Zeitlin, J., Manktelow, B. N., Piedvache, A., Cuttini, M., Boyle, E., Van Heijst, A., ... & Schmidt, S. (2016). Use of evidence based practices to improve survival without severe morbidity for very preterm infants: Results from the EPICE population based cohort. *British Medical Journal, 354*, i2976.

24 FINAL COMMENTS AND ACKNOWLEDGEMENTS

Julia Petty and Lisa Kaiser

The rewriting and updating of this book has been a team effort. All the contributors are to be thanked and commended for their involvement while engaging in work responsibilities and busy personal lives and commitments. We would also like to acknowledge, where applicable, all previous contributors from the second edition of the book: namely in order of appearance in the second edition: Glenys Boxwell, the previous editor and originator of this book; Fiona Hutchinson; Tilly Reid; Yvonne Freer; Sue Turrill; Pauline Fellows; Simone Jollye; David Summers; Rosarie Lombard; Anja Hale; Jackie Dent; Katie McKenna; Dee Beresford; Elizabeth Harding; Beverley Guard; Rachel Homer; Stevie Boyd; Anne Aspin; Anne Mitchell; Catherine Hall; Peter Mullholland; Joan Cameron; Helen Frizell. Their contributions have formed a vital and valuable basis for this update.

Other specific acknowledgements from current contributors are as follows:

Chapter 2 The author Linda McDonald would like to acknowledge Susan Smith, Vicky Payne and Dr Michael Hall at the University of Southampton for imparting their knowledge on history taking. She would furthermore like to thank Bekki White and Christine Butt for contributing to the photos illustrating the Look-Listen-Feel approach.

Chapter 4 The author Liz Crathern would like to thank Bruce Holliday, Multimedia Developer, University of Leeds, for his vision and help in designing the pictorial representation of 'The whirlpool of parents' feelings'.

Chapter 16 The authors Alison Mitchell and Ella Porter, would like to thank Kath Holt and Mo Keane for their encouragement and advice to complete the chapter.

Chapter 18 Lisa Kaiser is grateful to Dr Tim Scorrer for kindling her interest in neonatal infection, to Dr Ramon Fernandez for nurturing it, and to Dr Mike Hall for teaching her all about it.

Chapter 20 Beverley Guard was the co-author of this chapter with Liam Brennan in the first edition.

APPENDIX

CoNS	coagulase-negative staphylococcus
CPAP	continuous positive airway pressure
CQC	Care Quality Commission
CRP	C-reactive protein
CRT	capillary refill time
CSF	cerebrospinal fluid
CTG	Cardiotocograph
CUSS	cranial ultrasound scan
CVC	central venous catheter
DAT	direct antiglobulin test
DA	ductus Arteriosus
DCC	delayed cord clamping
DIC	disseminated intravascular coagulation
DJF	duodenojejunal flexure
EBP	evidence-based practice
ECG	electrocardiogram
ECMO	extracorporeal membrane oxygenation
EEG	electroencephalogram
ELBW	extremely low birth weight
ENNP	Enhanced Neonatal Nurse Practitioner
EOS	early onset sepsis
ESA	erythropoiesis-stimulating agent
ETT	endotracheal tube
EXIT	ex utero intrapartum treatment
FFP	fresh frozen plasma
FiO_2	fractional inspired oxygen concentration
FO	foramen Ovale
FRC	functional residual capacity
G6PD	glucose-6-phosphate dehydrogenase
GA	gestational age
GBS	group B beta-haemolytic streptococcus
G-CSF	granulocyte colony-stimulating factor
GFR	glomerular filtration rate
GI	gastrointestinal
GMC	General Medical Council
GORD	gastro-oesophageal reflux disease
GOR	gastro-oesophageal reflux
GP	General Practitioner
Hb	haemoglobin
HDFN	haemolytic disease of the foetus and newborn

HDN	haemorrhagic disease of the newborn; also haemolytic disease of the newborn
HFOV	high frequency oscillation ventilation
HHFNC	humidified high flow nasal cannula
HIE	hypoxic-ischaemic encephalopathy
HIV	human immunodeficiency virus
HR	heart rate
HTA	Human Tissue Authority
IADH	inappropriate (secretion) antidiuretic hormone
IM	intramuscular
IMV	intermittent mandatory ventilation
iNO	inhaled nitric oxide
IPPV	intermittent positive-pressure ventilation
IUGR	intrauterine growth restriction
IV	intravenous
IVC	inferior vena cava
IVH	intraventricular haemorrhage
IVIG	intravenous immunoglobulin
IWL	insensible water losses
LBW	low birth weight
LMA	laryngeal mask airway
LNU	local Neonatal Unit
LOS	late onset sepsis
MAP	mean airway pressure
MAS	meconium aspiration syndrome
MDT	multidisciplinary team
MetHb	methaemoglobin
ml	millilitre(s)
MRI	magnetic resonance imaging
MSAF	meconium stained amniotic fluid
MV	minute volume
NAS	neonatal abstinence syndrome
NBAS	Neonatal Behavioural Assessment Scale
nCPAP	nasal CPAP
NEC	necrotising enterocolitis
NGT	nasogastric tube
NHS	National Health Service
NICE	National Institute for Health and Care Excellence
NICU	Neonatal Intensive Care Unit
NIDCAP	Neonatal Individualised Developmental Care and Assessment Programme
NIPE	newborn infant physical examination

NK	natural killer (cells)
NLS	Newborn Life Support
NMC	Nursing and Midwifery Council
NNA	Neonatal Nurses Association
NNAP	National Neonatal Audit Programme
NNS	non-nutritive sucking
NNU	Neonatal Unit
NO	nitric oxide
OA	oesophageal atresia
ODN	Operational Delivery Network
OI	oxygen index
OT	Occupational Therapist
$PaCO_2$	partial pressure of carbon dioxide (in arterial blood)
PaO_2	partial pressure of oxygen (in arterial blood)
PCV	packed cell volume
PD	peritoneal dialysis
PDA	patent ductus arteriosus
PEEP	positive end-expiratory pressure
PICC	peripherally inserted central catheter
PIE	pulmonary interstitial emphysema
PIP	peak inspiratory pressure
PN	parenteral nutrition
PPHN	persistent pulmonary hypertension of the newborn
PPROM	preterm pre-labour rupture of the membranes
PSV	pressure support ventilation
PTV	patient-triggered ventilation
PVHI	periventricular haemorrhagic infarction
PVL	periventricular leukomalacia
PVR	pulmonary vascular resistance
RBC	red blood cells
RCN	Royal College of Nursing
RCOG	Royal College of Obstetricians and Gynaecologists
RCPCH	Royal College of Paediatrics and Child Heath
RCT	randomised controlled trial
RDS	respiratory distress syndrome
ROP	retinopathy of prematurity
SaO_2	saturation of haemoglobin (oxygen)
RR	respiratory rate
SALT	Speech and Language Therapist
SBR	serum bilirubin
SCBU	special care baby unit

SGA	small for gestational age
SIMV	synchronised intermittent mandatory ventilation
SIPPV	synchronised intermittent positive-pressure ventilation
SNNG	Scottish Neonatal Nurses Group
SVC	superior vena cava
SNOD	Specialist Nurse in Organ Donation
SPA	suprapubic aspiration of the bladder
SV	stroke volume
SVT	supraventricular tachycardia
TAT	transanastomotic tube
TcB	transcutaneous bilirubinometer
TEWL	transepidermal water loss
TGA	transposition of the great arteries
TH	therapeutic hypothermia
TIS	transport incubator system
TOF	tracheo-oesophageal fistula
TORCH	Toxoplasmosis, Other (usually chickenpox), Rubella, Cytomegalovirus and Herpes
TSH	thyroid-stimulating hormone
TTN	transient tachypnoea of the newborn
UAC	umbilical arterial catheter
UVC	umbilical venous catheter
VACTERL	Vertebral, Anal, Tracheal, (O)Esophageal and Renal anomalies, plus Cardiac and Limb anomalies
VKDB	vitamin K deficiency bleeding
VLBW	very low birth weight
V/Q	ventilation/perfusion
VSD	ventricular septal defect
VT	tidal volume
VT	ventricular tachycardia
WBC	white blood cells
WCC	white cell count
WHO	World Health Organization

GLOSSARY

abduction	to move (a limb) away from the midline of the body
adduction	to draw (a limb) into the midline of the body
adenosine triphosphate (ATP)	organic molecule in body cells responsible for storage and release of energy
aganglionic	without ganglia (innervation)
amniocentesis	removal of amniotic fluid via the maternal abdominal wall for foetal diagnostic purposes
anabolism	building phase of metabolism
anastomosis	a connection between two passages
anion	ion carrying one or more negative charges
anterior	towards the front of the body
antibody	protein released by plasma cells in response to an antigen
antigen	substance recognised as foreign by the immune system
apoptosis	programmed cell death
atelectasis	alveolar collapse
atresia	absence of an opening/passage in the body
auscultation	the process of listening with a stethoscope
autoregulation	the automatic adjustment of blood flow to a particular body area in response to current need
B-cells	cells responsible for humoral (antibody-mediated) immunity
baroreceptors	receptors stimulated by pressure change
bradyarrhythmias	slow heart rate, usually due to extracardiac pathology
bradycardia	slow heart rate, less than 80bpm (term) and 100bpm (preterm)
brown adipose tissue (BAT)	specialised, strategically placed tissue (fat) which is capable of generating heat

cardiac output	amount of blood pumped from ventricles in one minute
carina	the keel-shaped cartilage at the bifurcation of the trachea into the two main bronchi
catecholamines	compounds that have the effect of sympathetic nerve stimulation
cation	a positively charged ion
caudal	relating to the tail end of the body
cell-mediated immunity	immunity conferred by activated T-cells
cephalad	towards the head
chemoreceptors	receptors sensitive to chemical change
choroid plexus	CSF producing capillary 'knot' within a brain ventricle
cytochrome	iron containing proteins found on inner mitochondrial layer which function as electron carriers during oxidative phosphorylation
diaphoresis	sweating
diastole	relaxation phase of the cardiac cycle
distal	further from the attached limb or the origin of a structure, e.g. the elbow is distal to the shoulder
dynamic precordium	visible heartbeat due to PDA
embolus (plural **emboli**)	obstruction of a blood vessel by particulate matter, e.g. blood clot or air
epiglottis	leaf-shaped cartilage at back of throat, covers the larynx during swallowing
erythropoietin	hormone released predominantly by the kidney which stimulates red blood cell production (erythropoiesis)
eventration	flattening and non-movement of the diaphragm following denervation – may be congenital or acquired
evidence-based (care)	the integration of best available clinical evidence with an individual's expertise
extravasation	leakage of fluid from a vessel into the surrounding tissue
extremely low birth weight	infant of less than or equal to 999g
facilitated tucking	supported positioning of a baby to contain a limb
fistula	unnatural connection between two structures or body cavities
flexed	to curl inwards

gestational age	period of time from the first date of last normal menstrual period to the date of birth. Expressed in number of completed weeks or days
glomerular filtration rate	rate of filtrate formation by the kidneys
gluconeogenesis	formation of glucose from a non-carbohydrate source, e.g. muscle
glycogen	stored carbohydrate predominantly in muscle
glycogenolysis	breakdown of glycogen to glucose
haemolysis	rupture of red blood cells
histamine	chemical substance which promotes vasodilatation and capillary permeability
holistic	encompassing all aspects of care
homeostasis	a state of equilibrium within the body
humeral immunity	immunity conferred by antibody production
hydrocephalus	an abnormal increase in the amount of cerebral spinal fluid within the ventricles of the brain
immunoglobulins	antibodies that bind to specific antigens
inferior	away from the head or towards the lower body or structures
interferon	chemical that provides some protection against a virus
isotonic	fluids that have the same osmotic pressure as cells
kernicterus	yellow staining of brain stem, cerebellum and hypocanthus with toxic degeneration of nerve cells due to hyperbilirubinaemia
lateral	away from the midline of the body
linea alba	fibrous structure connecting the abdominal muscles
low birth weight (LBW)	infant of less than or equal to 2499g
lymphocytes	white blood cells arising from bone marrow denoted T- or B-cells
macrophages	principal phagocytes found at specific sites or within bloodstream
malrotation	anomaly of foetal intestinal rotation and fixation resulting in intestinal obstruction
medial	towards the midline of the body
mesenteries	extensions of the peritoneum that support abdominal organs
mitochondria	organelles found in all cells responsible for production of adenosine triphosphate (ATP)

myelination	the formation of a fatty insulating sheath surrounding most nerve fibres
nephrotoxic	damaging to nephrons/kidneys
nociception	the perception by the nerve centres of painful stimulation. The term used in relation to pain perception in neonates
non-shivering thermogenesis	ability to produce heat by activation of BAT
nosocomial	an infection that develops within the hospital environment
oligohydramnios	reduction in liquor volume
oliguria	diminished urine output, e.g. $< 1\,ml/kg/hr$
opisthotonus	severe contraction of the back muscles causing the body to arch backwards
opsonisation	process whereby antigens are made more 'attractive' to phagocytes
ototoxic	damaging to the eighth cranial nerve/hearing
petechiae	small haemorrhages in the skin
phagocytes	white blood cells (leukocytes) that destroy pathogens by engulfment
pharmacodynamics	how drugs affect the body
pharmacokinetics	absorption, distribution, metabolism, excretion or what the body does to a drug
pleural effusion	the presence of fluid in the pleural space
pneumoperitoneum	free air in the peritoneal space
pneumothorax	free air in the pleural cavity
polyhydramnios	an excess of amniotic fluid
postconceptional age	current age calculated from date of conception
posterior	towards the back of the body
preterm	less than 37 completed weeks of gestation (259 days). Accounts for 7 per cent of births
processus vaginalis	outpouching of the peritoneum which forms during embryonic development
prokinetic	agent that increases gastric motility
proximal	closer to the body or origin of a structure, e.g. the knee is proximal to the ankle
small for gestational age (SGA)	infant with birth weight less than the 10th percentile
solute	substance dissolved in solution
stenosis	an abnormal narrowing
stroke volume	amount of blood pumped from the ventricles with each contraction

superior	towards the head or upper part of the body or a structure
supine	lying on back, face upwards
suprapubic	above the symphysis pubis
systole	contraction phase of the cardiac cycle
T-cells	cells responsible for cell-mediated immunity
tachycardia	heart rate greater than 160bpm (term) and 180bpm (preterm) at rest
tension pneumothorax	free air (under pressure) in the chest resulting in a shift in the mediastinum potentially reducing cardiac output
term	from 37 to 42 completed weeks of gestation (259–293 days); see also **preterm**
thermogenesis	production of heat
thrombus	a clot that develops and persists within a blood vessel
torsion	twisting, e.g. of gut
tracheomalacia	'floppy' trachea
turbidity	clouded with a suspension of particles
very low birth weight (VLBW)	infant of less than or equal to 1499g; see also **small for gestational age**
xiphisternum	the lower part of the breastbone

NORMAL VALUES IN THE NEONATE

Listed below are the 'average' normal values expected in the first days of life. However, the infant's gestational age and day of life and clinical condition need to be considered before treatment is instigated.

	Term	Preterm
Temperature (°C)		
Rectal	36.5–37.5	36.5–37.5
Axillary	36.5–37.5	36.5–37.5

* The toe-core temperature gap should not exceed 1.5°C.

	Term	Preterm
Apex beat (per minute)	90–160	120–180
Blood pressure (mmHg)		
Systolic	46–94	50–62
Diastolic	24–57	25–30
Mean	31–63	25–47
Blood		
pH	7.3–7.4	7.3–7.38
PCO2 (kPa)	4.5–6.0	4.5–6.5
PO2 (kPa)	8.0–12	7.5–10
Bicarbonate mmol/L	18–25	18–25
Base excess	− 7 to + 3	− 5 to + 5

* To convert kPa to mmHg multiply by 7.5.

	Term	Preterm
Creatinine micromol/L	37–113	39–156
Calcium (corrected) mmol/L	1.8–2.9	1.9–2.6
Glucose mmol/L	2.6–6.0	2.6–6.0
Lactate mmol/L	0.5–2.0	0.5–2.0
Magnesium mmol/L	0.7–1.0	0.7–1.0

Phosphate mmol/L	1.8–2.6	1.8–2.6
Potassium mmol/L	3.5–5.5	4.5–6.0
Sodium mmo/L	135–145	135–145
Urea mmol/L	0.5–4.2	1.0–5.0
Haemoglobin g/L	165–180	165–180
Packed cell volume	0.53–0.58	0.53–0.58
Platelets × 10^9/L	150–400	150–350
Prothrombin time (seconds)	10–16	13–16
White cell count × 10^9/L	9.0–30	9.0–35
Neutrophils	50–80%	50–80%
Lymphocytes	25–40%	25–40%
Monocytes	5–8%	5–8%
Urine		
Osmolality mosmol/L	100–300	50–300
Sodium mmol/L	1.0	1–15.0
Specific gravity	1006–1020	1006–1020
Cerebrospinal fluid		
Protein g/L	0.3–2.5	0.5–2.9
Glucose mmol/L	1.5–5.5	1.5–5.5
* CSF glucose should be approximately 80% of the serum level.		
Red cell count	0–50	0–70

INDEX